CAMBRIDGE PUBLIC HEALTH SERIES

UNDER THE EDITORSHIP OF

G. S. Graham-Smith, M.D. and   J. E. Purvis, M.A.

University Lecturer in Hygiene and Secretary to the Sub-Syndicate for Tropical Medicine

University Lecturer in Chemistry and Physics in their application to Hygiene and Preventive Medicine, and Secretary to the State Medicine Syndicate

T0372343

THE
CAUSES OF TUBERCULOSIS

THE
CAUSES OF TUBERCULOSIS

TOGETHER WITH SOME ACCOUNT OF THE PREVALENCE AND DISTRIBUTION OF THE DISEASE

BY

LOUIS COBBETT, M.D., F.R.C.S.

University Lecturer in Pathology, Cambridge

Cambridge :

at the University Press

1917

CAMBRIDGE
UNIVERSITY PRESS

University Printing House, Cambridge CB2 8BS, United Kingdom

Cambridge University Press is part of the University of Cambridge.

It furthers the University's mission by disseminating knowledge in the pursuit of education, learning and research at the highest international levels of excellence.

www.cambridge.org
Information on this title: www.cambridge.org/9781107456563

© Cambridge University Press 1917

First published 1917
First paperback edition 2014

A catalogue record for this publication is available from the British Library

ISBN 978-1-107-45656-3 Paperback

Cambridge University Press has no responsibility for the persistence or accuracy of URLs for external or third-party internet websites referred to in this publication, and does not guarantee that any content on such websites is, or will remain, accurate or appropriate.

. . . .

EDITOR'S PREFACE

IN view of the increasing importance of the study of public hygiene and the recognition by doctors, teachers, administrators and members of Public Health and Hygiene Committees alike that the *salus populi* must rest, in part at least, upon a scientific basis, the Syndics of the Cambridge University Press have decided to publish a series of volumes dealing with the various subjects connected with Public Health.

The books included in the Series present in a useful and handy form the knowledge now available in many branches of the subject. They are written by experts, and the authors are occupied, or have been occupied, either in investigations connected with the various themes or in their application and administration. They include the latest scientific and practical information offered in a manner which is not too technical. The bibliographies contain references to the literature of each subject which will ensure their utility to the specialist.

It has been the desire of the editors to arrange that the books should appeal to various classes of readers: and it is hoped that they will be useful to the medical profession at home and abroad, to bacteriologists and laboratory students, to municipal engineers and architects, to medical officers of health and sanitary inspectors and to teachers and administrators.

Many of the volumes will contain material which will be suggestive and instructive to members of Public Health and Hygiene Committees; and it is intended that they shall seek to influence the large body of educated and intelligent public opinion interested in the problems of public health.

AUTHOR'S PREFACE

THIS book is addressed mainly to those who are interested in the stamping out of tuberculosis. It makes no attempt to deal with the disease from its clinical aspect which has already been treated abundantly by many eminent writers.

The outlook of the author has been that of the experimental pathologist, and it is from this point of view mainly that the problem has been approached. This outlook, though it limits the field, has the compensating advantage that it opens up that aspect of it which is, perhaps, the least familiar.

It is hoped that the book will meet a demand for information on many points about which the author is frequently questioned. For, though notable advances have been made since the subject of the relation of animal to human tuberculosis was first brought prominently forward by Koch's adverse pronouncement at the London Congress in 1901, the researches which have led to these advances are, for the most part, buried in Blue Books or hidden in other official publications. It is, indeed, one of the principal objects of this book to bring together in a handy form these researches, and particularly those of the late Royal Commission on Tuberculosis and the Local Government Board in this country, the Department of Health of the City of New York and the Imperial Board of Health in Berlin.

The greater part of the book will be found to deal with the tubercle bacillus and its varieties, or "types," as they are more generally called. It treats of their distribution, cultural characters and comparative virulence for a number of animal species. In particular the sharpness of characterization of these types and their stability under conditions which, if any, might be supposed to conduce to modification, that is to say the evidence of their existence as distinct varieties, is inquired into at some length.

Such questions may appear to some to be merely of academic interest. But it is not so. In reality their solution is necessary before a true opinion can be formed of the relative importance of the different sources of infection in human tuberculosis, and they play a practical rôle in the campaign for the eradication of the disease.

This book is addressed, as we have said already, to those who are interested in the stamping out of tuberculosis. And, consequently, it is intended both for those who are and those who are not members of the medical profession. The language has therefore been kept simple and as free as possible from technical difficulties; at the same time it has seemed desirable, in the interest of those who are following, or about to follow, lines of research similar to those dealt with here, to review much original work in considerable detail. It is feared that this survey, extended as it is over many pages, may prove tedious; and for this reason some of it has been printed in small type. Such parts may be passed over without interfering with the thread of the argument. But, indeed, the main defence of a detailed treatment lies in the fact that it should enable the reader to arrive at his own conclusion; and the author is more concerned that he may be held to have presented the evidence fully, clearly, impartially and with criticism which is just, than that he should be pronounced to have dealt with the subject in an agreeable manner.

The earlier chapters of the book deal with the magnitude of the evil imposed by the tubercle bacillus upon mankind, and with its age and sex distribution in town and country. The changes in this distribution, which have been so remarkable a feature of the history of human tuberculosis in the last half century, are described, and attention called particularly to the great diminution of mortality which has occurred among women at certain periods of life. The causes of the wonderful decline in the mortality from tuberculosis which has occurred in these, and to only a lesser extent in all other, classes of the population is briefly touched upon; and evidence is assembled in the hope of giving credence to the vision which has already gladdened the eyes of some seers that at a day, not too far distant, the world may become rid of this incubus, or at least that tuberculosis shall have ceased to exact an exorbitant tribute and have become reduced to the status of one of the less common diseases.

The part played by personal contagion in the spread of the disease, and the relative importance of individual predisposition and opportunity for infection, or as we may say of "soil and seed," about which such curious fluctuations of opinion have occurred in the past is considered in Chapters IV and V.

On this ancient controversy it is hoped that a new point will be found to have been brought to bear, namely the influence of the *quantity* of bacilli in the infecting dose. This, though recognized, more or less clearly, by certain writers, has, in the main, been strangely neglected hitherto, and evidence of an experimental kind is here brought forward, it is believed for the first time, to establish its importance.

Next follows a consideration of the *portals* through which tubercle bacilli enter the body most commonly, about which erroneous opinions, quite recently, have prevailed in high places. The practical bearing of this question on the decision whether pulmonary discharges or contaminated milk are most to be guarded against is sufficient justification for dealing with this question at large.

The chapters which follow deal with the bacillus itself and its various types, as already indicated, and with the means which are available for their identification.

Chapters XVIII to XXIII treat of tuberculosis in animals. The remarkable difference in histological response to invasion by tubercle bacilli presented by different species is pointed out; but the chief interest is devoted to types of bacilli found in instances of naturally acquired tuberculosis in each animal species, and in the relative susceptibility of that species to infection with each of the three types as shown by artificial experiment. As will be seen, it is not always the type which is most virulent for a given species that is responsible for the majority of instances in it of naturally acquired disease.

Human tuberculosis is treated in Chapters XXIV and XXV from the same standpoint, but at greater length as its importance demands. Each kind of tuberculous disease is dealt with separately, and special attention is given to lupus, concerning which so many problems of interest arise.

Lastly, in the concluding chapter is summarized the evidence as to the comparative distribution of the three types of tubercle bacilli in various animal species and the part, if any, played by each in the various kinds of tuberculosis in man.

Such is the programme of the book. How far the author has succeeded in carrying it out it must be left to his critics to judge; he himself is not unaware of numerous shortcomings, and he would beg his judges to bear in mind the difficulties of the task. On one point especially he would ask indulgence, namely on the classification of atypical tubercle bacilli. For this the time was not fully ripe; fresh facts were coming to light while the book was being put together, so that place for some of them has had to be found in an appendix. This circumstance was however not without its recompense for it conveyed a stimulating sense of the fact that one was dealing with a living and developing problem.

In conclusion, the author hopes that this book may receive a welcome from those who have at heart the victory over disease. And he will feel that he has not laboured in vain if it should lead, in some degree, to a more general interest in the fundamental problems concerning that disease which, without exaggeration, may be described as the commonest, most fatal and, perhaps, as the saddest of those which oppress mankind.

The author's thanks are due to many helpers, and especially to Dr A. Stanley Griffith and to Lieut. C. F. Fox, whose intimate knowledge of the Reports of the Royal Commission has proved invaluable.

L. C.

CAMBRIDGE,
  January, 1917.

CONTENTS

LIST OF ILLUSTRATIONS

Available for download from www.cambridge.org/9781107456563

---

xvi LIST OF ILLUSTRATIONS

CHAPTER 1

THE TRIBUTE EXACTED BY TUBERCULOSIS

The Annual Mortality. Its Age and Sex Distribution and the changes which these have undergone in the last half-century.

Tuberculosis is the commonest of all the important diseases of civilized lands. Over 51,000 deaths were attributed to it in 1910 in England and Wales[1]. This number was the lowest ever recorded ; yet it accounted for more than one death in every ten, and was in the proportion of 1434 to every million persons living.

Large as is this mortality at home, in nearly all other countries it is larger still ; and in some much larger. In Scotland the death-rate from tuberculosis is a little higher than in England and Wales, and in Ireland half as high again[2]. In Prussia, in 1910, it was 1510 per million ; in Austria 2880 ; and in Hungary 3480. In the Balkan Peninsula tuberculosis is extremely rife[3]. In Paris too it is a frequent cause of death ; and in a report of the Préfet de la Seine, some few years ago, it was stated that one person in every four who died there was certified to have died of tuberculosis.

Belgium, alone of all countries of Europe, has a death-rate from pulmonary tuberculosis lower than that in England and Wales—and the difference is inconsiderable ; and a review of all the countries of the world for which figures are available shows that only in New Zealand, Australia, and Ontario is the

[1] 73rd *Rep. Reg. Gen. England and Wales* (1910), p. lv. The actual number was 51,317. In 1911 the deaths from tuberculosis of all kinds were slightly more numerous, and numbered 53,120.

[2] 2150 per million in 1912.

[3] In Servia, for example, in 1910 the death-rate from pulmonary tuberculosis was 3437 per million.

mortality from this cause substantially less than it is in this country[1].

But though the number of deaths certified to be caused by tuberculosis is large it probably falls short of the truth ; for there is reason to think that a good many deaths which are really due to that cause become included in bronchitis, pneumonia, or some other category. Both to bronchitis and pneumonia are assigned each year almost as many deaths as to pulmonary tuberculosis itself ; and there is considerable uncertainty as to the etiology of bronchitis, and of some kinds of pneumonia also. It seems not unlikely then that, in early life, a good many cases of pulmonary tuberculosis get returned under the latter, and still more, towards the end of life, under the former heading[2]. It has even been suggested that the diminution of the mortality from phthisis towards the latter end of life which appears in our records is not a real one, and would disappear if all deaths from senile phthisis were correctly reported ; and that the registered mortality from that cause

[1] The death-rates per million from pulmonary tuberculosis (which are probably more reliable than those for all kinds of tuberculosis) were, in 1910 (unless otherwise stated), as follows in some of the principal countries for which statistics are available.

France	1788	
Ireland	1716	(Excluding acute miliary tuberculosis)
Germany	1421	
Denmark	1201	(1912. Principal cities only)
Netherlands	1189	
Italy	1174	(Including general tuberculosis)
Scotland	1142	(Excluding acute miliary tuberculosis)
England and Wales	1015	
Belgium	972	
Ontario	932	(1911)
Australia	700	
New Zealand	587	

(Calculated from figures given in the 74th Report of the Registrar General for England and Wales (1911), pp. 105 et seq.)

These are crude death-rates, uncorrected for sex and age constitution of population, and are therefore only roughly comparable with one another. See also 73rd Rep. (1910), p. xcviii.

[2] It was observed in Sheffield, when compulsory notification was introduced, that some of those who had been notified as suffering from pulmonary tuberculosis came in the end to be certified as having died of some other cause. Matthew Hay also has called attention to the confusion of bronchitis and phthisis in Aberdeen (see footnote on p. 13).

would then increase right up to the end of life, as it does in New York[1].

I. *Age Distribution of the Mortality from Tuberculosis.*

In order to appreciate fully the economic importance of tuberculosis to the community, one must know at what period of life the deaths fall thickest ; for it is obvious that diseases which destroy infants on the threshold of life, as, for example, measles and whooping cough, and others which, like cancer, carry off for the most part those whose work is nearly done, are of less consequence to the well-being of the state than such as remove the young adult (after much expenditure of labour and money has been incurred in his upbringing) and many of those who are in the full tide of their activity and upon whom, very often, children and wife or husband are dependent. And tuberculosis does just this ; for though it is true that the disease is more fatal in infancy than at any other period of life, yet the great bulk of its mortality falls in middle life[2].

At the present day, in England and Wales, the incidence of the tuberculosis mortality on the different periods of life is as follows :

Infancy. As already mentioned, tuberculosis is more fatal in infancy than at any other time of life, and most of all in the latter part of the first year. In 1911 the deaths from this cause in the first year formed 6·3 per cent. of the total for the whole of life ; those in the second year 5 per cent., and those in the first five years taken together 16·7 per cent.

The distribution of this mortality throughout these five years is shown in the following table, from which it will be seen how greatly it is concentrated into the 18 months which immediately succeed the first half-year of life.

---

[1] Dr Glover Lyon, quoted by Newsholme in *The Prevention of Tuberculosis* on p. 24.

[2] More than one-half of all the deaths ascribed to tuberculosis fall between the twentieth and the fiftieth year of age.

The deaths in 1911 were actually as follows:

Ages	0–5	5–20	20–50	50+
	8877	8178	27,365	8700

DIAGRAM I. *The Incidence of the Mortality from Tuberculosis of all kinds and from Pulmonary Tuberculosis at Different Periods of Life, as shown by the mean annual mortality per million persons living at each age period in England and Wales, during the decade* 1901–10.

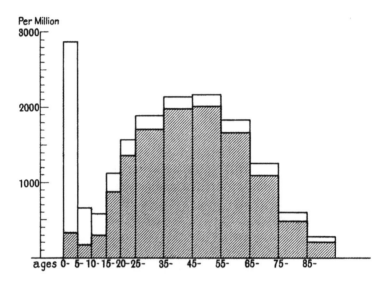

All Kinds of Tuberculosis.

Ages   0–   5–   10–   15–   20–   25–   35–   45–   55–   65–   75–   85– All ages
Males and
Females 2883 667 586 1125 1576 1892 2150 2163 1838 1246 602 280   1653

Pulmonary Tuberculosis only (shaded columns).
Males and
Females 327 166 283 873 1370 1708 1983 2004 1673 1095 477 180   1161

(Calculated from the figures published in the Annual Reports of the Registrar General, with the aid of a.table giving the mean annual population both male and female at various age periods, kindly supplied by him for the purpose.)

TABLE I. *Number of Deaths at Different Age Periods
in Early Life.* 1911.

	Months				Years					Total under 5	Total all ages
	0–1	1–3	3–6	6–12	0–1	1–2	2–3	3–4	4–5		
Pulmonary Tuberculosis *	8	16	63	219	306	356	198	138	123	1121	38,422
All other kinds	33	374	916	1724	3047	2284	1183	721	521	7756	14,698
Total (all kinds)	41	390	979	1943	3353	2640	1381	859	644	8877	53,120

* Pulmonary tuberculosis (not acute)+acute phthisis.
From figures in 74th *Rep. Reg. Gen. E. and W.* (1911), pp. 196, 197.

Childhood. What may be called the school age or, more precisely, that which extends from the fifth to the fifteenth birthday, is, if we except extreme old age (and here, as we have seen, the statistics are less reliable), the period of life when deaths from tuberculosis are least frequent. Indeed they are then, comparatively speaking, so uncommon that the death-rate from this cause is only about one-third as high as it is during the greater part of adult life.

Adolescence, Middle Life, and Old Age. After the school age the mortality from tuberculosis increases, rapidly at first, and afterwards more slowly, until it attains a second maximum between the ages of 35 and 55. It then again falls slowly, attaining the lowest point of all after 85.

Thus it may be said that the mortality from tuberculosis is concentrated about two distinct periods of life, namely infancy and maturity, culminating in the earlier period about the latter half of the first and the earlier part of the second year, and in the latter period about the very prime of life. Between the two is the school age when deaths from tuberculosis are comparatively rare.

The relative frequency of deaths from various kinds of tuberculosis at different periods of life. The type of tuberculous disease which prevails in each of the two periods of maximum fatality is distinct ; for, while all kinds of tuberculosis occur at both periods, some kinds preponderate greatly at the one period, and other kinds preponderate at the other. Thus in infancy the commonest type is tuberculous meningitis, followed, at an interval, by tuberculous peritonitis and general tuberculosis. At this early period pulmonary tuberculosis accounts for only 12·6 per cent. of all the deaths from tuberculosis[1]. After the 15th year, on the other hand, nearly 90 per cent. of the deaths from tuberculosis are caused by pulmonary disease, and there remains little more than 10 per cent. to include all other kinds of tuberculosis, a category which in infancy comprises 87·4 per cent. of the deaths from all kinds of tuberculosis.

II. *The Incidence of the Mortality from Tuberculosis on the Two Sexes.*

The extent to which the two sexes participate in the mortality from tuberculosis is very different to-day from what it has been in the past. Formerly the mortality was divided fairly evenly between the sexes, rather more women dying of tuberculosis than men. At the present day men suffer much more than women; taking all ages together, four males die from tuberculosis for every three females.

The following description is based on the figures of the first decade of this century.

In the first five years of life, taken as a whole, boys die of tuberculosis more frequently than girls, in the ratio, broadly speaking, of six to five. But after the fifth year the incidence on the sexes is reversed, and from 5 to 20 tuberculosis claims more victims among girls than boys. It may be said then that during childhood and adolescence girls suffer more than boys, the greatest difference between the sexes at that period occurring between 10 and 15, when the ratio of the

---

[1]   *Deaths from Tuberculosis under 5 years.* 1911.

Tuberculous Meningitis	3347
Tuberculosis of Peritoneum and Intestines	2700
Acute miliary Tuberculosis	327 ⎱ 1512
Disseminated Tuberculosis	1185 ⎰
Pulmonary Tuberculosis (not acute)	961 ⎱ 1121
Acute Phthisis	160 ⎰
All other kinds	197
Tuberculosis, all forms	8877

From the 74*th Ann. Rep. Reg. Gen. E. and W.* pp. 196 *et seq.*

tuberculosis mortality of females to that of males is about three to two.

From about the age of 20 onwards young men begin to die from tuberculosis more frequently than young women; and the difference increases and becomes very considerable as age

DIAGRAM II. *The mean annual Mortality from Tuberculosis of all kinds at different ages in Males and Females in England and Wales, 1901–10.*

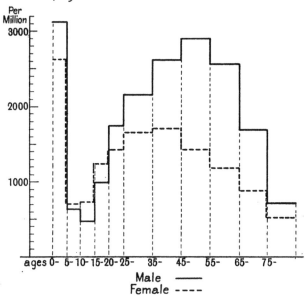

Male ——
Female - - - -

Ages	0–	5–	10–	15–	20–	25–	35–	45–	55–	65–	75–	85–	All ages
Males	3129	636	463	997	1774	2159	2622	2934	2574	1688	708	332	1902
Females	2636	698	710	1250	1425	1651	1710	1449	1186	894	529	250	1421

Ratio of the male to female death-rate from tuberculosis (the latter being taken as 100) at different ages.

118·7 91·1 65·2 79·8 122·4 130·8 153·3 202·5 217·0 188·8 133·8 132·8 133·8

advances, until the maximum disparity is reached between 45 and 65, when the mortality among men is twice as high as it is among women. In old age (if the figures for this period of life can be trusted) the disparity of the incidence diminishes and after 85 about four men are certified to die of tuberculosis for every three women.

The maximum mortality in adult life is attained considerably later among men than it is among women, occurring in the case of the former between 45 and 55, and in that of the latter between 25 and 45.

This was not always the case. In 1861–70 both maxima occurred earlier in life, and very much at the same period in the two sexes ; the maximum among women being then between 25 and 35 and that among men between 25 and 45. Thus we see that one of the important changes which have been taking place is the shifting of the maximum mortality from tuberculosis to a later period of life, and this to a greater extent among men than among women.

These and other changes which have taken place must be considered in greater detail in the following chapters.

CHAPTER II

THE DECLINE OF TUBERCULOSIS

At the present day, as we have seen, tuberculosis of all kinds claims rather more than 50,000 deaths per annum. Half a century ago the number was between 60,000 and 70,000. In *actual numbers* then, and not only in proportion to population, tuberculosis has declined, and the magnitude of that decline in the last fifty years has been, let us say, 20 per cent.[1]

The decline in the *death-rate* from this cause has, of course, been much greater, for the population has greatly increased during this period[2]. As we shall see, this decline, during the period under consideration, amounted to about 50 per cent.

---

[1] A decline in the number of deaths assigned to tuberculosis has occurred in other countries also. Thus Koch, in 1906, pointed out in his Nobel Lecture that the actual number of deaths from pulmonary tuberculosis in Prussia each year was then about 20,000 less than it was twenty years previously.

[2] For every 100 people living in England and Wales in 1851, there were estimated to be 197 in 1908. See *Public Health and Social Conditions*, p. 2, issued by the Local Government Board, 1909, Cd. 4671.

Can the Figures be Trusted?

This decline in the death-rate of tuberculosis is one of the most important and astonishing facts in medical history, and the question immediately arises whether it indicates a real decline of the disease, and how far the figures on which it rests can be trusted. The figures are based on death certificates; and these, as one knows, are likely too often to be the result of faulty or incomplete diagnosis. But when we are attempting to compare the records of the present day with those of previous times, it is perhaps not so much the mistakes due to human fallibility which concern us—for these are much the same in one period as in another—as the changes which the discoveries of recent times and the progress of medical education have deliberately wrought in the nomenclature of diseases—changes which have undoubtedly led to the attributing of many deaths at the present day to causes other than those to which they would have been assigned in the past.

We must therefore inquire how far the changes which have taken place in recent times invalidate a comparison of the records of the present day with those of a few decades ago.

It will be convenient to consider separately infantile and adult tuberculosis. Let us begin with the former.

The sum of infantile tuberculosis is, as we have seen, made up mainly of tuberculous meningitis, tuberculous peritonitis, and general tuberculosis. And to these must be added another category, namely tabes mesenterica, which formerly included a large number of deaths, but which is now comparatively unimportant. Pulmonary tuberculosis forms only about one-eighth of the whole.

It is in the large group of abdominal tuberculosis that most uncertainty is likely to be felt in diagnosis, and most change in the fashion of nomenclature has probably taken place. In 1891 over 7000 deaths were ascribed to tabes mesenterica in England alone. In 1910 there were less than 800 in England and Wales assigned to this cause. What has become of the others ? Surely they have not all found a haven in " tuberculous peritonitis " ? Is it not more probable that in the past, when there was less precision in diagnosis, many a case of wasting, associated with chronic diarrhœa or other abdominal symptoms, was put down to tabes mesenterica, and that now many such cases are recognized to have nothing to do with tuberculosis[1]?

If for this reason there is cause to think that the official figures may exaggerate the decline of infantile tuberculosis, there is yet another probable source of error which goes far to counteract this one, if not to overrule it altogether. For some authorities believe that tuberculosis is a much commoner cause of death among children than the death certificates show. Coates[2], for example, found that out of 77 children who died in Great Ormond Street Hospital in 1877, no less than 35 per cent. succumbed to some kind of tuberculosis. These were no doubt for the most part children of the poorer classes, among whom tuberculosis is very common, but Coates was of opinion that we might safely affirm that of

[1] See Tatham in the Supplement to the 65th *Annual Report of the Registrar General*, 1891–1900, Part I, p. lxxxiv. "It is reasonable to assume that in a considerable proportion of the deaths even now referred to 'tabes mesenterica' the tubercle bacillus would be sought for in vain." In this article the whole question of the comparability of the older with the recent statistics of tuberculosis, and of the reality in the decline in the mortality which they show, is briefly discussed.

On this subject see also Newsholme, *The Prevention of Tuberculosis*, Chap. III, " Are the statistics relating to tuberculosis trustworthy ? " Also in *The Relative Importance of the Constituent Factors involved in the Control of Pulmonary Tuberculosis*, Section headed " Can the Official Figures be Trusted ? " *Trans. Epidemiol. Soc.* xxv, p. 31. Newsholme is " not inclined to attach much value to the figures before 1870, or possibly 1866." Arthur Ransome, on the other hand, in " Phthisis Rates," *Trans. Epidemiol. Soc.* xxiv, is "inclined to think that it is not necessary entirely to reject the mortality figures during the thirty years preceding 1868." " There may be, and probably are," he adds, " inaccuracies in the returns for individual years ; but for the most part these inaccuracies will be in defect, not in exaggeration of the phthisis rate. It is more likely, for instance, that phthisis has been entered as bronchitis than that the converse has been the case. We may then, perhaps, accept the general outline of the curve " (showing the decline of phthisis from 1838) " as a fair representation of the truth " (*loc. cit.* pp. 261, 262).

See also Matthew Hay, quoted in footnote on p. 13, and Bulstrode, *loc. cit.* p. 32.
[2] Quoted by Newsholme, see *The Prevention of Tuberculosis*, 1908, p. 23.

the total deaths from all causes under 10 years of age among the masses of the people one-third are due to tuberculosis. Now if this is anywhere near the truth there must be an enormous number of deaths from tuberculosis among children which never get recorded as such, for in recent years only one-sixteenth of the total deaths from all causes under ten years were certified to be due to tuberculosis. Without doubt a very large diminution has taken place in the proportion of deaths from tuberculosis to those from all causes since Coates wrote, but after making the most liberal allowance for this it still seems certain that many deaths from tuberculosis get assigned to other causes. If this is the case at the present day it is probable that the error was still larger in the past, for it is reasonable to suppose that the progress of medical science and education has greatly increased the accuracy of diagnosis. The diminution of this source of error, by causing an ever increasing proportion of deaths from tuberculosis to be recognized as such, would by itself tend to raise the recorded death-rate from tuberculosis[1].

[1] Shennan (1909), who examined the post-mortem records, extending over the last 21 years, of the Royal Hospital for Sick Children in Edinburgh, found that out of 1085 children up to 13 years of age 421, or nearly 39 per cent., had died of tuberculosis (see p. 169).

More recently Eastwood and F. Griffith (1914) have published the results of an examination of the bodies of 150 children, aged from two to ten years, who died in general hospitals in London from all causes. There was no selection, the cases being taken as they came to the post-mortem room. Of these no less than 62·7 per cent. were found to be infected with tubercle bacilli, and in 40·7 per cent. death was considered to be due to tuberculosis, a proportion which agrees very closely with that found by Shennan.

On the other hand German investigations give a very different result. Thus Gaffky (1907), out of 300 unselected children examined post-mortem, found only 12 per cent. with more or less obvious tuberculosis. Rothe, out of 150, found only 9·3 per cent.

Ungermann (1912), working in the Gesundheitsamt, examined a series of unselected children who had died of any cause whatever in general hospitals in Berlin. The ages of the children varied from one month to 13 years. In 29, or 17 per cent., it is stated, tuberculosis was either the sole cause of death or a severe complication of some other disease.

Thus we see that the difference between the British and German figures is so great that it is quite clear that they cannot be relied upon to show, even very roughly, the relative importance of tuberculosis as a cause of death in childhood. For the Berlin figures give a ratio of considerably less than 17, and the London and Edinburgh figures one of 40, or thereabouts, of deaths

Thus it would seem that there have been two opposing changes in action, one tending to cause the returns based on death certificates to exaggerate, and the other tending to make them minimize, the real fall in the infantile mortality from tuberculosis.

In which direction is the resultant of these opposing tendencies ? It is difficult to say ; but one would be inclined to think that in the past the number of deaths from tuberculosis which were assigned to some other cause must have outnumbered those which were wrongly assigned to this cause, and that the effect of the progressive diminution of these mistakes has tended on the whole to increase the recorded mortality of the disease in question.

Turning now to tuberculosis in adult life, which, as we have seen, consists largely of pulmonary disease, we have to face a similar problem. Bronchitis and pneumonia are both of them diseases which, at times, are liable to be confounded with pulmonary tuberculosis, the former with the more chronic forms, especially in the latter part of life, the latter with the more acute forms, particularly among the young. Each of these categories is almost as large as pulmonary tuberculosis itself[1]

from tuberculosis to deaths from all causes in children dying in general hospitals, and yet the official death-rates show that tuberculosis is more rife in Berlin than in London. Clearly this ratio in hospitals is very different from what it is amongst the child population outside ; and in all probability the difference is caused by the methods adopted for selecting suitable cases for admission and for continued residence in the general hospitals, and the provision made for treating tuberculous cases in special institutions—factors which doubtless differ in the two countries.

While these figures, then, cannot be used to indicate the proportion of fatal cases of tuberculosis among children generally, the British ones at least show that death from tuberculosis is remarkably common among hospital children, and they lend some support to Coates' contention that tuberculosis is a commoner cause of death in the early part of life than the death-rates would lead us to suppose.

For references to the papers quoted in this note see list at the end of Chap. x.

For evidence on the degree of reliability of clinical diagnosis in America, a paper by Dr Horst Oertel in the *Lancet* (1914), I, p. 1150 may be consulted.

[1] In 1911 in England and Wales the death-rates from these causes were as follows :

Pulmonary tuberculosis		..	..	1080 per million.
Bronchitis	..	..	..	..	1010 ,,
Pneumonia	..	..	..	..	1040 ,,

and either of them therefore could absorb many cases of pulmonary tuberculosis without noticeable expansion ; we have therefore to enquire whether the fall in the recorded mortality from pulmonary tuberculosis has been caused to any serious extent by transference of deaths from the category of tuberculosis to that of bronchitis or pneumonia.

That this has not occurred on a large scale we may feel assured because while the mortality attributed to tuberculosis has been falling, that from bronchitis and pneumonia combined has not risen ; and indeed it is considerably lower at the present day than it was twenty years ago. Or if we do not consider this argument convincing we can at least feel certain that there has been a real and very substantial decline of all pulmonary diseases taken together[1].

The fall in the death-rate attributed to tuberculosis is so great that it seems very improbable that it can have been caused mainly by changes of nomenclature, or improvement in the accuracy of diagnosis. Some influence on the recorded rate such changes must, of course, have had, but it is impossible to say with certainty in which direction they have influenced it. Probably they have acted some in one way and some in another, and so, to a great extent, have neutralized one another. We may, therefore, feel some confidence that the record, as shown by official returns, based though these necessarily are on the shifting sands of death certificates, is a sufficiently close approximation to the truth.

[1] Matthew Hay, discussing the fall in the death-rate from phthisis in Aberdeen during the past fifty years, says, " It has not been due to changes in diagnosis or to the labelling, in recent years, as bronchitis or asthma cases that would formerly have been diagnosed as phthisis. The death-rate from bronchitis has fallen almost *pari passu* with that from phthisis. At the same time I am convinced, from observation of the nature of the illnesses met with in tuberculous families, that throughout the whole series of years under review, and right up to the present time, many cases of chronic phthisis have been wrongly spoken of as cases of bronchitis or asthmatic bronchitis. If there has been any change, it has rather been, by improved diagnosis, to transfer an increasing proportion of such cases to the tuberculous group, and thus to lessen rather than increase the apparent decline in pulmonary tuberculosis." " Tuberculosis in Aberdeen," p. 10, *Ann. Rep. City of Aberdeen for* 1909.

The Extent of the Decline of Tuberculosis.

Having seen good reason to accept the official returns of the mortality of tuberculosis as substantially trustworthy, let us proceed to examine them more closely.

The general death-rate from all causes has declined greatly in recent times, but the death-rate from tuberculosis has declined more than the general rate. Or, to put it another way, the proportion of people who die of tuberculosis is now considerably less than it used to be. Formerly more than one death in every eight was due to tuberculosis, now the proportion is about one in ten (100·6 in 1000 during 1911).

We have seen already that the actual number of deaths from tuberculosis has decreased by about 20 per cent. in the last half-century and that the death-rate has decreased far more owing to the growth of the population. The actual extent of the decrease in the death-rate from tuberculosis has been nearly 50 per cent. in 40 years, or more precisely 49 per cent. between the decade 1861–70 and the decade 1901–1910. And in 1911 the tuberculosis death-rate was lower than the mean annual rate of the earlier of these decades by 55 per cent.

If one looks at the " curve " formed by the annual death-rates from tuberculosis[1] for the 60 years or so since registration became general, one sees that from 1857 to 1867 the rate was practically stationary. Prior to that there seems to have been some slight fall (at least in the rate for phthisis alone)[2], but *since 1865 it has been falling steadily and with ever-increasing velocity.*

Irregularities in the curve have, of course, occurred from time to time owing to fluctuations in the conditions of life favourable or unfavourable to consumptive persons. Such fluctuations, no doubt, act as follows. In an unfavourable year, either from severity of the weather conditions, scarcity of work, rise of prices, prevalence of influenza or what not,

---

[1] See for example in the 69*th Ann. Rep. of the Reg. Gen.* 1906, p. xc.

[2] See chart in the Decennial Supplement to the 65*th Annual Report,* 1891–1900, Pt. I, p. xciv.

many phthisical persons, with lives hanging on a thread, die, who in more favourable times would have survived to the following year; and conversely in a favourable year many who, under normal conditions, would have died in that year, survive to swell the death-rate of a following year[1].

Such fortuitous variations interfere with the study of the curve, and, in order to eliminate them as far as possible, the following method has been adopted. The mean death-rate of each successive quinquennium has been calculated, and these have been represented in the form of a curve. These quinquennia then, it will be observed, do not run consecutively, but overlap one another. Thus the first includes the years 1860–64, the second 1861–65, the third 1862–66 and so on. The diagram may therefore be said to represent the mean death-rates of successive overlapping quinquennia. For the sake of brevity each column in the diagram is labelled with a single date which is that of the central year of the quinquennium it represents.

[1] An extreme example of this is furnished by the city of Paris, where the consumptives suffered severely in 1870 and 1871, during the siege and the disturbed times which followed it. The enormous mortality from tuberculosis during this period, and the temporary fall which followed it, is well shown in the following curve, which has been drawn from the official figures.

Death-rate from Phthisis in Paris.
1865–1905.

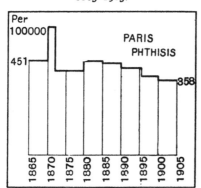

Arthur Ransome (see *Trans. Epidemiol. Soc.* XXIV, p. 262) called attention to periodic waves in the death-rate from phthisis, and noted faint indications of a rise in 1853, 1866, 1878 and 1890. Bulstrode, in referring

DIAGRAM III. *The Decline in the Mortality from Tuberculosis,
shown by the mean annual death-rate in successive (overlapping) quinquennia. [Based on the chart published by the
Registrar General, which is corrected for changes in the age
and sex distribution of the population.]*

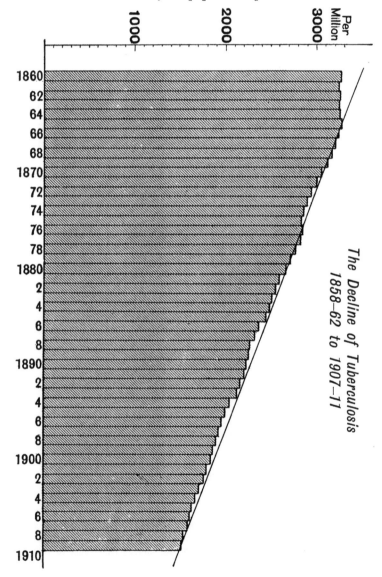

The Causes of the Decline.

Study of this diagram shows that the decline has been almost constant since 1863–67. A slight undulation is indeed just visible with crests rising every ten years or so, but no change in the general line of progress occurs anywhere to mark event or epoch. Thus there is nothing to indicate the effect of the discovery of the tubercle bacillus in 1882, or of the growth of the sanatorium movement which occurred about the beginning of the present century[1].

The causes of the decline, then, have evidently been acting continuously during the whole period under consideration. What are they? Is the tubercle bacillus undergoing a slowly progressive diminution of virulence? Is the intrinsic capacity for resistance of the race of men increasing? Or are the changes

to such rises, pointed out that there was an outbreak of influenza in 1855 which might possibly account for the increase of tuberculosis at that time. "In 1866 there was the cotton famine. In 1890 the recent prevalence of influenza began, but I find that in 1891 there was a much greater number of deaths from influenza than in 1890. There are many suggestions, but it does not seem to me that they fully explain the elevations" (*Ibid.* p. 293).

One would expect that severe winters would cause the death of many phthisical persons who otherwise would have lived longer, and that the curve of death-rates would show some correspondence with the meteorological records. To some extent it does so. The severe and prolonged frost which began in December, 1890, and lasted during the greater part of January, 1891, will be remembered by many. And the death-rate from phthisis during these years was conspicuously high. But the equally severe and prolonged frost of February, 1895, corresponds to only a small rise in the curve. The winter during the siege of Paris, 1870–71, was severe, and here again the curve rises. But with this the correspondence ceases. 1879–80 and 1880–81 were both severe winters, but the death-rate was low both in 1880 and 1881. The celebrated Crimean winter of 1854 corresponds to a slight depression in the curve, though the death-rate from phthisis was high in both 1853 and 1854. Moreover, the death-rate was high in 1875 and 1878, when the cold was not exceptional.

The fluctuations in unemployment (as shown in the *2nd Fiscal Blue Book*, Cd. 2337, 1904, p. 83) show very little correspondence with those of the death-rate from phthisis; the very worst year for employment, 1879, showing a rate which is not above the average for the time.

[1] Matthew Hay remarks, "The decline began before the germ origin had been demonstrated by Koch..." and "What is more remarkable, the rate of the decline was almost as great before any administrative attention was being paid to its infective character." "Tuberculosis in Aberdeen," p. 11, *Ann. Rep. City of Aberdeen for* 1909.

conveniently expressed by Ransome in the phrase " amelioration of social conditions " rendering the opportunities for infection fewer, and the mean level of health of the people higher,
so that, though their powers of defence are fundamentally
the same as before, they are better able to put them into
action ?

It is tempting to speculate on the possibility that the
virulence of the tubercle bacillus may have declined in recent
times[1]. This is not so inherently improbable as it may sound
at first ; for in the case of another disease, namely scarlet fever,
there is reason to think that the virulence of the causative
micro-organism, whatever that may be, has notably diminished.
At least there is no question whatever that the average severity
of the disease has decreased. The mortality is only one-tenth of
what it was fifty years ago, and prior to 1906 no year experienced
a mortality of less than double what it was in 1911[2]. Yet the
notification returns prove that scarlet fever is still widely
prevalent, " the diminished mortality corresponding with
extreme mildness of type[3]."

It is of course impossible to say to what extent this increasing mildness of type of scarlet fever has been due to changes in
the micro-organism on the one hand, and to changes in the
resistance of its host on the other. It is possible that the wide
prevalence of the disease has brought about an immunization
of the race, by a gradual elimination of the stocks most prone
to the disease. But this assumes an inheritable weakness
towards a particular parasite, a doctrine which, though probable
enough, has never been proved. Moreover in the case of a
disease which even in the past was relatively so seldom fatal
as scarlet fever, it would seem improbable that any widespread immunization could have been thus brought about ;
and the decline in the virulence of the disease seems to
have been altogether too rapid to be explained in this way.
There is therefore some reason for suspecting that the

[1] This was suggested by Sir Shirley Murphy, in a discussion on Dr Newsholme's paper read at the Epidemiological Society in December, 1905. See
Trans. Epidemiol. Soc. xxv, p. 120.

[2] T. H. C. Stevenson, Introduction to the 74*th Rep. Reg. Gen.* 1911, p. lix.

[3] *Ibid.* p. lx.

micro-organism of scarlet fever has suffered a loss of virulence in recent years, and it seems not impossible therefore that this may have occurred also with the tubercle bacillus.

There is, however, no positive evidence whatever to show that the tubercle bacillus has lost any of its virulence. Newsholme points out that there is nothing in the classical descriptions of the disease by Watson and Trousseau to make one suspect that phthisis, like scarlet fever, has greatly varied in virulence (*loc. cit.* 1905, p. 132). And the fact that the mortality from tuberculosis has been increasing in some countries (*e.g.* Norway and Ireland) while it has been diminishing in most other places does not, as Scurfield remarks, fit in very well with this view. Of course it is possible that the Irish bacillus may have been gaining virulence while the English bacillus, for example, was losing it, and if so a difference of virulence should exist at the present day, and ought to be capable of experimental demonstration. But it is not probable. The experience of the Royal Commission does not lend much support to the view that different strains of tubercle bacilli of one and the same type (bovine or human) differ from one another in virulence (certain strains from the surface of the body alone excepted); and the dominant impression made on those who worked out the question of stability for the Commission was that tubercle bacilli were remarkable among pathogenic bacteria for the stability of their virulence (see pp. 298 and 366).

We therefore cannot believe that tuberculosis is declining because the tubercle bacillus is becoming less virulent, but must seek for some other explanation.

There is rather more to be said for the view that the fundamental power of resistance to invasion by the tubercle bacillus has been increased among peoples who have long been subjected to tuberculosis by the slow but continuous elimination of the more susceptible families. This view assumes that high or low powers of resisting the disease are transmitted by inheritance, a view which is very generally held, but which, as we have remarked already, cannot be said to have been proved. Nevertheless there are strong reasons for believing that individuals belonging to races among whom tuberculosis was, until recently, unknown are peculiarly liable to become infected when brought to European countries, or when the disease is introduced into their own lands.   In this connection one recalls the well known susceptibility of the South Sea Islanders, of the North American Indians, and of the native races of South Africa.   Metchnikoff has called attention to the great susceptibility to tuberculosis of the Kalmuck students who come from Turkestan to be educated in Russia. And quite recently the writer has heard on good authority that certain natives of Arabia show a very high degree of susceptibility to tuberculosis when they come to reside in Jerusalem.

But while it is highly probable that for many centuries tuberculosis has been weeding out the more susceptible stocks among those races which have for ages been decimated by it, and has in this way materially raised the average resisting power of those races, yet at the same time it is clear that the process must have been very gradual in its action, and it seems inconceivable that it could have made such strides in recent times, and in countries like England where the disease has doubtless been established since the dawn of its history, as to have wiped out half the mortality from this cause in less than half a century.

There seems then no good reason to believe that racial immunization, by means of the gradual elimination of families who may be supposed to have transmitted an inheritable susceptibility to tuberculosis, can account for anything more than a very small part of the reduction in the mortality which has taken place in recent times.   Rather one must look for the explanation to other causes which have not been so long in operation.

But another kind of racial immunization not dependent on heredity has, not improbably, been going on, and more particularly in recent times, owing to the growth of our industries and the rapid increase of the urban population.   And the possibility that this may be playing a part in the decline of tuberculosis which is now taking place seems worthy of more consideration than it has received hitherto.

There is sure evidence, as will be pointed out fully in Chapter V (p. 69), that tuberculous infection is far more widely spread among the people than is indicated by the death-rate alone. We have seen that one person in ten dies of tuberculosis, but there is reason to think that one in two, if not more, is infected with tuberculosis which becomes arrested, usually without ever being suspected during life. Now we know that it is possible to immunize calves and other animals by means of sublethal injections of tubercle bacilli, and we may therefore fairly assume that those persons who are subjected to a tuberculous infection from which they recover, are to some extent immunized thereby, and possess a higher power of resistance to infection with the tubercle bacillus than they would otherwise have enjoyed. That this is no idle speculation is rendered probable by the observations of Naegeli who made a careful search for tuberculous lesions in five hundred autopsies at Zürich. Naegeli found, when he came to compare the numbers of those who had died of tuberculosis at each age period with the numbers of those in whose bodies he had found tuberculous lesions of all kinds at that age, that the fatality of tuberculous infection diminished as age advanced, and was inversely proportional to the frequency of tuberculous lesions. Thus in infancy but few bodies showed these lesions, but where they were present they had generally proved fatal. The frequency of tuberculous lesions increased rapidly with each succeeding age period until 18 when it amounted to 97 per cent. At the same time the proportion of fatal cases to those shown to have been thus infected fell quickly as age advanced, to about 29 per cent. about the 18th year, after which, with the exception of a small rise between 20 and 30, it continued to fall gradually until the end of life[1].

The lesser fatality of tuberculous infection as age advances, thus demonstrated by Naegeli, may of course be due to a gradual increase of the natural powers of resistance during the years of growth, caused by purely developmental changes, and quite independent of chance immunization. And this is rendered

---

[1] See especially the chart in Naegeli's paper, *Virchow's Archives*, CLX, 1900, p. 457.

more probable by the fact that the maximum powers of resistance (according to Naegeli) are nearly attained at the close of the period of adolescence. Nevertheless it would be rash to deny any immunizing influence to the increasing frequency of unprogressive tuberculous lesions as the early years of life advance, and we are obliged to credit them with some, possibly not inconsiderable, share in causing the resistance of the race.

If it be objected that artificial immunity is of short duration and lasts at most a year or perhaps two (as shown by calves which have been injected for the purpose), one may reply that opportunities for reinfection are constantly being afforded, and in this way the resistance of a large proportion of the population may be kept up to a high level.

Now we shall, in a future chapter, show cause for thinking that the reason the disease does not progress in such cases as those to which Naegeli drew attention is that the dose of tubercle bacilli which causes them is too small (one can produce such abortive infections at will in certain animals by employing small doses, even if the bacilli be the most highly virulent for the species in question). Now the liability to absorb small doses of tubercle bacilli must increase with the prevalence of the disease and the density of the population, and it is admitted that the growth of our towns which in the 19th century accompanied the rise of the great industries, by crowding the people together and thus increasing the risk of infection, greatly tended to spread consumption. Consumption, we know, declined in spite of the adverse influence of urbanization[1]. But the question may be asked did it decline *pari passu* with the rise of the towns? Was there not perhaps an increase of consumption in the early days of the movement[2] accompanied necessarily by a corresponding increase of minimal immunizing infections, which latter, by increasing the resisting power of the succeeding generation, so led in turn to a decrease in the

[1] See Newsholme, *loc. cit.* 1905, p. 109.

[2] This postulated increase in the prevalence of phthisis must, if it actually occurred, have taken place in England before registration of causes of death became general; but in Scotland where the industrial development started later, the records show that the death-rate from tuberculosis was rising up to 1870 (see Chambers, *Public Health*, 1913, xxv, p. 42).

fatality of tuberculosis ? Indeed it seems possible that we may now be reaping advantages which have followed, as a sort of reaction, after a period of great activity of the disease. If this is so the decline in the prevalence of pulmonary tuberculosis which is now going on may be leading to a slackening of the immunizing process ; and in time the mortality of the disease may rise again, unless some new factor intervenes. Thus the rate of mortality from tuberculosis may be subject to rhythmic changes, and the decline which we are now witnessing may be nothing more than a part of one of these waves.

These considerations seem to show that it would not be wise to be contented to allow things to go on as they are, satisfactory though the present rate of decline in the mortality may appear, but suggest that strenuous efforts should be made while the present comparatively low death-rate renders the problem capable of being dealt with. At the same time it would appear that great care must be taken lest things be made worse instead of better ; for if this general immunization by means of small doses of widely distributed tubercle bacilli is playing any important part in increasing the resistance of the present generation, it is just possible that by checking the distribution of bacilli, as for example by discouraging indiscriminate spitting, or by abolishing bovine tuberculosis from dairy cattle, we may actually be undermining the resistance of the race, and paving the way for a future increase in the severity of the disease. Probably our attention should rather be given in the first place to the prevention of massive infection.   To this point we shall return in Chapter XXVI.

These remarks are not intended to discourage the efforts which are now being made.   Some increase in the susceptibility of the people will, it seems, inevitably accompany any decline in the prevalence of tuberculosis, however brought about.   But the considerations put forward above will serve to show how complicated is the problem of the eradication of tuberculosis, and how necessary it is to study every aspect of the question in order that such efforts should be directed with sure aim.

But while speculations such as we have just been considering excite some little interest, they find few adherents as yet[1]. And nearly all authorities attribute the decline which has taken place in the death-rate from tuberculosis to the combined action of a number of causes which may be grouped together under the heading "improvement of social conditions"; though naturally all authorities do not agree as to the relative importance of these various causes.

Bowditch in America and Garvin Milroy in Scotland attributed considerable influence to drainage of the subsoil, a damp soil being held to predispose to consumption. A similar conclusion was arrived at quite independently by Buchanan, and the latter showed, in his well known researches, that in various towns where the laying of sewers had drained the subsoil a considerable improvement in the death-rate from phthisis had followed. But he was careful to point out several exceptions to the rule, and in Leicester and Stratford the improvement which was observed soon after the works were carried out was not fully maintained. The position taken up by Buchanan was supported by Thorne Thorne. On the other hand Dr Kelly, 1897, Medical Officer of Health for West Sussex, disagreed with Buchanan and pointed out that the death-rate from phthisis had been distinctly lowered in his district in recent years, while very little, if any, change had taken place in the same period in the drainage of the soil. Newsholme, from whose book, *The Prevention of Tuberculosis*, the preceding particulars are taken, does not attach much importance to subsoil drainage as a cause of the decline of tuberculosis[2].

---

[1] Dr Clive Riviere has recently argued strongly in favour of regarding infection with the bovine bacillus in childhood as having an important immunizing effect upon the people, and he goes so far as to say " I would put forward the proposition that until the human tubercle bacillus can be nearly eliminated from our midst, or artificial immunization becomes an accomplished fact, infection with the bovine bacillus through the use of a well-mixed milk, remains our best ally in the campaign against tuberculosis." At the same time he is careful to call attention to " the risk of massive tuberculous infection through the use of milk from a single cow or a small herd." *Brit. Med. Journ.* 1914, I, p. 221. Nathan Raw (*Tub. Year Book and Sanatorium Annual*, 1913–14) and William Muir of Glenafton (*Brit. Med. Journ.* 1914, I, p. 273) have expressed somewhat similar views. And the same position is maintained abroad by Much.

[2] See *The Prevention of Tuberculosis*, pp. 194 *et seq.*, and *Trans. Epidemiol. Soc.* xxv, pp. 51–52 and 132.

Thorne Thorne attached considerable importance to the removal of damp and otherwise insanitary houses, of narrow streets and alleys, of back to back houses and of *culs-de-sac*. Dampness and darkness and stagnation of air were, according to him, the enemies to be recognized and removed. This was the point of view of the sanitary engineer.

Others have attached more importance to the improvement of the food of the 'people. Sir Hugh Beevor held that " the British public eat more[1] " and pointed out that the successful treatment of consumption carried out at Nordrach was largely based upon extra feeding. Sir Shirley Murphy supported this view, and laid stress on the greater extent to which women have shared in the decline of tuberculosis as compared with men. This difference he explained on the grounds that women suffer more when food is short than men do, and conversely when food becomes more plentiful it is they who reap most benefit. The man is fed all the time, the women, sufficiently, only when food is plentiful[2].

That tuberculosis is closely associated with poverty, filth and overcrowding, there can be no doubt whatever ; though whether these act by favouring the spread of infection, or by diminishing the resistance of the individual, may still be a matter of opinion. Though it does not spare the rich, tuberculosis more than decimates the poor, and it is in the very lowest strata of society that its ravages are most serious. As evidence of this one may quote the following figures from a paper read by Sir Shirley Murphy before the British Congress on Tuberculosis (see Table II next page).

The close association of phthisis with overcrowding, and with poverty which naturally goes hand in hand with overcrowding, is strong evidence that tuberculosis can be spread by bad social conditions, and consequently lends strong support

[1] Hunterian Oration, *loc. cit.* p. 1008.

[2] " Now when a family is poor who is it that suffers most ? It is invariably the woman who goes without ; often indeed she starves herself. She feeds her husband, she feeds her children, but often she herself will go without. But with improved prosperity she comes in for her share ; and I think in all probability the people who have derived the most benefit from the improved conditions of recent years have been the women " (from the reply to Dr Ransome's paper in the *Trans. Epidemiol. Soc.* XXIV, p. 285).

TABLE II. *Overcrowding in London.*

Proportion of Total Population, living more than two in a room (in tenements of less than five rooms)	The Phthisis Death-rate per 1000 of Population in 1894–98, varied from
District with under 10 per cent.	1·07 to 1·18
,, ,, 10–15 ,, ,,	1·38 ,, 1·49
,, ,, 15–20 ,, ,,	1·57 ,, 1·64
,, ,, 20–25 ,, ,,	1·67 ,, 1·83
,, ,, 25–30 ,, ,,	2·06 ,, 2·11
,, ,, 30–35 ,, ,,	2·13 ,, 2·42
,, ,, over 35 ,,	2·46 ,, 2·66

From a paper read by Sir Shirley Murphy before the *Brit. Cong. on Tuberculosis*, Catalog. vol. 1901, p. 153.

to the view that the decline of the disease has been brought about largely by the amelioration of such conditions, to which end such great efforts have been devoted. Not in England only has the mortality from tuberculosis fallen greatly, but in all the most advanced countries for which statistics are available. Only in backward countries like Ireland or Norway has it increased[1].

There can be no doubt then that the changes which may be summed up in the phrase, amelioration of social conditions, have played a considerable part in the reduction of the death-rate from tuberculosis. There is no need to labour this point. It is admitted universally. Among such changes the improvement which has taken place in the manners of the people must not be overlooked[2]. The labouring man no longer spits on the floor in his home, as he used sometimes to

[1] In Ireland the highest point in the death-rate from tuberculosis was reached in 1904, when the rate was 2880 per million. Since that year there has been a gradual decline to a rate of 2150 in the year 1912, showing an improvement of more than 25 per cent., since attention was prominently called to the exceptional state of the country in respect to its tuberculous mortality. (See *Rep. of the Reg. Gen. for Ireland, for* 1912. Reviewed in the *Lancet*, 1913, II, p. 947.) Newsholme says there has been no reduction of phthisis in France (1905, *loc. cit.* p. 65). Complete phthisis statistics are available only for Paris, and it is doubtful whether these can be trusted. The most probable conclusion seems to be that in Paris the phthisis rate has declined little if at all (*ibid.* p. 56).

[2] See Dr Moore's contribution to the discussion on Newsholme's paper (1905) (*loc. cit.* p. 134).

do, and the children run so much the less risk of swallowing tubercle bacilli in the dirt which they suck off their fingers and toys. The standard of domestic cleanliness has no doubt improved in the poorer quarters of our great cities. Overcrowding especially is less common than it was; and it is to be hoped that consumptives are less frequently allowed to share a bed with a healthy person, or persons, than was formerly the case.

But it is held by some that such improvements as we have been considering are probably not sufficient by themselves to abolish consumption, otherwise, as Sir William Broadbent pointed out, it would have disappeared long ago from among the rich. It is probable therefore that some other, and more direct, factor also has been at work in reducing the death-rate from this cause. It has been rather the custom hitherto to disparage measures and tendencies which have combined to limit direct infection from the sick to the healthy; and this is not surprising, for, as we shall see in another chapter, the majority of authorities, in this country at least, have been inclined to belittle the direct infectiousness of phthisis.

Newsholme, however, after exhaustively investigating all the suggestions which have been brought forward to explain the fall in the death-rate from the cause in question arrived at the conclusion that "none of them sufficed to explain the experience of different civilized communities in regard to phthisis, both as to the epoch, and the extent of its decline; and the influence which, concurrently with all of these, has been exercising the predominant, though unrecognized, influence is the segregation of consumptives, especially of advanced cases, in general hospitals, infirmaries and asylums, as measured by the ratio of the respective amounts of total and institutional relief[1]." There has doubtless been a very large amount of segregation of consumptives going on, not indeed with the avowed object of diminishing infection, but for the purpose of treatment or the relief of destitution. The Rt Hon. John Burns[2], in an

---

[1] *Trans. Epidemiol. Soc.* 1905, xxv, p. 39. See also *Journ. of Hygiene,* 1906, vi, p. 373; *The Prevention of Tuberculosis,* p. 256.

[2] *Lancet,* 1913, ii, p. 459.

address read before the International Medical Congress in
London in 1913, gave some striking figures showing how segregation had increased in this country. Referring to deaths from
all causes these figures showed that the proportion which
occurred in public institutions had risen, in this country, from
one in nine in 1881 to one in five in 1910; while in London
it had risen from one in five in 1881 to two in five in 1910.
Concerning phthisis, he said that "in 1911, in the whole of
England and Wales, 34 per cent. of the male, and 22 per cent.
of the female deaths, and in London 59 per cent. of the male,
and 48 per cent. of the female occurred in institutions." So
great an amount of segregation, the growth, it need hardly
be said, of modern times, cannot have been without considerable effect on the death-rate from tuberculosis[1].

The Decline of Tuberculosis Accelerating.

Whatever be the causes of the decline, and they are without
doubt complex, one striking fact comes out from a study of the
chart, namely that *the rate of decline has been an ever-accelerating
one.* For surely we should judge of the relative rate of decline
at two given periods, not by comparing the actual annual
decrements at these periods, but the ratios which each of the
decrements bears to the mortality immediately preceding it.
That this is the right way to judge the rate of decline will be
evident if we consider a concrete example. Let us suppose
the mortality to fall in one year from 1000 to 990, and, at
another period, from 100 to 90 in the same space of time. In
each case the actual annual decrement is 10, but in the first
case the mortality has declined by $\frac{1}{100}$th, and in the second
by $\frac{1}{10}$th. Is not the rate of decline in the latter instance
ten times as great as in the former? If this is admitted then
we must define a constant rate of decline as one where the

---

[1] Koch, in 1906, in his Nobel Lecture, said that there had been a great decline
of tuberculosis in Prussia, and that in Berlin 40 per cent. of the cases of pulmonary tuberculosis died in hospital.
The influence of segregation is referred to more fully in Chap. v.

mortality each year is less than that of the year immediately preceding it by a constant fraction of the latter.

Again let us consider for example the case of a mortality which always declined at the rate of 1 per cent. per annum. In such a case the actual annual decrement, being by hypothesis a constant fraction of a diminishing quantity, will itself diminish in like proportion. The slope of the curve will therefore become less and less steep as time goes on; it will exhibit a convexity downwards ; and it will be continually approaching a direction parallel to the base line. It will, in fact, look very much like the lower half of a parabola or hyperbola drawn with its axis horizontal.

But this is not the case with the curve of the death-rate from tuberculosis in recent times. The " curve " in fact continues to approach the base in a nearly straight line, and from this it follows that the actual annual decrements have remained almost the same. They have not appreciably diminished, and consequently the ratio of the annual decrements to the mortality immediately preceding has been as constantly increasing, and the rate of decline has been an ever-accelerating one. This is important because it shows that the causes which have been producing this decline have been growing stronger every year; and it affords strong hope that the curve will actually some day reach the base line, a consummation which would never be reached if the rate were to fall by a constant percentage.

As a matter of fact if we compare the mean annual death-rates of successive decades with one another, we find the rate of decline from decade to decade has increased from 11·6 per cent. between 1861–70 and 1871–80, to 17·76 per cent. between 1891–1900 and 1901–10.

TABLE III.   *The Rate at which the Death-rate from*
Tuberculosis has Declined in Successive Decades.

Decades	Mean annual death-rate from tuberculosis of all kinds in England and Wales	Diminution each decade	Rate of decline between the decades as measured by the ratio of the decrement to the rate for the previous decade
1861–70	3239		
1871–80	2862	377	11·64
1881–90	2429	433	15·13
1891–1900	201c	419	17·25
1901–10	1653	357	17·76

This accelerating rate of decrease in the mortality raises
strong hopes that the disease will actually die out ; for if the
rate of acceleration in the decline, which has continued with
small fluctuations but without any real check for half a century,
were to go on undiminished in the future tuberculosis would
become extinct within the present century.

It seems too much to believe that this will be really
accomplished, and it may well be that the rate of acceleration
will slacken and that the last remnants of tuberculosis will be
slow in going. But while this is freely admitted, it nevertheless
seems probable that we are actually witnessing—unless the
present decline be merely the part of a wave such as we have
already seen some grounds for thinking is possible—the rapid
extinction of one of the greatest diseases which afflict mankind,
and that tuberculosis is going the same way as leprosy, ague,
black death, typhus, and may we add small-pox, and other of
the great scourges of the by-gone past.

Some there may be who will deplore such a prospect, on
the grounds that diseases are nature's means of removing the
unfit, and who will argue that if tuberculosis should become
extinct the necessary consequence will be a deterioration of the
race. But the great majority of sensible people will not take
this view. Even if it be granted that tuberculosis carries off
those who are less capable of resisting its attacks rather than
those who are most exposed to infection, it does not follow that
the particular weakness which such individuals possess will be
any detriment to them when tuberculosis is abolished, for there
is absolutely no reason to think that it is correlated with any

other weakness.   In this connection Scurfield remarks that he
has little faith in the tubercle bacillus as " an improver of the
race."   " Half the Sheffield grinders (he says) die from
tuberculosis of the lungs, but it would be absurd to say that
half the Sheffield grinders are therefore weaklings.   Athletes
as well as scholars die from tuberculosis.   The owner of a
pedigree bull does not consider the animal a weakling because
he has to take steps to protect it from tuberculosis."   " It is
the tuberculous who are the weaklings, not the tuberculizable[1]."
This view is completely borne out by the personal experience
of the present writer, who has been greatly struck by the fact
that among his friends and acquaintances who have been
attacked by tuberculosis many were physically considerably
above the average.

CHAPTER III

THE EXTENT TO WHICH EACH SEX HAS SHARED IN
THE DECLINE OF TUBERCULOSIS

We have already seen that, in the decline which has taken
place in the death-rate from tuberculosis, females have benefited
more than males.   It is proposed in the present chapter to
consider more closely the extent to which each sex has shared
in this decline.

The following diagrams, together with the accompanying
figures on which they are based, show, for each sex separately,
at various periods of life, the mean annual mortality from
tuberculosis during the decades 1861–70, 1891–1900, and
1901–10.   The intervening decades, 1871–80, 1881–90, might
have been given also, but it was thought better, for the sake
of clearness, to omit them, and to confine attention to the
changes which took place during the latter part of the 19th
century, and then see to what extent these changes have continued to act in recent years.

---

[1] "Tuberculosis in the British Isles," p. 16 of Reprint, *Public Health*,
June 1912.

DIAGRAM IV. *Mean annual death-rates from tuberculosis of each sex and at various age periods, for the selected decades[1].*

Decade	Sex	All ages	0-	5-	10-	15-	20-	25-	35-	45-	55-	65-	75-
1861–1870	M	3327	6018	1029	899	2382	4031	4206	4244	3969	3433	2174	740
	F	3156	4917	939	1300	3300	4087	4482	3988	2954	2178	1354	528
1891–1900	M	2265	4347	705	521	1234	2102	2541	3251	3296	2768	1706	629
	F	1771	3516	744	818	1555	1788	2086	2264	1753	1344	906	427
1901–1910	M	1902	3129	636	463	997	1744	2159	2622	2934	2574	1688	668
	F	1421	2636	698	716	1250	1425	1651	1710	1449	1186	894	494

It will be seen at once, on looking at the two diagrams, that both sexes have participated in the decline, but not to the same extent. At almost every age period the decline has been greater among females than males ; and in each sex the decline has been greater in adolescence and early adult life than at any other period. This will appear more clearly in the following analysis.

In order to facilitate a more exact comparison, the ratios which the rates of the two latter decades bear to those of the decade or decades which preceded them are set out as percentages in Table IV; and in Table V the percentage decline which took place in the intervals between these decades has been given. To these have been added the ratios which the decline (in each of the intervals) among females bears to that among males.

TABLE IV. *Comparing the death-rates from tuberculosis at the three selected decades, with those of the decade or decades preceding them.*

The rate for 1891–1900 expressed as a percentage of that for 1861–70.

	All ages	0-	5-	10-	15-	20-	25-	35-	45-	55-	65-	75-
Males	68	72	69	58	52	52	60	77	83	81	78	85
Females	56	72	79	63	47	44	47	57	59	62	67	81

The rate for 1901–10 expressed as a percentage of that for 1891–1900.

		0-	5-	10-	15-	20-	25-	35-	45-	55-	65-	75-
Males	84	72	90	89	81	83	85	81	89	93	99	106
Females	80	75	94	87	80	80	79	76	83	88	99	116

The rate for 1901–10 expressed as a percentage of that for 1861–70.

		0-	5-	10-	15-	20-	25-	35-	45-	55-	65-	75-
Males	57	52	62	52	42	43	51	62	74	75	78	90
Females	45	54	74	55	38	35	37	43	49	54	66	94

[1] The figures for 1861–70 and 1891–90 are taken from the *Supplement to the 65th Rep. of the Reg. Gen. E. and W.* Pt. I, p. cxciii, where may also be found the figures for the intervening decades. Those for 1901–10 have been calculated from the figures in the Annual Reports by the help of a table of the sex and age distribution of the population, kindly provided for the purpose by the Registrar General.

TABLE V. *Showing the decline in the mortality from tuberculosis for each sex at various age periods, during the intervals between the three selected decades; and further showing for each interval the ratio of the decline in the female mortality to that in the male mortality, the latter taken as 100.*

Decline between 1861–70 and 1891–1900.

	All ages	0–	5–	10–	15–	20–	25–	35–	45–	55–	65–	75–
Percentage decline in Male mortality	32	28	31	42	48	48	40	23	17	19	22	15
Percentage decline in Female mortality	44	28	21	37	53	56	53	43	41	38	33	19
Ratio of Female to Male decline	138	100	68	88	110	117	133	187	241	200	150	127

Decline between 1891–1900 and 1901–10.

	All ages	0–	5–	10–	15–	20–	25–	35–	45–	55–	65–	75–
Percentage decline in Male mortality	16	28	10	11	19	17	15	19	11	7	1	(increase) 6 %
Percentage decline in Female mortality	20	25	6	13	20	20	21	24	17	12	1	(increase) 16 %
Ratio of Female to Male decline	125	89	60	118	105	118	140	126	155	171	100	

Decline between 1861–70 and 1901–10.

	All ages	0–	5–	10–	15–	20–	25–	35–	45–	55–	65–	75–
Percentage decline in Male mortality	43	48	38	48	58	57	49	38	26	25	22	10
Percentage decline in Female mortality	55	46	26	45	62	65	63	57	51	46	34	4
Ratio of Female to Male decline	128	96	68	94	107	114	129	150	196	184	154	40

Let us first consider the decline which took place between the decades 1861–70 and 1891–1900, an interval which roughly corresponds to the latter third of the 19th century.

The first point to notice is that the decline in females of all ages exceeded that among males of all ages in a rather higher proportion than four to three.

The next point is that the reduction among males was very much greater in the earlier than in the latter half of life, amounting to 40 per cent. or more at each age period from 10 to 35, and being only about half as great at any age period afterwards. In other words youths and young men benefited twice as much as men of middle and old age.

Among females on the other hand the decline was more evenly distributed over the whole period of life. It was indeed greatest between 15 and 35, when it exceeded 50 per cent., but it continued to be over 40 per cent. up to 55 years, and even after that it fell off but slowly. The disparity in the benefit derived by the two sexes respectively was therefore greatest in the latter half of life.

Let us see more exactly how this disparity of benefit affected the two sexes at the different periods of life. In infancy the reduction in the mortality was equal in the two sexes. Between 5 and 10 it was considerably greater among boys than girls. Between 10 and 15 the difference was in the same direction but of less extent. Thus far only did the males benefit more than the females. At all other periods of life the reduction of the mortality of females exceeded that among males, and during a considerable portion of life it exceeded it greatly. Thus, during the whole period between 35 and 65 it was at least nearly twice as great among women as among men, and between 45 and 55 nearly two and a half times as great.

Thus, to sum up, the disparity in the reduction of the mortality from tuberculosis in the two sexes during the latter third of the 19th century was nil in infancy, and considerable in childhood when the reduction was greater among boys than girls. In adolescence the disparity was small, but was now in favour of the girls. Gradually, at each successive age period, the disparity advanced, becoming more and more in favour of females until it reached its maximum late in middle life, when nearly five men died of tuberculosis for every two women.

Turning now to the more recent period we find that very much the same changes went on. Again there was a great reduction in the tuberculosis mortality of both sexes, and at all ages (old age alone excepted)[1]. During this interval the greatest reduction occurred in infancy in either sex, and in

[1] This increase in old age may be due to a transference from bronchitis to phthisis as already explained in the last chapter.

The figures showing the decline at the various age periods are smaller than those which we have just been considering, and we must remember that we are now dealing with a period of 10 years whereas previously we were dealing with a period of 30 years.

each sex also the next greatest reduction occurred between 15 and 45.   Again we find that between 5 and 10 the reduction among males considerably exceeded that among females, and that at almost all periods of life after that the reduction among females considerably exceeded that among males.   But the disparity in the reduction among the two sexes respectively is not so great as before, and at no age period do we find a ratio of two to one.   The greatest disparity occurred again in the latter half of life, and corresponded to a ratio of 155 to 100 between 45 and 55, and to one of 171 to 100 between 55 and 65.

Taking all ages together the reduction among females to that among males was as five to four while in the earlier interval which we have been considering it was more than four to three.

Lastly let us look at the changes which have occurred during the whole period under review, namely between the decade 1861–70 and the decade 1901–10 (40 years).   We see that among males of all ages the reduction has been 43 per cent., and that during the first half of life (namely up to 35), excepting from 5 to 10 (when the mortality is very small), the reduction has either approximated to, or exceeded, 50 per cent., but that during the latter half of life it has been considerably less.

Among females the reduction at all ages was 55 per cent., and during nearly the whole of life up to 65, excepting only from 5 to 10 when the mortality was very low, the reduction either approximated to or exceeded (and often considerably exceeded) 50 per cent.   The greatest decline, namely 65 per cent., occurred between 20 and 25, but the decline was over 60 per cent. during the whole period from 15 to 35, and 57 per cent. from 35 to 45.

As to the *ratio* of the decline in the two sexes during the whole period under review, we find that the rate of decline among males exceeded that among females between 0 and 15 —considerably between 5 and 10, and very slightly between 0 and 5, and 10 and 15.   At all other age periods, extreme old age only excepted, the decline among females greatly exceeded that among males, and the disparity increased up to 45 to 55 years, when the decline among women was nearly twice as high as among men (196 per cent.), after which it diminished slightly.

It may be said in general terms, then, that during the latter half of life, namely from 35 to 75, the female mortality from tuberculosis declined at least half as much again, and from 45 to 55 nearly twice as much as the male mortality.

The changes which we have been considering in the incidence of the mortality on the two sexes may be shown in another way, namely by expressing the mortality of one sex as a percentage of that of the other, for each decade under consideration. This has been done in the following diagram which gives the ratio of the male mortality at each age period to the female at the same period, the latter being expressed as 100.

From this diagram we can easily see the unequal incidence of the mortality of the two sexes at different periods of life ; and how the inequality has increased or diminished, or in some cases become reversed, in the intervals under review.

In early life, between 5 and 10, where formerly rather more boys died than girls, the position has been reversed and the death-rate is now greater among girls than boys. Between 10 and 15, where the rate has always been much higher among the girls, the disparity has diminished slightly. Between 15 and 20, where the rate has always been somewhat higher among girls, the disparity has slightly increased. Between 20 and 35, the tables have been turned to the great advantage of women ; formerly the rate was rather higher among women than men, now it is very considerably higher among men. Between 35 and 45, the rate was formerly only a very little higher among men than women, now the male rate greatly exceeds the female. After 45 the male rate was formerly greatly higher than the female rate, and the disparity between the sexes has increased very considerably, so that at the present day, from that time of life up to old age, the death-rate from tuberculosis is twice as high among men as it is among women.

The Cause of the Unequal Sex Distribution of the Mortality

To what causes are these great differences in the respective liability of the two sexes to die of tuberculosis due ? The difference in the first few years of life is in accordance with the

DIAGRAM V. *Ratio of Male to Female Mortality from Tuberculosis.*

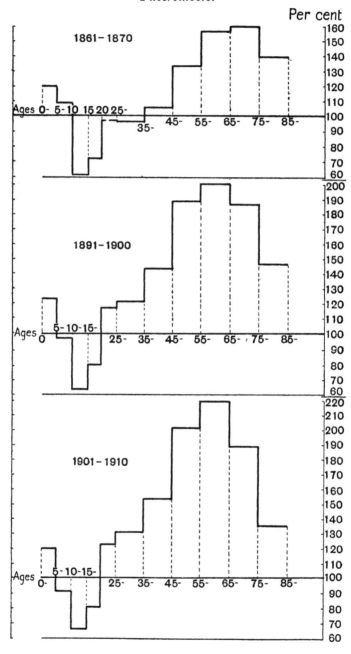

	All ages	0-	5-	10-	15-	20-	25-	35-	45-	55-	65-	75-
1861–1870	105·5	122·3	109·6	69·2	72·2	98·6	93·8	106·4	134·6	157·6	160·6	140·2
1891–1900	127·9	123 6	97·8	63·7	79·4	117·6	121·8	143·6	188·0	206	188·3	147·3
1901–1910	133·8	118·7	91·1	65·2	79·8	122·4	130·8	153·3	202·5	217·0	188·8	135·2

general rule that male infants are more delicate than female infants, for a similar difference is seen at this time of life in the mortality from all causes. It is difficult to say to what it is due.

After infancy the liability of girls to die of tuberculosis is, as we have seen, at the present day greater than that of boys, and this continues up to about the 20th year. Formerly the difference began at 10 and continued up to 35. Does this difference depend on some deep seated peculiarity of sex constitution which makes the tissues of the female at this time of life a more favourable soil for the development of the tubercle bacillus than those of the male, or is it simply dependent on differences in the habits of life of the two sexes? That the latter is the true reason would seem probable from the fact that the liability of the sexes between 5 and 10, and again between 20 and 35, has been reversed in comparatively recent times— for habits are more easily changed than differences of sex constitution. Sir Hugh Beevor[1] however takes the former view, and is inclined to see in the more rapid growth of girls than boys at this period of life, and more particularly of their lungs, an explanation of their greater liability to consumption ; for it should be pointed out that it is in a greater liability to pulmonary tuberculosis, and not to other forms of the disease, that the difference under consideration mainly lies.

The unequal incidence of the mortality on the two sexes at this period of life cannot have anything to do with the onset of puberty, because it is already well marked before puberty begins. Professor Hay suggests that it may be due to the larger amount of play and outdoor exercise enjoyed by the boys. But there is still another difference which may be more potent than any of those which we have considered so far. Upon the young girls of the poorer classes very often devolves the care of the younger children, and especially of

[1] " Sex Constitution and its Relation to Pulmonary Tuberculosis," *The Medical Magazine*, 1900.

the babies, who, as we have seen, often suffer from tuberculosis. But it is probably not so much to the increased opportunities for infection which are thus afforded—for infants seldom suffer from " open " tuberculosis—as to the interference with the freedom of respiration, and, consequently, to the development of the lungs, which is caused by the practice of carrying infants in the arms of children not yet strong enough to bear such burdens. While the girls are thus devotedly acting the part of little mothers, the boys are allowed far more freedom to play games out of doors, or are employed as errand boys, or in some other occupation in the open air. It would be interesting, as a means of testing the truth of this explanation, to know whether among the richer classes the same greater liability of the girls to suffer from tuberculosis than the boys prevails as is shown when all classes of the population are taken together; but the information, so far as the writer is aware, is not available.

After the age of adolescence, as we have seen, males die of tuberculosis much more frequently than females, and the disparity increases as life advances until the period 55 to 65 is reached, and only slightly diminishes in old age. It has been suggested that this difference, which at the present day prevails during the whole of adult life, may be accounted for, in part at least, on the ground that a larger proportion of females than males having died of tuberculosis in childhood and adolescence, the predisposed have become eliminated to a larger extent from the female than from the male sex, and the former consequently, when the years of maturity are reached, is the less susceptible sex. But while one must allow some difference of susceptibility on this account it is probable that it is only a very small one, and totally inadequate to account for a difference in the death-rate from tuberculosis which at certain periods of life is greater than two to one. It can hardly be doubted that this difference depends in the main on differences of occupation, for the great majority of the trades which predispose to consumption, in England at least, are followed almost exclusively by men[1]. This view of the case is supported by the fact that

[1] See p. 43.

DIAGRAM VI. *Incidence of the Death-rate from Phthisis on the Two Sexes.*

A. *In certain Industrial Towns.*

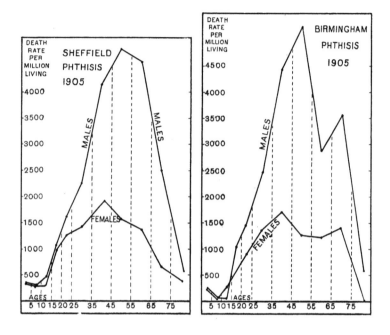

B. *In a Community mainly Rural.*

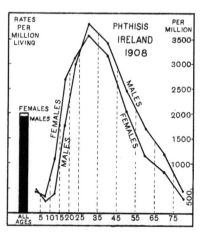

III] INFLUENCE OF THE GROWTH OF INDUSTRIES   41

the difference in the comparative liability of the two sexes to die of tuberculosis has increased greatly in modern times, that is to say *pari passu* with the continued growth of our industries.

It is a significant fact that the comparative prevalence of fatal tuberculosis in the sexes, taking all periods of life together, has been reversed since the modern development of industrialism, and that the change has occurred earlier in those countries which first developed their industries. In England and Wales the change occurred about 1868. In Scotland however it was delayed for nearly 25 years; while in those parts of the United States for which there is statistical information the change took place about the end of the seventies of the last century. In backward Ireland, on the other hand, females still continue to suffer from tuberculosis rather more than males.

In England and Wales the difference in the incidence of the tuberculosis mortality on the sexes is most marked in the urban counties, and least marked in the rural, and it reaches its maximum in such essentially industrial cities as Birmingham and Sheffield, where the dangerous occupation of grinding steel tools is largely carried on (see Diagram VI).

The great disparity which exists to-day in the comparative mortality of men and women during adult life has been brought about by a great decline in the mortality of women and not by an increase in the mortality of men. The mortality has, in fact, as we have seen, declined greatly in both sexes; and it is probable that both sexes would have shared equally in the improvement which has taken place, had it not been for the adverse influence of the rise of industrialism affecting, in the main, one sex only. Industrialism has not *increased* the mortality from tuberculosis of adult males, but, according to this view, it has *greatly retarded the decrease* which has been taking place. If this is so one of the most extraordinary facts about the decline of tuberculosis is that it has been taking place in spite of important and widespread changes which evidently by themselves tend to spread the disease[1].

---

[1] "The decline of the phthisis death-rate has been obtained in the face

In Scotland as a whole the disparity in the mortality from tuberculosis of the two sexes in adult life is not nearly so marked as in England and Wales, and in several of the Scotch towns the female mortality from tuberculosis of the lungs is almost as high, and in some even higher, than the male mortality.

TABLE VI. *Showing the mortality at all ages of tuberculosis of the lungs among males and females in certain towns and groups of towns in Scotland, 1901–7[1].*

Towns	Male per 10,000	Female per 10,000
Glasgow	16·84	15·22
Dundee	17·50	17·05
Aberdeen	13·52	12·97
Paisley	13·50	14·22
Paisley, Kilmarnock, Kirkcaldy and Perth ...	13·43	13·60
Coatbridge, Govan, Hamilton, and Motherwell	10·70	13·07

It is probable that the smaller difference in the mortality of the two sexes which obtains in Scotland, as compared with England and Wales, depends upon the fact that the occupations of males in Scotland are, as Scurfield points out, largely of an outdoor kind ; a larger proportion of occupied males in the latter country being engaged in agriculture, fishing, and coal mining (an occupation which curiously enough enjoys a markedly low rate of mortality from phthisis) than in England.

While Scurfield attributes the difference which we are now considering to a difference in the occupations of the men, Professor Hunter Stewart, on the other hand, considers that it is due to a difference in the occupations of the women, and he points out that the trades which women follow in Scotland are on the whole more phthisigenetic than those followed by women in England.   In Dundee for example the very high mortality from tuberculosis among women is probably attributable to the large numbers of them employed in the jute industry.   In

of the adverse influence of urbanization." Newsholme, *Trans. Epidemiol. Soc.* XXV, p. 109.
[1] From Professor Hunter Stewart's " Sex and Age Distribution of Mortality from Pulmonary Tuberculosis in Scotland, etc." *Proc. Roy. Soc. Edin.* 1911, p. 362.

England the conditions are different and, as a rule with but few exceptions, the industries which predispose to pulmonary tuberculosis are carried on by men.   As examples it will suffice to mention tin and copper mining, the various kinds of steel grinding and tool making, the manufacture of pottery and glass, and the trades of hairdresser, shoemaker, furrier and tailor. All these, for one reason or another, are associated with a high mortality from pulmonary tuberculosis.   On the other hand the kind of work at which women are employed in factories or elsewhere is not associated with a high mortality from phthisis. Female cotton operatives would seem, from such figures as are available, to be healthier at all age periods than other women, and the same is true of domestic servants; but statistics of female occupation mortality are unsatisfactory since a woman who has fallen ill and left her occupation may, if she comes to die, be returned as of no occupation[1].   It is true that among men the shop assistant suffers severely from phthisis, and that many women are employed in similar positions, but nevertheless it is abundantly clear that phthisis, as a disease of occupation in this country, affects men to a far greater extent than women.

But difference of occupation is probably not the sole explanation of the unequal distribution of the tuberculosis mortality during adult life ; for, as Dr Niven points out, there is great inequality in the phthisis death-rate of men and women working at the same occupation[2].   The concentration of population owing to the growth of towns must therefore have told more unfavourably upon the men than the women for other reasons besides that the urban occupations of the former are more phthisigenetic than those of the latter.   Niven points out that among the working classes men are more gregarious than women, they alone are apt to contaminate their workshops by spitting, and they spend far more time in public houses, which are notorious for being hotbeds of phthisis.

[1] See Dr Tatham's report on occupational mortality, which forms Part II of the *Supplement to the 65th Report of the Registrar General for England and Wales*, especially Table IV on pp. clviii *et seq.*, and the section on mortality among occupied females, *ibid.* p. cxxii.

[2] *Trans. Epidemiol. Soc.* xxv, p. 115.

Newsholme believes that the sex inequality of which we are speaking has been influenced greatly by segregation of the sick. He says " women have gained more than men from institutional segregation, (1) because the latter keep at work until disabled and infect factories and workshops more grossly than they would their own fireside ; and (2) because the men, when disabled from work and most likely to convey massive infection to wife and children, are segregated in the infirmary[1]."

But these two last-mentioned causes of the inequality are, one would think, of secondary importance; and it is probably not too much to say that it is the growth of certain of our industries and the change from rural to urban conditions generally which has been the chief cause in the change in sex incidence of phthisis.

We have seen that the difference in the mortality of the two sexes has been increasing right up to the present day; we must therefore conclude that the unfavourable influence of the growth of our industries and of the consequence which it entails is still at work. It is however some satisfaction to find that the rate of growth of disparity in the decline of the tuberculosis mortality in the two sexes during adult life was not so great during the period between 1890–1900 and 1901–10 as it was in the period which preceded it.

REFERENCES. I

(Chapters I, II and III)

Armstrong, H. (1902). A Note on the Infantile Mortality from Tuberculous Meningitis and Tabes Mesenterica. *Brit. Med. Journ.* II, p. 1024.
Beevor, Sir Hugh (1899). The Hunterian Lecture on the Declension of Phthisis. *Lancet*, I, p. 1005.
—— (1900). Sex Constitution and its Relation to Pulmonary Tuberculosis. *Medical Magazine*, June, 1900.
—— (1905). Discussion on Paper by Newsholme. *Trans. Epidemiol. Soc.* XXV, p. 129.
Broadbent, Sir William (1905). Discussion on Paper by Newsholme. *Trans. Epidemiol. Soc.* XXV, p. 117.

[1] *Trans. Epidemiol. Soc.* XXV, p. 132.

Bulstrode. See p. 96.

Burns, Rt Hon. John (1913). Address to International Medical Congress. *Lancet*, II, p. 459.

Chalmers, Dr A. K. (1913). A Page in the Natural History of Pulmonary Tuberculosis. *Public Health*, XXVII, p. 36.

Hay, Dr Matthew (1910). Tuberculosis in Aberdeen. *Ann. Rep. of Med. Off. of Health of Aberdeen for* 1909.

Koch, Dr Robert (1906). The Nobel Lecture. *Lancet*, I, p. 149.

Moore, Dr (1905). Discussion on Paper by Newsholme. *Trans. Epidemiol. Soc.* XXV, p. 124.

Muir, Dr W. (1914). *Brit. Med. Journ.* I, p. 221.

Murphy, Sir Shirley (1901). *Brit. Congress on Tub.* London. Catalogue vol. p. 153.

Naegeli, O. (1900). Ueber Häufigkeit, Lokalization, und Ausheilung der Tuberkulose. *Virchow's Archiv.* CLX, p. 426.

Newsholme, Dr A. (1905). Factors Involved in the Control of Pulmonary Tuberculosis. *Trans. Epidemiol. Soc.* XXV, p. 31.

—— (1906). An Inquiry into the Principal Causes of the Reduction of the Death-Rate from Phthisis, with special Reference to Segregation of Phthisical Patients in General Institutions. *Journ. of Hygiene*, VI, p. 304.

—— (1908). *The Prevention of Tuberculosis*. London. Methuen and Co.

Niven (1905). Discussion on Paper by Newsholme. *Trans. Epidemiol. Soc.* XXV, p. 112.

Public Health and Social Conditions (1909). *Local Government Board*, Cd. 4671.

Ransome, Dr A. (1905). Phthisis Rates, their Significance and Teaching. *Trans. Epidemiol. Soc.* XXIV, p. 259.

—— (1906). *Ibid.* XXV. p. 127.

Registrar General for England and Wales. *74th Annual Report, for* 1911.

Registrar General for Ireland. Report for 1912. *Lancet*, 1913.

Riviere, Dr Clive (1914). The Infection of Children with Bovine Tubercle Bacilli. *Brit. Med. Journ.* I, p. 221.

Scurfield, Dr H. (1910). Lung Diseases among Sheffield Grinders. *Public Health*, XXIII, p. 113.

—— (1912). Tuberculosis in the British Isles. *Public Health*, XXVI.

Stewart, Prof. C. Hunter (1911). Sex and Age Distribution of Mortality from Pulmonary Tuberculosis in Scotland. *Proc. Roy. Soc. Edin.* XXXI, Pt. III, p. 362.

Tatham. Report on Occupational Mortality. *Supplement to 65th Report, Reg. Gen. Eng. and Wales* (1901), Pt. II.

CHAPTER IV

THE ETIOLOGY OF TUBERCULOSIS

The Growth and Decline of the Doctrine of Contagion up to the time of the Discovery of the Tubercle Bacillus.

Tubercle bacilli are not known to grow outside the animal body, excepting of course in artificial cultures, and on these they do not grow very readily at least when first transferred from their living hosts; they are in fact " obligatory parasites." Yet like the mistletoe or the dodder they must of course have sprung from an ancestor which led an independent existence, and was incapable of causing disease. At what particular period of the world's development tubercle bacilli adopted the parasitic habit it is impossible to say, but at all events we know that tuberculosis was in existence at the very earliest period of which there is any documentary evidence; and it probably arose long before, for Elliot Smith and Ruffer[1] have described and figured the skeleton of an Egyptian mummy of about 1000 B.C. which appears without doubt to be affected with Pott's disease of the vertebral column, and they state that Dr Derry has more recently found a series of similar specimens belonging to the period 3000 to 2000 B.C. or even earlier. There can be no doubt that tuberculosis was well established as a human disease in the 5th century B.C., for it was well known to Hippocrates and probably to some of those who preceded him[2].

Hippocrates himself seems to have believed that consumption was due to some defect in the constitution of the individual. It is of course well known that he originated the idea of the

---

[1] G. E. Smith and M. A. Ruffer, 1910, "Pott'sche Krankheit an einer Ägyptischen Mumie," *Zur historischen Biologie der Krankheitserreger.*

[2] Sir William Osler suggests that one of the lost books of Democritus (460–370 B.C.) entitled " On those who are attacked with cough after illness " probably treated of phthisis. (Introductory chapter to Klebs' *Tuberculosis*, Arnold and Co. 1909.)

Plate I

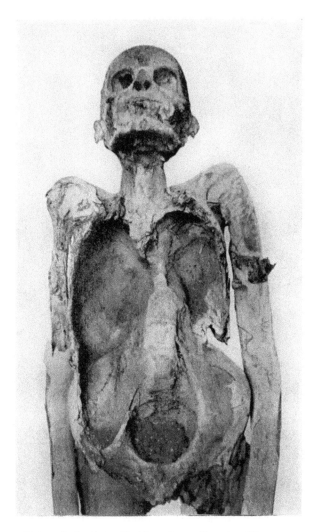

Tuberculosis of the Vertebræ in an Egyptian Mummy.

Reproduced by permission of Prof. Elliot Smith.

" phthisical diathesis," or peculiar constitution of body which predisposes to the disease, and which has survived in a more or less modified form to the present day. He does not seem to have considered that tuberculosis was contagious[1], although in his time the contagiousness of certain diseases, such as the plague which occurred at Athens, was well recognized by his contemporary Thucydides. That phthisis itself was contagious seems to have been held by Isocrates who lived about the same period; and in the following century Aristotle also seems to have believed that phthisis might be communicated to persons close at hand. Galen[2], Avicenna, and others among the ancients also held similar views. (Bulloch.)

With the passing of the classical period the development of medical science became suspended for centuries, until at the Renaissance it began to advance once more. But we find no progress in the pathology of tuberculosis until the 17th century, when the first accurate description of tubercles in the lung was given by Franciscus Silvius (1614–72). (Osler.)

At that period, and for a long time afterwards, extreme views were taken as to the infectiousness of phthisis in many parts of the continent of Europe, and especially in the south ; though the opinions held in England at the time were, for the most part, moderate[3]. In Spain, in the reign of Philip V (1700–24), a law was passed imposing on medical men the duty of

---

[1] Adams says (in his Translation of the Genuine Works of Hippocrates, *New Sydenham Soc.* 1849) : " There is not the least reference to contagion in any of the Hippocratic treatises ; and this is remarkable since the contagiousness of certain diseases would appear to have been the popular belief of the age."

[2] It is interesting to note that Galen prescribed a milk diet, and residence in a dry climate, for the disease; while Celsus particularly recommended Egypt, and long sea voyages.

[3] As an example Edward Mainwaring may be cited. In 1667 he wrote as follows : " Society also is to be regarded, and you must not frequently converse with a phthisical person, whose unwholesome breath may infect the sound, by drawing in the putrid vapours which the other breathes forth ; but above all a phthisical bed-fellow is most dangerous to affect a sound person, and chiefly to be avoided " (Bulstrode). Richard Morton (1697), too, held very similar views, for he stated that " a contagious principle also propagates the disease, for, as I have often found by experience, an affected person may poison a bed-fellow by a kind of miasm like that of a malignant fever " (quoted from *The Collective Investigation Record,* p. 29).

reporting deaths from phthisis; and at Valencia in 1738 compulsory notification of cases of the disease was enforced by the municipal authorities. (Bulstrode.) In Italy it was the custom, according to Morgagni (1765), to burn the bedding of persons who died of phthisis, and it is said that the great anatomist was afraid to make a post-mortem examination in a case of this disease, lest he should himself become infected. Valsalva also is reported to have shared these fears.

In Florence, in 1754, the infectiousness of tuberculosis was made the subject of a decree by the College of Physicians; and at Naples a royal edict of 1782 prescribed, under the most severe penalties for non-compliance, the isolation of consumptives, and the disinfection of the premises occupied by them and of their personal effects, by vinegar, lemon juice, brandy and fumigations; while the medical attendant had to notify the case to the authorities; and if he failed to do so was to be fined 300 ducats for the first offence, and to be banished for ten years for the second! (Straus.)

In France, in 1750, the magistrates of Nancy ordered to be publicly burnt in the market place the effects of a phthisical woman who was believed to have contracted the disease by sleeping with another suffering from consumption. (Straus.)

Portal states that in Spain and Portugal there was a law requiring the parents of a phthisical person to notify the authorities when the disease reached its last phase, in order that the clothes might be seized and burnt. It was the same, says Straus, in Languedoc.

Extreme views were still held on this question in these last-named countries as late as 1839; for Georges Sand describes how the musician Chopin, who had left Paris for Spain and Portugal, was turned out of the two small houses he was renting, because he was consumptive, and threatened with prosecution for infecting them[1].

---

[1] Georges Sand wrote: " At the end of a month poor Chopin, who since he left Paris has continued to cough, became ill. I called in a physician, two physicians, three physicians, each one a greater than the other, who spread abroad the tale that our patient was in the last stage of phthisis. There was immense excitement. Phthisis is seldom seen in those climates, and is so classed as a contagious disease. We were regarded as pest-breeders. The

In England such extreme views seem never to have gained ground, and at the beginning of the 19th century opinion on this question seems to have been moderate and sensible. The great Thomas Young (1773–1829) expressed himself in terms which would commend themselves to many at the present day. He protested against an exaggerated belief in the transmission of an inherited tendency to scrofula, and, while he admitted that it would be difficult to produce any demonstrative proof of the contagiousness of phthisis, he, nevertheless, brought forward strong presumptive evidence that it was so[1].

Heberden (1802) also held similar views. He had not seen proof enough to say that the breath of a consumptive was infectious, but he could not affirm the contrary, for he had "observed several die of consumption in whom infection seemed to be the most probable origin of their illness."

But belief in the contagiousness of phthisis was beginning to die away, and the inevitable reaction from the exaggerated views which were held on the Continent in the 18th century carried opinion in this and other countries to the opposite extreme in the 19th. Increasing importance came to be attached to the tuberculous diathesis, as for example by Bright

proprietors of two small houses which we had rented put us out of doors and threatened us with prosecution for infecting the houses." Bulstrode, Milroy Lecture, *Lancet*, 1903, II, p. 75.

[1] "It has been much disputed," he says, "whether or no consumption is capable of being communicated by contagion, and it must be allowed that it would be difficult to produce any strong demonstrative evidence of this fact." But he goes on to relate how a Dr Rush had "given an account of a consumption manifestly contagious, which spread from the proprietors of an estate among the negroes who were neither related to the first victims, nor had been subjected to fatigue or anxiety on their account." He himself had seen an "instance of a carpenter who died of laryngeal consumption, and whose wife died soon after of a disease precisely similar"; and he proceeds to state that he would "think it unjustifiable, from a full confidence in the absolute impossibility of infection, unnecessarily to expose any person who appeared to have the slightest predisposition to the disease to any intimate communication with a consumptive patient—as, for instance, to sleeping in the same bed, or living constantly in the same room, which is nearly the extent of the apprehension expressed by Galen himself, who observes that it is dangerous to pass the whole day with consumptive persons" (quoted from Bulloch and Greenwood, *loc. cit.* p. 16).

and Addison[1]. Graves[2] too attributed every form of consumption to the " scrofulous habit," which however, he thought, was not necessarily inherited. Dr Benjamin Rush (1808) and Sir Thomas Watson (1836–37) are said to have opposed the idea that consumption is contagious. Even Laennec[3] concluded from his great experience that consumption is not usually contagious, at least in France, though he admitted that it might become so under certain circumstances.

Sir James Clark[4] (1835), physician to the Duchess of Kent and the Princess Victoria, gives us a picture of the views held concerning pulmonary tuberculosis during his time. They seem to have been based in the main on the work of Todd who, studying the growth and organization of the chick *in ovo* and of the union of divided parts, etc., came to the conclusion that in development two processes are concerned, namely, first the secretion and deposition of a matrix, and secondly its conversion into organized tissue. In those predisposed to tuberculosis a general morbid constitution of the system caused the process

[1] *The Elements of the Practice of Clinical Medicine*, 1839, pp. 280 *et seq.*

[2] *A System of Medicine*, 1843, p. 279. Graves concluded that the " scrofulous habit " was not necessarily inherited because " a tiger, a monkey, or even a negro, brought to this country might fall ill of consumption, and yet be able to boast of a line of ancestors as free from phthisis as any of us."

[3] " Tuberculous phthisis," wrote Laennec, " has for a long time passed for a contagious disease, and it still passes for such in the eyes of the people, the magistrates, and some doctors, in certain countries especially in the southern parts of Europe. In France at least, it does not appear to be so. One often sees among the poor a large family sleeping in the same room as a phthisical person, or a husband sharing up to the last moment the same bed with his phthisical wife, without the disease being communicated. The woollen clothes and the mattresses of the phthisical, which they burn in certain countries, and which often they do not even wash in France, have never appeared to me to have communicated the disease to anybody. However that may be, prudence and propriety demands that one should take more precautions in the matter. Moreover many facts prove that the malady, which is not habitually contagious, can become so under certain conditions " (quoted by Straus, *La Tuberculose*, p. 124, from Laennec's *Traité de l'auscultation médiaté*. Édit. de la faculté de méd. de Paris, 1879). Laennec is said himself to have suffered from a growth which he regarded as tuberculous, and which had resulted from a scratch received when making an autopsy on a tuberculous subject. He died, as is well known, of phthisis, but whether as the result of this cutaneous infection or no is uncertain, since his death did not occur until twenty years after the accident.

[4] *A Treatise on Pulmonary Consumption*, 1835.

to stop short of organization. Thus we find Clark stating that " tubercle is now considered by the best pathologists as a morbid unorganizable product, having for its remote or pre-disposing cause a characteristic state of the general system, and for its immediate production some abnormal action of the vessels of the part in which it is deposited, but with the nature of which action we are not acquainted."

For Clark even Laennec, who, as we have seen, did not believe that phthisis was usually contagious, did not go far enough; and we find the English physician after bestowing a moderate meed of praise on the discoveries of the great French-man, objecting that " they had tended to keep up the idea that consumption is a local disease, referable to a local cause, and thus the investigation of the constitutional origin of tubercles—by far the most important part of the subject—has been neglected."

More and more, under the influence of the study of morbid histology, medical opinion tended to regard tuberculosis as due to a constitutional weakness which tended to prevent the organization of ordinary inflammatory material; and the disease came to be looked upon as caused by the presence of caseous or other inflammatory matter in the body of a person constitutionally incapable of bringing about its organization. Support for this view was claimed from the fact that miliary tuberculosis is often preceded by caseation elsewhere, and the truth was obscured, as we shall see, by the unlucky occurrence of spontaneous tuberculosis in the animals used in some of the early researches into the etiology of tuberculosis which made it appear that the disease might be induced by the introduction of ordinary inflammatory, or other non-tuberculous, foreign matter.

It is true that during the earlier half of the 19th century the researches of Villemin, Chauveau, Cohnheim, Klebs and others were demonstrating clearly, and for the first time, the fact that tuberculosis might be transmitted experimentally from one animal to another[1]; but these discoveries, momentous

---

[1] The earliest attempts to produce tuberculosis experimentally seem to have been made by Kortum in 1789, and by Cruveilheier in 1826. Apparently spontaneous tuberculosis in some of the research animals used proved a pitfall for the early researchers, no less than it has done for some of those of

though they subsequently proved, did not at the time greatly alter the course that medical opinion was pursuing, and although some men still continued to believe phthisis to be infectious, in general it may be said that as the century advanced this view of the etiology of tuberculosis receded more and more into the background until we find Dr (now Sir Clifford) Allbutt affirming, immediately after the discovery of the tubercle bacillus had been made known, that although his attention had been given for many years to this question he had never observed a case of even probable transmission of phthisis from one person to another[1].

While many of the more important authorities about this time held similar views—being probably influenced to a considerable extent by the great Laennec—there were others who were more impressed by the evidences of contagion.

In 1874 Hermann Weber[2] read a paper before the Clinical Society "On the Communicability of Consumption from Husband and Wife" in which he related from his own experience the history of 68 persons, male and female, who with a more or less pronounced consumptive taint had married healthy persons. The results were striking; for while "in 29 marriages between consumptive wives and healthy husbands only one husband became consumptive, in 51 marriages between consumptive husbands and healthy wives 18 wives became consumptive[3]."

to-day, and Cruveilheier was led to believe that tuberculosis was not a specific disease, and might result from the inoculation of various foreign substances. These unfortunate experiments left their mark for many years. More successful experiments were made by Klenke (1843) who was able to satisfy himself that tuberculosis was inoculable (Osler). It was however left to Villemin to demonstrate conclusively that tuberculosis is a specific infectious disease. Sir William Osler says of the *Études sur la Tuberculose*, published in 1868, that this "epoch-making work is one of the most remarkable contributions ever made to scientific medicine. The experiments were conducted with great care and accuracy, and his work everywhere shows the brilliant scientific investigator. For the period his conclusions were novel and far reaching, and it is not surprising they were received with a good deal of reserve."

[1] *The Collective Investigation Record.* Published by the British Medical Association, 1883, p. 91.

[2] *Trans. Clinical Society,* London, 1874, VII, p. 144.

[3] Weber afterwards communicated two more instances of apparent infection from husband to wife to the Collective Investigation Committee (see Report of that Committee, p. 45).

The following cases are of special interest.   One consumptive husband lost four wives in rapid succession from the disease, and another lost three, while four others lost two each, and three one apiece.   A striking feature of the cases referred to is that in all of them the husbands, nine in number, having been attacked when quite young men by hæmoptysis or some other manifestation of consumption, and having after a while recovered more or less completely, believed themselves to be sound when they married.   Their disease was chronic, stationary and apyretic, but all had some physical signs when Weber saw them, and all succumbed to phthisis in the end, save one who was living at the time of the communication.   Eight of the husbands came from consumptive families.   On the other hand the 18 wives who perished came from healthy families, and were quite well at the time of marriage.   The disease in them ran a very rapid course, not exceeding 18 months in any.   In all it was closely associated with pregnancy and parturition.

In 1883 the British Medical Association, at the instigation of its President, Professor (afterwards Sir George) Humphry, appointed a committee to conduct a collective investigation into the communicability of consumption.   This committee sent out a series of questions to the members of the Association, and the replies they received were published in a volume entitled *The Collective Investigation Record*.

The results of this investigation must be referred to again (on p. 80).   It will therefore be sufficient to state here that, though the total number of replies received was disappointing, nevertheless 192 cases of apparent transmission of tuberculous infection from one married partner to the other were communicated.

Among the replies was one from Dr Sprigge of Great Barford containing the following history, which is of considerable interest.   A consumptive dressmaker had three apprentices not in any way related to one another, and each coming from a different village.   These young girls, 17 to 19 years of age, took it in turn to remain in the house, and to sleep with their employer, one week at a time.   During their apprenticeship the dressmaker died of phthisis, and in less than two years all three apprentices were dead of this disease, although in the family history of each no trace of phthisis existed. (*loc. cit.* p. 82, see also *Brit. Med. Journ.* 1883, II, p. 983.)

The committee came to the conclusion "that if phthisis is a communicable disease it is so only under circumstances of extremely close personal intimacy, such as persons sharing the same bed or the same room, or shut up together in numbers in close, ill-ventilated apartments" (*loc. cit.* p. 41).

The replies received by the Collective Investigation Committee, disappointing though they were in number, probably afford a fair sample of the views held by the general practitioner at this time. But, though among the rank and file of the doctors there were many who recognized that consumption was communicable, the leaders of the profession for the most part held to the opinion of Laennec, and in 1884, shortly after the discovery of the tubercle bacillus, we find Henry Bennet[1], who had a very large experience of pulmonary tuberculosis, and who had himself suffered from the disease and recovered, striving to stem the tide of the growing belief in the infectivity of phthisis which had commenced to flow since the publication of Koch's discovery. Bennet said that "he did not deny the contagion of phthisis, far from it, he accepted it in certain conditions and limits, but he did not believe it to be the regular habitual cause of phthisis asserted by many"; on the contrary he attributed it either to an antecedent lowering of vitality or to hereditary predisposition. He admitted that phthisis had become more common among the inhabitants of Mentone since it had become a resort of consumptives, especially among the washer-women who handled the linen soiled by the sputa of the patients, but he was inclined to attribute "this undoubted increase of phthisis in a healthy southern locality" not to contagion but to a change from rural to urban conditions of life which had attended the growth of the community. "Times are changed" he wrote; "The Grimaldi girls" (who previously had been engaged in agricultural pursuits) "have all become town workers, washer-women, sempstresses, servants, and they begin

[1] "On the Contagion of Phthisis," by J. Henry Bennet. *Brit. Med. Journ.* 1884, II, p. 704.

to die of consumption." " Is it not," he asks, " because they work in close, badly ventilated, damp rooms, instead of in the open air ? Is it not again a question of pre-breathed air, not of contagion ? " Even the case of a young officer who, with no consumptive antecedents in his family, contracted phthisis whilst nursing a wife in the last stages of pulmonary tuberculosis during a four months voyage from New Zealand (though he points out that the man spent day and night with the patient in a small cabin only a few feet square, with the window generally shut) Bennet does not altogether admit to be a case of infection, but is inclined to attribute it to the undermining of the health caused by living in a vitiated atmosphere " which is calculated to produce that very condition of lowered vitality in which tubercular or caseous deposits appear in the lung tissues spontaneously, as believed until now, or under the provocation of accidental inflammatory conditions."

Such then we see was the opinion in England at the time of the discovery of the tubercle bacillus. Men like Bennet were striving to hold out against the new tendencies of thought which were already springing up from that discovery, while others like Weber were pleading for a fair hearing of the evidence of the infectivity of consumption.

The opinion in Germany at the time was summed up by Koch who said, in 1884, that " many practical men had no doubt kept in mind the possibility of infection, but with the medical profession generally phthisis is regarded as the result of constitutional peculiarities rather than of direct contagion[1]."

---

[1] " The Etiology of Tuberculosis," p. 67.

REFERENCES. II

(Chapter IV)

Adams. Translation of the Genuine Works of Hippocrates. *New Sydenham Society*, 1849.

Allbutt, Sir T. Clifford (1883). Quoted in *The Collective Investigation Record*, p. 91. Published by the British Medical Association.

Bennet, J. Henry (1884). On the Contagion of Phthisis. *Brit. Med. Journ.* II, p. 704.

Bright and Addison (1839). *The Elements of the Practice of Clinical Medicine*, p. 280.

Bulloch, Wm. (1910). The Problem of Pulmonary Tuberculosis considered from the standpoint of Infection. Horace Dobell Lecture. *Royal Coll. of Physicians.*

Bulloch and Greenwood. The Problem of Pulmonary Tuberculosis considered from the standpoint of Disposition. *Proc. Roy. Soc. of Medicine*, London.

Bulstrode (1903). The Milroy Lecture. *Lancet*, II.

—— (1905–6). 35*th Ann. Rep. Local Government Board*, p. 64.

Clark, Sir James (1835). *A Treatise on Pulmonary Consumption.*

Collective Investigation Record (1883). Published by the Brit. Med. Association.

Graves (1843). *A System of Medicine.*

Hippocrates, quoted by Adams.

Koch, R. (1884). The Etiology of Tuberculosis. *Microparasites in Disease.* New Sydenham Society, 1886.

Laennec (1879). *Traité de l'auscultation médiaté.* Édit. de la faculté de méd. de Paris. Quoted by Straus, p. 442.

Longstaff. Quoted in *The Collective Investigation Record.*

Osler, Sir William (1909). Introductory Chapter to Klebs' *Tuberculosis.* Arnold and Co.

Newsholme, A. (1905–6). *Trans. Epidemiol. Soc.* XXV.

Smith, G. Elliott and A. Ruffer (1910). Pott'sche Krankheit an einer Ägyptischen Mumie. *Zur historischen Biologie der Krankheitserreger* (Alfred Töpelmann, Giessen), Bd. i, Heft 3, p. 9.

Straus. *La Tuberculose.* Paris.

Villemin. Quoted by Osler.

Weber, Hermann (1874). On the Communicability of Consumption from Husband to Wife. *Trans. of the Clinical Society*, p. 144.

—— *The Collective Investigation Record*, p. 45.

Williams, C. Theodore (1882). The Contagion of Phthisis. *Brit. Med. Journ.* II, p. 619.

—— (1909). The Infection of Consumption. *Ibid.* II, p. 433.

CHAPTER V

THE ETIOLOGY OF TUBERCULOSIS (*continued*)

The discovery of the tubercle bacillus. The relative importance of seed and soil. The argument against contagiousness based on the frequency of infection. The influence of " dose " and of individual susceptibility, as shown by experiments on animals.

The modern era, so far as tuberculosis is concerned, may be said to have commenced with the discovery of the tubercle bacillus, first announced at a meeting of the Berlin Physiological Society on March 24, 1882[1]. Henceforward no one could any longer deny that tuberculosis is infectious in the true sense of the word, or cling, as we have seen Bennet did when the news was quite fresh, to the belief that caseous or tuberculous deposits might arise spontaneously in the lungs, or elsewhere, merely in consequence of a depressed condition of vitality.

All writers henceforth admit the rôle of the bacillus; but they differ as to the part played by personal contact with consumptive persons in the transmission of infection. The tendency to belittle the importance of contagion, which we have seen growing so strongly in the middle of the 19th century, did not die away; but, on the contrary, there arose a doctrine of susceptibility, of a special weakness of constitution, either inherited, or acquired as the result of ill health or privation, which rendered its possessor unable to resist the attack of a bacillus which had little power to affect normal persons. This doctrine has merely replaced the older one of a diathesis, or constitutional state, which made those who inherited or acquired it incapable of organizing inflammatory products.

[1] The earliest publication of the discovery of the tubercle bacillus was made in the *Berliner Klinische Wochenschrift* in 1882, and the full account of his researches Koch communicated in the *Mitteilungen aus dem Gesundheitsamte*, II, in 1884. This paper was translated by Stanley Boyd and the English version appeared in *Recent Essays on Bacteria in Relation to Disease*, published by the New Sydenham Society in 1886. In a recent article on Lister (*Cornhill Magazine*, Nov. 1913, p. 604), Stephen Paget relates that the news of Koch's discovery became known unofficially in London at the first International Medical Congress in 1881.

This is the view of the case which has been taken by most of the writers on the subject in this country, among whom may be mentioned Beevor, Bulstrode[1], Bulloch, Parsons and Karl Pearson. On the other hand there has not been wanting a growing conviction among all ranks of the medical profession that, in the spread of a disease caused by a bacillus which does not grow outside the animal body (except in our test-tubes), opportunities for acquiring infection in the immediate neighbourhood of those who are the main source of the dissemination of the bacilli must play an important part, even though evidence of contagiousness should not lie on the surface.

On the Continent both Koch and Behring, whose views on the etiology of tuberculosis differed widely in other important respects, agreed that direct infection plays the dominant part ; and in this country Broadbent and Newsholme have taken a similar view[2].

Those who are opposed to the view that tuberculosis is

[1] Bulstrode in the Milroy Lectures spoke on this point as follows: " While there can be no reasonable doubt that pulmonary tuberculosis is under certain conditions a communicable malady, there can equally be no question that its communicability is of a low order. The testimony of experience, which is a far more scientific test than the records of certain laboratory experiments, should I think be sufficient to satisfy us that the communicability of pulmonary tuberculosis can only be contrasted, not compared, with diseases such as smallpox, typhus fever, or whooping cough. It cannot indeed be compared with the communicability of enteric fever which is perhaps the least communicable of the diseases which are at present classed together as the infectious diseases, and concerning which preventive measures are taken " (*Lancet*, 1903, II, p. 75).

[2] Newsholme remarks that " having investigated nearly 1600 voluntarily notified cases of phthisis, as well as a much larger number of fatal cases of phthisis, from a public health standpoint, I do not conceive it to be possible that any physician having personally done similar work could fail to realize to the full extent the infectivity of this disease, when exposure to infection is protracted, and the dosage of infection is great : a state of matters which is the common domestic lot of most of the working classes, when tubercular infection attacks a member of the household. The evidence convincing one as to this does not lend itself to statistical statement, and when stated in print it may not be convincing ; but the steady succession of cases in infected households at intervals of one or two years, or longer, the intercurrent destruction of children by tubercular meningitis or ' broncho-pneumonia ' while their parents are suffering from chronic phthisis, and other similar evidence, can leave no doubts in the minds of those who come into continuous contact with the actual facts " (*Trans. Epidemiol. Soc.* xxv, p. 70).

contagious, or who hold that contagion plays only a small part in the matter of infection—and as we have seen they are both numerous and important—base their views mainly on the fact that the majority of persons who die of all sorts of causes, and whose bodies come to be examined after death, show more or less definite signs of past tuberculous infection, which has not progressed beyond a certain point, but which has remained quiescent or become healed. The existence of these old tuberculous lesions is not denied by anyone, and though the exact proportion of persons who carry in their bodies these unsuspected evidences of infection may be disputed, all are agreed that it is a high one, so high indeed that they are to be found in a majority of those who have passed the age of childhood; and since it is thus shown that very many persons become at some time infected with tuberculosis it is justly argued that opportunities for infection must be exceedingly common.

The views of the school we are now considering may be put somewhat as follows: Tubercle bacilli are so commonly present in the air we breathe and in the food we consume that opportunities for acquiring infection come to all of us, and indeed most of us do actually become infected at some time or other during our lives. But the disease soon becomes arrested in the majority of people, and leaves only a little scar in the lung, or a calcareous focus in some gland.

Opportunities for infection being so very common as these facts show them to be, it is manifest that they can count but little in the ultimate result. The determining cause whether we develop some unimportant lesion or a progressive and fatal disease must therefore depend on some other factor, and that factor can only be the power of resistance possessed by the individual.

This view of the case may be summed up in a single sentence: The seed comes to all; it is the soil which determines whether or no it shall germinate and grow to maturity[1].

---

[1] Cp. Pearson in "A First Study of the Statistics of Pulmonary Tuberculosis," 1907, p. 3. "The discovery of the possibility of phthisical infection has led, I think, to underestimation of the hereditary factor. Probably few individuals who lead a moderately active life can escape an almost daily risk

But this view neglects to take any account of the possibility that the severity of the results of infection may depend in no small part on the size of the infecting dose. What if the majority of the opportunities for infection which seem to be so common are opportunities for infection with quantities of bacilli so small as to be incapable of producing a progressive disease? And what if the severe infections are caused in the main by large doses, the opportunities for receiving which occur comparatively rarely, and only in close proximity with phthisical persons?

This possibility cannot be ignored, and it is worth closer consideration than it has received at the hands of most writers, though Robert Koch, Theobald Smith, Fowler, Newsholme and Latham have all referred to it.

" The Influence of Dose."

The influence on the severity of the disease of the number of bacilli which enter the body when infection takes place, or, as we say for the sake of brevity, "the influence of dose," can only be demonstrated by animal experiments in which the quantities of bacilli employed are accurately measured. Experiments of this kind have only been carried out in comparatively recent times, and it is no wonder then that their full significance has hardly as yet been recognized. The writer remembers well the strong impression which the result of such experiments made upon his mind when they were first performed in the laboratories of the Royal Commission.

The influence of dose has been seen at its best in the case of animals which, like the ox, possess a comparatively high power of resisting tuberculosis. In highly susceptible animals, on the other hand, as for example the rabbit whose power of resisting (bovine) tuberculosis is so small that even the smallest

of infection under urban conditions; but in the great bulk of cases a predisposition, a phthisical diathesis, must exist to render the risk a really great one. In this sense it is probably legitimate to speak of the inheritance of tuberculosis, and even of the inheritance of zymotic diseases, meaning thereby the inheritance of a constitutional condition favourable to the development of such diseases should a risk be run, which cannot in the ordinary course of life be wholly avoided."

possible doses of bovine tubercle bacilli suffice to produce a fatal infection, the difference in the severity of the disease caused by different doses of bacilli is not nearly so marked. In this latter class must be placed the Rhesus monkey and the chimpanzee[1]. Now we have just seen that man often successfully resists infection with tubercle bacilli. He must therefore be regarded as a comparatively resistant animal, and is probably in this respect on a par with the ox, and in no sense comparable to the animals which invariably succumb to the smallest possible doses. Therefore in attempting to arrive at a just estimation of the influence of dose in human tuberculosis it is to the comparatively resistant ox that we must go for experimental information, rather than to the highly susceptible rabbit, monkey, or even the chimpanzee.

The evidence that differences in the dose of tubercle bacilli injected into the ox play the dominant rôle in determining the severity of an experimental tuberculosis is given in full in Chap. XIII; and the diagrams which may be found opposite p. 364 will show in a graphic manner the difference in the result of injecting doses of 10 and 50 milligrammes respectively, and in the former place several examples are given of minimal retrogressive disease being set up in the calf by the subcutaneous injection of small doses of tubercle bacilli from strains which injected simultaneously in large doses into comparable animals produced rapidly fatal general tuberculosis.

It will be sufficient to summarize briefly the results here. Small doses of bovine tubercle bacilli, whose virulence was proved by control experiments, produced, when injected into calves, only localized or limited lesions which soon became fibrous and calcareous, and thus assumed a retrogressive type; while the animals themselves, after a transient disturbance of health, remained in excellent condition up to the time when they came to be slaughtered and examined. Medium doses

---

[1] The chimpanzee has shown a very high degree of susceptibility to experimental tuberculosis and has succumbed to an acute miliary form of the disease after so small a dose as one hundred thousandth of a milligramme subcutaneously injected, while one milligramme similarly injected would almost certainly be harmless to a small calf. (See Chimp. 7 and 24, *R.C.T. Final Report*, App. vol. I, p. 44.)

(10 mg.) on the other hand produced irregular results, while larger ones (50 mg.) invariably caused generalized tuberculosis which in all but a few animals (6 per cent.) proved fatal within a few weeks or months (17–76 days).

Some have questioned whether the disease found in the calves which received small doses of tubercle bacilli highly virulent for the species was really and finally arrested, or whether it might not have lighted up again at some future time if the animals had been allowed to live, and anything had happened to depress their vitality. But surely this is beyond the point we are considering? Possibly the disease would relapse in some of the more susceptible of such calves, or in others whose powers of resistance were temporarily lowered from one cause or another, but it is not likely that it would do so in the majority ; and the point of the matter, which probably no one will seriously question, is that a disease which becomes quiescent, if not arrested, at an early stage has a far better chance of becoming cured than one which is from the onset of the acute and actively progressive type. And the experiments show in no uncertain manner that the former type of disease is produced by small doses, and the latter type by large ones.

At first sight it is not easy to see why the size of the infecting dose should play so decisive a part in determining the severity of an experimental infection. For even with a relatively small dose, bovine tubercle bacilli multiply in the calf for a time, and the disease makes some progress at the start before it becomes quiescent or arrested. It may therefore be reasonably asked— " if the bacilli multiply, what can it matter how many we inject ? The small dose will soon grow to be as big as the large one. How then can there be all this difference in the result ? "

The answer to this question may not be easy to find, but the facts to be explained admit of no dispute : let us therefore see how the question can be met. In the case of an animal which, like the calf, can make a good fight against the infection of tuberculosis it is probably not easy for the bacillus to establish its hold at first. Certain special elements in the food which the microbes require are probably supplied more easily from the dead bodies of other tubercle bacilli than from the tissues and juices of the calf itself. Moreover in the large dose, by their very numbers, the bacilli protect one another mechanically from the bactericidal agents which their host can bring against them. We can therefore easily understand how in the case of the large dose the bacilli establish themselves, and grow and multiply, and manufacture their toxins, more easily than they do when the dose is small.

But this alone would not explain why the small dose is less effective than the large one in the long run ; for undoubtedly, as has been said, even in cases where the disease becomes quickly arrested, the bacilli may multiply for a time. This argument then only explains a temporary delay. Sooner or later the small dose becomes as large as the large one was originally, and what shall now prevent it from acting in the same way ? It can only be because the infected animal has by this delay been given time to mobilize and develop its protective forces. The small dose of bacilli now grown to be a large one finds itself in a very different environment from that in which the original large dose found itself when first it was injected. The bacilli are now no longer surrounded by normal, vulnerable, tissues, but by a special zone of highly resistant character, built around them by means of the protective reaction which the body of the invaded animal has been able to put into operation. In other words the bacilli are now walled up, and to a great extent deprived of their powers of harm. Possibly also the body fluids of the host have developed new bactericidal, opsonic, antitoxic or other protective powers.

One must admit, then, that immunity begins to develop from the very outset of infection, and *one must look for the explanation of the difference in the action of small and large doses of tubercle bacilli in experimental infections to the rapid augmentation of the local or general powers of resistance.*

This explanation is in harmony with the fact that differences in the dose of bacilli make far less difference in highly susceptible animals, such as the rabbit and monkey which succumb to the smallest possible doses, than they do in the case of the ox which can make a fair amount of resistance ; for we may suppose that those animals which are least capable of making resistance are also least capable of augmenting such resistance as they can make.   In other words *animals which succumb to the smallest doses are incapable of developing the apparatus of immunity fast enough to cope with the multiplication of the bacilli.*

Before we can apply the argument of the influence of dose, based, as it is, on experimental infections in the calf, to natural infections in man, we must show, not only that man is a resistant animal, and may therefore be expected to behave as the calf does—which we have already attempted to do—but also that it is permissible to apply to spontaneous or natural infections facts which have been elicited experimentally ; for it must be admitted that doses so large as those we use at the experimental station can never, by any stretch of imagination, be supposed to get into the body under natural circumstances.

It is found experimentally (see p. 266) that differences in the capacity for resistance of different individual calves come much more into evidence with smaller doses (10 mg.) of bacilli than with larger ones (50 mg.), and it may be freely admitted that this is probably the case (and even to a still greater extent) with natural infections, which are doubtless caused in the majority, if not in all cases, by quantities of bacilli far smaller than those which are commonly used in experimental investigations.   It is highly probable then that differences of dose do not play the dominant rôle in natural infections which they play in experiments ; at the same time it seems likely that even here they are not altogether without influence.   Whether the part they play is more, or less, important than that played by differences of individual resisting power would be hard to decide; and on this point there are likely to be considerable differences of opinion.   But probably few will be found to dispute the statement that both dose and resistance play an important part in determining the severity of an infection.

The most reasonable view of the case would seem to the writer to be somewhat as follows: The power of resistance of different individuals differs considerably, and that of any single individual varies from time to time.   A dose of tubercle bacilli, therefore, which would be harmless to one would seriously infect another, or even that one under certain circumstances. So much is admitted for differences of resistance.   On the other hand there are doses so small as to be incapable of infecting anybody, and others so large that no one, no matter how high their resisting power, can escape if they receive them.   Doses which lie between these limits produce results which vary according to the resisting power of the individual at the moment ;   for example parturition, or an attack of measles or influenza, might cause infections which otherwise would be trivial to become dangerous, while, if no such untoward circumstances should arise, similar doses might cause results limited to a few circumscribed lesions causing no very definite symptoms, and which would never become recognized during life.

The limit which divides the dangerous from the harmless doses then differs with every individual, and varies with circumstances, but *on the whole large doses are decidedly more dangerous than small ones. Very large doses are deadly and overcome the most resistant, while very small doses are harmless even to the most susceptible.*

If this is true of human beings it has a very important bearing on the question of the contagiousness of consumption. For where shall the large and deadly doses of bacilli be encountered except in close proximity to a consumptive patient whose cough is spraying tubercle bacilli into the atmosphere, or in a draught of milk from a cow with a tuberculous udder ? And where shall the small, and usually ineffective, doses, which produce the little lesions which are never suspected during life, and which may possibly even play a not unimportant part in immunizing against more serious infection afterwards, be met if it is not at a greater distance from the consumptive, the main source and fountain head from which tubercle bacilli are distributed, or in the much-mixed milk of the dairy in which the secretions from tuberculous udders are blended with those of normal ones ?

But we may go even further.   Those who admit that phthisis is contagious under the circumstances of closest personal intimacy, as for example when two persons share the same bed—and this we have seen was the opinion of many of the best authorities—are surely illogical if they deny that lesser degrees of intimacy with a phthisical patient are more likely to cause tuberculosis than no intercourse of any kind whatever. The truth would rather seem to be that very close personal intimacy with a phthisical patient who is disseminating bacilli may produce, in some cases, in consequence of the relatively large number of bacilli received, such immediate and acute disease that its origin in contagion is obvious, while lesser degrees of intimacy with such a person lead to the reception of smaller numbers of bacilli, and to disease of such slow and insidious onset that all evidence concerning the time and source of the infection is obscured, but which nevertheless may lead to a fatal termination in the end.

It was, the writer ventures to think, unfortunate that so much importance was attributed by Cornet, and even by Koch himself, to the danger of infection by means of tubercular sputum dried and pulverized and distributed in the streets and public places in the form of dust, since it has tended to foster the idea that everybody is continually being exposed to infection which may set up grave disease in the more susceptible. Possibly this source of infection may be serious where it is concentrated, as, at times, for example, in the public house; but elsewhere the quantity of such bacilli inhaled at any one time must be, one would think, as a rule exceedingly small, and not improbably harmless to ordinary people, or possibly even protective.

It is quite otherwise with the quantity of bacilli which may be taken in by those in close contact with a phthisical patient in the act of coughing, or perhaps even when he is speaking or laughing. It is in such situations that Flügge and his school believed that the majority of infections occur; and the recognition of the importance of dose would seem to strengthen greatly their position.

The question is of the greatest practical importance, and on the answer which is given to it will depend the measures which are taken to stamp out tuberculosis. For it is obvious that if everybody is exposed to the risk of serious infection, and whether he be exposed more or less, or to larger or smaller doses, matters not at all, it follows that it would be of little use to attempt to remove sources of infection by segregating consumptives who are expectorating bacilli, or by destroying cows with tuberculosis of the udder : one must rely in that case on such measures as are calculated to increase the powers of resistance.   But if, on the contrary, the views which have been put forward above are correct, there is more to be hoped from the segregation of consumptives and the destruction of cows which yield milk containing tubercle bacilli than from any other measure.

CHAPTER VI

THE ETIOLOGY OF TUBERCULOSIS (*continued*)

The Scanty Evidence of Contagion.
Latency.   The Comparative Immunity of Doctors and Nurses.
The Question of Marital Infection.   The Influence of
Heredity.

We have now to consider the argument which is often put forward, not without a considerable show of reason, that if tuberculosis is really a contagious disease we ought to see more evidence of direct transmission from the sick to the healthy : and this objection must be fairly met if such views as have just been expressed are to be maintained.   In the first place then it may be pointed out that perhaps after all there is more evidence of contagion than there is generally supposed to be ; and that we fail to see it because our eyes have been blinded by an unconscious prejudice in favour of the view that consumption depends in the main on inherited tendencies.   This view is so bound up with our traditions that it inevitably affects the unconscious reasoning, even of those who do not really believe it ; and so it comes about that when case after case occurs among the members of a certain family living together this seems so naturally the result of a family weakness of

constitution that it is hardly recognized that after all it may
be evidence of contagion.

But there is another and far more potent cause why the
evidence of contagion in tuberculosis is not more obvious.   The
disease is often a chronic one, and has usually a slow and
insidious onset, and its early symptoms are often mistaken
or overlooked.

And even when the apparent onset is well marked, it is
not by any means certain that the real commencement of the
infection was not many months, or perhaps years, earlier.   In
other words there are good reasons for thinking that the disease
is often temporarily arrested at an early stage and becomes
recognized for the first time only long afterwards when a serious
relapse occurs.   Many years ago it was remarked by Portal
that " in estimating the starting point of tuberculous disease
we have often to look or refer the patient back to early symptoms
long forgotten "; and since his time the evidence of latency has
been gaining steadily in strength.

In 1895 the Medical and Chirurgical Society of London held
a debate on latency in disease[1] in the course of which Dr Kingston Fowler[2], with Sir Jonathan Hutchinson in the chair,
introduced the subject of latency in tuberculosis, and in the
subsequent discussion Theodore Williams, Broadbent and others
joined.   The general consensus of opinion expressed seemed
to be that tuberculosis might remain latent for variable periods
of time in some small and unrecognized lesion.   Fowler was
inclined to believe that reactivation of such lesions was usually
brought about by local or accidental causes ;   and Broadbent
recalled the case of a young man whose disease, after tubercle
bacilli had been seen in the sputum, appeared to be arrested,
but in whom it was lighted up again by an accident.   The patient
had apparently recovered and was fat and well when a fall
from his horse was followed by an attack of acute tuberculosis
which proved fatal in about six weeks[3].

Latency was the corner stone of Baumgarten's theory of

[1] *Proc. Roy. Med..Chir. Soc. London*, 1896, N.S. III, p. 27.
[2] *Ibid.* p. 46.
[3] *Ibid.* p. 82.   With this case may be compared one reported by Hermann
Weber (see footnote, page 80).

congenital infection, and also of that put forward by von Behring[1] in his memorable address at Cassel in 1903. According to the latter, infection occurs in infancy, but the disease does not necessarily develop at once, and indeed as a rule remains dormant, until a depression of the powers of resistance, due to some cause, such as puberty, parturition, lactation, malnutrition, over exertion, or one of the acute infective disorders such as measles, kindles the latent disease into activity. " Then we have the beginning of phthisis, but the true commencement of the tuberculous infection dates from long before."

The frequency with which old tuberculous lesions, quiescent or healed, and which for the most part have been entirely unsuspected during life, have been found after death from other causes is one of the most surprising facts about tuberculosis, at one time thought to be an incurable disease. All who have had any extensive experience of post-mortem examination and who have sought carefully for evidence of tuberculosis admit that such lesions are exceedingly common in the bodies which they examine. Naegeli[2] who carefully looked for such lesions in a series of 500 autopsies made at Zürich found them in no less than 97 per cent. of all persons who had died during adult life, and after the age of 30 practically everybody showed some signs of tuberculous infection. There is therefore some justification for the saying " Jedermann hat am Ende ein Bischen Tuberculose."

Naturally all pathologists do not take quite the same view of what constitutes sure evidence of old tuberculous disease, and some observers have arrived at conclusions much more moderate than those of Naegeli[2]. But, as Naegeli pointed out,

[1] *Deutsch. med. Wochenschr.* 1903, p. 689 ; also *Lancet,* 1903, II, p. 1199.

[2] Bulstrode in his Milroy Lecture quotes the following records: Guillot in 1860 found tuberculous lesions in 60 per cent. of necropsies made upon old people. Ribart found them in 50 per cent. Litulle out of 189 adult bodies found only 76 quite free from tubercle. Bronardel at the Morgue found that 50 per cent. of those who had lived for 12 years in Paris were more or less tuberculous. Lubarsh in a Report on the Pathological Department of the Royal Hygienic Institute of Posen states that of 800 bodies which were dissected 61 per cent. showed tuberculous lesions, and if the observation was confined to those over 16 years of age 88·5 were found to be tuberculous. More recently Beitzke in a critical review has estimated the frequency of tuberculous lesions in adults at 70 per cent.

estimates of the frequency of tuberculous infection based on post-mortem records are bound to be too low unless the observer has devoted special attention to seeking for such lesions as are easily overlooked.

On the other hand it is probable that estimates based on post-mortem records are too high if applied to the general community, for such examinations are seldom made on those who have lived in comfortable circumstances, and among the poor tuberculosis is far commoner than it is among those who are better off. Some allowance therefore must be made for this difference. But even if that allowance be made in the most liberal manner, it still remains abundantly clear that some degree of tuberculous disease which has been arrested at an early stage is exceedingly common, and Sir Clifford Allbutt does not seem to have overstated the case when in an address to the British Congress on Tuberculosis in 1901 he said, " I am guilty of no exaggeration when I suggest that one-third of you who hear me, wittingly or unwittingly are, or have been, infected with tuberculosis."

The significance of these quiescent tuberculous lesions as evidence of latency depends of course on whether they contain living tubercle bacilli or no, for it is obvious that if they do not do so they can never become reactivated. In this connection Cornet stated that inoculation tests had shown that when the foci were caseous they always contained living bacilli[1]. This remark undoubtedly overstates the case. The writer[2] found, when working for the Royal Commission, that definitely caseous nodules taken from the lymphatic glands of children might be quite incapable of setting up tuberculosis when emulsified and injected into animals, even when the injections were made in such a susceptible animal as the guinea-pig. This was surprising, but what was more surprising still, the caseous matter thus shown to be totally devoid of infective power might contain plenty of well-formed tubercle bacilli, easily visible under the microscope. At first one could scarcely believe it to be true,

---

[1] Quoted by Newsholme, *loc. cit.* 1908, p. 78.
[2] *R.C.T. Int. Rep.* 1907, App. vol. II, p. 17, " Viruses which failed to produce Tuberculosis."

and suspected some mistake of technique, but the experience was repeated, and by and by one found that other observers were obtaining similar results. Thus A. S. Griffith met with several instances in which the injection into guinea-pigs of emulsions of caseo-calcareous glands failed to provoke tuberculosis[1]. Most of these glands came from adults, but in two cases in which the ages of the patients were five and ten and a half years, respectively, tubercle bacilli (numerous in one of them) were seen in the emulsions injected into the animals.

Similar observations were made at the Gesundheitsamt, and Weber[2] reported 17 cases in which caseo-calcareous glands found in children which had died of causes other than tuberculosis were injected into guinea-pigs without causing tuberculosis. In eight of the emulsions the microscope revealed tubercle bacilli.

A. S. Griffith (1914), who has recently examined a series of unselected bronchial and mesenteric glands obtained post-mortem from children who died in a general hospital, has met with five more cases in which the injection of emulsions made from caseous or calcareous material has failed to produce tuberculosis in guinea-pigs. And Eastwood and F. Griffith (1914) who made a similar investigation on 150 children had similar experience, and from 16 of their cases lesions which to the naked eye appeared tuberculous failed, on injection, to infect the guinea-pig though tubercle bacilli were seen in nine of them[3].

On the result of these investigations, then, one must freely admit that many of the lesions believed on anatomical grounds to be tuberculous, but which are found in persons who have died of other causes than tuberculosis, do not contain living, or at least virulent bacilli, and that therefore there is no reason to believe that they can ever be reactivated. But this is not the case with all, or indeed, probably, with the majority. Many

[1] R.C.T. Final Report, App. vol. 1, p. 18, "Seven cases which did not produce tuberculosis in guinea-pigs."

[2] Weber, 1906, "Die Infection des Menschen mit den Tuberkelbazillen des Rindes," Deutsch. med. Wochenschr. No. 49, p. 1980 (see p. 1982).

[3] A. S. Griffith, Supplement to the 42nd Annual Report of the Local Government Board, N.S. No. 88, p. 115. Eastwood and F. Griffith, ibid. p. 3. See also ibid. Table IV, p. 56.

such have been proved by those who worked for the Gesundheitsamt and the Royal Commission to be capable of transmitting tuberculosis to animals ; and even completely calcified
glands in which no tubercle bacilli can be found on microscopic examination may be still capable of causing infection
on injection. Four instances of this have been recorded by
Rabinowitsch[1].

The existence of old caseous and calcareous lesions, containing living tubercle bacilli, in a considerable proportion of
those who have never had any suspicion that they were infected
with tuberculosis may therefore be held to be proved.

Some authorities write as though they thought that the
term "latency" strictly speaking should be limited to instances
in which living bacilli are found in tissues which show no
histological changes whatever. Whether they are right or wrong
we need not stop to consider, since for the purpose of our
argument it is quite unimportant. Nevertheless it is interesting to know that there are numerous instances recorded
where this has occurred, and since this evidence also supports
the doctrine of latency it will be given in this place.

In 1876 Professor Orth drew attention to the fact that lymph glands which
appeared to the naked eye perfectly normal might reveal under the microscope histological changes characteristic of tubercle. Loomis (1891) was the
first to undertake the investigation of apparently normal glands by their injection into animals (rabbits). This was followed by a similar investigation by
Pizzini in 1892 who used guinea-pigs. These authors showed that apparently
normal lymph glands might sometimes cause tuberculosis when injected into
animals. But they did not show that the histological structure of the infective glands was unchanged. This, according to Rabinowitsch, was first done
by Kälble (1899) who was able to prove in two cases that tubercle bacilli
were present in certain bronchial glands which showed no histological changes
whatever.

In 1903 Alan Macfadyen and MacConkey inoculated into guinea-pigs the
substance of the mesenteric glands of 20 young children who had died of
causes other than tuberculosis. In five cases the guinea-pigs developed
tuberculosis. In four of these the glands which had thus been shown to
contain tubercle bacilli were examined microscopically, and in two no alteration of structure was detected. By the same method tonsils from 34 cases
and adenoids from 44 cases, obtained by operation from persons aged from

[1] *Berl. Klin. Wochenschr.* 1907, p. 37.

two to twenty-one years, were examined, but in no case did the injection cause tuberculosis in the guinea-pigs.

In a monograph published in Christiania in 1905 Harbitz collected the following results from various sources : Glands obtained post-mortem from 142 children were injected into guinea-pigs. In 91 cases there was no trace of tuberculous change either macroscopic or microscopic in the glands. In 18 of these latter cases, that is to say in no less than 20 per cent., the injection of the glandular material revealed the presence of tubercle bacilli.

Weichselbaum and Bartel, 1905, by means of inoculation of guinea-pigs, demonstrated the presence of tubercle bacilli in the apparently normal glands of eight children who had died of one of the infectious fevers, and in whose bodies the most careful anatomical examination failed to find any evidence of tuberculous changes. The bacilli were shown to be present in cervical, bronchial or mesenteric glands, and in some cases in the tonsils.

Rosenberger, 1905, using similar methods, found among 21 non-tuberculous persons six (two children and four adults) whose apparently normal glands provoked tuberculosis when injected into guinea-pigs.

Ipsen, 1906, had a similar experience in one case.

Calmette, Guérin and Deléarde, 1906, injected into guinea-pigs the mesenteric and bronchial glands taken post-mortem from 20 children whose bodies showed no sign of tuberculosis. In three cases tuberculosis was set up.

Goodale, 1906, examined by similar means a number of tonsils removed by operation, and found one, from a child two years of age, which caused tuberculosis when injected into the guinea-pig, but which showed on microscopic examination no sign of tuberculosis. In this case the type of tubercle bacillus found was investigated, and shown, to the satisfaction of Theobald Smith, to be bovine.

L. Rabinowitsch, 1907, obtained cultures of tubercle bacilli of the human type from guinea-pigs injected with the cervical and mesenteric glands of a child, 14 months old, who had died of broncho-pneumonia, but who showed no sign of tuberculosis.

Weber and Baginsky, 1907, tested by means of guinea-pig inoculations the cervical, bronchial and mesenteric glands, and the tonsils of 26 children, aged from three months to 12 years, who showed on post-mortem examination no trace of tuberculosis. Only in one case, however, did the injected material prove infectious to the guinea-pig which received it. In this case the material injected was obtained from the cervical glands of a child, two and a half years of age, and who had been reared on cow's milk. The strain of tubercle bacilli was found to be of the bovine type. No histological changes were found in the glands reserved for microscopic examination.

Gaffky, 1907, examined the bronchial and mesenteric glands obtained post-mortem from 300 unselected children. Among them were 264 in whom there was no macroscopic evidence of tuberculosis, and in 30 of these cases (11 per cent.) injection into guinea-pigs caused tuberculosis.

Eastwood and F. Griffith, 1914, investigated the bronchial and mesenteric glands, taken post-mortem without selection from 150 children, aged from two to ten years, and who had died in hospitals not specially devoted to tuberculosis. Among these there were five who showed no visible lesions, but from whom tubercle bacilli were recovered from apparently normal tissues.

A. S. Griffith, 1914, examined the glands of 72 children. Thirty-four of these were apparently non-tuberculous, and from the bronchial glands of two of these tubercle bacilli of the human type were cultivated. The ages of these two children were one year and nine months and five years respectively.

Instances such as these prove beyond doubt that tubercle bacilli may sometimes be present in lymphatic glands and tonsils of children and others whose bodies show no tuberculous changes, even in the glands themselves which prove infective to guinea-pigs. Of course the material actually injected cannot be subjected to histological examination, but the corresponding halves of the glands injected may be examined in this way, as was actually done by some of these observers, and this leaves no doubt that tubercle bacilli may be present in histologically unaltered tissues.

But a question which cannot be answered in these cases is— how long have the bacilli been there ? and this is very pertinent to the problem of latency. For it is possible that in such cases where they have been found in normal glands or tonsils they may have got there only recently, and may indeed be on the point of being destroyed, or of developing immediate disease. In either case they would afford no support to the doctrine of latency. If it be said that such cases are too numerous to be accounted for in this way (since the chances of finding in a living and virulent condition bacilli which are readily destroyed in the living tissues must be very small) one must ask in reply how frequently and in what numbers do tubercle bacilli gain access to such situations, and how long do they remain virulent while the process of destruction is going on. For it is obvious that if their entry, even in small numbers, is not a rare occurrence, and there is a delay of some days or even weeks before they are destroyed, there would be a fair chance of their discovery by such means as have been employed to search for them. It therefore seems that it has not been proved that the latency of tubercle bacilli in unaltered tissues is of long duration.

On the whole then, while admitting that the discovery of tubercle bacilli in apparently unaltered tissues is additional evidence of the doctrine of latency of tuberculous disease, we nevertheless think that the strongest support of that doctrine

is afforded by the frequent presence in the human body of old
and quiescent or partly healed lesions, obvious enough on post-
mortem examination, but which probably gave little or no
definite sign of their presence during life.   Such lesions, as we
have seen, are found with remarkable frequency in persons of
almost all ages, and in many cases they have been shown to be
capable of infecting the guinea-pig when injected.   It requires
no stretch of the imagination to believe that these are, in a
proportion of cases, capable of being reactivated should circumstances favourable thereto occur, as indeed seems actually to
have occurred in Broadbent's case already alluded to.

Our conclusion then, after considering the evidence as to
latency, must be that it is highly probable that tuberculous
disease when it has advanced enough to be obvious and
diagnosable is, in many cases, the result of infection received
some long time before.   If this be so then contagion may after
all be playing a great part in the spread of infection, though in
many a case the evidence of this may have become so obscured
by the lapse of time that some of the ablest physicians have not
been able to see any sign of it.

The Alleged Immunity of Doctors and Nurses in Hospitals for Consumption.

Yet another argument which has been urged against the
view that tuberculosis is contagious is based upon the experience
that the doctors, nurses, and other attendants in special hospitals
for consumption do not suffer from tuberculosis more than other
persons of like age who are not specially exposed to risks of
infection.   Such persons as are brought into close contact
with phthisical patients, ought, it is argued, if the disease is
really contagious, to contract the disease relatively frequently,
and yet the records of our hospitals and sanatoria do not show
that this is the case.

This argument was put forward by Theodore Williams
in 1882, and was based on the experience of the staff of
Brompton Hospital.   The hospital had grown in 36 years from
90 to 200 beds, and three-quarters of the patients were suffering
from phthisis.   The opportunities for infection should have been

ample, if such occurs, and yet the amount of phthisis among the resident doctors and nurses was no more than might be found in any large institution not specially devoted to consumption.   Consumption, therefore, was not a distinctly infective disease like a zymotic fever.

Williams returned to the subject in 1909, and reviewed the further evidence afforded by the hospital during the previous 18 years.   "There were," he says, "among the resident medical officers no cases of consumption.   Among the assistant medical officers one (from inoculation), and among the house physicians none, were affected during residence.   Two subsequently died of acute phthisis, when holding resident appointments in hospitals where cases of consumption were admitted, and one was attacked by consumption 14 years after he left the hospital, and recovered."   There were 57 resident and 79 non-resident porters since 1882, and of this number six became affected with consumption, and three of these died.

"These figures," he says, "do not testify to much danger of infection to those who have the care of consumptives, but show that with proper precautions such service is quite safe. At the same time the occurrence of tuberculosis among the porters, especially among those who handle the sputum, demonstrates where the true danger lies."

Thus we see that Theodore Williams did not entirely deny the infectiveness of phthisis, but maintained that with reasonable precautions it was not great   Under conditions where filth and overcrowding prevail he seems to have thought that it might be infectious, for he quotes the account of Dr Querli of Tacoma of the appalling spread of tuberculosis among the American Indians living under conditions extraordinarily favourable to the spread of infection.

The evidence of Brompton Hospital was supported by that of the Victoria Park Hospital for Diseases of the Chest and the Ventnor Hospital for Consumption, investigated by Drs Andrews and Robertson respectively, as well as by that of other hospitals and sanatoria both here and abroad[1].

---

[1] Bulstrode cites Falkenstein, Görbersdorf, the Friedrichsheim Hospital, Berlin, Saranack Lake in America and Crooksbury Sanatorium in this country, loc. cit. p. 58.

Newsholme criticizes the evidence, so far as it refers to Brompton, Ventnor and Victoria Park, and points out that it is incomplete and scanty. "The experiences of these places," he says, "are usually quoted as instances of non-infection in hospitals. They should rather be described as examples of investigations in which the data are, possibly owing to insuperable difficulties, incomplete and insufficient to justify any dogmatic treatment[1]."

But even if we accept the evidence, as showing that consumption is no commoner among the members of the staffs of consumption hospitals[2] than it is among members of the general community of similar age and social condition, it does not prove that, under domestic conditions, especially among the poorer classes, consumption is not contagious, for domestic and hospital conditions are apt to be very different. As Allbutt pointed out, similar testimony might be given with regard to typhoid fever. How often, he asked, does this spread in a general hospital to neighbouring patients or attendants, and yet who would deny its infectiousness? Professor B. Moore[3] also has criticized the inferences which have been drawn from the comparative immunity from phthisis of doctors and attendants in hospitals for consumption, and has attributed that immunity to the strict sanitary regime followed in such places. In hospitals "the whole life is different from the patient's home life, and the relations to him of doctor and nurse are essentially different from the relations of his relatives, friends and co-workers."

The evidence then, even if it is sound, only shows that consumption is not contagious under the special conditions of a well regulated hospital, and this is all that Williams claimed. We have seen that he admitted that the porters who had to wash the sputum pots, and who were probably not subjected

---

[1] *The Prevention of Tuberculosis*, p. 154.

[2] Doctors as a class suffer very little from phthisis in this country, coming with coal-miners, engine-drivers and clergymen at the very bottom of the list. Their comparative mortality from this cause in 1900, 1901, 1902 was only 65, while that of all occupied males was 175, and that of tin-miners 838, *Supplement to the 65th Rep. of the Reg. Gen.* 1908, Pt. III, p. clxxxvii.

[3] *The Dawn of the Health Age*, p. 152.

to the same strict discipline as the other members of the staff were sometimes infected, and in this connection one remembers the Grimaldi girls who washed the consumptive's linen in Mentone, so well described by Bennet (though Bennet himself did not see in this any evidence of infection).

But while the experience of English and some foreign hospitals has been that the members of their medical and nursing staffs do not suffer excessively from phthisis, this has by no means been the universal experience on the Continent. Long ago attention was drawn to the high mortality from phthisis in military infirmaries, monasteries, and other institutions, and this was well known to Laennec.

In 1889 Cornet, examining the official returns, for 25 years, of the religious orders of Prussia who attended on the sick, found that the death-rate from tuberculosis among them was actually two-thirds of that from all causes. Comparing the death-rate from tuberculosis of the sisters of charity with those of the rest of the population of equal ages, it appeared that from 15 to 20 years of age the former was four times as high, from 20 to 30 three times, and from 30 to 40 twice as high as that of the rest of the community[1].

The conclusions which Cornet drew from this investigation as to the infectivity of phthisis have been adversely criticized by Bulstrode[2] aided by a statistical examination to which they were put by Hamar. But the figures are striking, and the difference in the death-rate from phthisis among the nursing sisters and that of the general population of equal age is so great that it is not easy to believe that it can be due to the fact that many women join these religious orders because ill health has already turned their affections away from worldly things, or because, as Laennec suggested, the sad nature of their lives undermines their powers of resistance[3].

It seems far more likely that the nursing sisters abroad have suffered so greatly from tuberculosis in the past because they were brought into contact with phthisical patients, and

---

[1] Straus, *La Tuberculose*, p. 452.
[2] *Supplement to the Local Government Board Reports*, 1905–6, p. 64.
[3] Laennec, *loc. cit.* p. 423.   Quoted by Straus, *loc. cit.* p. 451.

because the precautions which alone would make such a life reasonably safe were neglected. This assumption is not entirely unwarranted because we know that in the comparatively recent past the general condition of many French hospitals was far below the standard of the English ones at the same period.

The difference between the English and the foreign records of those who are brought into professional relationship with persons suffering from consumption would seem, then, to be explicable on two grounds: (1) The members of the staffs of the English hospitals were at most temporarily resident there and not very easily traced after they had left, while the sisters of charity, having embraced the nursing profession for life, could not be so easily lost sight of; and (2) that the general sanitary routine and discipline of the English hospitals was greatly in advance of those on the Continent.

Marital Infection.

If pulmonary tuberculosis is contagious we ought to see many instances of it in both husband and wife. Some striking examples of this, brought forward by Hermann Weber in 1874, were mentioned in the last chapter[1]. We have now

---

[1] One was the case of a man, himself suffering from quiescent phthisis, who lost four wives in succession from pulmonary tuberculosis. The history is as follows: J. had lost his mother, two brothers and one sister from consumption; had twice himself had hæmoptysis when about 20 and 21 years of age; became afterwards a sailor; felt perfectly well after his 25th year; and married when 27—

1. A woman, belonging to a healthy family, who herself enjoyed good health till towards the end of her third pregnancy, when she began to cough and emaciate. She died from consumption after her third confinement.

2. After a year he married again, an apparently healthy woman who, after the first year of married life, began to cough, had hæmoptysis, and died from galloping consumption.

3. The third wife belonged to an exceptionally healthy family, having both her parents, four brothers and two sisters living, and in good health. She was 25 when she married and continued to enjoy good health until her second pregnancy, when she began to cough, became feverish, and twice had hæmoptysis. When Weber first saw her after the second confinement she had extensive affection of the upper portion of both lungs, hectic fever and profuse perspiration. A month later she had serious pulmonary hæmorrhages

to see how far these are representative and how far exceptional.

In 1883, nine years after Weber's paper, the Collective Investigation Committee of the British Medical Association issued to its members, as we have seen already, some questions concerning marital infection. Replies were received reporting 192 cases of apparent transmission of tuberculosis from one partner to the other; and in 130 of these it is expressly stated that no family history of the disease existed in the person to whom the disease was believed to have been transmitted. Taking only those cases where the history is sufficiently definite[1], the writer finds that 87 of these were instances of supposed infection of wife from husband, while 49 only were instances of supposed infection of husband from wife[2]. Weber discussed this point in relation to his own series of cases without coming to any definite conclusion. But it seems reasonable to believe that a wife is more liable than a husband to become infected from a diseased partner because she is likely to be much more in the atmosphere of the sick room than he is, and also because the exhaustion due to childbearing is a great cause of predisposition in the women, while no commensurate cause is present in the case of the man.

and died soon after, about eight months from the appearance of the first symptoms.

4. The fourth wife had no indication of phthisis in her family, and was, at the age of 23 when she married, in perfect health. About thirteen months later, three months after her first confinement, which had passed off quite well, she began to cough and nine months later she died of pneumonia and tubercular affection of both lungs, and with tubercles in the intestine, spleen and liver.

The man was afraid to marry again, thinking it certain death for any woman who mated with him. He continued in good health in his seafaring occupation until, through a severe fracture, he was laid up several months. He then began to cough ; the formerly healthy right apex became affected ; and consumption regularly developed itself, leading to death, when the post-mortem examination disclosed the cicatricized condition of the former seat of the disease, and also the recent affection (*Trans. Clin. Soc.* VII, p. 145).

[1] In many instances, where both husband and wife had died of phthisis, it was not certain which of the partners had been the first to develop definite symptoms of the disease.

[2] Cp. similar evidence from German data in Pope and Pearson, 1908, *loc. cit.* p. 15.

Weber was careful not to draw far-reaching conclusions from his own experience, but it is clear that it impressed him greatly. Indeed his cases, and many of those brought to light by the Collective Investigation, seem to be as clear instances of contagion as any one can expect to obtain.

The evidence however has been adversely criticized by statisticians, including Longstaff who contributed a communication to *The Collective Investigation Record* (p. 139) in which he calculated the chances that both husband and wife should die of consumption within a short time of one another, apart altogether from the question of personal contagion. This was afterwards expanded in his *Studies in Statistics*. Longstaff was led to conclude that " if the results are anywhere near the truth they show that a far greater number of coincidences of the death of both husband and wife from phthisis, within a short period of one another, would be required to prove that one had contracted the disease from the other by infection."

In recent years E. G. Pope (1908) in America has investigated by modern statistical methods the problem of marital infection in tuberculosis. His memoir was nearly, but not entirely, finished when he died, and his work has been edited and completed by Professor Karl Pearson.

The material for this investigation consisted of 37 reports from various sources, mostly German, and contained information concerning over 40,000 couples. One group consisted of the married population of two entire villages, another of the parents of non-tuberculous children, but the greater part dealt with the parents of tuberculous children who were being treated in sanatoria or hospitals. This distinction is of importance only if we assume the existence of a tuberculous diathesis.

The great majority of the reports show a very considerable excess of instances of tuberculosis in both husband and wife beyond what chance alone would have caused[1]. But it is pointed out that this excess may be due, in part at least,

---

[1] See Table I, *loc. cit.* p. 8. Out of a total of 10,980 couples in which at least one partner was tuberculous, both husband and wife were tuberculous in 1296 couples, that is to say in one couple out of 8·4.

to assortative mating. "The constitution which is peculiarly liable to tuberculosis [the tuberculous diathesis] is not unfrequently associated with certain mental and physical traits, which present undoubted sexual attraction. It is conceivable accordingly that the resemblance in phthisical character between husband and wife may be, wholly or in part, due to the tendency of like to mate with like, and not at all, or not wholly, to post-marital infection" (Pope and Pearson, p. 3).

In allowing for this tendency Pearson relied upon data which had been collected by Miss Elderton who worked out the coefficients of assortative mating for a number of cases of health, temperament and intelligence, and which are published as an Appendix to his paper.

Pearson tells us that Pope " had demonstrated that there was a sensible correlation between the presence of tuberculosis in husband and wife, and had reached the interpretation that this result depended upon the extent that assortative mating prevailed with regard to what we may term the tuberculous diathesis " (loc. cit. p. 3).

Pearson himself arrived at the following conclusion, which he expresses " in words slightly modified from those of Pope," " It would seem probable (1) that there is some sensible but slight infection between married couples, (2) that this is largely obscured or forestalled by the fact of infection from outside sources, (3) that the liability to infection depends upon the necessary diathesis, (4) that assortative mating probably accounts for at least two-thirds and infective action for not more than one-third of the whole correlation observed in these cases " (loc. cit. p. 15).

The reader will form his own opinion concerning the importance of the part played by assortative mating. The data for calculating the effect of such mating must necessarily be most uncertain, and even the existence of an inheritable tuberculous diathesis, probable as this may be, has never been proved. The fact remains that a considerable proportion of wives and husbands are both of them tuberculous beyond what chance alone would account for.

Even if we conclude that the evidence of marital infection in pulmonary tuberculosis is much smaller than might be expected by one who believed the disease to be distinctly contagious, this may be because the period of life when infection is most liable to occur is already passed at the time of marriage[1].   For we have seen, from the investigations of Naegeli and others as to the frequency of tuberculous lesions at different ages, reason to think that infection is most frequent in infancy and adolescence.

One of the objections which have been brought against the view that tuberculosis is contagious is based upon the comparative immunity of the wives of tin-miners, steel-grinders, stonemasons and others who in the course of their occupations inhale much stone dust and as a consequence are liable to suffer severely from consumption.   This subject will be treated fully in the next chapter, but it may be pointed out in the present connection that there is reason to believe that the type of pulmonary tuberculosis in these cases is peculiar, and that the low degree of infectiousness which they undoubtedly show is correlated with a paucity of tubercle bacilli in the expectoration.

The Influence of Heredity.

Tuberculosis is, of course, well known to run in certain families, but whether this is due to hereditary influences or to opportunities for infection is a very difficult question to decide.   The very existence of an inheritable weakness of constitution which predisposes to tuberculosis, though highly probable, is very difficult to establish conclusively[2], while it cannot be denied that if one member of a family has pulmonary tuberculosis, the other members are more exposed to infection than are those who belong to families where no such disease exists.

---

[1] Parturition and lactation have undoubtedly an unfavourable influence on the *course* of tuberculosis, and may possibly be the occasion of re-awakening a quiescent infection, but it is by no means certain that they predispose to *infection*.

[2] Among the conclusions which Pearson considers appear highly probable from his own " preliminary " investigation of the question is the following:

" What I have spoken of as the diathesis of pulmonary tuberculosis is certainly inherited, and the intensity of the inheritance is sensibly the same as that of any normal physical character yet investigated in man."   "A First Study of the Statistics of Pulmonary Tuberculosis," 1907, p. 24.

The relative importance of these two factors will be differently
viewed by different observers according to their bias, and
hence much that has been written on the subject in the past is
quite inconclusive.

More recently the question has been carefully considered
by Karl Pearson (1907) who made a statistical study of the
records of Crossley Sanatorium, Frodsham, which included
383 stocks in which cases of pulmonary tuberculosis had
occurred. It would be impossible to do justice to this study
in an abstract, and no more than a brief statement of the
conclusions arrived at will be attempted. Pearson convinced
himself that the diathesis of pulmonary tuberculosis is inherited[1].
" Infection," he says, " probably plays a necessary part, but
in the artizan class of the urban populations of this country it
is doubtful if their members can escape the risk of infection
except by the absence of the diathesis, *i.e.* the inheritance of
what amounts to a counter disposition " (*loc. cit.* p. 24). The
argument on which this conclusion is based cannot be summarized briefly, but it is evident that it takes no account of
the difference in the result of exposure to large and small
doses of tubercle bacilli respectively. This is pointed out by
Newsholme, who adds that Pearson's results depend in part
upon hypotheses which may not be accepted generally as
justified, and upon ascertained data which may be regarded
as too few to warrant conclusive inferences. Indeed Pearson
himself states " This investigation does not profess to be more
than preliminary, and its results need confirmation when much
more numerous data are available[2]."

Dr Emmanuel (1909), in a Presidential Address to the
Medical Society of Birmingham, has recorded some interesting
histories in which consumption appeared to spread to persons
not connected by blood with the original case. In one of these
a lady, with no history of consumption in her family, married

[1] See footnote 2 on previous page.
[2] A very curious point noticed by Pearson is thus stated by him: " Whether
we deal with all tuberculous stocks, or only with those having no parental
history (of tuberculosis), the elder offspring, especially the first and the second,
appear subject to tuberculosis at a very much higher rate than the younger
members " (*loc. cit.* 1907, p. 25).

a man with pulmonary tuberculosis, and then herself fell ill of the disease. She bore three children all of whom died of tuberculosis; her brother, who was much with her, died of hæmoptysis; and his wife also became consumptive. In another case a lady became consumptive after associating freely with an acquaintance who died of pulmonary tuberculosis; she was nursed by her mother who afterwards became infected. Emmanuel did not deny that heredity and infection play their respective rôles in the spread of consumption, but was inclined to think that, for all practical purposes, it is the infectiousness of consumption we have to deal with, and that we may, for the most part, disregard hereditary predisposition.

CHAPTER VII

THE ETIOLOGY OF TUBERCULOSIS (*continued*)

Variation in the Relative Fatality of Tuberculosis in Men, Women, and Children in Different Localities.

The Alleged Escape of the Wives and Children of Men who suffer from certain forms of Occupational Phthisis.

The Nature of the " Phthisis " which is Associated with certain Dusty Trades.

The Prevention of Tuberculosis. The Relative Value of Measures based upon Treatment of Early Cases, and those which aim at Limiting the Spread of Infection.

There now remains for consideration an important argument, against the view that contagion plays a prominent part in the spread of tuberculosis, based upon the great variations in the mortality from tuberculosis which occur among men, women and children respectively in different localities. The argument may be put somewhat as follows: If the men suffer severely from pulmonary tuberculosis in certain places owing to the nature of their occupations, then one would expect to find that their wives and children also would suffer to a greater extent than those of other men who follow ordinary occupations; and since, as is alleged, this is not the case, tuberculosis cannot be contagious.

The examples generally put forward in support of this argument are the grinders of Sheffield, the tin-miners of Cornwall (Haldane, Martin and Thomas), the stone-workers of Grinshill quarries in Shropshire (Wheatley), and the flint-workers of Brandon in Suffolk (Collis). These will be considered in their place ; but before proceeding to discuss special instances, which is rendered difficult by the scarcity of reliable statistics, it will be well to consider the relative mortality of men, women and children in certain towns and country districts for which official returns are available. And first we will consider the relation of the female to the male mortality from pulmonary tuberculosis, and afterwards the relation of the mortality from tuberculosis of children to that of adults.

The Relation of Female to Male Death-rate from Phthisis in Different Localities.

In order that the statistics of one place should be strictly comparable with those of another, it is necessary to make allowance for differences in the proportion of males and females in the different places, and in the relative number of persons of different ages living in them, or, in other words, the statistics of each district must be corrected for variations in the sex and age distribution of the population, and reduced to what they would have been had the population in the district in question corresponded in these respects exactly with a certain normal standard population. This has been done in the office of the Registrar General, and in the Report of the Medical Officer of the Local Government Board (1914)[1] will be found the death-rates thus " standardized " of males and females respectively from pulmonary and other forms of tuberculosis for the Administrative Counties, and County and Metropolitan Boroughs, of England and Wales.

In that Report the Medical Officer points out that—" In towns the standardized male death-rate " (from phthisis) " is nearly always much higher than the standardized female death-rate. In most administrative counties the female is

[1] *Supplement to the 42nd Annual Report,* see pp. xxvii *et seq.,* and Tables I–VI, pp. 234 *et seq.*

lower than the male phthisis death-rate. The ratio of female to male death-rate (male = 100) varies from 53 in Cambridgeshire, 58 in Surrey, 61 in Cornwall, 62 in Gloucestershire and 65 in Hertfordshire, to 109 in the North Riding, 111 in Norfolk, 117 in Cumberland, 120 in Monmouthshire and the East Riding, 135 in Herefordshire, 145 in Glamorganshire and 228 in Anglesey. These differences in the male and female death-rates call for detailed local inquiry, both as to the possible influence of migration of the sick and healthy, and as to the influence of local sanitary and social conditions " (*loc. cit.* p. xxxiii).

The writer can make no claim to have made any such inquiry, but a few remarks may perhaps be hazarded. It is, of course, evident that differences in the conditions of life and occupations of the people must largely influence the ratio of the female to male mortality from tuberculosis, and that such differences are not necessarily inconsistent with the view that the germs of tuberculosis are acquired by contagion. For home conditions influence the women mainly, while the conditions of labour mainly react on the men. If the housing conditions are poor and the men work largely at healthy outdoor occupations, one would expect this ratio to be relatively high, and, conversely, if the men work in factories where the conditions are favourable to the spread of phthisis, while their homes are of a good type, one would expect this ratio to be low. As a matter of fact in towns generally, and in manufacturing towns especially, it is low, and in country districts it is high[1].

In Scotland, as we have already seen, the ratio of female to male death-rate from phthisis is much higher than in England and Wales. This appears, at first sight, to be because in England and Wales a much higher proportion of occupied males are engaged in factories than is the case in Scotland, where relatively larger numbers follow outdoor occupations such as farming or fishing, or are employed in coal-mining. This explanation was offered by Scurfield. On the other hand Hunter Stewart attributed the high female to male ratio in Scotland to exhaustion entailed by agricultural work and the

---

[1] See *loc. cit.* p. xxxii, also Diag. VI opposite p. 41 of this book.

phthisigenetic nature of the occupations followed by many of the women of that country, as for example in Dundee where women are largely employed in the jute trade[1], an occupation which seems to predispose to pulmonary tuberculosis. It appears probable that both the causes suggested contribute to produce the result in question.

Analogous causes may be expected to produce similar discrepancies in the ratio of the female to male death-rates from phthisis in different counties and county boroughs. The case of Anglesey, as we have seen, is extreme. There the standardized death-rate of females from pulmonary tuberculosis is almost the highest on the list (namely 1·69 per 1000 living at all ages), while the corresponding male death-rate is very low (0·74). The lowness of the male rate, agreeing as it does with that for Herefordshire and Norfolk, and, very nearly, with that for the East Riding of Yorkshire, is probably attributable to the fact that almost the only industry of the island is agriculture[2]; but the very high female rate would seem to be inexplicable, unless indeed it be the case that there, more than elsewhere, many women, who have left their homes, when young, for service or other work elsewhere, return when attacked by phthisis to die in their native place.

Another interesting case is that of Glamorganshire, where the ratio of the female to the male death-rate from pulmonary tuberculosis is second only to that of Anglesey. Here again the death-rate of the males from pulmonary tuberculosis is very low (0·74), but for a different reason. Thirty-five per cent. of the occupied males are engaged in coal and shale mining[3], an occupation which elsewhere is associated with a low mortality from phthisis[4].

---

[1] In that industry, the Medical Officer of Health for the town states, that " 51 per cent. of the employees are women over 20 years of age, 22 per cent. are girls under 20, 11 per cent. are boys under 20, and only 16 per cent. are men." C. Templeman, *Public Health*, 1909, p. 385.

[2] Copper, lead, silver, marble, asbestos, lime and sandstone, marl, zinc and coal have all been worked in Anglesey. *Ency. Brit.*

[3] *Supp. to 42nd Rep. Loc. Gov. Board*, 1914, p. xxxi.

[4] The mortality of coal-miners from phthisis varies in different districts, probably with differences in the quantity and quality of the stone which has to be removed in getting out the coal; but everywhere it is considerably below

The contrast in the ratio in question which prevails in the neighbouring agricultural counties of Cambridgeshire and Norfolk is striking. In Cambridgeshire, in 1911, this ratio (53 : 100) was the lowest recorded in any county. In Norfolk it was high (111 : 100). The lowness of this ratio in Cambridgeshire was due to an excessively low mortality from pulmonary tuberculosis among women (0·54 per 1000), while the corresponding male rate was not abnormal (1·01). In Norfolk, on the other hand, the female rate (0·82) was near the average, while the male rate (0·74) was low. It is difficult to say what was the cause of the extremely low female rate in Cambridge, but the low male rate in Norfolk may, perhaps, be ascribed to the large proportion of males employed in fishing in addition to those who follow agriculture.

The case of Sheffield demands special consideration, since it is referred to in support of the argument urged against the contagiousness of phthisis. In that city the male mortality from this disease is high, in the ratio of 122 to 100 for England and Wales as a whole, while the female mortality from the same cause is low, 74 to 100 for England and Wales. The great departure from the average ratio of female to male mortality from phthisis which these figures imply needs careful investigation. It is explained by the Medical Officer of the City, Dr Scurfield, on the following grounds: Sheffield is naturally a healthy place. It is built on hills which allow the fresh air from the moors to circulate round the houses. The hills, again, enable the subsoil to be readily drained, and exercise beneficially the lungs of the inhabitants. Hence the death-rate from pulmonary tuberculosis among the women is low. Among the men, on the other hand, phthisis is frequent because of the occupations which some of them follow. " The great discrepancy between the male and female tuberculosis

the average for all occupied males. Thus, if we take the comparative phthisis mortality figure for the latter as 100, the following figures represent the mortality from this cause of miners in different districts of England and Wales: Monmouthshire and South Wales 58, Lancashire 55, Durham and Northumberland 51, Staffordshire 45, Derbyshire and Nottingham 37. With these may be compared the corresponding figures of the occupations which stand at the top and bottom of the list; namely, hotel and inn-servants (London) 328, tin-miners 275 and clergymen 36. (Calculated from Table V, *Supplement to 55th Ann. Rep. Reg. Gen.* 1897 (Cd. 8503), p. clxi.)

death-rates in Sheffield is due to the large amount of phthisis among the grinders, and, one might add, cutlers." It is true that the grinders (and cutlers) form only a small part of the adult male population of Sheffield—there were in 1908 nearly 4000 grinders and almost as many cutlers in a total population approaching half a million[1]—but nearly half the grinders and a large proportion of the cutlers die of phthisis, and "if the 4000 grinders with their 60 deaths annually from phthisis be subtracted from the population of Sheffield, the Sheffield tuberculosis statistics would resemble those of an ordinary English town as regards the discrepancy between the male and female death-rates[2]."

The lowness of the female death-rate from tuberculosis in Sheffield as a whole is sometimes assumed to extend to the wives and daughters of those engaged in the cutlery trade, and used as an argument against the contagiousness of phthisis. The argument one hears runs somewhat as follows : "Half the grinders die of phthisis, why do not their women-folk suffer in proportion if the disease is contagious?" Well this is just where information fails us. There are no statistics at present which show whether the wives and daughters of grinders and cutlers do, or do not, suffer from phthisis more than the rest of the women of Sheffield. It is however relevant to point out that the phthisis which the grinder dies of is peculiar. Probably, as we shall see reason to think, it is not tuberculous at all for a considerable part of its course (see p. 96). And when tubercle bacilli are at length implanted on a pulmonary fibrosis, they do not cause the same destruction of lung tissue and consequent dissemination of infection as occurs in advanced cases of ordinary pulmonary tuberculosis. But as this type of disease is common to all those who suffer in consequence of inhaling continually certain kinds of stone dust its further consideration must be deferred for the moment.

The Relation of the Death-rate of Children from Tuberculosis to that of Males and Females of all ages from Pulmonary Tuberculosis in Various Places.

In the Report of the Medical Officer to the Local Government Board which has been quoted in the previous section,

[1] *Public Health*, 1910, XXIII, p. 114.   [2] *Ibid.* 1912, p. 12.

the death-rate of children from tuberculosis in various districts is not given. Sufficient information for our present purpose, however, has been collected by Scurfield from local sources, and published (1909) in a paper in which he analysed the relative mortality from tuberculosis in a number of English and Scottish towns. From this paper[1] certain towns—or, in the case of London, districts—have been selected to the number of 17, and the death-rates of males and females from pulmonary tuberculosis and of children from all other kinds of tuberculosis transcribed. And from these figures have been calculated the ratios which these death-rates bear to the corresponding rates of England and Wales as a whole, in order that it may be seen at a glance how far they depart from the average.

TABLE VII.   *Average annual death-rates from Tuberculosis 1898–1907 (except where otherwise stated).*

(Arranged in the order of the female rate.)

| | Pulmonary Tuberculosis | | | | Other forms of Tuberculosis | |
| | Males (all ages) | | Females (all ages) | | Children (under 5) | |
Town or District	Per million males living	Ratio	Per million females living	Ratio	Per million children living	Ratio
England and Wales	1445	100	1033	100	2839	100
Dundee	1785	124	1834	178	4647	164
Glasgow	1856	129	1665	161	4377	154
Shoreditch	2588	179	1512	147	5191	183
Manchester	2433	168	1425	138	4265	150
Liverpool	2055	142	1361	132	3239	114
Bermondsey[2]	2417	167	1364	132	4561	161
Birkenhead	1611	111	1240	120	1820	64
Edinburgh	1753	121	1239	120	4360	154
Hull	1287	89	997	97	1990	70
Bristol[3]	1233	85	981	95	1681	59
Birmingham[4]	1818	129	886	86	2354	83
Blackburn	1330	92	883	86	3956	139
Kensington	1703	117	883	86	4081	159
Sheffield	1756	122	769	74	3721	131
Leyton[5]	1161	80	745	72	2191	77·2
East Ham[6]	827	57	718	70	2070	73
Lewisham[7]	1118	77	685	66	2181	77
Wolverhampton[8]	1162	80	643	62	2406	85

[1] *Brit. Med. Journ.* 1909, II, p. 462.   [2] 4 years, 1904–1907.
[3] 3 years, 1905–1907.   [4] 4 years, 1904–1907.   [5] 5 years, 1902–3, 1906–7.
[6] 7 years, 1901–1907.   [7] 6 years, 1902–1907.   [8] 5 years, 1902–1906.

From this table we can get a sufficiently close approximation to what we require for the purpose of comparing the
death-rate of children from tuberculosis with the number of
possible human sources of infection.   For it is obvious that
only " open " cases of tuberculosis can be regarded as sources
of infection, and such are confined almost entirely to pulmonary
tuberculosis.   Moreover we can obtain a rough approximation
to the death-rate of all persons from pulmonary tuberculosis
in the different localities by taking the mean of the male and
female rates[1].   Again the number of deaths attributed to
pulmonary tuberculosis in childhood is small, so that the
death-rate from all other kinds of tuberculosis gives us a fair
measure of the total fatal tuberculosis at this time of life.

From the preceding table therefore has been calculated
the ratio which the death-rate of children under five years
of age from other kinds of tuberculosis bears to that of all
persons from pulmonary tuberculosis.

TABLE VIII. *Ratio of the Death-rate of Children (under 5) from
"other forms" of Tuberculosis to the mean of the Male and
Female rates from Pulmonary Tuberculosis.*

Town or District	Ratios as stated above	Comparison of the ratios with one another. England and Wales taken as 100
Blackburn	358	*156*
Kensington	316	*138*
Sheffield	294	*128*
Edinburgh	291	*127*
East Ham	268	*117*
Wolverhampton	267	*117*
Dundee	257	*112*
Shoreditch	253	*110*
Glasgow	248	*108*
Lewisham	242	*106*
Bermondsey	241	*105*
Leyton	230	*100*
England and Wales	229	*100*
Manchester	221	*97*
Liverpool	190	*83*
Birmingham	174	*76*
Hull	174	*76*
Bristol	152	*66*
Birkenhead	128	*56*

[1] The figures thus obtained are of course not strictly comparable owing to
the varying proportion of males and females in different places, but they
will suffice for our present purpose which only aims at considering very
large departures from the average of the country as a whole.

This table shows how greatly the ratio of the tuberculosis mortality of children to the number of possible human sources of infection differs in different localities.   In Blackburn, for instance, it is half as high again as the average for England and Wales, while in Birkenhead it is scarcely more than half as great as the average ; thus in one town this ratio is nearly three times as large as it is in another.

In the great towns of Scotland, Edinburgh, Dundee, Glasgow, the ratio is greatly above the average, but Kensington, curiously enough, comes, second only to Blackburn, at the top of the list[1].

But there are good reasons why the ratio of the children's mortality from tuberculosis to that of all persons from phthisis should vary greatly in different places.   Not only are there domestic and economic causes, which will be considered in a moment, but there is the disturbing factor that tuberculosis in young children is attributable, not only to infection derived

[1] One would naturally suppose that if tuberculosis is contagious, the death-rate among children would show a closer relationship to that among females than to that among males, for children come into closer relationship with their mothers and sisters than with their fathers and brothers ; but it must be admitted that our figures do not show that such is the case.

Ratio of the death-rate of Children (under 5) from " other forms " of Tuberculosis to that of Males and Females respectively from Pulmonary Tuberculosis. The corresponding ratios for England and Wales being taken as 100.

Town or District	Ratio of Children's rate to Male rate	Ratio of Children's rate to Female rate
England and Wales	100	100
Blackburn ..	148	163
Kensington	122	168
Sheffield	108	176
Edinburgh ..	127	128
East Ham ..	129	105
Wolverhampton	106	136
Dundee	133	92
Shoreditch ..	103	127
Glasgow	120	96
Lewisham ..	99	116
Bermondsey	97	121
Leyton	96	107
Manchester ..	89	109
Liverpool ..	80	85
Birmingham	66	97
Hull	80	73
Bristol	69	62
Birkenhead ..	58	53

from human sources, but to a considerable extent also to that derived from the cow. It is clear then that this ratio in a given district will depend partly on the prevalence of bovine tuberculosis there, and the extent to which the babies are fed on unboiled milk. It is not improbable that these conditions vary greatly in different parts of the country; for example, infection with the bovine type of bacillus seems to be exceptionally prevalent in Edinburgh, if we can accept the opinion of Maxwell Williams, the Medical Officer of Health[1], supported as it is by the recent work of Fraser and Mitchell[2]. Variations in the local prevalence of tuberculosis among the cattle, and in the manner of feeding infants, then, would seem to be capable of accounting for many of the anomalies in the ratio of the tuberculosis death-rate in children and adults respectively. But, unfortunately, with the exception of London, Berlin, Edinburgh and New York, there is but scant material for estimating, even roughly, the relative fatality due to infection of children from bovine sources in different places.

Again, the ratio in question is affected by many other conditions besides the variations in the prevalence of bovine tuberculosis and of the practice of feeding infants. The occupations and the mode of life of the people, and the climate, must be taken into consideration. It is not proposed to examine these factors in great detail. That would require an amount of local knowledge which we make no claim to possess. But in the case of some of the towns we are fortunately in possession of the considered opinions of their Medical Officers of Health, for Scurfield in his paper invited them to express their views on any peculiarities which were shown by the figures of their district, and some of them responded to the invitation. The following remarks are based mainly on their replies[3]. Immunity of children from tuberculosis, as indeed from other causes of death also, must depend to a great extent on the amount of time and care which their mothers are able to spend upon them. Where a considerable proportion of the women, including the mothers, go out to work in factories

---

[1] *Public Health*, 1909, XXII, p. 385.   [2] See Chapter XXIV.
[3] *Public Health*, 1909, XXII, p. 378.

or elsewhere, the infants must be left to a great extent neglected at home, in the care of older children, or carried in the
cold of the early morning, perhaps insufficiently clothed, and
for a considerable distance, to be cared for by other women
who have only a pecuniary interest in them (Alfred Greenwood,
M.O.H., Blackburn). This is the case in Dundee, where it is
said that "something like 50 per cent. of all females over ten
are at work, and where 74 per cent. of all ' occupied ' women
work in mills or factories[1]," and where too the children die
of tuberculosis to a greater extent than in any other place
mentioned in Scurfield's tables, Shoreditch alone excepted.

A similar explanation of the high tuberculosis death-rate
among children in Blackburn and Kensington[2] is offered by
the Medical Officers of these places; while it is suggested
that the high rates in Edinburgh and Glasgow may partly be
due to the custom, common among the poorer classes there,
of living in flats several stories high, which places an obstacle
in the way of the children obtaining the same amount of outdoor life which others are accustomed to get elsewhere (Scurfield).

Many anomalies remain unexplained on social grounds, as
for example the contrast presented by Liverpool and Birkenhead, or by Sheffield and Birmingham. In the first of these cases,
while the female rate is only one tenth higher, and the male
rate one fourth higher in Liverpool than in Birkenhead, the
children's rate in the former town is nearly double that in the
latter, and yet the social conditions are said to be very similar[3].

[1] C. Templeman, M.O.H. for Dundee, *Public Health*, 1909, XXII, p. 385. In
Dundee the female death-rate from pulmonary tuberculosis also is, as we have
seen, extraordinarily high. The opportunities for the children to become
infected from their mothers must therefore be very great.

[2] J. E. Sandilands, M.O.H. for Kensington, wrote as follows : " A large
percentage of the mothers in my district go out to work early in the mornings
and do not return to their homes until late at night. Their children in the
meantime are left in crèches or minded by a neighbour...the children of
mothers who go out to work are likely to be badly fed and underfed, and
so might acquire, through a general lowering of resistance to disease, a special
liability to tuberculosis."

[3] The M.O.H. for Birkenhead writes: " Why should Liverpool and
Birkenhead be so different ? We have very similar populations engaged in
similar work and living under similar conditions—practically we are parts
of one great population." *Public Health*, 1909, XXII, p. 383.

In Birkenhead indeed the children's rate is, with the exception of Bristol, the lowest in our table.

In both Birmingham and Sheffield the male death-rate from pulmonary tuberculosis is abnormally high (129 and 122 respectively, E. and W. = 100) "no doubt owing to the grinding trades" (Scurfield), and the female death-rate from the same disease is abnormally low (86 and 74 respectively, E. and W. = 100), and yet in spite of this similarity both in the male and in the female rates of the two places, the children's rate in Birmingham is much lower than in Sheffield (83 and 131 respectively, E. and W. = 100). As Dr R. Sydney Marsden, M.O.H. for Birkenhead, writes[1]: "It is obvious that these tuberculosis rates are the result of many factors...of some of which we have no knowledge, and which require to be further sought for."

We have only touched the fringe of the matter, but perhaps enough has been said to show that the unequal incidence of the tuberculosis death-rate on children and older persons respectively in different places cannot be accepted, without detailed inquiry, as evidence of the lack of contagiousness of the disease in question. As the Medical Officer of the Local Government Board points out "Tuberculosis is not only an infectious but also a chronic disease, which, on the average, probably extends over years, and often escapes recognition during a large part of the time. Fallacy is almost inevitable in such a case if inferences as to causation are sought from individual groups of local statistics[2]."

The Infectivity of Certain Forms of Occupational Phthisis.

Let us now turn to the consideration of the alleged low degree of infectiousness shown by the phthisis which is so very common among those whose occupations cause them to inhale large amounts of stone dust, and let us inquire whether there may not be some peculiarity in the type of their disease which would account for a comparatively low infectivity[3].

---

[1] *Public Health*, 1909, XXII, p. 379.   [2] 1914, *loc. cit.* p. xxx.
[3] The mortality from phthisis among occupied males who follow certain trades and occupations may be found in the *Supplement to the 55th Report*

The Relation of Pulmonary Tuberculosis to Silicosis.

The Nature of Dangerous Dusts. It is well known that only certain kinds of dust are liable, when inhaled for long periods, to predispose to pulmonary tuberculosis. The dust caused by blasting or working certain kinds of stones is held to produce this effect, while dust of many other kinds, even when inhaled in enormous quantities, is considered not to do so. Coal-miners get their lungs choked with coal dust, and may even suffer to a certain extent from pulmonary fibrosis, but they are even less liable to die of pulmonary tuberculosis than most men[1]. Ironstone-miners too are exposed to dust, and yet enjoy a comparative immunity from this disease[2], while those employed in Portland cement works do not suffer more than the average males of Great Britain of like age, although their occupation is an exceedingly dusty one[3].

of the Registrar General, Part II, p. clxi. The deviation from the normal in each case must not entirely be attributed to the nature of the occupation in question, since certain occupations attract the strong and others the weak. Thus hotel servants come at the very top of the list with the highest mortality from phthisis. This may be not only because the work is indoors, and those employed in it are liable to be injured by drink, but because the work, being light, attracts those whose health prevents them from taking up more strenuous occupations, and thus the trade gets an undue proportion of those already tuberculous. Conversely the coal-miners of Derbyshire and Nottingham, who come, with clergymen, at the bottom of the list, probably owe some of their immunity to the fact that their occupation is not one for weaklings. But selection of this kind will not explain the high mortality from phthisis among the grinders of Sheffield, who, as Scurfield has pointed out, are by no means weaklings, but above the average in physique. And the same, one would suppose, is true also of the tin-miners of Cornwall. The fact that tin-miners and lead-miners on the one hand present such an extraordinary contrast in their liability to die of phthisis to coal-miners and ironstone-miners on the other, shows as clearly as possible that in many cases the nature of the occupation itself is the preponderating cause.

　　[1] See footnote 4 on p. 88.

　　[2] Haldane, Martin and Thomas, speaking of the tin-miners of Cornwall, state that the death-rate among machine men from respiratory diseases was about 30 times as great as that among colliers or ironstone-miners of the same age. (*loc. cit.* p. 14.)

　　[3] See Collis, *loc. cit.* Lime indeed has even been supposed by some to protect those who inhale it against infection with the tubercle bacillus (see W. J. Burns, Selkirk, "Tuberculosis in Lime workers," *Brit. Med. Journ.* 1908) and coal dust, and even coal smoke, have been credited with protective or curative properties,

It has always been recognized that the dust which is liable to predispose to pulmonary tuberculosis is that which comes from hard stones, which split, when broken, into sharp angular fragments. Masons and quarrymen are said to regard sandstones as dangerous, while limestones they look upon as harmless (Collis). The worst kind of stone is probably flint, which has so disastrous an effect upon the knappers of Brandon, and on many of those engaged in the pottery trade. Buhr-stone, which is built up into millstones in France, and largely used, until recently, in this country, has a bad reputation[1], as also has ganister, employed for making a fire-resisting material for lining crucibles, etc. Millstone grit and other hard stones (not including emery) used for making grindstones are little better (Collis).

It is commonly believed that the kinds of stone dusts which predispose to pulmonary tuberculosis owe their dangerous qualities to their mechanical properties, and act either as inoculating needles, making punctures which admit tubercle bacilli, or else by means of their sharp corners causing a constant irritation which leads eventually to the replacement of the normal lung tissue in the neighbourhood of the particles by fibrous tissue, upon which the tubercle bacillus gets subsequently implanted.

I am unable to find the reference but I well remember that the Chairman of the old underground railway in London, before it was electrified, once remarked at a meeting of shareholders, that the stations of Portland Road and Gower Street which, as everybody knows, are entirely below the surface of the ground, and which were formerly notorious for their mephitic vapours, were regarded by the management as particularly favourable places for consumptives, and as a matter of fact, he said, they were in the habit of transferring to these places any of their servants who showed signs of incipient phthisis.

Sulphur too has been credited with the power of preventing or curing pulmonary tuberculosis, especially in Italy. Some observations of Prof. Carozzi, of Milan, and of Dr Alfonso Giordano on the alleged immunity of the sulphur workers in Sicily are referred to in an Annotation in the *Lancet* of Oct. 18, 1913, p. 1134, and a letter from R. C. Hutchinson on the popular belief in the curative powers of sulphur will be found in the same volume (p. 1439).

[1] Millers formerly suffered greatly from phthisis in the days when old fashioned millstones were in universal use and the millers were frequently obliged to redress their stones, being greatly exposed to dust while doing so. That the flour dust was not responsible for the mischief is shown by the fact that miller's phthisis has almost disappeared since modern steel rollers have replaced the old stones (Collis).

It is tempting to embrace the inoculating-needle hypothesis, and to believe that the sharp particles predispose to tuberculous infection, by causing minute apertures in the bronchial mucous membrane through which the bacilli may easily penetrate, just as wounds of the skin open the door to pyogenic and other infections.   The mucous membranes, from this point of view, are part of the external covering of the body. They are freely exposed to bacteria, and doubtless have, when intact, good powers of resisting their penetration.   One recalls an old experiment which Pasteur made in the early days of bacteriology.   Attempting to prove that the spores of *B. anthracis*, when given with food, were capable of causing anthrax in the sheep, he at first met with ill success.   But when the animals were given along with the spores some hay which was full of the prickles of dried thistles, he found no difficulty in thus communicating the disease[1].   Typhoid fever has been thought by some to predispose to tuberculosis, and it is well known that measles and influenza do so.   It is possible that these diseases act in this way by causing little focal lesions in the mucous membranes, through which tubercle bacilli gain a ready entrance into the living tissues of the body.

But against the view that the inhalation of stone dust predisposes to tuberculosis in this manner, is the fact that the majority of miners, grinders, masons and others, who suffer from the effects of dust, do not generally develop their peculiar form of phthisis until they have been exposed for several years at least to the conditions of their dangerous occupation. And there is good reason to think that in such cases true tuberculosis only begins after pulmonary fibrosis has become well established.   This is the opinion of some of those best able to judge (Haldane, Oliver, Andrews).   We must therefore either believe that the tubercle bacillus remains a long time latent in such cases, or else conclude that infection takes place, as a rule, long after the patient has commenced to be exposed to the constant prickings of the sharp particles.

Dr Collis, H.M. Medical Inspector of Factories, indeed, thinks that it is not to its mechanical properties at all that

---

[1] *Life of Pasteur*, by Vallery Radot.   English translation, p. 264.

stone dust owes its dangerous quality, but rather to its chemical nature, and he has come to the conclusion that it is dangerous in proportion to the amount of silica it contains, and that it is silica, or some derivative of silica, which is the dangerous element[1].

The Low Degree of Infectiousness shown by that form of Phthisis which is common among persons whose work compels them to Inhale the Dust of Hard Silicious Stones.

It is probably true that the high death-rate from " phthisis " which occurs among the grinders and ganister-workers of Sheffield, the stone-workers of Grinshill and elsewhere, the flint-knappers of Brandon and the tin-miners of Cornwall is not accompanied by a correspondingly high death-rate from this cause among their women-folk and children. This, as we shall see, was the opinion of many of those best able to form an opinion, and there is no good reason to doubt its accuracy.

Wheatley (1911) tells us that in the parishes of Clive and Grinshill of Shropshire where there are quarries, half the stone-workers die of phthisis, yet there is no excess of phthisis among women and young persons in the parish. He investigated the 59 deaths from tuberculous diseases which had taken place there during the last 30 years, and found only five instances in which two or more relatives were affected. He adds " considering that 50 per cent. of the deaths of stoneworkers were from phthisis, the number of families with more than one death from this cause does not appear more than one would expect apart from home infection, and there appears to be no grounds for thinking that home infection or family susceptibility has played any considerable part in the causation of the disease[2]."

Haldane, Martin and Thomas, 1904, in their Report on the Health of Cornish Miners, say very little about the infectivity of the phthisis from which these men suffer so

[1] " The Effect of Dust in Producing Diseases of the Lungs." Paper read at the International Medical Congress, London, 1913.

[2] *loc. cit.* p. 13.

severely. They merely remark that " as there is no hospital in Cornwall where cases of miner's phthisis are treated, so that all the affected men remain in their homes, it is evident that they must tend to spread tubercular infection in the community. To what extent there is evidence of such spread (they say) we have not inquired. The very low death-rate from lung diseases among Cornish miners under the age of 25, seems, however, to exclude the idea that tubercular infection in the families of miners has been widespread hitherto[1]."

Collis (1913) inquired into the tuberculosis which causes the death of nearly 78 per cent. of the flint-knappers in the little community in Brandon, where this interesting and dangerous occupation is still carried on. He speaks of " the immunity from phthisis of the wives and widows of the flint-knappers," and adds that " during the last 25 years only one child of a flint-knapper has died from phthisis, and inquiry locally established the facts that (i) although ten flint-workers (males) in one family died from phthisis there are 13 females in the same family alive, and only three males (two flint-workers, and one not a flint-worker) ; (ii) of six males in another family, two out of three who became flint-workers died from phthisis, while the remaining three in other occupations are alive ; and (iii) two out of six brothers in another family became flint-workers, one of whom died of phthisis, while the four in other occupations are alive. I therefore conclude that, as far as this small industry is concerned, exposure to fine dust of pure silica causes an excessive mortality from phthisis, not found in the neighbourhood in which the industry is carried on, nor among the workers' relatives who do not follow the industry[2]."

Now as to the cause of the low degree of infectivity of the form of phthisis caused by stone dust, various opinions have been offered. Wheatley suggests the following reasons.

(1) " Many of the cases returned as phthisis may have been non-tuberculous lithosis.

(2) Those cases in which infection with tubercle intervened may have been of a type with little breaking down of the lung, and consequently little infection given off.

---

[1] *loc. cit.* p. 20.   [2] *loc. cit* p. 23.

(3)   The home conditions and general surroundings may be unfavourable to the spread of consumption.

(4)   Consumption under fairly good conditions may have even a much less degree of infection than is generally supposed[1]."

Collis (1913) appears to suggest that tubercle bacilli after growing in lungs which have been modified by silica dust become less virulent[2]. This seems very improbable. Do tubercle bacilli learn to assimilate silica when grown in its presence, and become unable to flourish afterwards without it? It may be so; but, on the other hand, there seems to be a simpler explanation, for there is reason to suppose that in this form of phthisis there is a scarcity of bacilli expectorated.

Thus Ritchie[3], when working for a Departmental Committee of the Home Office, examined the sputa of 23 Cornish miners who were suffering from phthisis. In 14 only were tubercle bacilli found by means of microscopic examination. Even when guinea-pigs were inoculated, only 15 out of 21 sputums caused tuberculosis in these highly susceptible animals. Taking the two tests together, tubercle bacilli were proved to exist in 17 out of 23 cases. Dr Tonking[4] of Camborne informed the same committee that he had frequently examined the sputum from cases of phthisis in miners, and had nearly always succeeded in finding tubercle bacilli in advanced cases, although sometimes repeated examination of the sputum was necessary to find the bacilli.

Tubercle bacilli would seem to be remarkably scanty in the sputum of South African gold-miners who suffer from phthisis ; for in a Report of the Committee of the Transvaal Medical Society which studied the disease, it is stated " that out of a series of over thirty sputa from cases of disease

[1] *loc. cit.* p. 13.
[2] " Silica dust then seems to modify the lungs so that they become more liable to disease in general, and specially liable to be invaded by the tubercle bacillus, which bacillus, after growing in such lungs, is less liable to attack normal human beings," *loc. cit.* p. 30.
[3] *Report on the Health of Cornish Miners*, 1904.   Eyre and Spottiswoode, pp. 19, 20.
[4] *Ibid.* p. 20.

of the lung of miners examined by a member of the Committee, only two or three were found to contain tubercle bacilli[1]."

Arlidge states that " In cases of potters consumption from inhaled dust, occurring under my own observation, bacilli have been sought for in vain."

It is, indeed, by no means certain that the " phthisis " which is so frequent a disease among the classes of workmen which we are now considering is always a manifestation of tuberculosis. In its earlier stages at least it is probably not so. But in fatal cases, which alone are relevant to the question which we are now considering, it is commonly held, by those best qualified to form an opinion, that the tubercle bacillus is the cause, at least in the final stages, of the mischief. Thus Ritchie, speaking of the phthisical Cornish miners, says : " Whether there exist certain cases of a true non-tubercular fibroid phthisis, which may ultimately cause death by acute or chronic bronchitis, is a question, but there is no doubt that in the majority of cases...death is due to tubercle[2]." The committee appointed to inquire into the health of Cornish miners themselves concluded that " it seems evident enough that the stone dust which the Cornish miners inhale produces permanent injury of the lungs...and that this injury, while it is apparently capable of gradually producing by itself great impairment of the respiratory function, and indirectly of the general health, also predisposes enormously to tuberculosis of the lungs, so that a large proportion of miners die from tubercular phthisis[3]."

Collis[4], in giving evidence before a Royal Commission, stated that amongst the Sheffield grinders he recognized " a distinct form of cirrhosis of the lung uncomplicated by tubercle."

Wheatley (1911)[5], after reviewing the question, says: " the balance of evidence appears to show that, apart from tuberculous infection, the inhalation of stone dust may produce

[1] Quoted in *The Health of Cornish Miners, loc. cit.* p. 24.
[2] *Ibid.* p. 20.
[3] *Ibid.* p. 21.
[4] Quoted by Wheatley.
[5] " Report on Lung Disease at Grinshill, Quarries," p. 13.

very serious incapacity, and even a fatal result, but whether
the proportion of deaths so resulting is large or small has not
been worked out."

The subject was discussed at the meeting of the British
Medical Association in 1903 by Sir Thomas Oliver and Professor Hamilton. Oliver attributed little importance to
tubercle, in connection with the disease, while Hamilton laid
stress on the tubercular complication[1].

Oliver (1902), in his *Dangerous Trades* (p. 272), when discussing the types of lung disease produced by dusty occupations, says : " the affected workman is regarded as the victim
of consumption, but the disease is not necessarily *tuberculous.*
Under these circumstances, where a lung has become altered
in structure, and its vital resistance diminished, it becomes
an easy matter for true tuberculosis, as the result of its specific
bacillus, to become grafted on to a pneumokoniosis, or dust
lung disease." This account was probably based largely on
the report of Dr Andrews (1900), on the examination of the
lungs of two ganister-miners who had died of " phthisis[2]."
In writing of the first of these cases Andrews emphasizes the
fact that there was no naked-eye evidence of tubercle ; and
after describing the fibrosis which he attributes directly to
the dust " and is most positively non-tubercular in origin "
he says that he found histological evidence of tuberculosis in
at least one of the seven blocks of tissue which were selected
for microscopic examination. This evidence consisted of " the
presence of small miliary tubercles embedded in the fibrous
tissues, and showing the characteristic structure of tubercles,
with typical giant cells. Even in these no tubercle bacilli
can be demonstrated." The tuberculosis he regarded " as
a recent and accessory phenomenon." One is struck in this description by the very small amount of evidence of tuberculosis,
and wonders whether the " characteristic structure of tubercles "
and the " giant cells " are really to be taken as conclusive

[1] *Brit. Med. Journ.* 1903, II, p. 268. The report of this discussion is
exceedingly brief. The allusion to it quoted above is from Haldane, Martin
and Thomas.

[2] *Ann. Rep. Chief Inspector of Factories and Workshops for* 1900–1901
(Cd. 668), p. 487.

evidence of the work of tubercle bacilli, or whether such structures may not be developed as the response to any sufficiently persistent irritant. A further systematic examination of such lungs accompanied by the inoculation of guinea-pigs is much to be desired.

In the second of Dr Andrews' cases, of which the immediate cause of death appears to have been acute pleurisy and pericarditis, there was extensive fibrosis, and the rest of the lungs were emphysematous. In addition the apex of the right lung was riddled with numerous small smooth-walled cavities. Among these were some small caseous areas of tubercle. The precise nature of these cavities could not be determined. The bronchial glands were not much enlarged, but some were caseating, as if from the presence of chronic tubercular infiltration. No tubercle bacilli were found. " But," Andrews remarks, " the difficulty of demonstrating tubercle bacilli in young tubercles is so great that no surprise need be felt at the fact." Finally he concluded " from an examination of these lungs, that the primary changes are dependent upon the chronic irritation of an inhaled mineral dust, which being absorbed by the lymphatics gave rise to a fibrosis....Upon the fibrosis a secondary tuberculosis has been grafted."

In ganister-miner's " phthisis " the clinical aspect of the case is very different from that of pulmonary tuberculosis. The Chief Inspector of Factories, Dr T. M. Legge, who inquired into this disease in 1900, remarked that the physical development of the affected men was surprisingly good, and conveyed no idea of the extent to which the lungs might be damaged by dust. "In five men" who were incapacitated from work on account of lung disease, " there was wasting, in two great dyspnœa, in one only was there a history of hæmoptysis ; all showed more or less physical signs of tubercular phthisis on auscultation. The typical condition noted in fibroid phthisis, no night sweats, no hæmoptysis, and no temperature, distinguishing it from tubercular phthisis has, however, been frequently observed by the medical practitioners of the district."

The special character of the pulmonary disease induced by

dust was noticed also by Arlidge (1892), who remarks that
" It must be accepted as a fact that dust induces a malady
bearing a strong similitude to tuberculous phthisis, and yet
that the malady is *not* tubercular in its actual nature."

Tatham (1897), too, referring to another variety of this
disease, said " It is certain that much of the so-called ' potter's
phthisis ' ought properly to be designated non-tubercular
cirrhosis of the lung[1]."

Again, Arlidge[2], referring to Cornish miners, says: " The
startling proportion in which phthisis figures as the cause of
mortality cannot be accepted as entirely correct ; for in this
class of workers especially, the returns made of the causes of
death are seriously vitiated by the popular nosology, which...
assigns the majority of deaths of miners to consumption, a
term which, in the hands of registrars, will often be transformed
into phthisis ; whereas in a true pathology the fatal lesion
should be entered as pulmonary cirrhosis or fibrosis."

The Committee of the Transvaal Medical Society, already
referred to, speaking of the phthisis so frequent in the miners
of that country, came to the conclusion " that while in some
cases a true tubercular phthisis may co-exist, or may be super-
added, the conjunction is only seen in a minority of cases,"
and they recognized " the pure fibroid non-tubercular type " as
" the commonest and most characteristic form of the disease."

Dr Summons stated that only 47 per cent. of miner's
phthisis amongst the workers in the gold mines of Bendigo
is tuberculous[3].

After reviewing the evidence summarized above, one must
still regard it as an open question how far the excessive
mortality from " phthisis " and other forms of pulmonary
disease which undoubtedly exists among those who are exposed
to certain kinds of stone dust is caused by the tubercle bacillus.
But whatever view one takes on this question there seems
good reason to think that in such cases tubercle bacilli are

---

[1] *Suppl. 55th Ann. Rep. Reg. Gen.* Pt. II, p. xcvii.
[2] *loc. cit.* p. 289.
[3] Quoted by Wheatley, *loc. cit.* p. 12.

not as a rule present in anything like the numbers which are found in ordinary cases of pulmonary tuberculosis.

If then a certain proportion of cases of grinder's, miner's, potter's, knapper's phthisis and the like are not tuberculous, and if in those which are, as there is reason to think, tubercle bacilli are scanty, an easy explanation is afforded of the absence of evidence of transmission of infection from the men so affected to their wives and children.

It is possible that tuberculous grinders, etc. give off sufficient bacilli to infect a certain proportion of their fellow workmen, whose lungs are especially disposed, by the nature of their occupation, to the attack of these parasites, but not sufficient, as a rule, to infect their wives and children (living under normal or, as Scurfield suggests, under specially favourable conditions) to an extent greater than is the case among other persons of similar age and sex in England and Wales as a whole.

The Prevention of Tuberculosis. The Relative Value of Measures based upon Treatment and those which Aim more directly at Limiting the Spread of Infection.

To return to the question of contagion, let us briefly summarize the argument set out in the preceding pages. We have tried to show that the difficulties are not insuperable of accepting the view that tuberculosis is not merely an infectious but a contagious disease; and by this is meant that the tubercle bacilli which cause the really serious forms of the disease are acquired, as a rule, in the close proximity of a phthisical patient, and not picked up at a distance, as for example in the street.

The objection, often raised against this theory on the ground that nearly everybody suffers, either consciously or unconsciously, from tuberculosis at some time or another, and that therefore the serious forms of the disease can have nothing to do with opportunities for contracting infection, since these must be so common, has been met by the experimental demonstration of the great influence on the severity of the disease exerted by differences in the numbers of infecting bacilli ; for it is obvious that large numbers of tubercle bacilli are more liable to be taken in the near neighbourhood of one who is disseminating them than at a distance from all the sources of infection.

The alleged scarcity of evidence of direct personal infection in individual cases has been accounted for partly on the ground that much of the evidence which exists is of the nature of family infection, and, being in accordance with preconceived ideas as to the importance of the part played by inheritable predisposition, is misinterpreted ; and partly by the fact that the disease is often very slow in developing so that the time when infection took place is liable to be misjudged, or the circumstances forgotten.

The argument based upon the comparative rarity of infection spreading from husband to wife, or vice versa, has been met partly by showing that such infection is, probably, much more common than can be accounted for by mere chance, and partly by evidence that in adult life susceptibility is not nearly so great as in infancy and adolescence.

Finally the small degree of infectiousness shown by that form of phthisis which is so common a cause of death in men whose occupations cause them to inhale continually certain kinds of stone dust has been attributed to the relatively small numbers of bacilli in the sputum of those who suffer from this form of the disease, and to the fact that some of them, very possibly, die of pulmonary fibrosis uncomplicated by tubercle.

Defence of the doctrine that opportunities for acquiring massive infection play a dominant part in the graver forms of tuberculosis has occupied the greater part of the section dealing with the causation of tuberculosis. This has been necessary because that doctrine has been so strongly opposed by many high authorities.

Far less has been said about the influence of differences in the resisting power of individuals, not because its importance is held to be small, but because, being admitted by all, it needs no defence.

The two main conditions, then, necessary for the causation

of tuberculosis are opportunity for acquiring the bacilli in numbers, and weakness in the powers of resisting their further invasion and multiplication. To these two factors, which for brevity may be spoken of as Seed and Soil, different observers will attach different relative values.

But while pathologists, in which term we include those who study the nature of diseases by any method whatever, differ as to the relative importance of seed or soil, there is another and more practical aspect of the question, namely, which of these two indispensable factors is the easier to control? This is a most important question, for, as Newsholme has justly pointed out, the available amount of energy and money which can be applied to the extermination of tuberculosis is not unlimited, and so much of it as is spent on measures which are less likely to yield results than others must be considered, to some extent, to be wasted. It is therefore highly important to know what kind of measures have yielded the best results in the past, and can be trusted to be fruitful in the future.

The methods available for stamping out tuberculosis may be grouped under four heads, according to the general principle involved :

I. The removal of predisposing causes which lower the individual's powers of resisting infection, such as poverty, ignorance, and dirt, bad housing, poor feeding, the specific fevers and insanitary conditions generally.

II. The removal, or prevention, of sources of infection by rapid cure, especially of early cases.

III. The removal of the more dangerous sources of infection by segregation.

IV. The eradication of bovine tuberculosis.

The first of these methods is the one which has been mainly relied upon in the past. And, it must be confessed, it has been used with conspicuous success; tuberculosis has diminished greatly; but something more is needed if tuberculosis is to be blotted out. The predisposing causes of tuberculosis, be their relative importance as compared with opportunities for infection what they may, are not easily controlled. And the movement directed towards abolishing that hydra, which, under the general term "insanitary conditions predisposing to tuberculosis," includes poverty, ignorance and dirt, bad housing, poor feeding and the existence of the specific fevers, will, though it continues to progress in the future, as it has in the past, with ever increasing momentum, require unceasing efforts for many years before it has reduced the mortality from tuberculosis to small dimensions; and eradication, by such means alone, will only be accomplished at the advent of the millenium.

But more amenable to control than the predisposing conditions are the exciting causes of tuberculosis. It is easier to restrict opportunities for infection, especially opportunities for infection with large numbers of bacilli, which we have reason to think are the most really dangerous, than to cure poverty. This aspect of the case was well put by Broadbent (1905). "With regard to poverty and all the conditions pertaining to it," he said, " to deal with that is an enormous question. To attain the ameliorations that are required for the general elevation of the lower classes, for the general improvement of their surroundings, and also in their disposition and morality —all this is a too gigantic task. No one would wish public attention to be drawn from it, but it will demand a long time and enormous cost would be involved. But here is a factor " (referring to segregation which Newsholme had just been advocating) " which can be dealt with much more effectually and at far less expenditure : the disease may be intercepted at its source by the isolation of advanced cases, and the prevention of the production and dissemination of the infective material. This is a much simpler task[1]."

Newsholme also made some remarks to the same effect : " If the control of tuberculosis must await the general perfection of sanitary conditions, including the economic and moral circumstances which form an essential part of them, no reasonable limit could be put to the time which must elapse before tuberculosis disappears[2]." No one denies that the great achievements in sanitation which have been made in the past have

---

[1] *Trans. Epidemiol. Soc.* xxv, p. 118.
[2] *The Prevention of Tuberculosis*, p. 211.

been extraordinarily successful in preventing disease, and have
been largely responsible for the decline of tuberculosis. No
one desires that the efforts which are being made in this
direction should be slackened; for, even if it could be shown
that there are other and better methods of preventing tuberculosis, they are abundantly justified by their other results. By
all means allow them to go on unabated, and let them continue
in the future to exercise the beneficial influence on tuberculosis
which they have done in the past.

But tuberculosis in spite of its decline still claims an
enormous number of victims, many of them in the prime of
life, and the time has come to consider whether a more direct
attack may not profitably be made on this most potent cause
of premature death. Up to the present moment efforts to dry
up the sources of infection by the segregation of those who are
excreting bacilli have not been deliberately made. But, as
Newsholme has shown, a good deal of segregation of consumptives has been effected already, not indeed with the direct
object of preventing infection, but in the ordinary operation
of the poor law; and he came to the conclusion, after exhaustive
inquiry, that this had been one of the principal causes of the
decline of the disease. "Institutional segregation," he said,
"notably of advanced cases, is the most powerful single means
available for controlling phthisis[1]."

Koch, in his Nobel Lecture in 1906, strongly advocated
segregation of advanced cases. His opinion on this point was,
he said, strongly supported by the behaviour of tuberculosis
in Stockholm, where a large proportion of the cases of phthisis
are cared for in hospital and where the death-rate from this
cause had gone down by 38 per cent.[2]

The importance attached by each student of the problem
to segregation as a means of eradicating tuberculosis will, of
course, depend on the view which he takes of the part played
by contagion in the spread of the disease. It is precisely
because they held that tuberculosis is not contagious that so
many of the greatest authorities on the subject have opposed
the policy of segregation. Bulstrode (1903) who made a most

[1] *Trans. Epidemiol. Soc.* xxv, p. 111.   [2] *Lancet*, 1906, 1, p. 1449.

careful study of the problem in his well known Milroy Lectures strongly maintained that the disease was not contagious, and pointed out that it had been rapidly dying out in England in the entire absence of any direct control, and in the presence of a belief in its non-communicability, and he advocated reliance upon general measures, among which he selected as the most hopeful, and in the following order: (1) the education of older children in hygiene, together with the physical examination of all children with a view to improving the health of those prone to tuberculosis, (2) compulsory insurance against sickness and invalidity, making for the provision of sanatoria, the support of those threatened with illness, and the general well-being of the poorer classes, and (3) improved measures of general sanitation. The recommendation of means for controlling the spread of infection is pointedly omitted[1].

Ransome too opposed segregation on the ground that it was unnecessary. " No attempt at isolation has been made in this country," he wrote in 1896, " and yet the disease is gradually disappearing." The true remedies, according to him, are free ventilation, good drainage, sunshine and abundance of good food and clothing.

But it cannot be doubted that segregation, if it were possible to carry it out on any complete scale, would be effective. It is hardly necessary to point out that if all persons infected with tubercle bacilli were to be entirely removed from the community there would be no more tuberculosis, except such as is of bovine origin. So much would be granted doubtless, but the objection would at once be raised that it could not be done. That no doubt is true under present conditions, and the question perhaps is not so much whether segregation is right in principle, but whether so much segregation as might be effected is worth having at the cost of the expense and disturbance of domestic relationships which it would cause.

But there is good authority for thinking that partial segregation would be effective very much in proportion to the extent to which it was carried out. Koch, in his Nobel Lecture already referred to, has called attention to what partial isolation

[1] *Lancet*, 1903, II, p. 442.

of infected cases has accomplished in the case of leprosy in Norway. " There they have not isolated all the lepers, but only a fraction of them, including however just the most dangerous ; and the result has been that the number of lepers, which in 1856 still amounted to nearly 3000, has now gone down to about 150. This is the example," he said, " to be followed in the combating of tuberculosis, and if all cases of pulmonary tuberculosis cannot be provided for, at least as many as possible, including the most dangerous, *i.e.* those in the last stage of the disease, ought to be lodged in hospital." Newsholme also, in *The Prevention of Tuberculosis* (p. 265), has referred to the example of leprosy in Norway, where, he says, the disease has been rapidly disappearing in consequence of a system of segregation " at no time amounting to a total segregation of all known cases " and " almost entirely without compulsion."

It seems not improbable that the attitude assumed by many persons towards the question of the contagiousness of consumption has been influenced, perhaps unconsciously, by a dread of inflicting additional hardship on those who already have plenty of trouble to bear in that they have been struck down by an incapacitating and probably fatal disease. It is so natural to feel sympathy with the sufferer whom we see, so difficult to do justice to those who, as yet unhurt, need to be protected. But which is the greater evil : that the present generation of consumptives should suffer additional hardships, or that an unending succession of persons as yet in sound health, or still unborn, should be struck down in turn ? It cannot be doubted what answer would be given by any sound minded person who really believed that a reasonable measure of segregation was likely to help materially to rid the world of this incubus.

It is said that anything like a general adoption of a policy of segregation would increase the alarm already felt at the presence of phthisical persons. The writer hears that the working classes are beginning to recognize the danger of associating in their occupations with consumptive fellow-workers. The men may say : "we don't so much care for

ourselves ; as to that we would take the risk ; but we have
to consider our wives and children." And so the consumptive
workman may be driven from his occupation a few months
earlier than he otherwise would have been by ill-health
alone, and he and his family may be reduced to penury. Be
it so! It is for the good of the community. The authorities
must see to it that the men so driven out in the interest of
public health, are assisted out of public funds. In some
cases even workshops might be instituted where the consumptive workmen could be segregated and continue to work at
their occupation without risk to their fellows. It is necessary
that public opinion, goaded by fear of infection, should bring
pressure to bear on Public Authorities before any general
policy of segregation can be adopted. Until then there is every
prospect that all available funds will be spent on attempts
at cure rather than prevention.

Too much has been, and still is, expected from measures
based on treatment. It may be doubted whether sanatoria
have contributed much to the stamping out of the disease,
successful though they have been in patching up cases, and
in prolonging life ; for they have, thereby, prolonged the
period of infectivity of many of the cases they have benefited.
Admitting that some patients have been cured outright, and that
others have received rudimentary notions of sanitary discipline,
is not this advantage more than counterbalanced by the number
of those who would otherwise have quickly died, but who,
through the help of the sanatoria, have continued to live for
years to be a danger to their neighbours, just as the husband
in one of Weber's cases referred to in an earlier chapter, who
though believing himself to have been cured, infected four
wives in succession with fatal tuberculosis, and himself succumbed to the disease in the end ?

Sanatoria, then, take away with one hand what they give
with the other. The remedy is to be looked for, not in attempting
to cure, but in trying to prevent. Segregation of dangerous cases
must somehow be effected. Compulsion should be avoided.
The writer is inclined to think that public opinion should
be encouraged to look upon consumption as contagious, and

that provision for segregation and relief should go hand in hand with the progress of public opinion in this direction, and so meet half way the hardships which would otherwise arise.

The principle of segregation, he ventures to suggest, should be adopted as a policy, but it is not necessary to segregate every case of consumption, nor in the present state of public opinion would that be possible. All that it seems practicable to do at present is to augment as far as possible the segregation now going on in hospitals and infirmaries by means of the provision of (*a*) industrial colonies for those who are still able to do some work; and (*b*) for those who are not, homes, under a not too rigid supervision, and imposing a minimal amount of restraint. Much might be done without using compulsion, if no effort were spared to make such homes and colonies attractive. For it is not so much in the ranks of the rich and prosperous who live in large houses that any organized system of segregation is desirable, but among the poor whose conditions of life are most favourable to the spread of infection ; and especially among those of the lowest strata of society, in which, in consequence of ignorance, overcrowding and filthy habits, it were a miracle if any child living with a phthisical patient escaped infection[1]. It is during the later stages of illness when the patient is expectorating large numbers of tubercle bacilli, and his frequent cough is repeatedly spraying them into the air, when, rendered helpless by his increasing weakness, he is gradually relinquishing one by one the ideas of decency which he once possessed, when, possibly, poverty caused by the incapacitating of the bread-winner has led to overcrowding, so that, perhaps, several children are sharing the same bed as the sufferer—it is under such circumstances that the disease is most contagious and the need for segregation most urgent. Fortunately it is under such circumstances also that it is least unacceptable.

Segregation is no doubt often desirable at a much earlier stage, and this will probably be more difficult to secure in the present state of public opinion. The prospect of cure may be

---

[1] For the relative incidence of tuberculosis among rich and poor see Newsholme, *The Prevention of Tuberculosis*, Chaps. XXXI and XXXII.

expected to prove an inducement to persons in this stage to enter institutions under medical supervision. It will be more difficult to keep them there. Compulsion, we have ventured to insist, except in very exceptional cases, must be renounced. The people must be behind the movement, or it cannot succeed. But probably public enlightenment on the question will proceed quite as fast as accommodation can be provided.

The Stamping out of Bovine Tuberculosis.

As for the eradication of bovine tuberculosis, that is a perfectly practicable matter, but one which would probably involve enormous expense. The question before the authorities is How far is it desirable to go in this direction? As we shall see later on, it is difficult to form an estimate of the number of human lives claimed by this form of the disease. Possibly it differs greatly in different places ; and there are those who would have us believe that it is extraordinarily great in Edinburgh. If this is so then the suppression of bovine tuberculosis should be attempted locally, in the worst centres, and gradually extended as experience is gained. To attempt to abolish bovine tuberculosis at a stroke would be a mistake. It would cost so much money as to cripple all efforts in other directions. It would stir up bitter enmity against sanitary legislation in general, and perhaps after all we should lose as much as we should gain, for who can say whether the frequent swallowing of bovine tubercle bacilli in numbers too small to cause grave infection in ordinary people does not exert a widespread influence in protecting the people against more serious infection from other sources? At present at all events it would seem wise to leave the mixed milk of the large dairy much as it is, trusting intelligent inspection for removing such cows as have obvious disease of the udder, and concentrating attention upon the small herds and single cows, with the aim of preventing milk rich in tubercle bacilli from being consumed undiluted, or only slightly diluted, with the milk of normal animals.

As to the condemnation of the carcases of infected animals the present state of practice is absurd. If an animal has

" generalized " tuberculosis its flesh is condemned, although it is almost certainly free from tubercle bacilli, is not given to infants (that is to say to persons at the age most susceptible of infection with tubercle) and is never consumed raw. On the other hand, the law allows enormous quantities of milk full of tubercle bacilli, and which is consumed uncooked, to be sold and given to babies. Could anything be more illogical? The money now wasted on the confiscation of tuberculous carcases might with advantage be devoted to the inspection and testing of dairy cattle. But the public is shocked to think of the flesh of obviously diseased animals being eaten, even though it can be shown to be harmless, while it contemplates with equanimity the consumption of milk full of tubercle bacilli, because its appearance is not repulsive.

REFERENCES. III

(Chapters v, vi, and vii)

Allbutt, Sir T. Clifford (1902). *Trans. Brit. Cong. on Tuberculosis,* London.

Andrews (1901). A Case of Ganister Miner's Disease. *Ann. Rep. Chief Inspector of Factories,* Cd. 668, p. 487.

Arlidge (1902). *The Hygiene, Disease, and Mortality of Occupations.* Percival & Co., London.

Baumgarten (1909). *Deutsch. med. Wochenschr.* p. 1729.

Behring (1903). *Deutsch. med. Wochenschr.* p. 689.

—— (1903). *Lancet,* II, p. 1199.

Broadbent (1896). *Proc. Med. Chir. Soc. London.* N.S. vol. III, p. 27.

—— (1905). See discussion at end of Newsholme's paper. *Tr. Epidem. Soc.* vol. XXV, p. 117.

Bulstrode (1903). The Milroy Lectures. *Lancet,* II, pp. 73, 206, 297, 361 and 437.

—— (1908). On Sanatoria for Consumption, and certain other Aspects of the Tuberculosis Question. *Supplement to the 35th Ann. Rep. Loc. Govt. Board for* 1905–6.

Burckhardt (1906). Ueber Häufigkeit und Ursache menschlicher Tuberkulose. *Zeitsch. f. Hygiene,* vol. LIII, p. 139.

Calmette, Guérin and Deléarde (1906). Origine intestinale des Adénopathies trachéo-bronchiques tuberculoses. *Acad. de Scien.* May, 1906.

Chalmers, A. K. (1913). A Page in the Natural History of Pulmonary Tuberculosis. *Public Health,* vol. XXVII, p. 36.

Cobbett (1907).   Report on the Influence of Individual Susceptibility and Dose on the Severity of Experimental Infection
by Tubercle Bacilli.   *R.C.T. 2 Int. Rep.* App. vol. III,
p. 247.
Collis (1913).   The Effect of Dust in Producing Disease of the Lung.
Henry Frowde.   Oxford Univ.   Press.   xvIIIth *Internat. Med.
Cong. London.*
Eastwood and Griffith, F. (1914).   *Reports to the Local Government Board
on Public Health and Medical Subjects.*   N.S. No. 88.
Emmanuel, J. E. (1909).   On the Spread of Tuberculosis, Heredity
or Infection.   *Lancet,* I, p. 1369.
Esslemont, J. E. (1913).   Tuberculosis : Its Eradication.   *Medical
World,* p. 8.
Fowler, Kingston (1896).   On Latency in Tuberculosis.   *Proc. Roy.
Med. Chir. Soc. London.*   N.S. vol. III, p. 27.
Goodale (1906).   An Examination of the Throat in Chronic Systemic
Infections.   *Boston Med. and Surg. Journ.* Nov. 1906.
Griffith, A. S. (1911).   *R.C.T. Fin. Rep.* App. vol. I, p. 18, "seven cases
which did not produce tuberculosis in guinea-pigs."
——— (1914).   *Reports to the Local Government Board on Public Health
and Medical Subjects.*   N.S. No. 88.
Haldane, Martin and Thomas (1904).   *The Health of Cornish Miners.
Rep. to Sec. of State.*   Eyre and Spottiswoode, London.
Hamilton (1903).   *Brit. Med. Journ.* II, p. 268.
Harbitz (1905).   *Untersuchungen über die Häufigkeit, Lokalization,
und Ausbreitungsweise der Tuberkulose,* Christiania.
Hay, Matthew (1909).   Notes on Tuberculosis in Aberdeen.   *Ann.
Rep. of Med. Off. of Health of City.*
Heller (1902).   Kleine Beiträge zur Tuberkulosefrage.   *Münch. med.
Wochenschr.* p. 1003.
Ipsen (1906).   Untersuchungen über primäre Tuberkulose im Verdau-
ungskanal.   *Berl. klin. Wochenschr.* No. 24.
Kälble (1899).   Untersuchungen über die Keimheit normaler Bron-
chialdrüsen Nichttuberkulose.   *Münch. med. Wochenschr.* p. 622.
Koch, R. (1884).   The Etiology of Tuberculosis.   *Microparasites and
Disease.*   New Syd. Soc.
——— (1906).   The Nobel Lecture.   How the Fight against Tuber-
culosis Now Stands.   *Lancet,* I, p. 1449.
Latham, A. and Garland (1911).   *The Conquest of Consumption.*
Fisher Unwin, London.
Legge, T. M. (1901).   *Ann. Rep. H.M. Chief Inspector of Factories
for* 1900.   Eyre and Spottiswoode.   (See p. 484.)
Macfadyen and MacConkey (1903).   An Experimental Examination of
Mesenteric Glands, Tonsils and Adenoids.   *Brit. Med. Journ.* II,
p. 129.
Moore, B. (1911)   *The Dawn of the Health Age.*   J. and A. Churchill,
London.

Naegeli, O. (1900). Ueber Häufigkeit, Localization und Ausheilung der Tuberkulose. *Virchow's Archiv*, vol. 160, p. 426.

Newsholme, A. (1905–6). The Relative Importance of the Constituent Factors involved in the Control of Pulmonary Tuberculosis. *Trans. Epidemiol. Soc.* vol. xxv, p. 31.

—— (1906). An Inquiry into the Principal Causes of the Reduction of the Death-Rate from Phthisis during the last 40 years with special Reference to the Segregation of Phthisical Patients in General Institutions. *Journ. of Hygiene*, vol. vi.

—— (1908). *The Prevention of Tuberculosis.* Methuen and Co.

Oliver, Prof. Sir T. (1908). *Dangerous Trades.* John Murray, London.

—— (1903). *Brit. Med. Journ.* ii, p. 268.

Orth. Quoted by Rabinowitsch, 1907.

Pasteur. *Life*, by Vallery Radot.

Pearson, Prof. K. (1907). A First Study of the Statistics of Pulmonary Tuberculosis. *Drapers' Comp. Research Memoirs.* Dulau and Co. London.

Pizzini (1892). Tuberkelbazillen in den Lymphdrüsen Nichttuberkulose. *Zeitsch. f. klin. Med.* vol. xxi.

Pope, E. G. and Pearson, Prof. K. (1908). A Second Study of the Statistics of Pulmonary Tuberculosis. Marital Infection. *Drapers' Comp. Research Memoirs.* Dulau and Co. London.

Rabinowitsch, Lydia (1907). Zur Frage latenter Tuberkelbazillen. *Berl. klin. Wochenschr.* Jan. p. 35.

Ransome, A. (1896). Tuberculosis and Leprosy. *Lancet*, ii, p. 16.

—— (1897). Researches on Tuberculosis. The Weber-Parkes Prize Essay.

—— (1904–5). Phthisis Rates. *Trans. Epidemiol. Soc.* vol. xxiv, p. 259.

Report of the Medical Officer of the Local Government Board, 1914. *Supplement to 42nd Annual Report.*

Report of the Transvaal Medical Society. Quoted by Haldane, Martin and Thomas.

Ritchie (1904). See Haldane, Martin and Thomas, p. 19.

Rosenberger (1905). A Study of the Mesenteric Glands in Relation to Tuberculosis. *Journ. of American Sciences.*

Scurfield (1912). Tuberculosis in the British Isles. (Report prepared for the International Tuberculosis Congress at Rome.) *Public Health*, June, 1912.

—— (1909). Notification of Tuberculosis of the Lung in Sheffield, and the Incidence of Tuberculosis in Males, Females, and Children in Various Towns. *Brit. Med. Journ.* 1909, ii, p. 462.

—— (1909). *Public Health*, vol. xxii, p. 378.

—— (1909). Lung Diseases among Sheffield Grinders. *Journ. of the Roy. Sanit. Inst.* vol. xxx, p. 458, and *Public Health*, vol. xxiii, 1910, p. 113.

Stewart, Prof. C. Hunter (1911). The Sex and Age Incidence of Mortality from Pulmonary Tuberculosis in Scotland, etc. *Proc. Roy. Soc. Edinburgh*, vol. xxxi, Part iii, No. 22, p. 352.

Tatham (1897). *Supplement to the 55th Annual Report of the Registrar General for England and Wales*, Part II, p. xcvii.

Tonking. Quoted by Haldane, Martin and Thomas.

Weber (1906). Die Infection des Menschen mit den Tuberkelbazillen des Rindes. *Deutsch. med. Wochenschr.* No. 49, p. 1982.

Weber and Baginsky (1907). Untersuchungen über das Vorkommen von Tuberkelbazillen in Drüsen und Tonsillen von Kindern welche sich bei der Obduction als frei von Tuberkulose erwiesen hatten. *Tub. Arbeit. a. d. Kaiserl. Gesundheitsamte*, Heft 7, p. 102.

Weichselbaum and Bartel (1905). Zur Frage der Latenz der Tuberkulose. *Wien. klin. Wochenschr.* No. 10, p. 241.

Wheatley (1911). Report on the Prevalence of Lung Disease amongst the workers at Grinshill Quarries. *Report to the Public Health and Housing Committee.*

Williams, Theodore (1882). The Contagion of Phthisis. *Brit. Med. Journ.* II, p. 619.

—— (1909). The Infection of Consumption. *Ibid.* II, p. 433.

CHAPTER VIII

PORTALS OF ENTRY OF TUBERCLE BACILLI.
PRE-NATAL INFECTION

That the seeds of tuberculosis may be acquired before birth, either through the ovum or spermatozoon, or by trans-placental infection, was at one time widely believed; but at the present time this view finds little favour. Yet the possibility of such infection must not be dismissed too summarily; for it is probable that the opinions of to-day are founded partly on conceptions which are slowly changing; and among these one must count the possibility of latency of tuberculous infection, a conception which, if accepted, is bound to influence our views concerning pre-natal infection, and which, as we have seen, appears to be gaining ground.

Infection of the Ovum. Pre-natal Infection in Birds. The evidence concerning the possibility of infection of the ovum is, as is natural, derived mainly from the study of birds. It has long been suspected that tuberculosis in domestic fowls is commonly transmitted through the egg; but this, as we shall see reason to think, is probably a mistake. Infection through the egg is certainly not the usual way in which these creatures acquire tuberculosis; for there can be no doubt now that the disease, in the main, is a feeding infection. The possibility of infection through the egg has, indeed, been proved experimentally, but this is a very different thing from showing that this mode of infection occurs commonly under natural conditions.

The idea that congenital infection with tubercle is common in birds has, very likely, been fostered by the fact that the most important tuberculous lesions found in domestic fowls usually occur in the liver. If this be so the line of reasoning is unsound, for it has been shown conclusively that the most conspicuous lesions which commonly arise as the result of experimental feeding with tubercle bacilli also are in this situation.

It is certainly against the view that avian tuberculosis is commonly congenital that the disease is relatively rare in young birds. M. Koch and Lydia Rabinowitsch, 1907, who examined a large number of birds of different species which died in the Zoological Gardens in Berlin, reported that they found no example of the disease in very young birds; and in the writer's own poultry yard, where about half-a-dozen cases of tuberculosis have occurred among the older fowls in the last few years, no disease has been seen in the young chickens killed for the table. These facts can be made to fit in with the theory of congenital transmission only on the assumption that the germs acquired by the egg may remain latent in the bird for many months.

Baumgarten and also Pfander[1], in 1892, rejected the view which is now generally held, that tuberculous infection in the domestic fowl commonly occurs through the alimentary canal. They pointed out that the bird does not emit any sputum. Tubercle bacilli, they (erroneously) maintained, cannot as a rule be found in the excreta. They could find no ulcers in the intestine[2]; and since it had been shown that fowls could not be infected by feeding them on tuberculous sputum there seemed to be no other possibility but that the disease was hereditary[3]. This reasoning is now known to be false; but it probably

---

[1] Quoted by Koch and Rabinowitsch, *loc. cit.* p. 268.

[2] Ulcers are not uncommon (see p. 532).

[3] Weber and Bofinger, *loc. cit.* p. 99.

lay at the root of many of the opinions held on this subject twenty-five years ago. For until the clear distinction between the different types of tubercle bacilli had come to light, and the impossibility of infecting the birds commonly used in laboratory experiments with the human type of bacillus had been discovered, the universal failure of the numerous attempts to infect fowls by feeding them with the expectoration of consumptives naturally carried much weight, and led to erroneous conclusions.

On the other hand we shall see that tubercle bacilli, when artificially injected into eggs, remain alive (though they do not thrive there) and that a few successful experiments have been made in which tuberculous chickens were produced from artificially infected eggs. The experiments of Baumgarten, Maffucci, Gärtner and, more recently, those of M. Koch and Lydia Rabinowitsch and of Weber and Bofinger have established the *possibility* of this way of infection.

Among the first to attempt to cause tuberculosis in birds by artificially infecting their eggs was Maffucci, 1889. He observed that the disease made no progress whatever in the chick so long as the latter was in the egg ; the tissues of the embryo appearing to be resistant to the growth of the bacillus. Indeed, in the egg the bacteria did not seem to multiply at all ; but, on the contrary, soon lost their characteristic form, and were converted into little coccoid bodies.

Several other observers have noticed the peculiar resistance of living eggs to the growth of tubercle bacilli[1]. Koch and Rabinowitsch, 1907, could find no tubercle bacilli, as such, in eggs which they had previously inoculated, but they saw, here and there, little rounded bodies, stainable by carbol-fuchsin, which may have been the coccoid forms described by Maffucci.

Weber and Bofinger also noticed the resistance of the avian embryo to tuberculous infection. Having inoculated hens' eggs with avian tubercle bacilli, they removed the embryos twenty-six days later and having emulsified them, made injections into mice. The mice developed tuberculosis, indeed,

---

[1] Egg substance, however, when suitably diluted and coagulated by heat forms an excellent medium for tubercle bacilli of all types.

showing that the bacilli were present in some form or another, but the microbes could not be seen in microscopic preparations of the embryo livers.

Tubercle bacilli then may remain alive in the egg, though they do not develop there ; they seem to be changed in form and to remain latent. After the chickens are hatched the bacilli may again become active and cause tuberculous disease, and this happened in several of Maffucci's experiments.

The results which Maffucci obtained from chickens which hatched out of artificially infected eggs were as follows : in one chick which died shortly after it was hatched and in another which succumbed when 42 days old no tuberculous lesions were found ; in two killed when respectively 20 and 32 days old only microscopic tubercles were seen in the liver ; in two others killed when 40 and 47 days old microscopic lesions were seen in liver and lungs ; the first tubercles visible to the naked eye were seen in chickens killed when 78 days and $4\frac{1}{2}$ months old (Koch and Rabinowitsch, *loc. cit.* p. 421).

Baumgarten obtained the following results : from 12 eggs which he had infected with avian bacilli two chicks were hatched out, and these, when killed 4 and $4\frac{1}{2}$ months later, showed tuberculous lesions in the spleen and liver but not in the intestine (Koch and Rabinowitsch, *loc. cit.* p. 422).

Koch and Rabinowitsch (*loc. cit.* p. 426) infected hens' eggs and ducks' eggs with various kinds of tubercle bacilli. The microbes were introduced into the white in doses of 1 mg., contained in as small a volume of fluid as possible. From 12 fertile eggs infected with avian bacilli only one chick came out alive. It did not appear to differ at first in any way from normal chicks just hatched, but it grew very little and died of tuberculosis after 75 days. From ten fertile eggs infected with human tubercle bacilli, one chicken and two ducklings were born. They grew quite normally, and when killed about four months afterwards showed no trace of tuberculosis. From seven eggs infected with bovine bacilli four chicks hatched out. All these showed, when killed some months later, some traces of tuberculosis.

These experiments go but a little way towards proving the existence of hereditary transmission of tuberculosis. They show, indeed, that tubercle bacilli do not get destroyed in the egg, and may persist to cause disease after birth, but they do not prove that these bacilli ever, under natural conditions, get into the egg in sufficient numbers to produce this effect. Gärtner's[1] experiments go a little further, and show that tubercle bacilli may, under experimental conditions, pass from

---

[1] Experiments with hens failed Of nine eggs obtained from canaries infected intraperitoneally two produced tuberculosis when injected into guinea-pigs ; and, in a second series of experiments, out of 24 eggs obtained from these birds after they had been infected by intraperitoneal injection two produced tuberculosis in guinea-pigs. (Koch and Rabinowitsch, *loc. cit.* p. 422.)

the hen to the egg ; for he has demonstrated the presence of
tubercle bacilli in the eggs of canaries which had been
infected artificially by intraperitoneal injection of human
tubercle bacilli. Koch and Rabinowitsch[1] state that they
have seen on several occasions tubercle bacilli in the egg
within the ovary and that too when there was neither severe
disease of the ovary itself or tuberculosis of the peritoneum ;
and F. Griffith[2] has found tubercle bacilli in the dried up yolk
of an egg found in the oviduct of a fowl infected 254 days
previously with avian tuberculous material injected subcutaneously. In this bird the ovary itself was tuberculous.

These latter experiments though they distinctly increase the
probability of hereditary transmission of tuberculosis in the bird,
are far from proving that this is the common way of infection.
Koch and Rabinowitsch clearly recognize this, and state that
they believe that this mode of transmission is quite insignificant as compared with infection through feeding[3].

The majority of writers on this subject also, including
Weber and Bofinger, agree that " tuberculosis in the bird is in
the main a feeding infection[4]."

*Transmission of Infection from the Male Parent to the Ovum,
in Man.* No one, so far as the writer is aware, has ever seen
tubercle bacilli within spermatozoa. That tubercle bacilli may
be present in the semen from tuberculous testes is however
true ; for its injection into animals has produced tuberculosis.
Calmette, 1913, after mentioning this fact, says that clinical
observers are aware that it is a somewhat rare occurrence

---

[1] *Virchow's Archiv*, Beiheft zum Band 190, p. 313.
[2] *R.C.T. Final Rep.* 1911, vol. IV, p. 220 (Fowl 250).
[3] The possibility of hereditary transmission they admit, but what part it
plays in nature they do not venture to estimate. In the Zoological Gardens
in Berlin at least (from which the numerous tuberculous birds which they
examined were obtained) it plays, they say, as good as none (*loc. cit.* p. 487.
See also pp. 310, 313).
[4] Weber and Bofinger regard the hereditary transmission of tuberculosis
in the bird as a rare occurrence, and scarcely of practical importance as compared with infection through food contaminated with bacilli contained in the
droppings of tuberculous birds. They themselves found bacilli in the excreta
of fowls as Mohler and Washbourn had done before them. F. Griffith found
no difficulty in infecting birds by feeding them with food containing avian
tubercle bacilli.

for infection to be transmitted by this means from husband to wife. He can, moreover, affirm that in certain families the children born of a healthy mother and a father suffering from tuberculosis of the epididymis have remained unaffected. One may search in vain, he adds, in the literature for observations proving the infection of the ovum from a paternal urogenital tuberculosis ; and he concludes as follows : " Nous sommes donc fondés à admettre *qu'il n'existe pas de fait positif établissant qu'un enfant puisse être procréé tuberculeux par son père* " (*loc. cit.* p. 2).

Pre-natal Infection in the Ox and other Animals. Congenital tuberculosis is believed to be rare in the ox. In 1894, at the International Congress for Hygiene and Demography held at Budapest, Prof. Bang of Copenhagen, in bringing forward a scheme for combating tuberculosis in cattle, said : " Congenital tuberculosis in the calf is a rare occurrence, and is only to be apprehended when the cow has very wide-spread tuberculosis, and especially when the uterus is affected. The immense majority of tuberculous cows bear healthy calves, and these would remain healthy if protected from infection[1]." The collected experience of the *abattoirs* shows that tuberculosis is relatively seldom seen in the calf ; as an example Bang cites the experience gained at the small slaughter-house in Aarhus, where the observations were very carefully made, and where bovine tuberculosis was very rife. In the year 1903, out of 6765 calves which were slaughtered and examined there, 100 (or 1·48 per cent.) were tuberculous. Among these were 14 new-born calves, in which the disease was obviously congenital. On the other hand, of the adult cattle 51 per cent. were tuberculous.

In the experience of the present writer tuberculosis, visible to the naked eye, has never been seen in guinea-pigs or rabbits born of tuberculous dams, though very many such animals, killed soon after birth or taken from the uterus, have been examined by him[2].

---

[1] " Bekämpfung der Tuberkulose der Haustiere." *International Veterinary Congress in Budapest,* 1905.

[2] Wilson Fox reported a case of inherited tuberculosis in the guinea-pig ; but the animal was not killed until it was eight months old, and the evidence of inheritance does not seem quite conclusive (see *Trans. Path. Soc. Lond.* 1869, p. 442).

The writer's very limited experience of congenital tuberculosis in the ox is possibly quite exceptional[1], and since it concerns three calves only, and these born of cows which had not contracted tuberculosis naturally, but which had been infected experimentally, the experience must not be taken as representative, and considerable caution is necessary in drawing any conclusion from it. But since it is not without interest, a brief account will be given.

In the experimental station of the Royal Commission on Tuberculosis at Blythwood Farm six calves were born of heifers which some time before had been artificially infected with tuberculosis, five by subcutaneous and one by intramammary injection. No less than three of the calves were born tuberculous. In every one of the three heifers which bore a tuberculous calf the uterus was the seat of tuberculous changes. In none of them was there general tuberculosis. Two had extensive and advanced tuberculosis of the lungs of the *perlsucht* type, and the third had tuberculosis of the mammary gland, as well as of the uterus, but there was no tuberculosis elsewhere, except a lesion at the seat of injection and a few little retrogressive foci in the prescapular gland of the same side and in the thoracic glands. The heifers were inoculated when pregnant, and gave birth to their calves 5, 6 and 4 months respectively after subcutaneous inoculation[2].

The first of these calves was killed 26 days after birth. It was found to have caseous patches in the portal lymphatic glands, and a suspicious focus in the lungs. An emulsion of a portion of the lung, and also one made from a part of the apparently normal liver, caused tuberculosis in guinea-pigs into which they were injected. A tuberculin test made on the day of its birth showed that this calf was tuberculous at that early stage of its existence; for it then gave a slight but definite reaction (rise of $1\cdot1°$ C. to $39\cdot9°$ C.). Twelve days later it was again tested and gave a good reaction (rise $= 1\cdot8°$); and a week after this, tested a third time, it gave another good reaction (rise $= 1\cdot8°$);

[1] *R.C.T. Int. Rep.* 1907, vol. III, p. 261. Report on Congenital Tuberculosis at Blythwood Farm.

[2] Of the three heifers which gave birth to *healthy* calves, two had been injected with very small quantities of tubercle bacilli, namely one and two millions respectively, one of them received an intramammary, the other a subcutaneous injection. The third heifer was injected subcutaneously with 53 million bacilli. None of these animals had anything more than minimal and retrogressive lesions when they came to be killed.

and after another three days it received a fourth injection and gave a reaction (rise = 1°). (A chart illustrating these reactions may be seen in a supplementary volume to the Report of the Royal Commission, dealing with Tuberculin Tests, 1913; see calf 327, p. 107.)

The second calf was killed when five days old. A few tubercles were found in its portal lymphatic glands.

The third calf was killed when six days old. In its portal lymphatic glands numerous early caseating foci were found, and there were a few early tubercles in the lungs, liver, spleen and kidneys, and in the thoracic and lumbar glands.

These instances of congenital tuberculosis in the ox must not, as we have said before, be accepted as representative without considerable reserve, and for the following reason. The mothers had all been injected subcutaneously, and with quantities of bacilli estimated at 4½, 157, and 2800 million bacilli respectively. Now it has been shown that when tubercle bacilli are injected in large quantities (50 mg.) into calves and other animals some of them get carried in a few days, or perhaps hours, all over the body; they have been found wherever they were looked for; not in the great organs only and in the lymphatic glands, but in the bone marrow, the blood, and even, in small numbers, in skeletal muscle[1]. Unfortunately it did not occur to us at the time to see whether they reached the uterus, but it can scarcely be doubted that they did so. Now it is unlikely that anything like this general distribution commonly occurs in natural infections, which must be determined by far smaller numbers of bacilli; and therefore it seems only reasonable to expect that tubercle bacilli would reach the uterus after subcutaneous injection more readily and in larger numbers than occurs in cases of natural infection.

But while for this reason the fact that three calves, out of six born of tuberculous cows in the experimental stations of the Royal Commission, had congenital tuberculosis cannot be accepted as in any way representative of what occurs under natural conditions; another fact which was brought to light by these investigations is not without significance in this connection. This is the enormous difference in susceptibility of the pregnant and the virgin uterus. The latter, like the skeletal

[1] R.C.T. Int. Rep. vol. III, pp. 219 and 235. Reports on the Dissemination of Tubercle Bacilli after Subcutaneous Injection. See also App. I, p. 472 of this volume.

muscles, is very insusceptible to tuberculosis; several hundred heifer calves, many of them suffering from the most acute and generalized forms of experimental tuberculosis, were examined for the Royal Commission without in a single instance tuberculosis being seen in the uterus, although this was always looked for. On the other hand among six cows similarly infected, and examined after calving, three were found with tuberculosis of this organ.   There can therefore be scarcely any doubt that the uterus of the cow, when pregnant, is far more liable to tuberculosis than the virgin uterus of the calf.   Now if a similar increase of susceptibility occurs in the human uterus during pregnancy the possibility of congenital tuberculosis in man would not seem to be so remote as it is often supposed to be.

Pre-natal Infection in Man.   The view that human tuberculosis is commonly due to inherited infection—at one time very widely accepted, and vigorously upheld by Baumgarten in comparatively recent times—has few advocates at the present day.   Possibly the pendulum has swung too far in the other direction, and the opinion now generally held is too extreme; for cases of congenital tuberculosis in man certainly do occur, though demonstrable instances may be rare; and if we are prepared to believe that tuberculosis may remain latent for long periods before developing into evident disease, pre-natal infection may be more frequent than is generally supposed.

The mortality from tuberculosis, as we have seen, is higher in infancy than at any other time of life, and falls with special severity on children aged from six months to two years; a period when congenital infection, if it occurs, might be expected to bear most of its fruit (see p. 5).

On the other hand such evidence as can be collected from post-mortem records does not support the view that congenital tuberculosis is common.   Naegeli, 1900, examined the bodies of twelve new-born infants without finding tuberculosis in any.

Ungermann, 1912, examined very carefully the glands of 14 children under two months of age who died from various causes.   The most delicate method of detecting living tubercle bacilli in these organs, namely the injection of emulsions into guinea-pigs, was employed, and yet no trace of tuberculosis was found.

Gaffky, 1907, who made a similar investigation on a larger scale found on one occasion tubercle bacilli in the mesenteric glands of a child who died of atrophy when one day old.

Macfadyen and MacConkey, 1903, also reported a similar case, in which injection of the mesenteric glands of a still-born infant into guinea-pigs caused tuberculosis. In neither this nor in Gaffky's case are any particulars given about the parents.

Such instances are not sufficient to be of great value, neither is the negative evidence enough to carry much weight. What is wanted to settle definitely the question of congenital tuberculosis is a systematic investigation (by injection of guinea-pigs) of the glands and organs, particularly the portal glands and the liver, of still-born children of tuberculous parents. Such an investigation has hitherto not been made on any sufficient scale, doubtless on account of the difficulty of collecting the material. But the difficulty ought not to prove insurmountable, especially if the investigation were to be taken up by some well-organized authoritative body which could obtain the co-operation of the maternity departments of several of our large hospitals.

Post-mortem Evidence bearing on the Question of Congenital Tuberculosis. The Age at which Infection commonly occurs. So far as post-mortem evidence can tell us, infection seems to occur after birth, mainly during the early period of infancy and during adolescence. Thus Naegeli, 1900, as we have seen, found no tuberculosis in 12 newly-born infants, nor did he find any in 16 children who died under one year of age. From this point the proportion of children which showed more or less evidence of tuberculous infection rose rapidly; from one to five years the proportion found in his investigations to be infected was 17 per cent.; about the 14th year 50 per cent.; and at 18 there was a sudden rise to 96 per cent.

Ganghofner of Prag has recorded as follows the result of 1800 autopsies on children dying in that city from causes other than tuberculosis, and presenting no clinical symptoms of that disease.

Age	Number	Proportion with tuberculous lesions
0–1	460	7·1 per cent.
1–2	536	16·0 ,,
2–4	476	24·5 ,,
4–6	271	26·9 ,,
6–8	123	26·8 ,,

Ungermann[1] quotes the following additional investigations. Sehlbach among 1157 bodies of children under one year found tuberculosis in 7·8 per cent. The percentages of those found with lesions in the different quarters of the first year of life were as follows: 1–3 months, 2·1 per cent.; 4–6 months, 10·8 per cent.; 7–12 months, 19·4 per cent.

Hamburger found the following proportion affected in the early months of life: 1–3 months, 4 per cent.; 4–6 months, 18 per cent.; 7–12 months, 23 per cent. In the second year of life the proportion of those infected rose to 40 per cent. and in the third and fourth years to 60 per cent. Albrecht found among 3213 children whose bodies were examined after death, 14·6 per cent. tuberculous in the first year, 44·3 tuberculous in the second to sixth year, and 50·1 per cent. in the sixth to twelfth year.

Ungermann himself made a very careful search for tubercle bacilli in the lymphatic glands of 171 young children who had died from various causes, using the method of guinea-pig inoculation. Even by this means he could find, as we have seen, no evidence of tuberculous infection in children (14 in number) up to two months of age; but in those aged from two to six months, 10 per cent. were found to be infected, and of those who died in the second half of the first year, 23 per cent. were found to be harbouring tubercle bacilli.

The frequency with which tubercle bacilli were found by Ungermann in the different periods of early life will be seen in the following table:

Ungermann.

Age	Number examined	Percentage in which tubercle bacilli were found
0–1 month	5	0
1–2 months	9	0
2–6 ,,	38	10·5
6–12 ,,	39	23·1
1–2 years	24	37·5
2–3 ,,	11	38·2
3–5 ,,	} 42	33·3
5–10 ,,		23·8
10–13 ,,	3	33·3
Total	171	22·8

[1] 1912, p. 118.

The material, obtained from a general hospital, was entirely unselected. In 39 cases, tubercle bacilli were proved to be present. In 29 tuberculosis was either the sole cause of death or a severe complication of some other disease. In ten the tuberculous infection was of slight severity, and in four of these no anatomical changes could be found, although the glands when injected produced tuberculosis in guinea-pigs.

Eastwood and F. Griffith, 1914, and A. S. Griffith, 1914, made independent investigations for the Local Government Board of the glands and organs of 195 unselected children, aged from two to ten years, dying from all causes in general hospitals. The combined results of these investigations show the following proportion of tuberculous infection at different ages[1].

Age	Number infected	Percentage infected	
2–3 years	20 out of 47	43	51
3–4 ,,	23 ,, 35	66	
4–5 ,,	18 ,, 32	56	58
5–6 ,,	18 ,, 30	60	
6–7 ,,	19 ,, 20	95	
7–8 ,,	4 ,, 7	57	77
8–9 ,,	6 ,, 10	60	
9–10 ,,	10 ,, 14	71	

The results of all these researches are gathered together in the following table :

	Months			Years				
	0—3	—6	—12	—2	—3	—4	—6	—12
Naegeli	0			17				50
Ganghofner		7·1		16	24·5		26·9	26·8
Sehlbach	2·1	10·8	19·4					
Hamburger	4	18	23	40	60			
Albrecht		14		44·3			50·1	
Ungermann	0	10·5	23	37·5	38·2	33·3	23·8	33·3
Eastwood, F. Griffith and A. S. Griffith				43	66	58	77	

[1] *loc. cit.* p. 1. Prefatory Note by the Medical Officer of the Board.

It will be seen that there is a good deal of discrepancy between the figures given by different authors ; those of the English investigators being particularly high. This is not completely explained by the fact that eight of A. S. Griffith's cases came from institutions where tuberculous cases alone were investigated, because Eastwood and F. Griffith found an even higher proportion of infections than did A. S. Griffith. Probably the results depend more on the principles governing the admissions to the hospitals. While the results of different observers do not entirely agree with one another as to the general frequency of tuberculous disease, they all concur in showing that the *relative* frequency of infection is low in the first few months of life and increases very rapidly during the first few years. And there seems no reason to hesitate to conclude from this that very few children are born with tuberculous lesions in their bodies, and that infection, if acquired before birth, remains, in the great majority of cases, latent.

Many cases of alleged, or probable, congenital tuberculosis have been recorded from time to time, but only such as have been thoroughly investigated by modern methods can, at the present day, be accepted as evidence. Auché and Chambrelent, 1899, could only find records of 20 which satisfied their requirements ; and they concluded that transmission of tuberculosis from mother to fœtus through the placenta is rarely observed. When it is transmitted in this way, they say, the placenta itself is always tuberculous. It is curious that among the 20 cases which they collected there were no less than 12 in which there were no tuberculous lesions, either macroscopic or microscopic, in the fœtus, the evidence of transmission of tubercle bacilli resting solely on the results of infecting guinea-pigs with blood from the umbilical vein, or with portions of one or other of the fœtal organs. This fact, at first sight, seems to support Baumgarten's view that fœtal tissues do not permit of the growth of the bacillus and the development of lesions at this stage, and that it is only at a later period that disease becomes evident. But we must remember that this kind of evidence has in the past led to erroneous conclusions[1]. The remaining eight cases showed definite lesions, and in these, with one exception, tubercle bacilli were very numerous, showing, as Auché and Chambrelent point out, that human fœtal tissues are not unfavourable to their development.

Warthin and Cowie, 1904, submitted the collected evidence of the existence of congenital tuberculosis to a searching investigation, and contributed several cases which they had themselves observed. They assumed a cautious attitude towards this question, but concluded " that the dictum, accepted by most writers at the time, that intra-uterine transmission is possible but extremely rare, needs to be supported by further research before it can be taken as final."

These authors remarked that the cases of supposed congenital tuberculosis reported from time to time have been collected by several writers, among them being Gärtner, Hauser, D'Arrigo and Cornet, a more or less complete list being given by each author ; but they very justly point out that many of the cases regarded as undoubted examples of congenital tuberculosis have been accepted as such on insufficient grounds. For this reason they submitted all the known cases to a rigorous examination, admitting as undoubted only those which showed characteristic anatomical changes and tubercle bacilli, and in which the lesions were found within so short a period after birth as to exclude the possibility of post-natal infection, and those in which congenital syphilis could be excluded.

In 1904 they could only find five cases recorded which fulfilled their requirements, and to these they themselves added one other. But they pointed out that among the cases, 37 in number, which they had to exclude as failing to satisfy their rigorous standard of certainty, were, very probably, a certain number of instances of congenital tuberculosis. They also found eight cases of placental tuberculosis which they admit into this category without reservation, and to these they added another of their own; and they admitted twelve cases in which tubercle bacilli were proved to be present in the placenta and in the fœtus, but without histological changes.

[1] See footnote, p. 51.

Among the conclusions arrived at in this paper is the following : " the fœtal blood may contain great numbers of tubercle bacilli without changes, other than small agglutination thrombi, being seen. Inoculation shows these bacilli to retain their virulence. From this it may be assumed that the fœtal tissues are relatively immune to the action of the tubercle bacillus. Granting such an immunity it is possible that tubercle bacilli may be present in the fœtus and new-born child without exciting histological changes ; and, developing some time after birth, may then give rise to characteristic tuberculous lesions. A true latent tuberculosis is therefore both possible and probable ; but additional investigations are necessary to settle the question of the frequency of such an event. The commonly accepted dicta regarding congenital tuberculosis are probably extreme. It is not at all unlikely that it is of much more common occurence than is generally supposed."

In 1907 Warthin returned to the subject. He had in the meantime been able to collect another twelve cases of tuberculosis of the placenta from the literature. The rapidity with which the recorded cases had increased, together with the small number of observers who had recorded them, Warthin held to be in favour of the view that congenital tuberculosis is commoner than it is usually believed to be. Two observers, namely Schmorl and Geipel, had actually found nine placentas tuberculous out of sixteen taken from tuberculous mothers.

Conclusion.

There seems no reason to doubt that cases of congenital tuberculosis occur. How frequent they are cannot be determined without further investigation ; but they are probably uncommon. The conclusions which are arrived at concerning the latency of tuberculous infection in general may perhaps modify our opinion concerning the frequency of congenital infection ; and it is possible that Warthin and Cowie may be right when they say that " the commonly accepted dicta regarding congenital tuberculosis are probably extreme." On the other hand infection experiments, so far as they go, seem to show that the presence of tubercle bacilli in the bodies of very young infants is rare. In order to clear up the question more investigations of this kind are needed, especially on the bodies of children of tuberculous parents.

REFERENCES. IV

(Chapter VIII)

Congenital Tuberculosis.

D'Arrigo (1900). *Centralb. f. Bakteriol.* vol. XXVIII, p. 683.

Auché and Chambrelent (1899). De la Transmission à travers le Placenta du Bacille de la Tuberculose. *Archiv. de Méd. expérim. et d'Anatom. pathol.* vol. XI, p. 521.

Bang, Prof. B. (1905). Bekämpfung der Tuberkulose der Haustiere. *7th Internat. Veterin. Cong.*, Budapest.

Baumgarten (1891–2). Ueber experimentelle kongenitale Tuberkulose.

—— (1909). *Deutsch. med. Wochenschr.* vol. II, p. 1729.

—— (1911). *Lehrbuch der pathogenen Micro-organismen,* Leipzig.

Beitzke (1910). *Ergebnisse der Pathologie,* vol. XXIV, p. 169.

Cobbett (1907). Report on Congenital Tuberculosis at Blythwood Farm. *Roy. Com. Tub. Int. Rep.* App. vol. III, p. 261.

Dietrich (1912). Ueber kongenitale Tuberkulose. *Berl. klin. Wochenschr.* p. 877.

Gaffky (1907). Zur Frage der Infectionswege der Tuberkulose. *Tuberculosis,* vol. VI, p. 437. Reference to Congenital Tuberculosis, p. 445.

Ganghofner. Quoted by Bulstrode, 1908, *Supp. to 35th Rep. Loc. Gov. Bd.* p. 106.

Gärtner (1891). Ueber die Erblichkeit der Tuberkulose. *Zeitsch. f. Hygiene,* vol. XIII, p. 101.

—— (1893). *Ibid.* vol. XIII, pp. 101–250.

Hauser (1898). *Deutsch. Archiv. f. klin. Med* vol. LXI, p. 221.

Koch, M. and Rabinowitsch (1907). Die Tuberkulose der Vögel und ihre Beziehung zur Säugetier Tuberculose. *Virchow's Archiv,* Beiheft zum Band 190, p. 246.

Lehmann (1893). *Deutsch. med. Wochenschr.* vol. XIX, p. 200.

Macfadyen and McConkey (1903). *Brit. Med. Journ.* II, p. 129.

Maffucci (1889). Tuberkulöse Infection der Hühner-embryonen. *Centralb. f. Bakteriol. etc.* vol. V, and many other communications for which see Koch and Rabinowitsch.

Naegeli (1900). *Virchow's Archiv,* vol. 160, p. 426.

Nothnagel (1900). *Spec. Pathol. u. Therap.* vol. XIV, 2 Abt.

Novak and Ranzel. Placentar Tuberkulose. *Zeitsch. f. Gynækologie,* vol. LXVII, p. 719.

Pfander (1892). Beitrag zur Histologie der Hühnertuberkulose. *Arbeit. auf den Gebiete der pathol. Anat. und Bakteriol. von Baumgarten,* Bd. 4.

Rietschel (1909). *Jahrb f. Kinderh.* vol. LXX.

Runge (1903). *Archiv. f. Gynækol.* vol. LXVIII, p. 388.

Schmorl and Geipel (1904). *Münch. med. Wochenschr.* vol. I, p. 676.

Sitzenfrey (1909). *Die Lehre von der kongenitalen Tuberkulose.* Berlin, 1909.

Warthin and Cowie (1904). A Contribution to the Casuistry of Placental and Congenital Tuberculosis. *Journ. of Infectious Diseases,* vol. I, p. 140.

Warthin (1907). *Ibid.* vol. IV, p. 347. A Histological Study : with especial Reference to the Nature of the Earliest Lesions produced by the Tubercle Bacillus

Weber and Bofinger (1904). *Tub Arbeit. a. d. Kaiserl. Gesundheitsamte,* Heft I, p. 83.

Westenhoefer (1903). *Deutsch. med. Wochenschr.* vol. XXIX, p. 221.

Wolf (1912). Die Kindertuberkulose und ihre Bekämpfung. *Ref. Münch. med. Wochenschr.* No. 6.

Wollstein (1905). *Archives of Pediatrics,* vol. XXII, p. 321.

For other literature see list at end of next chapter.

CHAPTER IX

PORTALS OF ENTRY (*contd*). POST-NATAL INFECTION

Invasion through the Skin and Respiratory and Alimentary Mucous Membranes. The relative Number of Bacilli which Suffice to Infect in Inhalation and Feeding Experiments. The Body's Three Lines of Defence. Question of the Permeability of the Second Line. The Relative Frequency with which the Various Portals Act as Transmitters of Tubercle Bacilli. Conclusion as to the Probable Portal of Entry in Various Forms of Tuberculosis.

The tubercle bacilli which cause the various kinds of tuber-culosis must, if they enter the body after birth, pass through one or other of its surfaces. And in this connection we must regard as surfaces not the skin only, or indeed principally, but the mucous membranes also which line the cavities and passages which communicate freely with the exterior. Among these the most important are those which line the respiratory passages and the alimentary canal, for they are freely accessible to micro-organisms which come from without.   Possibly one ought to include also among the surfaces liable to be penetrated by bacteria, the surface of the eyeball, and the mucous membranes which line the urinary and genital passages, though to what extent these are actually penetrated, or indeed how far the latter are accessible at all to micro-organisms coming from without, would be difficult to decide.   But even if we grant that in all probability tubercle bacilli may enter through these portals and set up disease, yet the amount of tuberculosis caused in this way must be insignificant as compared with that caused by bacilli which enter through the respiratory or alimentary mucous membranes or through the skin, and we shall therefore be wise if we confine our attention at present to those main frontiers of the body which lie most exposed to the enemy.

Invasion through the Skin.

The skin, as the least important of the three main portals of invasion by tubercle bacilli, may be disposed of first.   The intact skin is, no doubt, capable of being infected by micro-organisms, but it is through wounds, either trivial or severe, that that infection takes place most commonly.   In tuberculosis cases demonstrably due to wound infection certainly occur, but they are comparatively rare, and·usually unimportant.   They are for the most part confined to butchers and pathologists.   It is probable that the disease seldom spreads in such cases to internal organs, though the nearest glands are not unfrequently affected.

Invasion of the intact skin may possibly occur in lupus, but it is more likely that this affection takes place—if indeed it be due to direct infection—in consequence of inoculation of small scratches or abrasions.   There are not wanting those who maintain that lupus is not a primary infection of the skin at all.   It is true, they say, that the fact that lupus is so often limited to the skin, or only involves deeper structures by direct extension, seems at first sight to be in favour of a local origin, but it might equally well be explained as an infection through the blood stream by a particular variety of bacillus specially adapted to live in the skin, or on the assumption of a peculiar susceptibility to tuberculosis in the skins of certain individuals.

The great majority of strains of tubercle bacilli which, in this country at least, have been isolated from cases of lupus, are, as a matter of fact, peculiar in that their virulence for various species of animals is more or less, and often considerably, attenuated[1]; and this peculiarity may of course be correlated with others, such as a special capacity for living in the skin. But whether this peculiarity existed in the strains of bacilli at the time when they invaded the patient's skin, or was acquired afterwards, perhaps as a consequence of living in that environment, is not known.

The fact that tubercle bacilli both of human and bovine type take part in the causation of lupus is perhaps rather against the view that the disease is caused by a specially adapted bacillus, and seems rather in favour of a peculiar weakness in the skin of those who suffer from lupus. Moreover, the fact that many of the strains of tubercle bacilli found in lupus seem, though attenuated, to belong to the bovine type may be held to be rather against the view that this disease is the result of direct infection of the skin ; for bovine bacilli, one would suppose, are more likely to be swallowed than brought into direct contact with the surface of the body.

Lupus is certainly sometimes secondary to tuberculous disease elsewhere, and occurs not rarely as an extension from tuberculous glands in the neck. In such cases it seems almost certain that the bacilli must have entered through the mucous membrane of the mouth or pharynx. On the other hand, in the somewhat uncommon co-existence of pulmonary tuberculosis and lupus in the same individual, it is by no means certain that the two affections have not resulted from independent invasions of tubercle bacilli[2].

---

[1] The careful and extensive work of A. S. Griffith leaves, as we shall see further on (Chap. xxv), no doubt whatever about this point.

[2] A. Latham once communicated a case to the Cambridge Medical Society in which a medical student about to enter for his final examination, and who previously had suffered from pulmonary tuberculosis, developed tuberculous

Post-mortem examinations in cases of lupus are rare. Eastwood and Griffith, 1914 (case 89, *loc. cit.* p. 32), describe the principal organs of a child in whose case there was a history of lupus. Both bronchial and mesenteric glands contained tubercle bacilli and there was miliary tuberculosis of the lung. The authors regarded the origin of the lesions which they examined as probably respiratory. It seems likely that the skin affection had a similar origin ; but no opinion was expressed on this point.

Invasion through the Respiratory and Alimentary Mucous Membranes.

Let us turn now to the mucous membranes which line the respiratory and alimentary tracts, through one or other of which the penetration of the tubercle bacilli which cause the immense majority of cases of tuberculosis undoubtedly occurs.

The question through which of these portals tubercle bacilli most commonly enter the body in numbers sufficient to cause serious disease is not of academic interest only, but is also of great practical importance; for on its solution must depend, in the main, the judgment arrived at as to the relative importance of contaminated air and contaminated food, and consequently the shaping of the preventive measures selected to stamp out the disease. For though the bacilli which enter the body through some part of the alimentary canal, even if it be the intestine, need not necessarily have reached the body in its food (for air-borne bacilli may become arrested in the mouth or pharynx and subsequently swallowed), and though those which enter through the bronchial mucous membrane need not in every case have been carried there by the air (for, as we shall see, there is reason to believe that infective material in food and drink may slip through the glottis oftener than is commonly supposed), yet we shall probably not err greatly if

---

lesions in the skin on various parts of the body, namely face, arms and legs. In this case there may have been opportunity for direct infection of the skin in the post-mortem room ; but the multiplicity of the cutaneous lesions is at least suggestive of a central origin. (See also pp. 616 and 654, footnote 2.)

we assume that, in the great majority of cases of natural tuberculosis, air-borne bacilli enter through the respiratory mucous membrane and food-borne bacilli through that which lines the alimentary canal.

The Portals of Invasion in Pulmonary Tuberculosis. The theories of von Behring and Calmette.

Phthisis, that is to say tuberculosis affecting principally the lungs, is by far the most important variety of tuberculosis in man, accounting in this country for 74 per cent. of all the deaths attributed to the tubercle bacillus[1]. It is concerning the mode of infection in this disease that the most diverse opinions have been held, and controversy has been keenest. Until the last few years phthisis was believed, almost universally, to be caused by tubercle bacilli which entered with the inspired air and produced their lesions wherever they came to rest in the lungs. This view was maintained by Koch in 1884, and strongly reaffirmed by him in 1901. For many years it found almost universal acceptance. Keenly as the rival schools of Cornet and Flügge might dispute as to whether dry and pulverized sputum, or the fluid droplets freshly expelled from the mouths of phthisical patients, played

---

[1] This was the ratio in England and Wales in 1911. Phthisis as now defined by the Registrar General includes acute miliary tuberculosis, previously classed with general tuberculosis. This transference, made to bring our returns into line with International Statistics, only affected 810 cases in 1911, and the total deaths from phthisis amounted to 39,232. Of these, 20,730 were returned as " pulmonary tuberculosis," 15,132 as " phthisis," 2560 as " acute phthisis " or " acute pulmonary tuberculosis," and 810, as we have seen, as "acute miliary tuberculosis." (74th Rep. Reg. Gen. E. and W. 1911, p. lxx.)

The proportion which deaths from phthisis bear to deaths from all kinds of tuberculosis differs greatly in different countries. Thus in Scotland they form only 61·8 per cent. of the total, while in Prussia they form 89·6 per cent. The following figures are taken from a paper on the Tuberculosis Death Rate in Switzerland by Schmidt, in the Report of the 20th International Tuberculosis Congress held in Rome in 1912 (p. 436).

	Phthisis	All other kinds of tuberculosis
England and Wales	70·8 per cent.	29·2 per cent.
Scotland	61·8 ,,	38·2 ,,
Italy	62·1 ,,	37·9 ,,
Prussia	89·6 ,,	10·4 ,,

the more important part in propagating the disease, they were of one accord in believing that the air passages afforded the highway of entrance. So universal at one time was this opinion that Cornet spoke of it as " the common possession of all physicians."

But here and there a voice was raised in protest ; Chauveau indeed, in 1868, long before the discovery of the tubercle bacillus, held that the alimentary canal might be the portal of entry in tuberculosis even more frequently than the air passages ; but for a long time no one of importance seems to have followed him. Woodhead, it is true, drew attention in 1894 to the evidence of intestinal origin in many cases of pulmonary tuberculosis, but this applied mainly to children[1]. But von Behring was the first who uncompromisingly maintained the intestinal origin of pulmonary tuberculosis irrespective of age, in his address at Cassel in 1903. According to him tubercle bacilli received in infancy may pass through the wall of the intestine and through the mesenteric glands and so reach the lungs, without leaving in the abdominal cavity any lesion which might serve to indicate the route by which they have passed. Calmette relates with what disfavour this view was received at the time, and how, when put forward again in the following year at Berlin, it was met with vigorous protests from Fraenkel, Baginsky and other eminent authorities.

[1] Woodhead upheld the view that many cases of phthisis are of abdominal origin. He freely admitted that inhalation accounted for a large number of cases, but as this was not seriously disputed at the time he devoted the greater part of an address given to the N. London Med. and Chirurg. Society to a defence of the doctrine of infection through some part of the alimentary tract. He pointed out the frequency with which pulmonary tuberculosis seems to be secondary to disease of some of the glands of the neck or abdomen, both in the hospital post-mortem room, and in the experimental laboratory. " I have seen," he said, " in case after case in children, and in animals fed on tuberculous material, the lung markedly affected, but in a large proportion of these cases it has been possible to trace the course of invasion back from a caseous or old calcareous mesenteric gland, through the chain of retro-peritoneal glands, up through the diaphragm to the posterior-mediastinal and bronchial glands, and so to the lung. I have seen this not in a few cases only, but in dozens of children, in a few adults, and in many animals." Furthermore, from experiments made on pigs, he considered that tuberculosis might follow an analogous course from the pharyngeal tonsil, through the chain of cervical to the bronchial glands and so to the lungs. *Lancet*, 1894, II, p. 957.

Nevertheless this view gained ground in France, where Vallée of Alfort supported it, following the traditions not only of Chauveau, but of Nocard, his own immediate master, who had long before convinced himself that the normal intestinal mucosa is penetrable by bacteria; and he concluded from his own investigations that ingestion of dust or food infected with tubercle bacilli is the quickest and surest method of pulmonary infection.

Calmette, in 1905, strongly supported the theory of the intestinal origin of phthisis, though he did not agree with Behring in thinking that infection occurs commonly in infancy. On the contrary, he believed that the lymphatic glands are more permeable in the adult than in the child, and consequently that infective germs may pass through them, from the intestines to the lungs by way of the thoracic duct, more readily in the former than in the latter[1]. Calmette's views were based on his own experimental investigations and on those of his pupils. He came to the conclusion that the air passages offer an effective resistance to the entry of bacteria into the lungs, and that of all the methods of communicating the disease, infection by the digestive tract is at once the most efficacious, and the one in closest accord with the conditions of natural infection. He even went so far as to declare that the immense majority of cases of pulmonary tuberculosis in man are caused by the ingestion, and not by the inhalation of tubercle bacilli[2].

This astonishing generalization was supported by Sir William Whitla and Professor Symmers of Belfast (1908) on the grounds of their own experimental researches; and Dr Theodore Williams (1909) and, more recently, Sir Thomas Oliver (1912) have accepted this view. But the majority of observers have not been converted, and many have adversely criticized Calmette's conclusions, and have been unable to confirm his observations.

Von Behring's theory contains three propositions: first, that infection occurs commonly in infancy; second, that it is caused by bacilli which are ingested; and third, that the bacilli themselves come from cow's milk. This last proposition

[1] *Ann. Past.* 1905, p. 618.   [2] *Ibid.* p. 617.

is no longer tenable, since recent discoveries have clearly proved that bovine tubercle bacilli are accountable for only a small part of the total of human tuberculosis. The first seems unlikely to be true of the great majority of cases, though, as we have tried to show in an earlier chapter, latency probably plays a greater part in the etiology of tuberculosis than was at one time supposed. It is the second proposition that more particularly concerns us now, and in respect of this Calmette's views are in agreement with those of Behring.

Calmette's conclusions were based upon the experimental infection of goats and cattle carried out by himself and Guérin, and on the investigations of his pupils, van Steenberghe and Grysez, concerning the origin of pulmonary anthracosis.

The infection experiments were few in number, and the results did not differ, as a rule, from those of other observers. Feeding with tubercle bacilli resulted in almost all his cases in intestinal or mesenteric tuberculosis, and lung disease, when it occurred at all, was in almost all cases secondary and of no great severity.

Calmette himself admits that when *young* goats were experimentally infected with tuberculosis by allowing them to feed, in the natural way, from mothers into whose udders tubercle bacilli had been introduced artificially, lesions always appeared first in the mesenteric glands[1].

Even with adult goats, when fed naturally, no tuberculosis of any kind was induced though enormous quantities of bovine tubercle bacilli were administered between slices of bread[2]. It seems that it was only when the bacilli were introduced by means of an œsophageal tube that any tuberculosis of the lungs without obvious involvement of the mesenteric glands occurred[3].

---

[1] *Ann. Past.* 1905, p. 607.

[2] *Ibid.* p. 612. 20 grammes of fresh bacilli from glycerine-broth cultures were administered to four animals !

[3] Calmette tells us that he used the œsophageal tube in his feeding experiments on cattle, because *he found it difficult* to infect them when they were allowed to swallow the bacilli in the natural way. Under the latter conditions, he says, the bacilli find their way into the rumen where the conditions are unfavourable to them; but if introduced by a tube, the end of which stops short of the rumen, the liquid in which they are suspended escapes the first and second stomachs and falls directly into the third and thence into the

In one goat, however, the pulmonary disease was severe ; and since the experiment on this animal lends more support to Calmette's views than any of the others it deserves to be mentioned in detail. This animal was an adult, two years old. It was fed with bovine tubercle bacilli by means of the œsophageal tube on each of four successive days, receiving each time 50 mg. of fresh tubercle culture finely divided and suspended in 10 c.c. of water. When the animal was killed three months later the lungs were found to be filled with tubercles in all stages of evolution, and there were enormous cavities ; on the other hand the mesenteric glands were normal in size and showed no obvious lesions though microscopic sections revealed small tubercles with calcareous centres[1].

Here then was a case of severe pulmonary disease following an experimental feeding with tubercle bacilli, and one without obvious disease in the mesenteric glands. It is by no means certain, however, that the pulmonary disease in this goat was caused by bacilli absorbed from the intestine. Apart from the possibility that it may have been due to an independent and antecedent infection—a possibility which must always be considered in such cases—there is the chance that it was caused by bacilli aspirated into the trachea.

That such aspiration is by no means an improbable accident in feeding experiments the writer is firmly convinced from evidence which will presently be adduced[2]. Moreover, the use of the œsophageal tube does not avoid this danger, but rather perhaps, as Beitzke has suggested, aggravates it. From his own, possibly clumsy, attempts to feed guinea-pigs and rabbits by means of such a tube, the writer is not inclined to regard it as a satisfactory means of insuring that the infective material goes exactly where one intends it to go[3].

fourth stomach. McFadyean, who has tested this assumption experimentally, says that it is entirely erroneous. When coloured liquids were administered by him in this manner and the animals killed immediately after he generally found that not a drop of liquid had reached the fourth stomach. (See McFadyean, *loc. cit.* 1910, p. 244.)

[1] *loc. cit.* p. 613.   [2] See p. 165.

[3] The principal trouble in the author's experience with the guinea-pig was regurgitation while the tube was in the stomach, and when the mechanism of the glóttis was probably being interfered with.

Sir John McFadyean has criticized this work very severely (*loc. cit.* p. 246). Referring to those experiments in which some tuberculosis of the lung resulted together with lesions in the mesenteric glands, he says, Calmette "must have entirely misunderstood the position of those who maintain that inhalation is the commonest method of natural infection in human and bovine tuberculosis, and have thought it necessary to prove, what no one has ever denied, viz. that an animal infected with tuberculosis by ingestion may, when it is killed or when it dies, be found to have intra-thoracic lesions." This indeed is all that Calmette's experiments prove. No one doubts but that tuberculous infection is sometimes caused by bacilli which have been swallowed, but that phthisis, or tuberculosis which is mainly pulmonary, can be caused in this way his experiments, with the exception of that made on goat 10, already referred to, afford no semblance of evidence. McFadyean sums up his criticism as follows : "Reviewing the whole of these experiments by Calmette and Guérin, one cannot fail to be struck with their absolute inefficiency to prove, or even make probable, the point which the authors are seeking to establish. In reality the experiments were too few in number to justify any very sweeping conclusions, but so far as they go they indicate that the usual result of infection by ingestion is the development of a tuberculosis which primarily involves the mesenteric glands. It is true that some of them showed that when animals are infected by causing them to swallow doses of bacilli, which must be considered enormous as compared with those that are commonly in operation in natural circumstances, the disease may become rapidly generalized, with the result that tubercle bacilli, or even definite tuberculous lesions may be found in the lungs or thoracic glands within a few weeks after the act of infection. But that falls far short of proof that a tuberculosis with well defined macroscopic lesions confined to the thorax can be set up by introducing tubercle bacilli into the alimentary canal."

Experiments designed to show the Channels of Access to the Lungs. Experimental Anthracosis. Part of Calmette's case was, as we have said, based on the experimental production of pigmentation in the lungs of guinea-pigs which had been fed with Chinese ink ; and this must now be considered. The investigations were conducted under Calmette's direction by van Steenberghe and Grysez at Lille, and they have been repeated with almost identical results by Sir William Whitla and Professor Symmers in Belfast.

These observers, when they introduced Chinese ink into the stomachs of adult guinea-pigs by means of the œsophageal tube, found, a few hours later, that the lungs were pigmented, while the mesenteric glands remained free from carbon. None of the observers found pigment in the lungs of young guinea-pigs which had been fed with the ink ; but with regard to the mesenteric glands of animals of this age the results differed, for while van Steenberghe and Grysez found these glands pigmented, Whitla and Symmers say that they remained free from carbon.

None of the observers found it easy to cause pulmonary anthracosis by causing the animals to breathe air ladened with soot from a smoking lamp, unless the dose was excessive ; and they all found that pulmonary anthracosis did not occur under these circumstances if the œsophagus was previously ligatured.

From these experiments it was concluded that anthracosis of the lungs is the result of *swallowing* particles of carbon, and is not caused by particles suspended in the air finding their way *by inhalation* into these organs.

This conclusion is directly opposed to that reached in his well known researches by J. Arnold in 1885, and, since the appearance of the work of the Lille and Belfast schools, many good observers have re-investigated the subject experimentally and have been unable to get results similar to those claimed by Calmette and his followers. Like many others, the present writer made careful experiments in order to satisfy his own curiosity and he found that he was entirely unable to produce any pigmentation, either of lungs or mesenteric glands, by feeding with Indian or Chinese ink, or with soot, though much larger quantities were used than those employed in Lille or Belfast, and the pigment was administered, not once only, but many times, and in some cases daily for one or more weeks[1].

Sometimes, indeed, the writer found, in the older animals, some amount of pigmentation of lungs ; but he was careful to examine a large number of control animals (a precaution which seems to have been omitted by Calmette and the others, for they make no mention of it), and he found just as much pigmentation in them, and just as often, as in those animals which had been fed with carbon.

This then was the case with adult guinea-pigs bred in Cambridge.   Some amount of pulmonary pigmentation was the rule.   In young animals pigment was not seen, whether they had been fed with carbon or not.   It was clear that some amount of pigmentation of lungs was to be reckoned with in the older town-bred animals, and the author remembered that he was accustomed to see a considerable amount of carbonization in the lungs of adult guinea-pigs when he was working in Sheffield.   It was therefore decided to repeat the experiments with country-bred animals ; and when this was done no pulmonary pigmentation was seen in any of the animals, whether they had been made to swallow the ink or not.

Now Lille, like Sheffield, is a manufacturing town, and so is Belfast, and if one finds, not unfrequently, some pigment in the lungs of normal guinea-pigs in Cambridge, shall we not find it also in those of Lille and Belfast ? Yet, as already pointed out, the observers whose work we are considering make no mention of what they found in control animals, indeed they do not seem to have thought it necessary to examine controls.   It is therefore conceivable that the anthracosis which they saw in guinea-pigs which had swallowed Chinese ink was nothing more than the pigmentation natural in animals which had lived for some time in a smoky town. This explanation is in harmony with the fact that Calmette's pupils could produce no pigmentation in the lungs of young animals but only in adults.   Indeed it seems incredible that the "ebony-like blackness" of the lungs described by Whitla and

---

[1] *Journ. of Pathol. and Bact.* 1910, vol. XIV, p. 563.

Symmers could have resulted, as they believed, in a few hours from a single feeding with Chinese ink, unless indeed they had poured the ink into the animals' lungs, for, surely, anthracosis is the result of a chronic process to be measured in years rather than hours ?

One experience, several times repeated, impressed the present writer very much. Guinea-pigs were made to swallow several cubic centimetres of an emulsion of cream and Indian ink. The mixture was black as pitch ; yet, when the animals were killed a few hours later, the lacteals in the mesentery stood out clearly as ivory-white lines, evidently filled with the cream ; and no perceptible portion of ink could be detected in the chyle by microscopic examination, so complete had been the separation effected in the process of absorption (*loc. cit.* p. 586).

Calmette, in supporting his case, denied that air-borne bacteria can readily enter the lungs with the air stream owing to the effective filtering action of the nasal and buccal mucous membranes. But there is abundant evidence to prove that such filtration is very far from being complete even in such nose-breathers as guinea-pigs and rabbits. The author has been for some years investigating the content of bacteria, if any, in the organs of normal animals. In this respect, he finds, the lungs present a marked contrast to other organs in that they invariably yield copious cultures of bacteria, including moulds, streptothrices, spore-bearing bacilli, sarcinæ and cocci. Even the marginal portions of these organs (in the guinea-pig and rabbit) reveal the presence of these micro-organisms. On the other hand, the other great organs, as well as the lungs of *fœtal* guinea-pigs, are either entirely sterile or yield, at most, an occasional, and possibly accidental, colony.

That these bacteria really get into the lungs with the inspired air there can be no doubt. If proof were needed it is afforded by experiments with *B. prodigiosus*. This micro-organism is not found in normal lungs, nor in the air under ordinary circumstances; but if ever so small a quantity be gently sprayed into the air by an " atomiser " and guinea-pigs be allowed to breathe this air, the bacilli penetrate to the furthest parts of the lungs of the animals, as is easily shown by killing them and making cultures from the margins of these organs. In such cultures the characteristic sealing-wax red colonies invariably appear, even though the animals have breathed their last within five minutes of the commencement of exposure to the infected atmosphere, or even when the œsophagus has been previously ligatured (*loc. cit.* p. 588).

Similar results have been obtained by many observers; moreover, several of them, including Findlay, have produced pigmentation of the lungs by causing animals to breathe a soot-laden atmosphere. To produce this result, no doubt, the air has to be densely contaminated with smoke; and even then the distribution of pigment, as pointed out by Calmette, is different from that seen in normal cases of anthracosis. Of course it is! The time factor is so different. In such experiments what time is there for leucocytes to clear away the pigment and store it in the interstices of the tissues and in the lymph glands? The pigment, as is only natural, is mostly in the air cells, and not incorporated with their walls; but the point is that it is in the lungs, that is to say it has passed the alleged barrier of the nasal and buccal mucous membrane.

Calmette's pupils, as we have seen, were entirely unable to produce pulmonary pigmentation by inhalation in an animal whose œsophagus had been ligatured, and they concluded that such pulmonary anthracosis as they were able to cause by this means in animals who had not been subjected to this operation was caused by particles of soot which were swallowed. But one would have thought that the failure to produce pulmonary pigmentation by inhalation in a guinea-pig with the œsophagus ligatured would have been interpreted otherwise by anyone who was familiar with the excessive salivation and consequent respiratory distress which is caused by this operation. The air passages indeed become so choked with fluid that respiration becomes very difficult. Under these circumstances, as we have seen, it is true that *B. prodigiosus* may get into the lungs, and so, presumably, may fine particles of carbon also, but it takes very few bacilli to yield a culture, whereas it requires far larger particles of carbon to become visible, and it is not surprising that the carbon which enters in such experiments is not sufficient to be seen, though *B. prodigiosus* under similar circumstances can readily be demonstrated.

Inhalation and Feeding Experiments with B. tuberculosis. The Relative Number of Bacilli which suffice to Infect by each of these methods. Calmette, and Vallée also, maintain that ingestion is the easiest way to produce pulmonary infection in animals. Almost all other observers who have investigated the question experimentally hold that it is the most difficult. The writer, judging from experience gained when working for the Royal Commission, cannot understand how anyone can hold the former opinion. In some experiments of his made subsequently, guinea-pigs were fed with tubercle bacilli while others were infected by inhalation, and the animals were killed in series after increasing intervals of time, and the march of the bacilli and lesions followed. In those animals which were fed the earliest lesions were found in the cervical glands, and the lungs became affected only when the disease became completely generalized[1]. On the other hand, when the guinea-pigs were infected by inhalation[2], lesions appeared in the lungs first, long before they were seen anywhere else, the mesenteric and ileo-colic glands never became affected, and the cervicals only at a comparatively late stage, when the disease had reached the spleen.

Many observers have made careful experiments with measured doses of bacilli in order to ascertain whether it is easier to infect by inhalation or ingestion. All, without exception, from Flügge downwards, have found that it requires much larger doses to infect when the bacilli are swallowed than when they are inhaled. Thus Gebhardt, 1890, working with diluted sputum, found that 800 bacilli sufficed to infect guinea-pigs when administered with the inhaled air, while 10,000,000 or 20,000,000 failed to do so when swallowed.

Preyss, 1891, who worked in a similar manner, was able to infect guinea-pigs by inhalation with 40 bacilli. Kossel, Weber and Heuss, 1905, working for the Gesundheitsamt in Berlin,

---

[1] *Journ. of Pathol. and Bact.* vol. XIV, 1900, see Table IX, p. 600.
[2] *Ibid.* see Table VII, p. 596.

Plate II

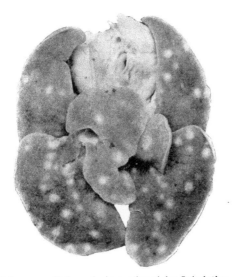

Pulmonary Tuberculosis produced by Inhalation.

Lungs and bronchial glands of a guinea-pig killed 28 days after inhaling
tubercle bacilli (Guinea-pig No. 46, *loc. cit.* p. 596).

found that 1 mg. would infect calves by inhalation while 1000 times this dose given by feeding produced little more than minimal lesions[1]. More recently, Weber and Titze, 1910, have shown that it requires at least 10 mg. of bacilli to infect a calf by feeding, while $\frac{1}{100}$ mg. will infect by inhalation. Reichenbach, 1909, found that he could infect goats with $\frac{1}{100}$ mg. by inhalation, while 500 times this amount by ingestion only produced minimal lesions. Findel, 1907, has been able to infect dogs by inhalation with doses down to 0·14 mg., while feeding with doses up to 63 mg. produced no effect whatever. In numerous and very careful experiments with guinea-pigs he found that 62 bacilli would certainly infect by inhalation, 20 sufficing in some cases, and in very young animals even 5 bacilli, while, on the other hand, doses up to 20,000 given by feeding failed to infect. Findel's results with guinea-pigs have been controlled and confirmed by Pfeiffer and Friedberghe; and Laffert has shown that it requires comparatively large doses of tubercle bacilli to infect these animals by feeding. Without wishing to insist on the strict accuracy of the numbers quoted above, which from the necessity of the case must be estimates only, it is abundantly clear that inhalation is a much more certain method of infection than ingestion, in a number of animal species including the ox, goat, dog and guinea-pig, and it presumably is so in man also. We must therefore hold that Calmette and his followers have failed to make out their case. The old theory of the origin of phthisis then would seem to be unshaken, and indeed to have emerged greatly supported by results obtained experimentally in consequence of the attacks which in recent years have been made upon it.

The Three Lines of Defence of the Animal Body.

It will be admitted, probably by everybody, that the interior parts of the body (and in this expression one does not include the lining of the hollow viscera which communicate freely with the exterior, but all living tissues other than the skin and mucous membranes) are guarded against invasion by

---

[1] *Tub. Arbeit. a. d. kaiserl. Gesundheitsamte,* Heft 3, p. 20 (calf 18) and p. 40. Compare also calf 14, p. 26.

bacteria by means of lymphatic glands and other aggregations of lymphoid tissue. Following Prof. Adami[1] one may regard this lymphoid tissue as arranged in two lines of defence; the one situated at the front, so to speak, that is to say in the mucous membrane itself, close to the frontier to be defended; and the other at a greater distance, aggregated into groups of glands, each group receiving the lymph from a definite territory. There is doubtless also a third line of defence constituted by the phagocytic leucocytes of the blood and the endothelium of certain of the capillaries.

It is, no doubt, not very easy to see how the lymphoid tissue of the first line performs the function of arresting bacteria that penetrate the surface near which it is situated, for it is not spread out as a continuous layer, but scattered in Peyer's patches, agminated follicles and the like. It is difficult, for example, to understand what good the tonsil can exert in this direction; judging from clinical experience alone it would seem rather to be a source of weakness than of protection. Possibly that is because it possesses the defects of its merits; and being a defender is the more liable to be injured; just as a policeman is more liable to have his head broken than an ordinary mortal.

On the other hand one may observe that the lymphoid tissue of what we have called the first line is developed in proportion to the local need for defence; for example, in the bronchial mucous membrane, which, as we have seen, is indeed constantly exposed to bacteria, though to a far lesser extent than that of the alimentary canal, it is far less abundant than in the intestine.

But, be the function of the lymphoid tissues of the mucous membranes what it may, there can be no doubt that these latter offer a considerable, though not an absolute, barrier to the penetration of bacteria. If evidence of this were needed it would be found in the fact that injury to the mucous membranes enormously increases the number of bacteria to be found in the blood and interior tissues of the body. An example of this is afforded by the grouse badly infested with intestinal

[1] *Principles of Pathology*, 1908, p. 291.

worms[1], by the young rabbit whose intestine is damaged by coccidia, and by lambs whose stomachs are infested by nematodes. In all these cases the author has found numerous intestinal bacteria in the blood and internal tissues, in marked contrast to the sterility, or approximate sterility, of the tissues of normal animals.

One need not insist on the protective nature of the lymphatic glands. That one of their principal functions is to arrest and destroy micro-organisms carried to them in the lymph, probably no one would deny. The only question is to what extent they succeed in carrying out this function completely.

The Penetrability of the First Line of Defence. It is probable that bacteria in small numbers are constantly invading the lymph through the mucous surfaces. The writer in an experimental investigation of the question whether bacteria are present in the tissues and fluids of the normal living body, which has been already alluded to, found bacteria almost constantly present in mesenteric glands and bronchial glands, and in the latter situation in animals which had inhaled *B. prodigiosus* that micro-organism was found. These results are in harmony, as we shall see, with those of Ravenel, and also of A. S. Griffith, who, having fed dogs with *B. tuberculosis*, found these organisms in the mesenteric glands. The amount of penetration in perfect health is probably small. Griffith, in the experiments alluded to, found the tubercle bacilli in the mesenteric glands of only half the dogs which had been fed with them, though they were sought for by the extremely delicate method of guinea-pig inoculation. On the other hand, as we have seen in the case of the grouse, etc., if the mucous membrane be injured the number of bacteria which enter the body is greatly increased.

The Penetrability of the Second Line of Defence. While there can be little doubt that tubercle bacilli and other bacteria do to some extent and in small numbers, even under normal conditions, penetrate the mucous membranes and reach the nearest lymphatic glands, it seems probable that the latter

---

[1] *The Grouse in Health and Disease,* 1911, Smith, Elder & Co. The Final Report of the Committee of Inquiry on Grouse Disease, see p. 289.

form, as long as they are themselves intact, an almost insuper-able barrier to the further progress of the bacteria.

Nevertheless opinion on this point has been much divided, some holding, with Nocard and his followers, that the blood and internal organs normally contain bacteria, especially after a meal rich in fat, others maintaining, with Neisser, that the blood and tissues are normally sterile. In Canada Ford, working in the school of Professor Adami, supports Nocard's position, while in Cambridge the writer, who has investigated the question independently, inclines rather to the side of Neisser, though he does not deny the occasional penetration of microbes.

Nocard's views seem to have been based largely on some experiments carried out under his direction by Porcher and Desoubrey in 1895. These experiments seem to us very unsatisfactory at the present day[1], yet at one time they were widely accepted, and they have had considerable effect upon opinion in the past. Nocard tells us how he came to suspect the entry of bacteria into the blood during digestion. He was in the habit of using as a culture medium horse serum which was not subjected to any sterilizing process. Usually this proved quite satisfactory, but on one occasion a whole batch of tubes was found to be contaminated. On inquiry he found that the animal had been bled soon after feeding, and he set Porcher and Desoubrey to work to see if the bacteria in the blood of animals were increased after a meal. These observers, as is too common, seem to have found just what they were led to anticipate. At the present day, when so much horse serum is used for

[1] Porcher and Desoubrey (1895, No. 1) communicated their experiments —twenty in number—to the Société de Biologie. Chyle was taken from dogs killed, some fasting, others after a meal, and several drops were sown on gelatin plates. Colonies appeared in all cases when the chyle was taken after a meal of milk or fat. The authors add that in several of their earlier experiments they sowed the blood from the portal vein, and were able to demonstrate the presence of microbes there also.

In a later communication (1895, No. 2) they describe how they made cultures from the blood of dogs, both fasting and after a meal, and were careful to compare those from the right and left sides of the heart with one another, that is to say, cultures from the blood before and after it had been subjected to the filtering action of the lungs. They reported fifteen experiments. Colonies were commonly obtained, often in large numbers. They were relatively few in the cultures made from the blood of fasting dogs, and they were almost constantly more numerous in those made from the blood of the right side than in those made from that of the left side of the heart. The work, however, is vitiated by their method of making the cultures. The plates do not seem to have been sown directly with the blood, but the latter was first incubated in broth, and the plates sown from these young fluid cultures, thus gratuitously opening the door to errors caused by chance contaminations.

therapeutic purposes, and experience consequently has enormously increased, it is hardly necessary to point out that serum properly taken is almost invariably sterile, or, at most, contains only an occasional stray microbe.

The Montreal School has, in the main, followed Nocard, though recently its views have been expressed with great moderation.   The history of the Canadian observations bearing on this question are briefly as follows :   Adami, in 1894–5, when he was investigating the " Picton disease " of cattle in a district of Nova Scotia of that name, found little coccoid bodies in the livers of diseased animals.   These bodies were thought to be either diplococci, or bacilli which stained mainly at the poles.   Not long afterwards Nicholls, also of the Montreal School, found similar bodies in human livers, both in cases of cirrhosis and afterwards in those who had died of other causes. These granules he took to be *B. coli*, and from his observations he concluded that bacteria are constantly passing into the body tissues through its various epithelial surfaces.   This opinion was cautiously endorsed by Adami in his *Principles of Pathology*, where, referring to the resistance offered by the body to the entrance of bacteria into its tissues, he says: " It is wrong to imagine, as is too often taught, that the hindrance to the entrance of bacteria into the tissues is, under all circumstances, complete in the healthy individual.   *A certain number of microbes is always gaining admission*—nay, is being actively introduced by the cells of the organism[1].   *But under such circumstances they do not cause infection.   In health they tend to be destroyed very soon after their reception.*   The evidence that this is the case is now overwhelming.   It is true of the lower respiratory tract....It is true also of the intestines " (*loc. cit.* p. 290).

The position taken up by the Montreal School is based partly also on the researches of Ford on the bacteriology of normal tissues.   Ford obtained cultures of various micro-organisms by planting portions of the organs of animals, taken with all possible precautions, into solid nutrient jelly and incubating for a considerable time.   He explained the failure of other observers

---

[1] Referring to the leucocytes which are said to be " constantly passing out between the epithelial cells to gain the surface," some of which are said to "find their way back" after having acted as "scavengers and cleansers" (*loc. cit.* p. 289)

to obtain similar evidence of bacteria in normal tissues on the
ground that they had not incubated their culture tubes long
enough.   Referring to this work, Adami says, " Ford's cultures
proved that over 70 per cent. of the livers and kidneys of these
animals...yield cultures of various forms of pathogenic and
non-pathogenic microbes, such as are found in the intestinal
contents.   The interesting point is that the growth of these
forms is peculiarly slow.   Ford, in general, obtained no growth
within three days, but, keeping (his cultures) for several days, he
obtained positive results.   Evidently (1) the bacteria are attenuated so that their growth is feeble, and (2) it is arrested until
the bactericidal substances of the organs have become inert."

A few lines further on, after alluding to some experiments
by Wrosczek, he adds, " These observations then prove conclusively that bacteria are constantly entering the organism "
(*loc. cit.* p. 292).   But he goes on to say that the bacteria
are very rapidly removed from the blood and destroyed by the
endothelial cells which line the blood vessels, more especially of
the liver, kidneys and spleen, so that " *while the tissues of the
healthy body are not necessarily free from micro-organisms they
are potentially sterile* " (p. 293).

The present writer, founding his opinions on his own hitherto
unpublished experiments, agrees in the main with Adami that
the tissues of the healthy body are substantially sterile, though
in the production of this result he is inclined to attribute more
importance to the barrier offered by the lymphatic glands and
relatively less to the bactericidal action of the other tissues.

His own experimental results differed from those of Ford, for he found
that the cultures from the blood and principal organs (lungs excepted) remained
as a rule sterile though kept under careful observation and incubated for more
than a week. In a certain percentage of the tubes one or more colonies appeared,
though whether these were due to bacteria which were present in the tissues
during life, or were caused by accidental contamination during the necessary
manipulations, could not be ascertained with certainty. It is at least probable
that some were of this latter kind, since with all possible precautions it is
impossible to be sure that every chance of contamination is absolutely excluded,
but at the same time the writer was inclined to believe that some of them
were produced by bacteria actually in the tissues during life. It is not possible
to go fully into the reasons for this conclusion here ; it must suffice to say
(1) that the increase of skill and rapidity acquired as the result of experience and practice, as well as the adoption of fresh precautions which took

place from time to time, did little or nothing to diminish the frequency with which these occasional colonies occurred : (2) that the colonies were commoner in cultures made from the liver than in those made from the spleen, although there was just as much risk of accidental contamination in dealing with the latter as with the former : (3) the bacteria which grew on the cultures sown from the organs did not correspond with those found on agar plates exposed to the air during the experiments ; in particular, segmented bacilli, somewhat resembling *B. diphtheriæ*, were relatively common in cultures from the organs but were hardly ever seen on the air plates.   And lastly (4) colonies occurred from time to time on blood cultures, the blood being taken directly from the heart by means of a sterile pipette, a method which should be free from almost all risk of accidental contamination.

It has already been mentioned that cultivations from the lungs of various animals, even from the marginal portions of the lobes, always gave colonies of a large variety of micro-organisms, including, in the case of the guinea-pig and rabbit at least, moulds, streptothrices, spore-bearing bacilli and cocci The contrast between the cultivations from these and other organs was absolute.   The former always showed numerous colonies, the latter seldom showed any.   Cultivations from the mesenteric and bronchial glands nearly always yielded colonies. In the case of the former spore-bearing bacilli were preponderant and colonies of non-spore-bearing intestinal bacteria were rarely seen ; a fact which affords strong evidence of the bactericidal power of these glands.

From these experiments the writer was led to conclude that the tissues and fluids of the body (lungs excepted) are almost entirely free from living bacteria, and that the lymphatic glands, the body's second line of defence, as Adami aptly calls them, offer an exceedingly efficient (though not an absolutely perfect) barrier to the passage of micro-organisms, and that the number that pass them depends largely on the number brought to them, that is to say, on the condition of the first line of defence at the epithelial surfaces.

The Bearing of the preceding Conclusions on the Possibility of Detecting by Anatomical Evidence the Portals of Entry of Tubercle Bacilli.   The bearing of these conclusions on the question by what means we can detect the portal of entry of the tubercle bacilli which have set up tuberculosis will be evident.   For, if the lymph glands are such efficient filters as we have seen reason to believe, it seems probable that they will seldom, if ever, let a tubercle bacillus through their meshes without retaining in their substance a number of others sufficient to cause disease there and produce obvious lesions which will serve to mark the path along which the invaders penetrated into the body, and to point to the portal through which they entered. In other words it seems probable that those bacilli which get through the barrier are only stray members of a crowd, the great majority of which remain behind in the gland. Now the glands have, no doubt, greater powers of destroying bacteria than other organs. Yet it seems almost certain that their power of dealing with tubercle bacilli, as compared with that of other tissues, can scarcely be so great that they themselves can escape disease when sufficient bacilli are brought to them for some of the latter to get through their meshes and cause disease in the lungs or elsewhere. Thus, it seems probable, that, whatever happens at the first line of defence, tuberculous disease is almost always developed at the second, in the glands which guard the portal of entry, before it appears in parts of the body on the further side of those defences.

Experimental Investigation of the Question of the Permeability of Lymphatic Glands by Tubercle Bacilli. Having now considered the question of the permeability of the normal lymph glands by bacteria in general, and discussed the bearing of the conclusions arrived at on the question of their probable permeability by tubercle bacilli in particular, let us turn to the consideration of experiments designed expressly to test this more limited aspect of the matter.

The permeability of healthy mesenteric glands by tubercle bacilli was investigated by Schlossmann and Engel, who injected tubercle bacilli directly into the stomachs of young guinea-pigs through an incision in the abdominal wall, and, having killed the animals six hours later, demonstrated the presence of tubercle bacilli in the lungs by injecting cultures of these organs into other guinea-pigs. The operative interference was severe and it seems possible that the bacilli may have been regurgitated into the mouth with some of the other contents of the stomach, and have become aspirated into the air passages, for it has been observed that regurgitation is very easily provoked in these animals.

Ravenel and Reichel, 1908, made similar experiments on 50 young guinea-pigs. In 28 of these animals tubercle bacilli were proved to be present in the lungs within twenty-four hours of the operation; from 22 they were absent. In another 10 guinea-pigs, which were infected by the same method but allowed to live for several weeks, tuberculous lesions were found in those organs. The authors were convinced that the tubercle bacilli which they found in the lungs had been absorbed from the intestine, but they admitted that this was not proved conclusively, and they refrained from drawing any positive conclusions. This cautious attitude was adopted because in all the ten animals which were allowed to live some weeks after the injections tuberculous lesions were found, not, as we have seen, in the lungs only, but in the omentum also and in the abdominal wall at the seat of operation, thus showing that the investigators had not succeeded completely in avoiding direct infection of these parts, and in thus excluding the possibility of all absorption except through the abdominal mucosa.

In some earlier experiments Ravenel (1903) fed dogs with cultures of tubercle bacilli, and, having killed the animals after a short interval, injected emulsions of their mesenteric glands together with as much chyle as he could obtain from the thoracic ducts into guinea-pigs. In ten out of twelve experiments tuberculosis resulted from these injections, thus proving the absorption of bacilli from the intestine, but throwing, of course, no light on the question whether the bacilli had passed beyond the glands into the thoracic duct.

A. S. Griffith[1] repeated these experiments for the Royal Commission, injecting glands and chyle separately. Dogs, both young and old, were fed with large quantities of culture of tubercle bacilli and killed after intervals of several hours. The mesenteric glands of these animals, emulsified and injected into guinea-pigs, caused tuberculosis in six out of twelve experiments. The chyle of eleven of these dogs was collected during life from

[1] *R.C.T. 2nd Int. Rep.* vol. I, p. 696.

the terminal portion of the thoracic duct in the neck, and as large a quantity as possible (in one case 8 c.c.) was injected into guinea-pigs. But in no case was tuberculosis caused by these injections. Equally without result was a chyle experiment made in a similar manner on a monkey.

Some support, however, was lent by these experiments to the view that some tubercle bacilli fed to dogs get past the mesenteric glands and reach the blood stream; for from four of the dogs already referred to portions of lung were taken, emulsified, and injected into guinea-pigs, and in two cases tuberculosis resulted. This may have been because some bacilli had been *aspirated* into the lungs during the experimental feeding, an accident which we shall see reason to believe is not improbable[1]. It is only fair, however, to add that the positive results were obtained in experiments where the time allowed for passage through the glands was considerable, namely in two dogs which were killed 31 and 96 hours respectively after swallowing the bacilli, while the negative results were obtained in the case of animals killed 3 and 24 hours respectively after feeding.

A. S. Griffith afterwards fed nine pigs, three monkeys, a goat and a cat with tubercle bacilli, and killed and examined them after intervals of some days, with the object of finding out whether, and if so how soon, the bacilli get through to the lungs. The following table is compiled from his report[2].

Animal	Interval between Feeding and Examination	Result of Inoculating Tissues into guinea-pigs			
		Mesenteric glands	Lungs	Liver	Spleen
Pig	2 days	+	o	–	o
,,	4 ,,	+	o	o	o
,,	5 ,,	+	o	o	o
,,	7 ,,	+	o	o	o
,,	7 .,	+	+	o	o
,,	7 ,,	+	+	o	o
,,	7 ,,	+	+	o	o
,,	12 ,,	+	o	o	o
,,	13 ,,	+	+	o	o
Rhesus Monkey	2 ,,	o	o	o	o
,,	4 ,,	+	+	+	+
,,	6 ,,	+	–	o	+
Goat	8 ,,	+	+	o	o
Cat	9 .,	+	+	+	+

[1] See p. 162.   [2] *R.C.T. Final Rep.* vol. I, p. 52.

From this table it will be seen that tubercle bacilli were present in the mesenteric glands of every animal, one monkey alone excepted. Among the pigs tubercle bacilli were present in the lungs also in four of the nine animals, namely in four out of the six examined a week or more after the experimental feeding, while they were absent from the lungs of those killed at an earlier period. In two of the three monkeys also, and in the goat and the cat, the bacilli were found in one or more of the great organs after intervals of 4 to 9 days.

Many continental observers have obtained similar results, among whom von Behring and Roemer, Nicolas and Descos, Bisanti and Panisset, Ficker, Oberwarth, and L. Rabinowitsch, are mentioned by Calmette[1].

Nicolas and Descos are said to have fed dogs with fatty soup, and to have killed them three hours afterwards, in the period of full digestion. The chyle, taken from the receptaculum, was injected into guinea-pigs in doses of 5 to 10 c.c., and shown by the results of these injections to contain tubercle bacilli.

Bisanti and Panisset carried out similar experiments, also on dogs, and found tubercle bacilli in the organs in four out of six, and in one case in the chyle also.

Some of the results obtained by foreign investigators are so contrary to the experience of the present writer that he is unable to accept them. Thus Plate is said to have found tubercle bacilli *constantly* in the blood, spleen, and liver of guinea-pigs, both young and old, within an hour and a half of their having been fed with tubercle bacilli.

The present writer's experiments never produced any such results. The following are some of his experiences:

Guinea-pigs and rabbits were fed with large doses of tubercle bacilli from culture, and the animals were killed after intervals of from 17–42 hours. The blood and various organs were tested for the presence of tubercle bacilli by injection into guinea-pigs. The injections of blood (five in number) and of liver (five in number) never produced tuberculosis. Injections of mesenteric glands produced tuberculosis twice out of seven times. Injections of right lung (six in number) never produced tuberculosis, but injections of left lung (seven in number) produced tuberculosis in one of the two animals injected no less than three times. This difference between the infectivity of the two

[1] *Les Voies d'Infection Tuberculeuse,* 1913, p. 22.

lungs seems to be more than a mere coincidence, and to be more explicable on the hypothesis that the bacilli were aspirated into the lung, rather than that they were carried there by the blood stream[1].

In the experiments of some of the numerous continental observers mentioned above, the passage into the blood of tubercle bacilli introduced into the alimentary canal did not occur by any means constantly. Thus in the experiments of Orth and Rabinowitsch, in which tubercle bacilli were administered to rabbits and guinea-pigs per rectum, and their blood and organs examined after several days, in five only out of 42 experiments was it shown that tubercle bacilli had found their way into the blood stream.

Experiments with tubercle bacilli, such as we are now considering, are difficult to carry out successfully. The guinea-pig is so susceptible to tuberculosis that probably a very few bacilli will suffice to cause disease if they are injected. In spite of great care in dealing with the bodies of animals which have been fed recently with large numbers of tubercle bacilli, and whose intestines probably still contain many millions, the risk of accidental contamination is always imminent. Under these circumstances, and when the results of different observers are at variance with one another, experiments which have given negative results are, to say the least of it, as convincing as those which have yielded positive results. It will not do to accept all results as equally reliable without critical inquiry. It is absolutely necessary to attempt to discriminate between the sound and the unsound.

The reasonable conclusion to be drawn from these experiments would seem to be that *tubercle bacilli do occasionally pass through the intact mesenteric or cervical glands when animals are made to swallow very large quantities of these micro-organisms, but that they do so without leaving behind sufficient numbers to produce obvious lesions in those glands has not been established.*

But there is a special source of fallacy with regard to the lungs, in such feeding experiments, which it seems well nigh impossible to exclude entirely, namely the danger of some of the bacilli which are intended to be swallowed gaining, accidentally,

[1] *Journ. of Pathol.* 1910, vol. XIV, see Table VIII, p. 598.

direct access to those organs by aspiration into the trachea. The possibility of this accident was forced upon the attention of the writer some years ago when making feeding experiments with *B. prodigiosus*. However carefully the feeding was conducted, and whether artificially contaminated food was consumed in the natural manner, or minute quantities of emulsified bacilli were introduced into the animals' mouths by means of a platinum loop, the bacilli were invariably found in the lungs. Since this was the case when the animals were killed *immediately* after such feeding, it was quite certain that the bacilli could not have reached the lungs after being absorbed from some part of the alimentary canal, for there was no time for such absorption ; they must have gained *direct* access to the lungs. It was, of course, felt to be possible that the bacilli might have been aspirated into the lung in consequence of convulsive inspirations during the death struggle, and that they would never have got there, by that route, if the animals had been allowed to continue living. Various methods therefore were tried of killing the animals in such a way as to avoid convulsive or gasping respiration, but these were not very successful in their object. Finally a clamp was constructed by means of which a suitable ligature round the neck could be suddenly tightened so as to occlude the trachea completely, the animal being killed by a blow on the head almost simultaneous with the tightening of the ligature. After death the completeness of the occlusion of the trachea was tested by trying to force air through it with a bicycle pump while the body of the animal was held under water. Even when this severe test proved the completeness of the occlusion, cultures from the lungs still yielded colonies of *B. prodigiosus*. It seemed evident then that the bacilli had gained direct access to the lung while the animals were alive and under perfectly normal conditions[1].

If such an accident is liable to happen when animals are fed with *B. prodigiosus*, it must also occur sometimes when

---

[1] The writer was very reluctant to accept a conclusion which seems so improbable, and it was only after numerous experiments, varied in many ways, that he felt at last compelled to do so.

they are fed with *B. tuberculosis*. One can then no longer accept the presence of tubercle bacilli in the lungs of animals which have been artificially fed with copious doses of this microbe as conclusive evidence of their absorption through the lymphatic system of the alimentary canal.

It must, however, be added that, in all probability, the bacilli which enter the lungs directly when these organisms are placed in the mouth, either deliberately in experiments, or accidentally when contained in food, are as a rule very few in number[1]; for one must remember that the methods of detecting them (cultivation in the case of *B. prodigiosus*, injection of tissue emulsions into guinea-pigs in the case of tubercle bacilli) are exceedingly delicate. It seems probable, therefore, that in the case of animals which possess a fair amount of power of destroying tubercle bacilli, such as the ox, or man, the tubercle bacilli which enter the lungs in this way are commonly insufficient in number to produce disease.

The possibility of error due to accidental aspiration into the lungs of bacilli administered in feeding experiments has not escaped the attention of other observers. It was for this reason that Orth and Rabinowitsch, in the experiments which have just been quoted, made use of rectal injections; and, as we shall see, A. S. Griffith accepted it as the most probable explanation of some of his results. This observer made a large number of feeding experiments, besides those already referred to, and these must now be briefly considered[2]. They lend but slight support to the view that tubercle bacilli can be absorbed from the gut and infect the lungs without causing lesions in the mesenteric glands. Those made upon cattle at least (22 in number) show, as McFadyean has pointed out[3], that "the almost invariable result of infection by ingestion is a tuberculosis with more or less conspicuous lesions in the abdominal cavity, and

---

[1] Cp. the very minimal results of injecting lung emulsions of guinea-pigs and rabbits fed with *B. tuberculosis* in the course of the writer's own experiments. *Journ. of Pathol.* vol. xiv, Table IX, p. 598.

[2] *R.C.T. Int. Rep.* 1907, App. vol. i, pp. 499–708.

A summary of these experiments is given by McFadyean in the *Journ. of Comp. Pathol., etc.*, 1910.

[3] 1910, *loc. cit.* p. 250.

especially in the mesenteric glands." In dogs and monkeys however, as we shall see, this was not always the case ; and Griffith
himself at one time concluded from the whole series of feeding
experiments now under consideration that " the experiments
have conclusively shown that tubercle bacilli which have been
ingested, may, within a very short time, find their way into
the lungs, where they set up tuberculous lesions. Pulmonary
tuberculosis so induced may or may not be accompanied by
lesions in the mucous membrane of the alimentary tract, or
glands connected with it[1]." This opinion was, as we shall see
in a moment, somewhat modified later.

The author is given to understand that in making this
statement Griffith relied largely upon the results obtained in
dogs. These latter experiments, therefore, demand more particular attention.

Eleven dogs were fed with cultures of tubercle bacilli in
doses of from 1 to 100 milligrammes. Three of the animals
remained free from tuberculosis ; three developed more or
less tuberculosis in the lungs, with lesions in the glands of the
alimentary canal ; and " in the other five there was no disease
of the alimentary tract or glands in connection with it, but in
each one or two small tubercles in the lungs[2]."

This then is the evidence, but it is by no means convincing,
and Griffith himself seems to have recognized that, for in a letter
to the writer written in 1912 he said : "there is a goodly number of
animals " (other than those mentioned above) " fed with tubercle
bacilli which showed at the post-mortem examination tuberculosis of the lungs without alimentary lesions, but I am of opinion
that in all these cases the pulmonary disease was produced by
inhaled or insufflated bacilli." And, he concludes, " there is
little comfort for those who hold that pulmonary tuberculosis is
of alimentary origin in the feeding experiments of Volume I[3]."

We shall see how Griffith was led to this belief in the possibility of accidental insufflation into the lungs complicating
feeding experiments. Fourteen monkeys were fed with tubercle

---

[1] 1907, *loc. cit.* p. 706. For Griffith's more mature opinion see p. 173 of
this book.

[2] *Ibid. loc. cit.* p. 632.   [3] *I.e.* vol. I of App. to the *Fin. Rep. R.C.T.*

bacilli[1], three of these animals were found after death to have
developed no abdominal lesions, but in all there was more or
less tuberculosis in the lungs. The pulmonary disease in the
three animals specially mentioned may have been spontaneous,
for these animals frequently suffer naturally from tuberculosis,
and it is very difficult to be certain that monkeys used for
experiment are free from antecedent disease of this kind since,
when known to be infected, they react very badly to tuberculin[2].
Griffith, however, considered the possibility of spontaneous
infection, and rejected it on grounds which need not now
detain us. He inclined rather to the view that the pulmonary
disease was due to insufflation. His own account is as follows :
" In five of the experiments...the disease appeared to have
originated in the thorax, the type of disease presented being
that of an inhalation tuberculosis[3]." " Four of the monkeys
were fed by means of a pipette, the culture suspension being
allowed to trickle slowly on to their tongues ; the fluid appeared
to be swallowed in a natural manner and there was no choking,
yet there can be little doubt that in all these cases some of the
material gained direct access to the lung alveoli by way of the
bronchial tubes[4]."

Another monkey was fed daily with the milk of a cow with
tuberculosis of the udder. This animal was allowed to drink
the milk out of a small vessel, " and in this case also, as will be
seen from the history of the monkey's habits and manner of
drinking, there is the possibility that the bacilli were insufflated
or inhaled[5]." " The milk was given to the monkey in a small
trough, and his affection for the latter became so great that he
became inconsolable whenever it was taken away from him ;
he was allowed to have it constantly in his cage, and he was
accustomed to sleep curled up in it at night." "The monkey
very greedily drank the infected milk, plunging mouth and nos-
trils into the fluid and consuming sometimes the whole quantity
given to him, 75 to 100 c.c., without taking breath ; as a result

---

[1] *loc. cit.* p. 628.

[2] Cobbett and A. S. Griffith, 1913. *R.C.T.*, Supplemental Volume on
Tuberculin Tests. For monkeys, see pp. 50, 78 *et seq.*

[3] Griffith, 1907, *loc. cit.* p. 629.   [4] *Ibid.* p. 630.

[5] *Ibid.* pp. 629, 630 and 651.

on several occasions he was observed to cough and choke as if some of the fluid had been drawn into the larynx." " These details in the history of the animal are given to show that there is the possibility that tubercle bacilli may have got to the lungs by way of the bronchi either by insufflation or inhalation[1]."

It is only right to add that " in other cases " which developed lesions in the lungs " the distribution of the disease was such that there could be little doubt that the tuberculosis was caused by the bacilli ingested[2]." " Bacilli can undoubtedly pass through the alimentary mucous membrane and affect the lungs directly, as was shown in the series of monkeys included in the third special feeding experiment[3]; but in these cases the lesions in the lungs were few and discrete, and the intestines and mesenteric glands were tuberculous in every case[4]."

This is the gist of the matter : " the mesenteric glands were tuberculous in every case." For, as McFadyean pointed out, the question is not so much whether tubercle bacilli can pass through intact mesenteric glands, as whether they can pass these glands without causing obvious lesions there which may serve to mark the portal by which they entered.

General Conclusion as to the Penetrability of the Second Line of Defence. The bearing of the Results arrived at on the Determination of the Portal of Entry in Individual Cases of Tuberculosis. After considering the large mass of evidence referred to above, and indeed much more for which room can not be found, it seems reasonable to conclude that what we have called the body's second line of defence, the lymphatic glands, are very efficient bacterial filters at all ages, and that they retain the immense majority of bacteria which are brought to them, and prevent their getting into the blood. Like all bodily mechanisms, they are good enough for their purpose, but they fall short of perfection. They probably allow some bacilli to pass through them, especially when defects in the mucous membranes cause large numbers of bacteria to be carried to the glands. But it seems probable that, as a general rule, if tubercle bacilli pass

---

[1] Griffith, 1907, *loc. cit.* p. 651.   Cp. Titze and Weidanz, *postea,* p. 500.
[2] *Ibid.* p. 629.   [3] *Ibid.* p. 591.   [4] *Ibid.* p. 630.

through the lymphatic glands in sufficient numbers to cause disease elsewhere, enough will have been retained in the glands themselves to cause disease there also, and thus to indicate the portal of entry. This has sometimes been called Cohnheim's law ; and it seems as true to-day as when he enunciated it.

If this be allowed, but not otherwise, we may reasonably seek to discover the portal of entry in any given case of tuberculosis by seeking for early lesions in the various sets of lymphatic glands through one or more of which the infecting virus must have passed, and we may pass on to a consideration of the anatomical evidence bearing on the question of the portals of origin of the different clinical manifestations of tuberculosis.

It is no exception to this law that tuberculous lesions may occur on the *proximal* side of the glands without these structures being affected. This is often the case in adults in whom primary tuberculosis of the lung is seen without obvious disease in the bronchial glands, and ulceration of intestine (due to swallowing sputum) without marked tuberculosis of the mesenteric glands.

On the other hand it is admitted that the first line of defence—the mucous membranes—may be penetrated by tubercle bacilli without tuberculous lesions necessarily arising there. This seems to occur not unfrequently in young children in whom it is common to find tuberculous disease in the bronchial, cervical, or mesenteric glands without any obvious tuberculous lesions in the lungs, buccal cavity or intestines respectively.

The Relative Frequency with which the Intestinal and Respiratory Portals act as Transmitters of Tubercle Bacilli.

In considering this question the truth is assumed of what we have hitherto endeavoured to establish, namely, that the presence of old tuberculous lesions in a given set of glands may, as a general rule, be taken as indicating that the bacilli have entered through the surface whose lymph drains away towards the glands in question, and if there is disease on the *distal* side of these glands that the bacilli which caused it have passed through those structures.

Only three groups of glands need be considered in detail, the cervical, the mesenteric, and the bronchial.   The inguinal and axillary need not concern us now, since no one believes that internal tuberculosis caused by bacilli which have entered through the skin is anything but a rare and exceptional occurrence.

Shennan has repeatedly analysed the records of the post-mortem room of the Royal Edinburgh Hospital for Sick Children going back for the last 21 years.   His last report, in 1909, deals with 1085 post-mortem examinations made on unselected cases dying in the hospital from various causes. The results showed that 421 children (38·8 per cent.) had died of tuberculosis.   Of these the records were sufficiently definite for analysis in 413 cases.   They are divided into two series; one including 250 cases, aged from one to 13 years, examined prior to 1888, up to which time infants under one year of age were not admitted to the hospital; the other including 308 cases of all ages from birth to 13 years.

In these 413 fatal cases of tuberculosis in childhood it was found that the lymphatic glands were tuberculous in 92·4 per cent. in the first series, and 78·8 per cent. in the second series. " The mediastinal glands were more affected than the abdominal glands ; and dissemination took place more frequently, apparently, from the former group."   " Tuberculosis of the mediastinal glands was commonly unaccompanied by primary tuberculosis of the lungs, but was frequently associated with recent tuberculosis of those organs, in many cases evidently secondary to the glandular tuberculosis."   " In nearly half the cases of Tabes Mesenterica there was no ulceration of the intestines."

In recent years some very complete researches have been carried out on consecutive and unselected cases from the post-mortem rooms of general hospitals.   Not only has very careful search for all tuberculous lesions been made in these cases, but the glands, whether they appeared normal or not, have been emulsified and injected into guinea-pigs ; cultures have been raised from the infected parts, and the type of bacillus concerned determined by suitable experiments.   Only the more recent and important of these investigations will be reviewed here[1].

Gaffky, 1907, in the series of researches already referred to in connection with the problem of latency, examined the bronchial and mesenteric glands of 300 children between the ages of a few weeks to 13 years. Among them were 36 with more or less obvious tuberculosis, and in 27 of these the glands were found to contain tubercle bacilli capable of infecting guinea-pigs. In addition, the apparently normal glands of 30 children who showed no signs of tuberculosis proved to be infective. Adding these two classes together there were in all 57 children, some of whose glands were proved to contain tubercle bacilli. Of these both the bronchial and mesenteric glands contained tubercle bacilli in 29 cases; the bronchials alone contained them in 17, and the mesenterics alone in 11.

The investigation was continued by Rothe, 1911, on similar lines, the bodies of 150 children who had died under the age of five being examined. In 14 of them there were tuberculous lesions of some kind and in all of these living tubercle bacilli were proved to be present, in one gland or another, by injection into guinea-pigs. Eight had suspicious lesions, and in two of these the glands were found to be infectious. Among the remaining 128 children were five from whom apparently normal glands caused tuberculosis on inoculation.

Taking together all the 21 children whose glands were thus proved to contain tubercle bacilli, we find that there were 13 with tubercle bacilli present both in the bronchial and mesenteric glands; five with these bacilli present in the bronchials alone ; and three with the bacilli in the mesenterics alone.

From these researches it begins to appear that the bronchial glands are more liable to be injured by tubercle bacilli or to contain tubercle bacilli than the mesenteric, even in children ; a fact which, as we shall see, is confirmed by subsequent researches.

Ungermann, 1912, working in the Gesundheitsamt, Berlin, examined the glands of 171 children aged from three weeks to 12 years. The material came from a general hospital and was,

---

[1] For further evidence on this question see Ungermann, 1912.

like that of Gaffky and Rothe, entirely unselected. The examination in this research was not confined to the bronchial and mesenteric glands but was extended to the cervical glands also.

In 39 cases some of the glands proved to be infectious to guinea-pigs. In 29 of these cases tuberculosis had been either the sole cause of death or a severe complication. In six the tuberculosis was of slight extent; and in four there were no macroscopic lesions[1].

The distribution of the bacilli in the various glands in these 39 cases was as follows: In 30, all three sets of glands were infected. In the remaining nine, six of whom died of causes other than tuberculosis, the mesenterics alone were infected in two, the bronchials alone in one, and the cervicals alone in none. Bronchials and mesenterics were infected together in four, and bronchials and cervicals together in two.

It is surprising how often two or more sets of glands are found to be infected. In some of these cases it is quite probable that the bacilli had entered through two or more portals, but this is not necessarily the case since the infection of one set of glands may have been secondary to that of another. When this has occurred one would expect to find that the lesions in one set of glands were decidedly more advanced than those in the other, or others. In many of Ungermann's cases this was certainly the case, and he states definitely that " in a preponderating majority of cases the oldest lesions were in the bronchial glands." This fact is clearly revealed by the following analysis, copied from Ungermann's paper (p. 155), which shows that caseation, partial or total, was much commoner in the bronchial than in the other glands.

Glands	No. of cases in which the glands mentioned were infectious	Appearance of gland normal	Suspicion of tubercle in gland	Definite early tubercle	Caseation of part of gland	Almost total caseation
Cervical	32	7	11	7	5	2
Bronchial	37	3	2	3	17	12
Mesenteric	36	10	5	5	13	3

[1] There were several instances of apparently normal glands, taken from children with tuberculosis elsewhere, proving infective to guinea-pigs.

Two more papers dealing with this subject in a comprehensive manner have just been published by the Local Government Board ; one from the Pathological Laboratory of the Board, by A. Eastwood and F. Griffith, and the other from the Field Laboratories of the University of Cambridge, by A. S. Griffith.

Eastwood and F. Griffith, 1914, examined the glands and organs obtained *post-mortem* from 150 unselected children who had died of various causes in general hospitals, and found tubercle bacilli in 94 (62·7 per cent.). They draw the following conclusions as to the portals of entry in these cases. " In 22 the anatomical evidence was strongly in favour of the glands draining the alimentary tract as being primarily affected."... " In 52 the anatomical evidence was definitely in favour of primary infection through the respiratory tract....In 20 the anatomical evidence as to portal of entry was inconclusive." In addition there were five children whose bodies presented no macroscopic evidence of tuberculosis, and yet their glands contained tubercle bacilli (as shown by guinea-pig inoculations). In three of these the mesenteric glands alone were affected[1]. In one the bronchial glands alone[2], and in one the cervical, bronchial and mesenteric yielded bacilli[3] (*loc. cit.* p. 5).

Thus the evidence was very much in favour of the respiratory mucous membrane being the commoner portal of entry than the alimentary (ratio = 53 : 25) even in children.

A. S. Griffith, 1914, examined material derived from unselected autopsies of 73 children under 12 years of age, who had

---

[1] Human type of bacillus in one, bovine type in two cases.
[2] Bovine type.
[3] Human type.

In the 22 cases in which the authors concluded that the portal of entry was probably intestinal, the bacilli were of the bovine type in 12 (including H 99, in which the strain had low virulence for rabbits coupled with dysgonic characters of growth) : in three they were of human type : in seven they were apparently dead and the type could not be determined.

In the 52 cases in which the anatomical evidence was definitely in favour of primary infection through the respiratory tract the bacilli were of the human type in 43 : and in one only were they of the bovine type : in eight they were apparently dead.

died from any cause whatever in general hospitals[1]. As to the
portal of entry of the tubercle bacilli in these cases, he draws
the following conclusion : " The great majority of the tuberculous cases can be readily classified, according to the localization of the oldest and most severe tuberculous lesions, in one
or other of two groups ; one in which the lesions are in the
thorax, the other in which they are in the abdomen." In eight
cases " the intestines or mesenteric glands (in one the pharynx
as well) were the seat of the primary manifestations of the
disease." In 22 cases " the lungs or bronchial glands showed
more extensive and more advanced caseation than any other
organ or glands of the body[2]."

A. S. Griffith's mature opinion on the vexed question of
the common portal of entry in pulmonary tuberculosis may
be gathered from the following quotation :

" While there can be no doubt but that the tubercle bacilli
in the first class of case (abdominal) entered the body through
the mucous membrane of the alimentary tract, it cannot be
asserted with equal confidence that the invasion in the second
group (thoracic) was by way of the respiratory tract " (loc. cit.
p. 120).

" Is it possible in man for single bacilli which have passed
through the alimentary mucous membrane to be carried with
the lymph stream direct to the lungs and set up primary
thoracic tuberculosis ? Whilst experiments on animals have
not provided a conclusive answer to this question, the following
considerations, which have arisen as a result of this study of
anatomical distribution of disease in relation to type of infecting
organism, go, in my opinion, to support the view that direct

[1] Except in eight cases provided by two of the institutions which aided
the research, from which alone cases recognizable at autopsy as tuberculous
were investigated.

[2] Of the eight cases in which the portal of entry was probably abdominal
six were caused by the bovine type of bacillus and two by the human type.
Of the 22 in which the lungs or bronchial glands showed more extensive or
more advanced caseation than any other organs or glands of the body, the
tuberculosis was in every instance caused by the human type of bacillus ;
and Griffith adds, " this class of tuberculosis has not, to my knowledge,
ever been associated with the bovine type of tubercle bacillus." (loc. cit.
p. 120.)

infection of the thoracic organs by way of the alimentary tract is exceedingly infrequent."

" A common form of fatal tuberculosis in childhood is that in which the disease is most severe in the thorax (primary in lungs and bronchial glands). If the portal of entry of the ba-cilli in these cases be the alimentary tract then human tubercle bacilli behave differently in the body from bovine tubercle bacilli. For it is perhaps exclusively by way of the alimentary tract that bovine tubercle bacilli gain access to the tissues of children, yet there is no recorded instance in childhood of primary thoracic tuberculosis due to the bovine tubercle bacillus, though bovine tubercle bacilli must frequently enter the alimentary tract and be absorbed from it in small numbers " (*loc. cit.* p. 121).

Other Channels of Infection in Pulmonary Tuberculosis. From the evidence already examined it may be concluded that when pulmonary tuberculosis is unaccompanied by disease of the glands in the neck and abdomen, there exists a strong pre-sumption that the bacilli which caused the disease have reached the lungs by the air passages. But it may be questioned whether these conditions are commonly fulfilled in phthisis, for possibly lesions in the glands of the alimentary canal may be present unnoticed. Primary lesions in glands need not be con-spicuous ; the disease may even become arrested there at an early stage while it advances beyond; in one of A. S. Griffith's cases this was found to be the case (see p. 180).

Walsham, 1903, examined 27 fatal cases of phthisis, with the express object of seeing how often the cervical and bronchial glands were involved, with the " remarkable result that these glands (and in one instance the axillary glands likewise) were found tuberculous in all with one exception and that was a case of fibroid disease of the lung " (*loc. cit.* p. 6). But it does not follow that these glandular lesions were primary.

Several instances of disease of mesenteric glands were met with among the small number of cases of phthisis investigated by the Royal Commission.

T.C., H 49, died of phthisis at the age of 18. At the post-mortem examin-ation several calcareous nodules as hard as stones, but containing living tubercle bacilli, were found in the mesenteric glands[1].

[1] *R.C.T. Int. Rep.* vol. II, p. 839.

P.W., H 81, and E.R., H 104, died of "chronic ulcerative phthisis," aged 33 years and 31 years respectively.   In the mesenteric glands of each were some stony-hard calcareous nodules[1].

It cannot be denied that in such cases the pulmonary disease may have arisen from tubercle bacilli swallowed and absorbed from the intestine and passed through the mesenteric glands and thoracic duct, but this is by no means certain, for in such cases the disease both of lungs and glands is often of old standing, and it is impossible to say which is primary ; the glandular lesion may after all be secondary to that in the lungs, or, as is not improbable, each may be the result of an independent infection.

Woodhead, 1894, was convinced, as we have seen already, that many cases of phthisis, especially in children, were of abdominal origin.   He had been struck by observing in the post-mortem room the frequency with which pulmonary disease appeared to be secondary to disease in the mesenteric or some other glands.   He apparently did not attach much importance to the passage of tubercle bacilli into the thoracic duct, and so through the right side of the heart to the lungs, but he believed that tuberculous disease was apt to track from gland to gland, from the mesenterics to the retroperitoneal, through the diaphragm to the mediastinal, and so to the bronchial glands and finally to the lungs.   An analogous course would convey bacilli from the pharyngeal tonsil through the cervical chain of glands to those in the thorax.

Walsham came to the conclusion that "tubercle may be primary in the tonsil"; and many thoughtful observers have maintained that tubercle bacilli may enter through some part of the mouth or pharynx, very possibly through a decayed tooth or through the tonsil, and track from gland to gland down to the root of the neck until the lung itself is affected by direct contact with a caseous gland; and in this explanation they find the solution of the curious problem why pulmonary tuberculosis begins so often in the apices.

Grober has recently attempted to support this view by experiments made upon dogs.   Injecting large quantities of Indian ink (10 c.c. !) into the tonsils, he found that the pigment tracked down the neck and reached the apical

[1] *R.C.T. Fin. Rep.* vol. I, pp. 8, 98, 126 and 141.

pleura, and the bronchial and mediastinal glands. It is not surprising. Any-one who has injected Indian ink will have been astonished to see how widely it spreads in loose connective tissue, and would be prepared to find it spreading in the tissues of the neck[1].   It is, of course, impossible that 10 c.c. could have been injected into the tonsil without much of it getting into the connective tissues around.   Once there it naturally worked its way to the thoracic opening. Beitzke, who repeated these experiments, thinks that the ink got to the lung by being expressed from the tonsils into the pharynx and then aspirated into the air passages.

Other observers believe, with Woodhead, that there is a direct lymphatic connection between the deep cervical and the bronchial glands, and that tubercle bacilli entering through the pharyngeal or nasal mucous membrane, or through carious teeth, may pass by this channel to the lungs.   Beitzke names Aufrecht, Bartel and Spieler, Batier, Beckmann, Behring, Cornet, Harbitz, Pattenger. Weichselbaum, Weismayr and Wele-minsky, as holding this opinion.   Aufrecht was struck by fre-quently seeing a complete chain of tuberculous glands extending from the neck to the root of the lung.   Beitzke thinks this only occurs when there is ulceration of the larynx and tracheal tuber-culosis.   In other cases, especially in children, he finds a tuber-culosis diminishing in severity from above downwards towards the opening of the thoracic duct, and a tuberculosis diminishing upwards from the bronchial and tracheal glands.   In such cases, he thinks, one has to do with an infection through two portals. He finds from his own experiments and observations no evidence of a direct lymphatic connection between the cervical and bronchial glands.

Summary of the Evidence of the Portal of Entry in Phthisis. The evidence upon which were based the views of von Behring, Calmette, and others who believe that phthisis is commonly of intestinal origin has been examined at some length in the earlier part of this chapter, and found to be unconvincing. Reasons, based largely upon experimental investigations, have been brought forward for believing that when tubercle bacilli

---

[1] When one considers the mechanics of the neck one cannot fail to notice that the tissue which binds together the various structures there must neces-sarily be very loosely developed because of the great flexibility of the part, and the consequent necessity for means of allowing one structure to slip easily over another.

pass through lymphatic glands on their way from the portals of entry in sufficient numbers to cause disease in the tissues beyond those glands, enough bacilli, in the great majority of cases, are retained in the latter situation to cause obvious tuberculosis there, and thus produce lesions which serve to indicate the portal of entry. In phthisis it is probably uncommon to find old lesions in the mesenteric glands. Such cases, however, exist and it is not denied that in them the disease may possibly have had such an origin as Calmette ascribes to the "immense majority of cases of pulmonary tuberculosis"; at the same time it is quite possible in such cases that the mesenteric disease may be secondary, or due to an independent infection.

Several careful investigations, carried out on modern lines, of unselected material provided by children dying in general hospitals, have shown, both in Germany and this country, that the bronchial glands are affected with tuberculosis, or tubercle bacilli, much more commonly than the cervical or mesenteric glands, and there can therefore be no longer any doubt that the lungs, even in young children, are a commoner portal of entry of tubercle bacilli in tuberculosis in general than the intestine or pharynx. The rarity of bovine bacilli in pulmonary tuberculosis is strong evidence that the latter is seldom caused by bacilli which enter through the alimentary canal.

Finally, many independent experimenters have found that far smaller numbers of tubercle bacilli suffice to infect animals when administered by inhalation than when passed into the intestine.

From the mass of investigation carried out in recent years, prompted by the theories of intestinal origin which have been put forward in various countries, the old theory of the inspiratory origin of pulmonary tuberculosis has emerged greatly strengthened. It is not denied that some cases of phthisis may be due to bacilli which entered through the pharyngeal or intestinal mucous membrane, and which have passed through the cervical or mesenteric glands (leaving some, possibly small, lesion there), and so have reached the lungs, either directly into the thoracic duct or by tracking from gland to gland; but it seems probable that such cases form only a small part of the whole.

If this conclusion be sound then one must agree with Koch, that the one important source of tuberculous infection is the phthisical patient, for, of course, only " open " cases of tuberculosis are a source of danger to others, and of open cases phthisis constitutes the immense majority. Bovine tubercle bacilli, as we shall see, seldom, if ever, cause phthisis even in children, and even of cases of primary abdominal tuberculosis many are caused by the human type of bacillus.

Some considerable number of cases of tuberculosis, especially in children, are caused by infection derived directly from the cow. These will have to be considered in the sequel, but, as we shall see, they form but a small part of the total.

Portals of Entry in Other Forms of Tuberculosis. Abdominal Tuberculosis. Tuberculous Peritonitis. Probably no one, at the present day, would be found to deny the existence of many cases of primary abdominal tuberculosis, nor to maintain that such have any other than an intestinal origin. When tubercle bacilli enter the tissues of the body from the intestine the mucous membrane, as we have seen, is not always visibly affected, but the abdominal lymphatic glands (mesenteric, ileocolic or retroperitoneal) probably never escape.

Tuberculosis of cervical glands. As in the abdomen, so in the neck the lymphatic glands may become the seat of tuberculosis without obvious disease in the corresponding mucous membranes, but there can be little doubt that in such cases the tubercle bacilli have entered through the latter (or through a carious tooth). Such infections may be caused by bacilli brought either in the air or in the food.

General Tuberculosis and Meningitis. General miliary tuberculosis sometimes arises in consequence of a tuberculous nodule in some gland or other part ulcerating, and discharging its bacilli into a vein. In this way a widespread massive hæmatogenous infection occurs. This had very obviously taken place in the case of a horse related by Koch[1], and is described by Weigert as occurring in the human subject.

[1] " The Etiology of Tuberculosis," Eng. trans. p. 126.

It seems probable, however, that, in childhood at least, the less acute forms of the disease are due to bacilli which simply pass through tuberculous lymphatic glands along the ordinary lymph channels into the blood stream. Tuberculosis occasionally occurs in the thoracic duct[1], and, in the experience of those who worked for the recent Tuberculosis Commission, little tubercles were quite common in the intima of the right auricle of calves which were affected by acute general tuberculosis as the result of experimental injections.

In 44 of Shennan's cases death was due to general tuberculosis. In these cases the dissemination had taken place apparently from caseous glands, and more often from the mediastinal than the abdominal.

To judge by the groups of glands found principally infected during recent investigations by Eastwood, Griffith, Ungermann and others, the disease would seem to be sometimes of intestinal origin, but the bronchial glands were more often the principal seat of primary disease than the mesenteric[2]. It must be granted, however, that in a very large proportion of cases both sets of glands are affected almost equally ; and it seems not unlikely that in these cases the bacilli have entered simultaneously through the alimentary and respiratory portals.

The same is true of meningitis, which is usually only the most conspicuous part of a more or less generalized tuberculosis. A. S. Griffith, 1914, investigated 18 cases of this disease in children aged from eight months to six years. Four only were definitely intestinal in origin. In nine the condition of the bronchial glands strongly indicated a thoracic origin. In four both sets of glands were affected but the lesions were considerably more advanced in the bronchials ; and in one the lesions were almost precisely similar in character and extent in the two groups of glands.

Eastwood and F. Griffith, 1914, examined 31 cases of meningitis in children. From the distribution of the lesions in the lymphatic glands they concluded that 22 were of respiratory and four of alimentary origin. In five the portal of entry could not be determined.

[1] See Walsham, 1903, p. 73.   [2] See p. 171.

Putting these investigations together we have 49 cases of meningitis in children, 31 of which were considered to be of thoracic and 8 of abdominal origin, while in 10 the evidence was not conclusive[1].

In *Tuberculosis of Bones and Joints* but little is known about the condition of the lymphatic glands which might point to the portal by which the bacilli entered. It is comparatively seldom in such cases that opportunity for making a post-mortem examination occurs, and in its absence it is often assumed that the disease is limited to such parts as clinical examination shows to be affected : but this is probably not the case.

A. S. Griffith, 1914, reported a case of death from caries of the spine in a boy of 8½ years. Mesenteric and bronchial glands contained several calcareous nodules of the size of peas. Cervical glands were enlarged but there was no sign of calcification or caseation. It was impossible to say where the portal of entry had been. It is interesting to observe that while the disease advanced in the vertebral column it apparently became arrested in the mesenteric and thoracic glands, for no tuberculosis was caused by injection of emulsions of the lesions in these organs into guinea-pigs (case 5, *loc. cit.* pp. 116 and 124).

Eastwood and Griffith, 1914[1], investigated seven cases of tuberculosis in children in which one or more bones or joints were affected. In all the bronchial or mesenteric glands showed evidence of tuberculosis. In two the condition of the bronchial glands was such that the authors considered that the portal of entry was probably respiratory, and in two they believed that it was probably mesenteric. In the other three they thought the evidence as to the portal of entry was inconclusive.

The author witnessed the post-mortem examination of the body of a man aged 60 who died in Addenbrooke's Hospital in Cambridge of tuberculosis of the spinal column. Careful

---

[1] It is true that of the cases investigated by the Royal Commission, five out of 12 were definitely abdominal in origin and only four definitely thoracic, while three were doubtful ; but it must be remembered that cases of probable abdominal origin were largely selected for investigation during the earlier part of the work.

search among the glands revealed a hard calcareous nodule as large as a pea in one of the mesenteric group. But whether this represented the primary focus of the disease which was the cause of death, or some entirely independent and possibly long antecedent infection, could not be determined.

In another case at Addenbrooke's Hospital in the body of a child four years of age who died of tuberculosis of the dorsal vertebrae, a hard mesenteric gland advanced in caseation was found.

Taking these ten cases together, if we may generalize at all from such a limited number, it would seem that in bone and joint tuberculosis, both the intestinal and respiratory portals may admit the bacilli, but there is nothing to show which of the two do so more frequently than the other.

REFERENCES. V

(Chapter IX)

Portals of Entry of Tubercle Bacilli. (Post-natal Infection.)

Adami (1908). *Principles of Pathology.* Lea and Febiger, New York.

Alexander (1908). Das Verhalten des Kaninchens gegenüber den verschiedenen Infektionswegen bei Tuberkulose und gegenüber den verschiedenen Typen des Tuberkelbacillus. *Zeitsch. f. Hyg.* vol. LX, p. 467.

Arloing and Fargeot. *Comp. Rend. Acad. des Scien.* vol. 144, p. 786.

Arnold, J. (1885). *Staubinhalation und Staubmetastase,* Leipzig.

Bartel and Neumann (1906). Ueber experimentelle Inhalationstuberkulose beim Meerschweinchen. *Wien. klin. Wochenschr.* vol. XIX, pp. 167, 213.

Basset (1907). A propos de la pathogénie de l'anthracose pulmonaire. *Comp. Rend. de la Soc. de Biol.* vol. I, p. 148.

Basset and Carré (1907). A propos de l'absorption intestinale des particles solides. *Ibid.* vol. I, p. 261.

—— A propos du passage dans le thorax des poussières introduites dans le péritoine et de leur localisation. *Ibid.* vol. I, p. 348.

—— Conditions dans lesquelles la muqueuse digestive est permeable aux microbes de l'intestin. *Ibid.* vol. I, p. 890.

Baumgarten (1909). Welche Ansteckungsweise spielt bei der Tuberkulose des Menschen die wichtigste Rolle? *Deutsch. med. Wochenschr.* No. 40, p. 1729. (Abstract of Address to 16th Internat. Med. Cong., Budapest.)

von Behring (1903). Address at Cassel. *Deutsch. med. Wochenschr.* Sept. 24. Summary in *Brit. Med. Journ.* 1903, II, p. 993.

—— (1907). Beitrag zur Lehre von den Infectionswegen der Tuberkulose. 6th Internat. Tuberculosis Conference. *Tuberculosis*, vol. VI, p. 423.

Beitzke, A. (1906). Ueber den Weg der Tuberkelbazillen von der Mund- und Rachen-höhle zu den Lungen, mit besonderer Berücksichtigung der Verhältnisse beim Kinde. *Virchow's Archiv*, vol. 184, p. 1.

—— (1907). Ueber den Ursprung der Lungenanthracose. *Virchow's Archiv*, vol. 187, p. 183.

—— (1910). Häufigkeit, Herkunft und Infectionswege der Tuberkulose beim Menschen. *Ergebnisse der Allgem. Pathol. u. Path. Anat. d. Mensch. u. d. Tiere*, XIV Jahrgang. (Contains a full list of literature.)

Bisanti and Panisset (1905). Le bacille tuberculeux dans le sang après un repas infectant. *Comp. Rend. Soc. der Biol.* vol. I, p. 91.

Bulloch (1909). Paths of Infection in Pulmonary Tuberculosis. *Allbutt's System of Medicine*, London, 1909, vol. V, p. 299.

Calmette et Guérin (1905). Origine Intestinale de la tuberculose pulmonaire. *Ann. de l'Inst. Pasteur Paris*, vol. XIX, p. 601.

—— (1906). *Ibid.* vol. XX, pp. 353 and 609.

Calmette, Van Steenberghe and Grysez (1906). Sur l'anthracose pulmonaire d'origine intestinale. *Comp. Rend Soc. de Biol. Paris*, vol. II, p. 548.

Calmette (1913). *Les Voies d'Infection Tuberculeuse.* Masson et Cie, Paris.

Cobbett (1910). The Portals of Entry of Tubercle Bacilli which cause Phthisis. *Journ. of Pathol. and Bacteriol.* vol. XIV, p. 563.

—— (1911). The Portals of Entry in Phthisis. *Proc. Roy. Soc. of Med.*

Cobbett and Graham-Smith (1911). The Pathology of " Grouse Disease." *The Grouse in Health and Disease*, Smith, Elder & Co. p. 273.

—— (1911). The Passage of Bacteria from the Mouth to the Lung. *Proc. Camb. Phil. Soc.* vol. XVI, Pt. II, p. 126.

Dieterlen (1908). Beitrag zur Frage der Infectionswege. *Tuberkul. Arbeit. a. d. Kaiserl. Gesundheitsamte*, Berlin, Heft 9, p. 93.

von Dungern and Smidt. Ueber die Wirkung der Tuberkelbazillenstämme des Menschen und des Rindes auf Anthrapoïde Affen. *Arbeit. a. d. Kaiserl. Gesundheitsamte*, Berlin, vol. XXII, p. 570.

Eastwood and F. Griffith (1914). The Incidence and Bacteriological Characteristics of Tuberculous Infection in Children. *Rep. to the Loc. Govt. Board on Public Health and Medical Subjects*, N.S. No. 88, p. 1.

Escherich and Pfaundler (1903). Article on *B. coli* in Kolle and Wassermann's *Handbuch der pathogenen Microorganismen.* (Discusses the penetrability of the gut wall by *B. coli* during the moments of death and immediately after.)

Ficker, M. (1905). Ueber die Keimdichte der normalen Schleimhaut des Intestinaltractus. *Archiv f. Hyg.* vol. LII, p. 179.

Ficker, M. (1905). Ueber die Aufnahme von Bakterien durch den Respirationsapparat. *Ibid.* vol. LIII, p. 50.
—— Ueber den Einfluss des Hungers auf die Bakteriendurchlässigkeit des Intestinaltractus. *Ibid.* vol. LIV, p. 354.
Findel (1907). Vergleichende Untersuchungen über Inhalations- und Fütterungstuberkulose. *Zeitsch. f. Hyg.* vol. LVII, p. 104.
Findlay (1911). Ueber den Ursprung der Anthracose der Lungen. *Arbeiten zum Zehnjährigen Bestehen des Kinderasyls der Stadt,* Berlin.
Ford (1900). The Bacteriology of Normal Organs. *Trans. Assoc. Amer. Phys.* vol. XV, p. 389.
Freeman, R. G. (1905). Infantile Tuberculosis. Its Portal of Entry, etc. *Medical News,* May, 1905.
Gaffky (1907). Zur Frage der Infectionswege der Tuberkulose. *Tuberculosis,* vol. VI.
Gebhardt (1890). Experimentelle Untersuchungen über den Einfluss der Verdünnung auf die Wirksamkeit des tuberkulösen Giftes. *Virchow's Archiv,* vol. 119, p. 127.
Gotschlich (1903). Article in Kolle and Wassermann's *Handbuch der pathogenen Microorganismen,* vol. I, p. 132. (Discusses the portals of entry in infections in general.)
Griffith, A. S. (1907). *Roy. Comm. Tub. Int. Rep.* vol. I.
—— (1911). *Ibid. Final Rep.* vol. I.
—— (1914). The occurrence and distribution of Tuberculous Infection in Children. *Loc. Govt. Rep. on Public Health and Medical Subjects,* N.S. No. 88, p. 105.
Hartl and Herrmann (1905). Zur Inhalation zerstäubter bakterienhaltiger Flüssigkeit. *Wien. klin. Wochenschr.* vol. XVIII, p. 798.
Heymann (1908). Versuche an Meerschweinchen über die Aufnahme inhalierter Tuberkelbazillen in die Lunge. *Zeitsch. f. Hyg.* vol. LX, p. 490.
Koch, R. (1902). *Trans. Brit. Cong. Tubercul. London,* vol. I, p. 23.
Kossel, Weber and Heuss (1905). Vergleichende Untersuchungen über Tuberkelbazillen verschiedener Herkunft. No. 2. *Tub. Arbeit. a. d. Kaiserl. Gesundheitsamte,* Berlin, Heft 3, p. 40.
Kuss and Lobstein (1907). Passage de poussières insolubles à travers l'intestine. *Comp. Rend. de la Soc. de Biol.* vol. I, p. 139.
McFadyean (1910). What is the Common Method of Infection in Tuberculosis? *Journ. Comp. Pathol. and Therap.* vol. XXIII, pp. 239 and 289.
Macfarlane Walker (1913). The Paths of Infection in Genito-urinary Tuberculosis. *Lancet,* vol. 184, Feb. p. 435.
Neisser (1896). Ueber die Durchgängigkeit der Darmwand. *Zeitsch. f. Hyg.* vol. XXII, p. 12.
Nenninger (1898). Ueber das Eindringen von Bakterien in die Lungen durch Einathmung von Tröpfchen und Staub. *Zeitsch. f. Hyg* vol. XXXVIII, p. 94.

184   PORTALS OF INFECTION (2)   [CH.

Nicholls (1904). A Simple Method of Demonstrating the Presence of Bacteria in the Mesentery of Normal Animals. *Journ. Med. Res. Boston, U.S.A.* vol. XI, p. 455.

Nieuwenhuyse (1907). On the Origin of Pulmonary Anthracosis. Refer. in *Bull. de l'Inst. Past.* vol. V, p. 472.

Nocard (1895). Influence des repas sur la pénétration des microbes dans le sang. *La Sem. Méd. Paris*, p. 63.

—— (1898). Sur les Relations qui existent entre la Tuberculose Humaine et la Tuberculose Aviaire. *Ann. de l'Inst. Past.* vol. XII, p. 561.

Ochlecker (1907). Untersuchungen über chirurgische Tuberkulosen. *Tub. Arbeit. a. d. Kaiserl. Gesundheitsamte*, Berlin, Heft 6, p. 88.

Oliver (1912). Dust and Fume. *Lancet*, II, p. 870.

Paul (1902). Ueber die Bedingungen des Eindringens der Bakterien der Inspirationsluft in die Lungen. *Zeitsch. f. Hyg.* vol. X, p. 468.

Porcher and Desoubry (1895). De la présence de microbes dans le chyle normal chez le chien. *Compt. Rend. Soc. de Biol. Paris*, pp. 101 and 344.

Preyss (1891). Ueber den Einfluss der Verdünnung und der künstlich erzeugten Disposition auf die Wirkung des inhalierten Tuberculösen Giftes. *Münch. med. Wochenschr.* Nos. 24 and 25, pp. 418 and 440.

Ravenel (1903). The Passage of Tubercle Bacilli through the Normal Intestinal Wall. *Journ. Med. Res.* vol. X, p. 460.

Ravenel and Reichel (1908). Tuberculous Infection through the Alimentary Canal. *Ibid.* vol. XVIII, p. 1.

Reichenbach (1909). Experimentelle Untersuchungen über die Eintrittswege des Tuberkelbacillus. *Zeitsch. f. Hyg.* vol. LX, p. 446.

Remlinger (1907). Sur la pathogénie de l'anthracose pulmonaire. *Comp. Rend. de la Soc. de Biol.* p. 202.

Rothe (1911). Untersuchungen über Tuberkulose Infection in Kindersalter. *Veröff. d. R. Koch Stiftung z. Bekämpfung der Tuberkul.*

Shennan (1909). Tuberculosis in Children, with Special Reference to Tuberculosis of Lymph Glands, and its importance in the Invasion and Dissemination of the Disease. *Lancet*, I, No. 5.

Still (1899). Observations on the Morbid Anatomy of Tuberculosis in Childhood. *Brit. Med. Journ.* II, p. 455.

Symes and Fisher (1904). An Enquiry into the Primary Seat of Infection in 500 Cases of Death from Tuberculosis. *Brit. Med. Journ.* I, p. 884.

Ungermann (1912). Untersuchungen über die Tuberkulose Infection der Lymphdrüsen in Kindersalter. Ein Beitrag zur Frage der Infectionswege, etc. *Tub. Arbeit. a. d. Kaiserl. Gesundheitsamte*, Berlin, Heft 12, p. 109.

Vallée (1905). Sur la Pathogénie de la Tuberculose. *Comp. Rend. Soc. de Biol. Paris*, vol. I, p. 568.

Van Steenberghe and Grysez (1905). Sur l'origine intestinale de l'Anthracose Pulmonaire. *Ann. de l'Inst. Past.* vol. XIX, p. 787.

Vincent (1907). Passage des poussières insolubles à travers la muqueuse intestinale. *Comp. Rend. Soc. de Biol.* vol. I, p. 664.

Walsham (1903). *The Channels of Infection in Tuberculosis.* Weber-Parkes Prize Essay. Bale and Danielson.

Weber and Titze (1910). Inhalations- und Fütterungs-versuche mit Perlsuchtbazillen an Rindern. Bestimmung der geringsten zur Infection notwendigen Bazillenmenge. *Tub. Arbeit. a. d. Kaiserl. Gesundheitsamte,* Berlin, Heft 10, p. 146.

Whitla (1908). The Etiology of Pulmonary Tuberculosis. The Cavendish Lecture. *Brit. Med. Journ.* II, p. 61.

Williams, C. Th. (1909). On the Infection of Consumption. *Brit. Med. Journ.* II, p. 433.

Woodhead (1894). The Channels of Infection in Tuberculosis. *Lancet,* II, p. 957.

CHAPTER X

THE RELATION BETWEEN ANIMAL AND HUMAN TUBERCULOSIS

I. *Early Investigations.*

The first suggestion that human tuberculosis differs etiologically from that which affects the lower animals is to be found in the writings of Villemin, 1868. In his *Études sur la Tuberculose* occurs this passage " We must remark that none of our rabbits inoculated with human tubercle have presented a tuberculization so rapid and generalized as that which we have obtained with material from the cow. At first we were inclined to regard this as fortuitous, but subsequent experiments led us to suppose that the tubercle of the bovine race inoculated into rabbits possesses a much greater activity than that obtained from man. It may be supposed that, like all virulent matter, the tuberculous matter is the more virulent the more the affinity of the animal supplying the virus and the animal receiving it[1]." Thus was foreshadowed half a century ago the

---

[1] *Études sur la Tuberculose,* p. 538.

recognition of the human and bovine types of tubercle-bacillus.

This statement, which seems to us, in the light of recently acquired knowledge, so significant, was completely overlooked at the time—though several other investigators made somewhat similar observations—and was even forgotten by Koch when he announced the discovery of the tubercle bacillus.

Koch, in 1884, succeeded in cultivating this organism not only from tuberculous lesions in man, but from those in many of the lower animals also, and, though he made numerous inoculation experiments on rabbits as well as on other animals, he does not seem to have noticed what Villemin observed. So similar did the various strains of bacilli isolated from these sources appear to him, and so like to one another the lesions caused by their inoculation into different kinds of animals, that he concluded that human and bovine tuberculosis were identical diseases[1]. At first he was inclined to regard avian tuberculosis

[1] See "The Etiology of Tuberculosis," Eng. trans., in *Microparasites in Disease*, New. Syd. Soc. 1886, p. 197. In his earliest publication concerning the etiology of tuberculosis Koch had stated that "Bovine tuberculosis is identical with that of man, and is therefore a disease transferable to man. It must consequently be treated in the same manner as other infectious diseases that are transferable from animal to man. Whether the danger resulting from the consumption of meat and milk from tuberculous cattle be ever so great, or ever so small, there is no doubt that it must be avoided." "Die Ätiologie der Tuberculose," *Berl. Klin. Wochenschr.* 1882, No. 5. Also in *Gesamte Werke von Robert Koch*, Georg Thienne, Leipzig, vol. 1, p. 445.

It is curious that Koch did not notice either the cultural or pathogenetic differences between human and bovine tubercle bacilli, for he appears to have been on the look out for such differences. He says that he examined a large number of cultures because "it seemed not improbable that, though the bacilli from various forms of tuberculosis, *perlsucht*, lupus, phthisis, etc., presented no difference microscopically, yet that in culture differences might become apparent between bacilli from different sources. But although I devoted the greatest attention to this point I could find nothing of the kind " (Eng. trans. p. 150). Again (p. 164), he says, " I was not able to distinguish any difference in the effect of inoculation with material derived from varieties of the tuberculous process, as miliary tuberculosis, phthisis, scrofula, fungus inflammation of joints, lupus, *perlsucht* and other forms of animal tuberculosis. So that in this respect also the different forms of tuberculosis resemble each other exactly." It is extraordinary that so acute an observer should have missed the striking difference in the effect of injecting the human and bovine tuberculosis virus respectively into the rabbit and cat, especially in such an experiment on the latter as is reported on p. 177 of the English translation.

as identical with these. He had not at the time been able to obtain cultures from fowls for want of fresh material, but as all other kinds of tuberculosis had yielded similar bacilli, and those of fowl tuberculosis, in their appearance and behaviour towards anilin dyes, completely agreed with them, he believed himself, in spite of gaps in the evidence, to be in a position to speak of the identity of tuberculosis in different species of animals. But he corrected his position with regard to avian tuberculosis quickly when he had an opportunity of becoming acquainted with cultures of tubercle bacilli obtained from birds. For soon after the discovery of the tubercle bacillus by Koch the study of the bacteriology of tuberculosis was taken up in Paris by Nocard and Roux, who obtained from a pheasant a strain of tubercle bacilli which differed culturally and pathogenetically from the bacilli which Koch had obtained from mammals. Koch himself received a culture of this strain, sent him by the French observers, and at once recognized that the differences between it and mammalian tubercle bacilli were fundamental; and he became convinced that the fowl-tubercle bacillus belongs to a species distinct from, though closely related to, that of mammals[1].

About the same time the Italian observers Rivolta and Maffucci had come to the same conclusion, and this view continued to gain adherents. But it was not at once accepted universally, and for a time those who took an active part in the study of the etiology of tuberculosis were divided into two opposing parties, one upholding the unity, and the other the duality of that disease[2].

Meanwhile, except for a single dissenting voice in England, the identity of the tuberculosis of man with that of the lower mammals was not questioned for many years.

The one dissenting voice was that of Klein (1883) who, in the year following the announcement of the discovery of the tubercle bacillus, pointed out that Koch's work had not clearly established the identity of human and bovine tuberculosis. Klein himself had noticed differences in form and arrangement

---

[1] See Weber and Bofinger, *loc. cit.* p. 86.
[2] See Koch and Rabinowitsch, *loc. cit.* p. 247.

of the bacilli found in human and bovine lesions, and in the relative numbers of these micro-organisms found in them respectively.

At his suggestion Heneage Gibbes made comparative inoculation experiments on small animals with tuberculous material taken from man and the ox, with the consequence that, for the second time, the important fact was brought to light that, while in the guinea-pig the disease could be reproduced by inoculating material from either of these sources, in the rabbit " no tuberculosis was produced when human tuberculous matter full of tubercle bacilli was injected, while the virus from the cow produced a very high degree of general tuberculosis."

Feeding experiments, carried out during the following year, confirmed the relative insusceptibility of the rabbit to human and its susceptibility to bovine tuberculosis.

From these experiments Klein concluded that " the tuberculous virus derived from the human subject is not exactly the same as that derived from the tubercles of the cow[1]."

Klein's work attracted little or no attention at the time. But it is remarkable in that it demonstrated, so very early, an important fact the significance of which was destined to be overlooked for many years, and which, followed up comparatively recently, has revolutionized the views held as to the relationship of animal and human tuberculosis.

In 1895 Sidney Martin, carrying out investigations for the Royal Commission on Tuberculosis appointed in the previous year, observed, as indeed others, for example Chauveau, Günther and Harms and Bollinger, had done before, differences in the severity of the action of human and bovine tubercle bacilli on the ox. In the course of his researches he fed ten calves, some with sputum, and others with an emulsion of the tuberculous udder of a cow. The former group developed only some slight tuberculosis of the intestines spreading in one case to the mesenteric glands, while of the latter, fed with the bovine material, all suffered from more or less widespread tuberculosis. Martin justly remarked that " it is evident that in the case of tuberculous sputum we are dealing with material

[1] 1883, 13th Rep. Loc. Gov. Bd. p. 185.

which is less infective to calves than bovine tuberculous material." But he seems to have missed the full significance of this, and to have regarded the difference as merely a difference in degree of virulence, for he adds " this lessened infectivity is possibly not merely a question of dosage, but one of diminished activity of the tubercle bacilli in sputum as compared with its activity in the tuberculous lesions of the cow[1]."

The next step towards the differentiation of human and bovine tuberculosis was taken in the United States in the following year when Theobald Smith (1896) published a comparative investigation of two strains of tubercle bacilli, one from a bovine source, and the other from a pet animal[2] believed to have contracted tuberculosis from its tuberculous master. In these researches, which mark the commencement of the modern views on the relationship between the bacilli of human and animal tuberculosis, decided differences in the virulence for the ox and rabbit of the two strains of bacilli, one presumably human, the other certainly bovine, came to light, and morphological peculiarities also were described.

Two years later (1898) Smith recorded the results of a thorough investigation of fifteen additional strains of tubercle bacilli[3] which led him to suggest the existence of " a distinctively

---

[1] *Loc. Gov. Bd. Reports*, 1895, p. 19. For particulars of the experiments referred to see table on p. 20.

[2] A coati, or *Nasua narica*, an animal described by Smith as belonging to the bear tribe.

[3] These included seven from sputum, five from the ox, and one each from the cat, horse and pig.

Smith, who drew his conclusions with great moderation, modestly said he had " presented nothing but problems to be solved, and doubts to be entertained " (1898, p. 511); but in reality he had laid a solid foundation upon which the modern views on this subject came to be built. His researches caused the problem to be followed up in America by a number of observers, among whom were Ravenel, Dinwiddie, Frothingham, Pearson and Lartigan, whose work tended on the whole to support the distinction tentatively drawn by Smith between the human and the bovine types of tubercle bacilli, and there can be little doubt that they were the cause of Koch's returning to the subject in 1901.

Some of these observers isolated strains of bovine tubercle bacilli from children (Ravenel, Dinwiddie, Lartigan), and Vagedes, in Germany, working under Koch's direction obtained a strain of bacilli from a case of human tuberculosis which in Smith's opinion was a bovine bacillus (*Journ. of Med. Research*, vol. XIII. 1904-5, p. 295).

human or sputum, and a bovine variety of tubercle bacillus "
while he continued to recognize the close relationship between
these varieties.

But on the whole little heed was paid to Smith's
discovery, and for some years more the general belief in
the identity of human and bovine tuberculosis remained
undisturbed, or, at most, it was thought that tubercle bacilli
from the ox were a little more virulent than those from
man. Consequently the scientific world was ill-prepared for
Koch's revolutionary statement, made in London in 1901
at the British Congress on Tuberculosis, to the effect that
"human tuberculosis differs from bovine and cannot be
transmitted to cattle[1]."

This conclusion was based upon inoculation experiments—
briefly reported to the Congress but fully described later[2]—
which he had been making during the preceding two years,
in conjunction with Schütz, upon cattle and swine with different
kinds of tubercular material. It was also supported by certain
observations gathered from the older literature of the subject,
in which it is recorded that a number of experimenters (among
whom were Chauveau, Günther and Harms and Bollinger)
had attempted to infect calves, pigs or goats by feeding them
with tuberculous material of various kinds, with the result
that animals which ingested tuberculous milk or pieces of the
lungs of tuberculous cattle always fell ill of tuberculosis, while
those which received tuberculous material from a human source
did not.

But Koch not only drew from these experiments the conclusion that human tuberculosis differs from bovine and cannot
be transmitted to cattle—a conclusion which, if we understand
by "human tuberculosis" that kind of tuberculosis which
is present in an overwhelming majority of the cases which
occur in man, has since been fully confirmed—but he went on to
deny that bovine tuberculosis is transmissible to man, or, he said,
is at least so rarely transmitted to him that the danger may be

---

[1] *Transact. Brit. Cong. on Tuberculosis* (1901), London, vol. I, p. 29.

[2] Koch and Schütz, *Archiv f. wissenschaftliche u. praktische Tierheilkunde,*
1902, Nos. 1 and 2.

safely ignored[1]. In this he was, doubtless, in error, as the very extensive researches carried out since have amply shown.

It will be observed that Koch went much further than Smith and his followers in America who, while distinguishing clearly between the human and bovine types of tubercle bacilli, never denied that the latter was pathogenic for man.

The announcement of the distinction between bovine and human tuberculosis, and the assertion that the latter is not transmissible to man, provoked at the time a storm of opposition, especially among those who were striving, in the interest of human public health, to eradicate tuberculosis from among cattle.. Nocard, Bang, Woodhead, McFadyean, Crookshank and Delépine all more or less strongly opposed Koch at the Congress. Nocard admitted that there was a tendency to exaggerate the danger of bovine tuberculosis to man, and he was glad that Koch had checked this movement. But he feared lest the reaction might go too far. " Bovine tuberculosis," he said, " plays a very secondary part in human tuberculosis, but as long as this danger exists at all it cannot be suppressed by denying it[2]."

Lord Lister, who presided on the occasion of this address, at once grasped with great precision both the strength and the weakness of Koch's position, and pointed out that, while the evidence which Koch had brought forward that human tuberculosis cannot be communicated to the bovine species was " exceedingly conclusive," the converse proposition that bovine tuberculosis is incapable of development in man was a totally different one ; it did not follow necessarily from the first, and the evidence of its truth which had been brought forward did not seem to him very conclusive[3].

---

[1] " Though the important question whether man is susceptible to bovine tuberculosis at all is not yet absolutely decided, and will not admit of absolute decision to-day or to-morrow, one is nevertheless already at liberty to say, that if such a susceptibility really exists, the infection of human beings is a very rare occurrence. I should estimate the extent of infection by the milk and flesh of tuberculous cattle, and the butter made from their milk, as hardly greater than that of hereditary transmission, and I therefore do not deem it advisable to take any measures against it " (Koch, *Trans. of the Congress*, vol. I, p. 30).

[2] *loc. cit.* p. 37.   [3] *loc. cit.* pp. 35, 36.

In drawing his conclusion concerning the transmissibility of bovine tuberculosis to man Koch was undoubtedly influenced by the alleged rarity of primary intestinal tuberculosis in Germany. He argued that if bovine tuberculosis is transmitted to man it must be through the tubercle bacilli contained in milk and butter, it must, in fact, in man be a food infection, and therefore should cause intestinal tuberculosis[1]. But cases of primary intestinal tuberculosis were rare; "Among 933 cases of tuberculosis of children at the Emperor and Empress Frederick's Hospital for Children (in Berlin) Baginsky never found tuberculosis of the intestine without simultaneous disease of the lungs and the bronchial glands"; and Biedert had observed only 16 cases of this kind among 3104 post-mortems on tuberculous children; consequently infection with bovine tubercle bacilli must be rare also[2]. He does not seem to have recognized the fact, now generally admitted, that tubercle bacilli may enter through the mucous membrane of the intestine, or of some other part of the alimentary tract, and set up primary tuberculosis in the lymphatic glands connected therewith without causing any visible lesions at the point of their entry, but producing in the glands themselves abundant evidence to indicate the route by which they had travelled and the surface through which they had penetrated.

It would be difficult to exaggerate the effect of Koch's announcement. It at once completely paralyzed all the many efforts which were then being made in the interest of human public health to stamp out tuberculosis from among the herds of cattle; and, on the other hand, it is probable that no single incident has ever done so much to stimulate experimental investigation. Great Britain appointed a Royal Commission which carried out on a liberal scale a long series of researches continued without interruption for nine years.

Equally thorough investigations were undertaken by the

---

[1] "That a case of tuberculosis has been caused by alimenta can be assumed with certainty only when the intestine suffers first...but such cases are extremely rare" (Koch, *loc. cit.* p. 29).

[2] *loc. cit.* p. 30.

Gesundheitsamt in Berlin, and elsewhere in Germany many valuable investigations were made.

In the United States, at Harvard University, Theobald Smith continued his researches, while for the Bureau of Animal Industry at Washington Mohler and Washburn, and for the Public Health Department of the City of New York Park, Krumwiede and others went to work on the problem of animal and human tuberculosis.

In France, Italy, Denmark, Holland, Sweden and Japan, important researches were undertaken.

The collective result of these investigations has been an enormous advance in the knowledge of tuberculosis, the consideration of which in detail will occupy many pages of the succeeding chapters. Meanwhile it may be permissible to anticipate a little in order to see to what extent the position taken up by Koch at the Congress of 1901 has been justified, and to what extent corrected.

On the one hand it has been proved conclusively that Koch was right in his contention that " human tuberculosis differs from bovine "—that is to say, if we understand by " human tuberculosis " the result of infection with that type of tubercle bacillus which is found in the overwhelming majority of cases of tuberculosis in man. Human tuberculosis, in this sense, cannot be transmitted to cattle.

On the other hand it has now become certain that Koch underestimated very greatly the danger of tuberculosis being transmitted from cattle to man. Many cases of tuberculosis in the human subject have since been proved conclusively to be caused by the bovine tubercle bacillus; and it cannot be doubted that these cases, with perhaps a rare exception here and there, have been derived directly from the cow. Such cases may now be regarded as instances of bovine tuberculosis occurring in man. But their number is, almost certainly, small compared with the great mass of cases caused by the human type of tubercle bacillus. And there is good reason to believe that they are mainly, if not almost entirely, confined to young children. What exactly is the proportion of bovine tuberculosis to the commoner kind of tuberculous infection in man it is impossible at present to say; in a subsequent chapter a rough estimate, based on such evidence as is available, will be given[1]. But the subject is complicated by the fact that some recent researches would seem to indicate that this proportion may be very different in different places. Of one thing, however, we may be sure : bovine tuberculosis is an insignificant cause of death in those who have passed the age of childhood[2].

Koch, therefore, while his characteristic impetuosity undoubtedly led him to overstate his case, is justified in the general object of his announcement, which was to turn the attention of public authorities from a too exclusive concentration on the animal sources of infection, the importance of which was being overestimated at the time, and to focus them once more on the phthisical human being, the one and only great source of human tuberculosis.

REFERENCES. VI

(Chapter x)

*The Relationship of Animal and Human Tuberculosis.
Early Investigations.*

Villemin (1868). *Études sur la Tuberculose ; preuves rationnelles et expérimentales de sa spécificité et de son inoculabilité.* Paris.
Koch (1882). Die Ätiologie der Tuberkulose. *Berl. klin. Wochenschr.* p. 221.
Koch (1884). Die Ätiologie der Tuberkulose. *Mitteilungen aus dem Gesundheitsamte,* vol. II, 1884. English translation by Stanley Boyd in *Recent Essays on Bacteria in Relation to Disease,* 1886, p. 67. New Sydenham Society.

[1] See p. 659. It is there estimated at six per cent.
[2] " Bovine tuberculosis is practically a negligible factor in adults.... In young children it becomes a menace to life, and causes from 6⅓ to 10 per cent. of the total fatalities from this disease." Park and Krumwiede, 1911, *Collected Studies from the Research Laboratory Dep. of Health,* City of New York, p. 88.

Speaking of the cases investigated by them the Royal Commission stated that " so far as these 128 cases have been examples of tuberculosis in the adult, and especially when they have been pulmonary tuberculosis, the lesions of the disease where fatal have been referable with few exceptions to human bacilli....Of young children dying from primary abdominal tuberculosis the fatal lesions could in nearly one half of the cases be referred to the bovine bacillus, and to that type alone." *R. C. T. Final Report,* 1911, p. 39.

Klein and Gibbes (1883). 13*th Rep. Loc. Gov. Bd.* p. 177.
—— (1884). 14*th Rep. Loc. Gov. Bd.* p. 169.
Nocard (1885). Recherches expérimentales sur la tuberculose des oiseaux; Culture du Bacille. *Compt. rendu de la Soc. de Biologie,* p. 601.
Nocard and Roux (1887). Sur la culture du bacille de la Tuberculose. *Annales de l'Institut Pasteur,* p. 19.
Yersin (1888). Étude sur le développement du tubercle expérimentale. *Annales de l'Institut Pasteur,* p. 245.
Rivolta (1889). Sulla tuberculosi degli uccelli. *Giorn. di Anatomia e Fisiologia,* fasc. I, p. 22. *Baumgarten's Jahresbericht,* 1899, p. 313.
Maffucci (1890). Contribuzione all' etiologia della tuberculosi (tuberculosi dei gallinacci). *Riforma Medica.*
—— (1892). Die Hühnertuberculose. *Zeitschr. für Hygiene, etc.* vol. XI, p. 445.
Martin, Sidney (1895). *Report of the Second Royal Commission on Tuberculosis* (1894), Appendix, Inquiry No. II, p. 9.
Smith, Theobald (1895-6). Two Varieties of Tubercle Bacilli from Mammals. *Ann. Rep. U.S. Bureau of Animal Industry,* p. 149. Also in *Transactions of Assoc. of American Physicians,* vol. XI, p. 76.
—— (1898). A Comparative Study of Bovine Tubercle Bacilli and of Human Tubercle Bacilli from Sputum. *Journ. of Experimental Medicine,* vol. III, p. 451.
Vagedes (1898). Experimentelle Prüfung der Virulenz von Tuberkelbazillen. *Zeitschr. f. Hygiene,* vol. XXVIII, p. 276.
Dinwiddie (1899). The Relative Virulence for the domestic animals of human and bovine tubercle. *The Veterinarian,* vol. LXXII, p. 53.
—— (1899). *Bulletin of the Arkansas Experimental Station,* No. 57. Quoted by Ravenel. See *Trans. Brit. Cong. on Tuberculosis,* 1902, vol. III, p. 553.
Koch (1901). Address to the British Congress on Tuberculosis, 1901. *Trans. Brit. Cong. on Tub.* (Clowes and Sons, 1902), vol. I, p. 23.
Koch and Schütz (1902). Menschliche Tuberkulose und Rindertuberculose. *Archiv für wissenschaftliche und praktische Tierheilkunde,* Nos. I and 2.
Lartigan (1901). *Journal of Medical Research,* vol. VI, p. 156.
Ravenel (1901 and 1902). The Intercommunicability of Human and Bovine Tuberculosis. *Univ. of Penn. Med. Bull.*
—— (1901). The Comparative virulence of the tubercle bacillus from human and bovine sources. *Trans. Brit. Cong. on Tuberculosis.* vol. III, p. 552.
Smith, Th. (1902). The Relation between Bovine and Human Tuberculosis. *Medical News,* vol. LXXX.
—— (1903). Studies in Mammalian Tubercle Bacilli. Description of a bovine bacillus from the human body. *Transact. Assoc. of American Physicians.* Also in *Journ. of Med. Research,* vol. XIII, p. 253.

Smith, Th. (1904). A Study of the Tubercle Bacilli Isolated from Three Cases of Tuberculosis of the Mesentèric Lymph Nodes (all belonged to the human type). *American Journal of Medical Science*, 1904.

Weber (1912). Zur Tuberkulose des Menschen und der Tiere. *Centralb. f. Bakteriol. etc.* Abt. 1, vol. LXIV, p. 243.

For a summary of the literature see :

Kossel, Weber and Heuss (1904). Vergleichende Untersuchungen über Tuberkelbazillen verschiedener Herkunft. *Tuberkel. Arbeiten a. d. Kaiserl. Gesundheitsamte*, Heft 1, p. 1. Also Weber and Bofinger. Die Hühnertuberculose, in the same volume, p. 83. See also Park and Krumwiede. The relative importance of bovine and human types of tubercle bacilli in the different forms of human tuberculosis. *Journal of Medical Research*, 1910, vol. XXIII, p. 205.

CHAPTER XI

THE RELATION BETWEEN ANIMAL AND HUMAN TUBERCULOSIS (*continued*)

II. *The Three Types of Tubercle Bacilli.*

Morphological and Bio-chemical Characters. Acid-fastness. Variation in length. Branched forms.

Cultural Characters. Eugonic and Dysgonic Strains. Adaptation to conditions of saprophytic life. Growth of the three types on various media.

Pathogenicity. The existence of specific differences and not mere variations of virulence.

Atypical Strains. Mixtures of Types, Attenuated Varieties, Transitional Forms.

Some Practical points concerning the Cultivation of Tubercle Bacilli. The Choice of culture media for primary cultures. The Antiformin method of raising cultures from sputum. The Length of Life of Cultures.

As the result mainly of the investigations of Theobald Smith, of Koch and Schütz, and of the researches which have been carried out since in response to Koch's announcement of 1901, three types of tubercle bacilli have come to light. These are named, after the hosts in which they commonly occur, *the human, the bovine* and *the avian types*[1].

That the three types exist there can be no doubt ; cultural differences are, as a rule, evident ; and there are well-marked distinctions of virulence for certain species of animals. On the other hand the resemblances are striking, and there can be no doubt that the types are nearly related. So much is admitted on all sides. But while some regard the types as clearly distinct and stable, others hold that they merge into one another, and find transitional forms[2]; and there are not wanting those who believe that, under favourable circumstances, a strain of a given type may be converted into one of another type.

Stability of type characters is the one condition upon which the existence of species among bacteria can be established, and until the vexed question of the stability of the three kinds of tubercle bacilli shall have been settled it is not admissible to apply to them any term of precise meaning such as "species,"

[1] A fourth type is sometimes recognized, and spoken of as the fish-tubercle bacillus, or, since it has been found in other of the lower vertebrates, as the tubercle bacillus of cold-blooded animals (Kaltblütertuberkelbazillus). It doubtless possesses some degree of pathogenic power, and it seems capable of producing tubercles in frogs when injected in sufficient quantity, but it is to be found in many cold-blooded animals which appear to be perfectly healthy, and it is by no means certain that the gross lesions which have sometimes been seen associated with it are really the result of its activity, and not of that of some other parasite. (See p. 302.)

[2] Thus, for example, Fibiger and Jensen, who, after giving in detail the conclusions which they drew from their extensive researches, sum up with reference to mammalian bacilli as follows : "There are therefore no characteristics of which one can say that they are absolutely distinctive of the alleged types, and which may serve as trustworthy diagnostic criteria. The unsoundness of the classification into two sharply opposed types comes out clearly when one compares a series of strains with respect to their various properties. One must, indeed, admit that the majority of strains isolated from the ox show those characters which are held to distinguish the bovine type, and also that the majority of strains isolated from human sputum may be brought, without much straining, within the conception of the human type ; there remain however certain strains which must be looked upon as intermediate because they possess one or more characters of the human type, and others of the bovine type." They then give nine examples of such intermediate strains. (*Berl. med. Wochenschr.* 1908, No. 45, p. 2031.)

"sub-species," or "varieties"; and one must be content, at least for the present, to speak of them as "types," an expression which does not connote any definite commitment as to the exact degree of relationship[1].

Morphological and Bio-chemical Characters.

General considerations. Tubercle bacilli are small motionless rods, rather irregular in outline, more or less segmented, and often showing polar bodies. They possess no flagella, and form no spores—or at least none of the usual type. They are probably related nearly to a number of other species which resemble them more or less closely in morphological, bio-chemical and cultural, and to a very slight degree in pathogenetic, properties. Since all these species have certain peculiarities of chemical composition, which render them, when once they are stained, more or less incapable of being decolorized by moderately strong acids—a treatment which instantly removes the colour from all other stained bacteria—they have been placed together in a class conveniently named the acid-fast group.

In their morphological characters tubercle bacilli, and other members of the acid-fast group, resemble the diphtheria bacillus and those other bacteria which constitute the so-called diphtheroid group. The following characters are common to all the bacteria placed in these two groups : The bacilli are somewhat irregular in·outline, more or less curved, and have rounded,

[1] These types of tubercle bacilli are not confined strictly to the hosts whose names they bear ; for, as we shall see, the human type of bacillus has been found in the monkey, the pig and the parrot, the bovine type in many other mammals besides the ox, and the avian type in the pig, the rabbit and the mouse, and possibly also in man ; nor is the susceptibility of a single species of animal necessarily limited to one type of bacillus, man, for example, as we shall see, being attacked both by the human and bovine types, and the pig, to a variable extent, by all three types. Nevertheless these names, human, bovine, and avian, as applied to the three types of tubercle bacilli, though perhaps not strictly accurate, are so firmly established by usage, and are on the whole so convenient, that they will probably continue to be employed.

It must be understood that when, in these pages, the terms *human, bovine,* or *avian* tubercle bacilli are mentioned, the type alone, and not the origin, is referred to.

and sometimes clubbed, ends. Irregular distribution, or segmentation, of the chromophil substance of the bacillus is usually a marked character, and polar bodies are often present. In both groups branching is sometimes, though rarely, seen.

This occasional branching has suggested a more distant relationship to the streptothrices, a view which is supported by the existence among these latter micro-organisms of acid-fast species.

In their manner of staining with anilin dyes the acid-fast bacteria differ from the diphtheroids, and from most of the streptothrices, in that they stain imperfectly and slowly with dyes which are successfully employed for staining other bacteria. Placed, for example, in Löffler's (alkaline) methylene blue for a few minutes tubercle bacilli remain almost unstained ; some individuals take up a little of the colour, but in none is the staining anything but very imperfect. If such staining, however, be prolonged for 24 hours or more, very fair results may be obtained. This was the method used by Koch when he first discovered the bacillus ; but it has given way to another, originally introduced by Ehrlich and since slightly modified, and this is now employed almost universally. It consists essentially in staining the bacilli for a few minutes in carbolfuchsin, or anilin-fuchsin, heated nearly to the boiling point. This powerful dye penetrates easily and quickly into the refractory bacilli, and when once the latter have taken up the colour they hold it firmly, so that the preparation may be washed freely in fairly strong solutions (20–30 %) of the mineral acids and also in alcohol, without losing the colour.

It must be added that there are degrees of acid-fastness among the members of the acid-fast group. The bacillus of leprosy is not so acid-fast as that of tubercle. Tubercle bacilli probably represent one extreme, and at the other are certain species of bacilli which are only acid-fast under certain conditions of culture. One of these the writer has isolated several times from cow's milk. This organism was acid-fast only when grown in the presence of fat (cream), and on ordinary media, such as nutrient agar, closely resembled the bacilli of the diphtheroid group. Such species form a true link between the acid-fast and the diphtheroid groups.

Morphological Characters of the Human and Bovine Types Compared. Tubercle bacilli of the mammalian types are very variable in length, being found sometimes as short as ·5 or ·75 μ, and at others attaining a length of 2 to 4 μ, or, according to Eastwood, 7 to 8 μ.

Forms as long or even much longer than this undoubtedly occur, but it is difficult to know whether we are dealing with single bacilli or with threads composed of a number of bacilli arranged end to end. Such threads sometimes occur in old potato cultures, and probably in those of the avian type more commonly than in those of the two mammalian types.

Too much has been made of the fact that bovine tubercle bacilli are shorter than human. There is, no doubt, some slight difference as a rule, but the longer forms of the bovine bacillus exceed in length the shorter forms of the human bacillus, and the difference on the whole is so small as to be of no practical value.

H. J. Hutchens, when working for the Royal Commission, made a series of very careful measurements of various strains of tubercle bacilli. The method consisted of measuring the length of 100 consecutive bacilli from a given source, care being taken to avoid, as far as possible, conscious or unconscious selection. The results were then set out graphically in order, a number of parallel lines being drawn at right angles to a common base, each line representing a single bacillus and being proportionate in length to that bacillus. In this way a number of graphic representations were obtained which could be readily compared with one another, and which possessed this advantage over numerical averages that they avoided the difficulty of deciding whether the long forms alluded to above should be treated each as a single bacillus or as a chain of several bacilli, for with the graphic method such forms could be included in the comparison or disregarded at will.

These diagrams are selected from a considerable number,

DIAGRAM VII.   *The Length of Human and Bovine Tubercle Bacilli under different Conditions of Growth.*

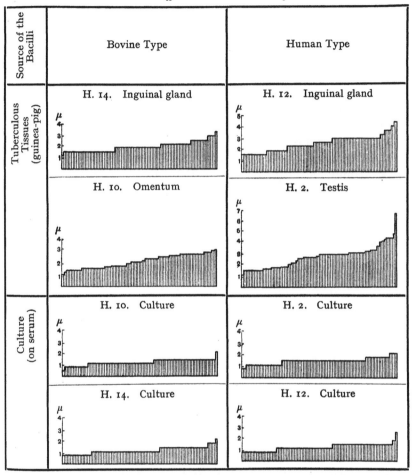

and are fair representations of differences and similarities which were constantly observed. They show clearly:

1. That tubercle bacilli whether they be of human or bovine type are much longer when they have grown in animal tissues than in artificial culture.

2. That tubercle bacilli of bovine and human type respectively differ very little in length when grown in pure culture on serum.

3. There is probably rather more difference between bovine and human bacilli when grown in animal tissues, but of this there is not sufficient evidence to make certain.

Other diagrams made on the same plan showed that both human and bovine tubercle bacilli when grown in broth culture are considerably longer than when grown on serum cultures, but not so long as when grown in animal tissues.

Morphological Characters of the Avian Type. Avian tubercle bacilli, though as a rule relatively short, are perhaps the most variable of the three types of tubercle bacilli, and quite long forms are seen, not uncommonly, both in the animal body and, sometimes, in cultures. In old cultures, for example on potato, extensive threads are, as has been said, sometimes seen. These are of two kinds, one indefinite in outline and staining badly, and the other thicker, extraordinarily sharply defined, and beautifully and regularly articulated. It is among such forms that the branched elements are seen. There can be no question that these represent true branching and not an appearance produced by the fortuitous arrangement of several bacilli lying in contiguity, for there is often a little thickening at the point where a branch leaves the parent stem, an appearance which could not possibly be simulated by two bacilli lying accidentally the one at an angle to the other, and moreover some of the branches appear as small buds. Sometimes the branched threads end in a slight club-like expansion.

Branched forms are said to occur in the two mammalian types of tubercle bacilli also, but they have never been seen by the writer.

Cultural Characters.

General considerations. Tubercle bacilli grow slowly. In primary cultures no growth is seen for, as a rule, nearly a fortnight, and even in the case of strains which have been growing on artificial media for a long time the first visible signs of multiplication do not appear for several days after sowing a subculture.

But though the growth of tubercle bacilli is slow, compared with that of other bacteria, it is long continued, and cultures which are doing well produce eventually a considerable mass of bacilli which forms a layer of some thickness.

But this is not the case with primary cultures. When first

isolated from animal tissues and planted on artificial media tubercle bacilli grow not only slowly, but with difficulty ; usually some of the attempted cultures fail altogether, and in others multiplication may cease after the formation of a few isolated colonies. At times, when the medium proves to be in particularly good condition, growth may proceed further, and raised colonies of some size develop, but even then they remain discrete[1].

On many of the usual culture media on which they afterwards do well tubercle bacilli in primary culture do not grow at all. Some preliminary adaptation on substances, such as egg or serum, which resemble as closely as may be the substance of the living body being necessary before these hitherto parasitic bacteria can be got to thrive on agar, potato, or broth[2].

Adaptation to new conditions of life outside the living animal body proceeds slowly, and it is not, as a rule, until a number of subcultures have been grown in a succession extending over many weeks that the maximum degree of luxuriance of which a given strain is capable is attained.

Eugonic and Dysgonic Strains. Now while this slowly-progressing adaptation to the conditions of a saprophytic existence occurs with all tubercle bacilli, it differs greatly in degree with the different types, and even to some extent with different strains of any one type. So much is this the case that one strain, after a few months, may grow so luxuriantly that a thick wrinkled cream-coloured layer is formed on glycerin-agar, a heaped-up nodular growth on glycerin-potato, and a continuous crêpe-like pellicle on glycerin-broth (a pellicle which soon covers the whole surface of the fluid, and even commences to climb up the sides of the vessel which contains it), while another will barely grow at all on such media, and on glycerin-broth forms at best only a delicate lace-like film or network which ceases to grow when it has covered a small portion of the surface.

Strains of tubercle bacilli which, after a reasonable period

---

[1] See photographs by A. S. Griffith n vol. I of the *Final Report Roy. Comm. on Tub.* 1911, p. 537, Primary Cultures on Egg medium.

[2] Primary cultures have been raised on glycerin-potato, but this method is difficult and uncertain, and is quite unsuited to the bovine type.

of repeated subcultivation on artificial media allowed for the earlier stages of adaptation, still grow feebly have been well described, by the Royal Commission, as *dysgonic*, and those which grow luxuriantly under such conditions as *eugonic*.

The Cultural Characters of the two Mammalian Types of Tubercle Bacilli. The human type of bacillus is eugonic, the bovine dysgonic. The difference is, on the whole, well marked; but it must be admitted that in each type different strains may differ considerably from one another at the start, while some adapt themselves more readily than others to the conditions of artificial cultivation. Thus there are different degrees of eugony and dysgony.

Eastwood, who examined for the Royal Commission a large number of strains of tubercle bacilli both of human and of bovine type, believed himself able to arrange them " according to their capacity for growth " on glycerin-broth, glycerin-agar, and glycerin-potato in "one continuous and absolutely unbroken series, passing by gradual and only just perceptible stages of transition from the top of the series which contains the strains which grow with greatest difficulty, down to the bottom of the series where are found the strains which grow with greatest luxuriance." This unbroken series he divided, merely for convenience, into five "arbitrary grades." But it is to be observed that while he did not admit any break in the series which would serve to divide the bovine from the human type, he nevertheless, on cultural grounds alone, placed all the strains which possessed the virulence of the bovine type above a certain point, and all those which showed the virulence of the human type below it. There was no exception, at that time, so that while the least dysgonic of the bovine type approximated very closely to the least eugonic of the human type there was no overlapping[1].

The view that a sufficient number of strains of mammalian tubercle bacilli arranged according to the luxuriance of their

---

[1] *R.C.T. Int. Rep.* 1907, App. vol. IV, p. xviii. Atypical strains which have the dysgonic characters of growth of the bovine type, and the low virulence for rabbits characteristic of the human type, as well as others which have the virulence of the bovine and the cultural characters of the human type, have since come to light.

cultural characters will form an unbroken series is perhaps an extreme view to take[1]. Other observers, particularly Kossel and Weber and their colleagues at the Gesundheitsamt, and Park and Krumwiede in America, as well as some of those who worked for the Royal Commission, see a more decided difference between the types. But the question is by no means easy, being, as we shall see, complicated by the difficulty of obtaining culture media of constant value, and by the varying degree of adaptation to the conditions of artificial cultivation attained by the various strains when they come to be tested. We shall have to return to these points again when we are considering differential diagnosis (p. 231); but we may perhaps venture to say now that we are inclined to think that the more successfully these difficulties are overcome the clearer the difference in the cultural characters of the two types will appear[2].

Cultural Characters on Various Media. On coagulated blood-serum both the human and bovine types form a thin uniform dull grey film with a surface like that of ground glass. This is the usual form; in badly-growing cultures, on the one hand, the growth may assume the form of small, more or less discrete, irregular, grey colonies, while in cultures which are doing unusually well the film may be thicker, whiter, and even slightly nodular or scaly. No very obvious difference in the mode of growth of the two types is evident on this medium[3]. On the

---

[1] M. Koch and Rabinowitsch hold very similar views about tubercle bacilli of avian origin. Referring to 95 strains, which they isolated from various birds in the zoological gardens in Berlin, and three of which they concluded belonged to the human type, they say: " These strains formed a complete scale, beginning with a typical moist slimy growth (*i.e.* typical of the avian type), and passing to the dry scaly vegetation distinctive of mammalian bacilli " (*loc. cit.* p. 332).

[2] On this point Park and Krumwiede, speaking only of the human and bovine types, say: " The number of viruses showing intermediate characteristics will vary with the technique employed. Our experience, as well as that of others, has shown that, the simpler the methods, the more ideal the medium, and the greater the number of tests to avoid irregularities not under our control but dependent on the material employed, the greater will be the difference shown by the two types, and the smaller the number of cultures showing intermediate characteristics." *Collected Studies, Res. Lab. City of N.Y.* vol. v, 1910, p. 41.

[3] Differences in pigmentation are described on pp. 209 and 682.

other hand, on serum to which 2–5 per cent. of glycerin has been added a marked difference is seen as a rule. The bovine strains grow on the glycerin medium much as on pure serum—some worse, a few a trifle better[1]—while the human strains grow decidedly better on the glycerin-serum and form much thicker and more opaque layers of growth[2].

The difference of growth in the bovine and the human types indeed appears to depend on the difference in their capacities for making use of glycerin. In the case of other media than serum, such as agar, potato and broth, glycerin is always added, and the human strains grow on them far better than the bovine. These media are seldom, if ever, used without glycerin even for the cultivation of tubercle bacilli of bovine type, because strains of this type, although they grow as a rule better without glycerin, nevertheless will not grow at all on

---

[1] *The Influence of Glycerin.* There seems to be a very general opinion that glycerin hinders the growth of all bovine tubercle bacilli, at least in early cultures. Thus Weber in 1912 said "I myself have gained the impression, in the course of my work on tuberculosis extending over years, that the addition of glycerin is favourable to the growth of the human tubercle bacillus, and obstructive to that of the bovine bacillus," and he adds that Beck, the English Commission, Moeller, Dorset, Park and Krumwiede and Jancsó and Elfer had come to the same conclusion. But he goes on to say that, in the case of serum media at least, this difference is not quite constant, and in some instances might even be reversed. It was his custom to sow primary cultures from tuberculous guinea-pigs on three tubes of glycerin-serum, and three of serum without glycerin. And while the difference described above occurred as a general rule, it was not very striking, and in many cases the raising of cultures of bovine bacilli from the guinea-pig succeeded easily on glycerin-serum and with difficulty on pure serum (*Centralb. f. Bakt. etc.* Orig. vol. LXIV, p. 254). At one time the writer thought that glycerin hindered the growth of all bovine bacilli, but more extended experience showed that while it does so in the case of many, and probably of the majority, of bovine strains, when freshly isolated, it does not do so in all. Some strains there undoubtedly are which are indifferent to glycerin and others which are slightly favoured by it, even in the early stage of artificial cultivation.

[2] Koch in his early work was quite unable to detect any difference in the cultural characters of strains of tubercle bacilli from bovine and human sources, although, as he says, he devoted the greatest attention to this point. This failure to detect differences now seen by everybody is to be explained by his use of solidified blood-serum as his usual culture medium; and, although he tried other media, such as broth, nutrient agar and potato, he seems to have had little success. He makes no mention anywhere of glycerin (*loc. cit.* 1884, Eng. trans. p. 150).

these media until they have become adapted to the saprophytic habit by continued cultivation on media, such as serum
or egg, which more nearly resemble their natural habitat ; and
during the process of adaptation they acquire the capacity of
utilizing glycerin.

On glycerin-agar. The human type of bacillus soon adapts
itself to this medium, and comes· to grow luxuriantly on it.
In cultures which are not doing well, growth may be confined
to several isolated patches, which then become nodular, and
may be surrounded by a thin radially folded margin ; but on
satisfactory media, and when well established, strains of this
type form a dense whitish or cream-coloured wrinkled layer.
The bovine type of bacillus, on the other hand, grows badly
on glycerin-agar. At first it will scarcely grow at all, and
frequently only a thin patchy film appears. At other times
little, more or less discrete, nodules may appear, or a delicate
wrinkled film resembling that of the human type only much
thinner.

On glycerin-potato. The human type of bacillus, when it
has accustomed itself to artificial cultivation, grows very
abundantly on glycerin-potato. The growth usually takes the
form of a thick cream-coloured layer covered with nodular or
warty elevations. These nodules when seen slightly magnified,
especially under the stereoscopic binocular microscope, present
a peculiar resemblance in form to worm casts, and their surfaces, which have a dull or " matt " appearance, may be seen
to be studded all over with little secondary elevations. The
bovine type of bacillus grows badly on this medium, and
seldom, even· after long-continued subcultivation, attains any
degree of luxuriance comparable to that of the human type.
Often it forms little else than a barely visible grey layer, best
seen on potato which has been coloured with litmus. At times
the margin of the grey patch may be a little thicker than the
middle, and, at the best, there may be some development of
nodular outgrowths.

On glycerin-broth. The human type of bacillus when doing
well begins to grow on this medium as a delicate greyish white
pellicle with, as a rule, one or more denser spots in the middle.

The film continues to spread, when the culture is growing strongly and the medium is proving favourable, until it covers the whole of the surface of the fluid, and even climbs to the height of a quarter or half an inch up the sides of the vessel which contains it. Meanwhile the pellicle thickens and becomes whiter or cream-coloured, and, expanding laterally, it grows too large for the surface and is thrown into innumerable deep wrinkles. The broth meanwhile remains quite clear, but there is usually a little granular deposit at the bottom due to pieces of growth which have fallen from the surface, or perhaps to a multiplication of bacilli which have settled there[1].

Frequently, however, when the medium is apparently some-what unfavourable, growth is checked for a while at an early stage, and instead of a thin spreading pellicle there is formed a little dense circumscribed island of bacilli, thick and granular and with abrupt margins. The islands may continue slowly to increase in thickness and area for some time until finally growth becomes arrested. But in other cases, after continuing to increase in this way for a longer or shorter period, a little thin grey film is seen one day extending from some portion of the thick raised margin, and after that the film quickly spreads, as described above, and is thrown into deep wrinkles which radiate out from the thickened patch in the middle[2].

[1] This description refers to cultures grown on broth made of veal, on beef or goat-flesh broth the human type of bacillus has sometimes been seen to grow in large cauliflower-like masses which dip down deeply into the fluid.

[2] In such cases it seems as if there was some condition which prevents the spread of the pellicle and forces the bacilli to grow only where, by massing together, they can render one another mutual assistance. What the nature of this inhibiting condition may be is not known. That it is not due to unfavourable degrees of acidity or alkalinity seems to be proved by some experiments undertaken to investigate this possibility. Experience shows that sometimes it disappears quite rapidly. On the whole it looks as if some of the food required by the bacilli for their normal growth is wanting, or insufficient, in certain samples of broth, and that the bacilli for a time can multiply only by living partly on the dead bodies of their predecessors, until the substance of these dead bodies shall have passed into solution. This explanation is in harmony with the observation that success in culti-vation is rendered more certain by transferring large quantities of bacteria when sowing a new culture; a remark which is true, not of broth cultures only, but of those on other media also; but naturally its truth is more

Large broth cultures have a very distinctive and not altogether unpleasant odour, which is difficult to describe.

The bovine type of tubercle bacillus grows, on the whole, badly on glycerin broth, and, for a long period after a strain of human type would have acquired the power of spreading over the surface as a thick wrinkled cream-coloured pellicle, it may form no more than a delicate lace-like grey film which stops growing when it has covered but a small portion of the surface. In time, however, and after repeated subcultivation on this medium, strains of bovine type, or some of them at least, may come to grow on broth as luxuriantly as the human type of tubercle bacillus. This has been demonstrated more than once by A. S. Griffith, and also by Grund, by weighing the bacilli removed from comparable cultures of the two types (see pp. 236 and 237).

Pigmentation. A yellowish or golden colour may often be observed in serum cultures of the human type of tubercle bacillus, especially when the serum is of an unusually rich colour. On potato the growth of this type may assume an orange yellow, or even a dull reddish colour. This phenomenon seems to depend more on the medium than on the particular strain of bacilli, for Duval[1] has observed it in one part of a potato culture while the other maintained a normal appearance, and the writer has more than once seen the same thing. When this has occurred it has been the growth on the upper part of the potato which has changed colour, a fact which suggests that reddish appearance is associated with a partial drying of the potato.

The diffuse violet coloration seen in glycerin-agar cultures of one of the streptothrices, and which is not uncommon in glycerin-potato cultures of the so-called fish-tubercle bacillus, has never been seen by the writer in cultures of true tubercle bacilli.

The Cultural Characters of the Avian Type of Tubercle Bacillus. The avian tubercle bacillus may be cultivated rather

apparent when dealing with strains which grow with difficulty than those which have more fully acquired the saprophytic habit.

[1] *Transactions of the Tuberculosis Congress in Washington*, vol. IV, Pt. II, p. 728.

C

more easily than either of the mammalian types. It grows copiously on all ordinary media, resembling the human more closely than the bovine type, except in that it does not form at all readily a pellicle on glycerin broth, and that on all media its growth tends to be moist and glistening instead of dull and dry. Like the human type it grows better in the presence of glycerin.

The cultural characters of the avian tubercle bacillus are however very variable, and while sometimes the cultures may be characteristically distinctive, at other times they may be practically indistinguishable from those of the human type. This is insisted on strongly by Max Koch and Rabinowitsch[1], who examined 92 strains of avian tubercle bacilli from 67 different birds, and arrived at the conclusion that the traditional characters which are supposed to distinguish this type from the others have been based on too limited an experience, and that they break down, as a means of distinguishing the types, when a sufficient number of strains are examined.

For his own part, the writer, while fully admitting that individual cultures of avian bacilli which he is unable to distinguish from those of human bacilli not unfrequently occur, nevertheless is of opinion that, if one does not rely too much on single cultures, but takes a general survey of the growth characters of a given strain extending over a reasonable period of time and including all the usual culture media, the generally recognized cultural distinctions hold good. He is not aware that any strain of avian bacilli will grow consistently like the human bacillus, no matter how closely certain individual cultures of the former may resemble those of the latter type.

Admitting then that the cultural characters of the avian tubercle bacillus may vary within rather wide limits, the following description, which is based on personal observation, but which corresponds closely with that of the majority of observers, may be taken as characteristic of this type.

On egg or glycerin-egg the avian tubercle bacillus when growing well tends to form a thick layer composed of prominent

---

[1] *loc. cit.* pp. 323 *et seq.*

nodules some of which may be spherical or umbilicated—like a glass bead—or even cup-shaped.

On glycerin-agar the growth may take the form of a smooth ivory-white plaque, which looks as though it were formed of confluent drops of thick white paint. At other times it is thinner, and more nearly resembles a layer of rich milk. Both these forms are characteristic, and are never seen in cultures of the human bacillus. Sometimes, however, the growth is wrinkled and has a dull surface, and then closely resembles the usual type of culture produced by the human bacillus.

On glycerin-potato the growth is copious and nodular. When most characteristic the surface appears moist and glistening, but this, though usual, is not always the case[1].

On glycerin-broth the avian bacillus grows as a rule only as a granular deposit at the bottom of the fluid. Pellicle formation is, in the experience of the writer at least, very imperfect, and rarely seen. O. Bang, however, states that all avian strains may be induced to grow sooner or later on the surface of the broth, and Koch and Rabinowitsch, though they do not go quite so far as this, state that two-thirds of their avian strains grew in this way.

Specific Pathogenicity.

The most important distinction between the three types of tubercle bacilli, as we have said already, lies in the difference in their power of causing disease in different species of animals.

The mammalian tubercle bacilli are pathogenic for many mammals, and for a few birds including those of the parrot tribe, but the common domestic fowl and the pigeon are almost entirely insusceptible to their attack, only the most trivial lesions, or more commonly none at all, being caused by subcutaneous or intraperitoneal injection. Intravenous injection, it is true, may cause death, but the signs are rather those of toxæmia than of a true infection, and the formation of tubercles does not occur. (See p. 541.)

---

[1] Horn-like outgrowths, hooks and loops are not uncommon, and when present are characteristic.

While the bovine type of bacillus is pathogenic for all mammals, the human type is incapable of producing progressive tuberculosis in many, including the ox, pig, goat, sheep, horse, cat and rabbit ; but it is highly virulent for the monkey, guinea-pig, and, of course, man.

The avian type of tubercle bacillus is virulent for all birds, so far as is known, but has very little pathogenic effect on most mammals. The rat, mouse and rabbit are, however, exceptions, and the guinea-pig may be killed with large doses, though typical anatomical lesions are absent (see p. 437). The pig is sometimes found to be suffering from a local form of tuberculosis caused by this type of bacillus (see p. 403).

The Difference in Virulence between the Human and Bovine Types of Tubercle Bacilli no Mere Difference of Degree. Some observers have thought that the virulence of the bovine bacillus differs from that of the human merely in degree, and not in its specific nature. Their case may be stated somewhat as follows : guinea-pigs and monkeys are so extremely susceptible to tuberculosis that they are affected by bacilli of low virulence almost to the same extent as they are by bacilli of high virulence, and the same is true of man. It is only when one comes to such comparatively resistant animals as the ox, goat, rabbit, etc., that the difference in virulence of the types becomes evident. These animals can resist the less virulent human, but fall victims to the more virulent bovine type. At the extreme end of the scale is the dog, whose resistance is so very high that neither type is able to exert any very marked effect. In harmony with this view is the fact that the less virulent (human) type grows on artificial culture more luxuriantly than the more virulent (bovine) type, that is to say, the degree of virulence is in relation to the strictness of the parasitic habit.

This view, which at one time seemed plausible enough, has had to give way with the advance of knowledge. Many facts clearly prove it to be untenable. It will suffice to refer to a few of them here. The rabbit which differentiates clearly between the two types of bacilli does not do so because it has a high degree of resisting power towards tuberculosis in general. It is true it resists infection with the human type of bacillus very well as a rule, but towards infection with the bovine type it is one of the most susceptible species known ; in this respect it is probably in no way inferior to the guinea-pig, an animal which is one of the few species capable of being seriously infected with human tubercle bacilli[1]. The dog alone is sufficient to upset the hypothesis. It is a fairly resistant animal no doubt, but not so resistant that it escapes tuberculosis altogether. As a matter of fact it suffers sometimes from spontaneous infection, and in such cases as have been observed the human type of bacillus has been found at least as often as the bovine[2]. The cat on the other hand, which probably suffers from tuberculosis about as frequently as the dog, is susceptible to the attack of the bovine bacillus only. Finally, while the chimpanzee, an extremely susceptible species, shows, so far as experiments have determined, absolutely no difference in its susceptibility to infection with the two types, and thereby conforms to the hypothesis, man, whose resistance is certainly much higher than that of the chimpanzee, is susceptible at all ages to infection with bacilli of the human type, while to that of the bovine type he is practically only susceptible in childhood.

It can no longer be doubted therefore that between the bovine and human types of tubercle bacilli there exist differences of virulence, which are not mere differences of degree, but are due to real differences of character, caused, almost certainly, by long-established adaptation to different hosts. Though why one species such as the dog should be equally liable to be attacked by both types of bacilli, while another closely allied species such as the cat is susceptible to one only, is difficult to explain[3].

[1] See p. 274.
[2] Schornagel, 1914, *Untersuchungen über elf Fälle von Hundetuberkulose*, Beijers., Utrecht. See also p. 496.
[3] P.S. Unless it be that the association of the dog with man is much older and more intimate than that of the cat.

Atypical Strains.

Many observers have described atypical strains of tubercle
bacilli, that is to say strains the particular degree of virulence
of which for certain animals would suggest one type while
their cultural characters would suggest another, or strains
possessing characters which in some other way depart from
those that are believed to belong to one or other of the types.
Apparent deviation from type may be due to faulty technique,
especially to unsatisfactory culture media, and it can hardly
be doubted that Park and Krumwiede are right when they
say that the better the technique the sharper will the distinction between the types appear.   Yet, after making all allow-
ances for bad technique, it cannot be doubted that atypical
strains of tubercle bacilli are sometimes met with.

Some of these have possessed the cultural characters of
the human type and the virulence, more or less, of the bovine.
Many such strains, as we shall see, have been proved to be
mixtures of human and bovine bacilli.   This has been done
in several ways, but particularly by cultivating typical bovine
and human strains from single colonies of the original strain
(p. 342).   Moreover, it has been shown that artificial mixtures
of bovine and human types behave exactly as these strains do.

Other strains, particularly many of those isolated by
A. S. Griffith from cases of lupus, have shown, together with
typical characters either of the bovine or human type, a
relative virulence for certain animals which, while more or less
resembling that of the type whose cultural characters they
possess, nevertheless fall, to a greater or lesser extent, below
the standard of virulence for that type.   Such strains will be
fully discussed in another chapter, and reason shown for considering them to be attenuated members of one or other type.

Possibly other kinds of atypical strains exist[1]; but if so it
seems not unlikely that they too will be found capable of

---

[1] A more or less dysgonic type with low virulence for the rabbit, etc. and
which perhaps we may regard as a variety of the human type with an unusually
small capacity for saprophytic growth has been described quite recently by
Eastwood and F. Griffith and by A. S. Griffith. (See Appendix, p. 680.)

some such simple explanation. At the same time it must be stated that not a few observers see in these atypical strains intermediate forms which represent links between the types. This is an important and much contested view, and its further consideration will have to be deferred to another chapter.

Summary and Conclusions.

1. Three types of tubercle bacilli exist, which differ sharply in their cultural and pathogenic properties, and slightly in their shape and size.

2. The types are distinct ; and while atypical strains undoubtedly exist, many of them can be resolved into mixtures of two or more of the types, or explained as attenuated members of one or other of the types.

3. It is doubtful whether transitional strains, which stand half-way between two types, have any real existence.

Some Practical Details concerning the Cultivation of Tubercle Bacilli.

Since the cultivation of tubercle bacilli, though not a difficult matter, cannot be attained by the methods which succeed well in the case of most other bacteria, it may not be out of place to touch here on a few points connected with the subject.

The Isolation of Tubercle Bacilli from Animal Tissues. Strains of tubercle bacilli which have adapted themselves to the conditions of artificial cultivation will, as we have said already, grow on a variety of culture media, including glycerin-agar, glycerin-potato, and glycerin-broth; but it is more difficult to obtain *primary* cultures, that is cultures directly from the animal body. A medium more closely resembling the substance of animal tissues is necessary for this purpose, and since the discovery of the bacillus by Koch some kind of serum, with or without glycerin, has been used almost universally for this purpose, until quite recently.

The serum of all animals is not equally favourable to the growth of the bacillus. Its value as a culture medium has nothing whatever to do with the susceptibility of the animal yielding the serum. Long ago Koch discovered that the serum of the dog, which is a particularly resistant animal to tuberculosis, is good for growing the tubercle bacillus, and the serum of this animal was particularly recommended for the purpose by Theobald Smith. A. S. Griffith, who tested a great many kinds of serum, thought that that of the cat gave the best results. But it is difficult to obtain serum from these two species in quantities sufficient for the needs of an active investigator, and one usually has to fall back on that of some larger animal. The serum of the horse seems to be particularly unsuitable, while that of the ox is very variable ; on the whole the serum of the adult ox gives better results than that of the calf and is to be recommended[1].

The serum should be collected in a sterile condition by allowing the blood to flow directly from the carotid artery through a cannula and rubber tube into a sterile bottle (Winchester quart). With a little tact and trouble blood may usually be obtained in this way at the slaughter-house. The serum, after distribution into test tubes, should be subjected only to the minimal amount of heating necessary to set it ; and it should be sealed with paraffin immediately after to prevent drying. When circumstances permit it is better to obtain the blood from the living animal, by inserting the cannula into the jugular vein, just as anti-diphtheria serum is obtained from the horse immunized for the purpose.

There is no doubt that the addition of killed tubercle bacilli, or other acid-fast bacteria, or of tuberculin or some other extract of these bacilli, according to the method introduced by Twort (and successfully applied by him and Ingram to the cultivation of Johne's bacillus, an acid-fast organism which had hitherto resisted all attempts to grow it), greatly increases the nutritive value of serum for tubercle bacilli unaccustomed to artificial media.

The difficulties of raising primary cultures of tubercle bacilli on serum having proved considerable in the past, and costly both in time and material, it is not surprising to find that efforts

---

[1] This opinion is held by Weber also (see *Centralb. f. Bakt.* Orig. vol. LXIV, p. 255).

have been made to find a more satisfactory medium.   This has
been successfully accomplished by Marion Dorset in the United
States who introduced coagulated egg for the purpose, a medium
which was re-discovered independently by A. S. Griffith, and
which has proved very useful in his hands.   Park and Krumwiede speak very highly of the medium.   It is made out of
both yolk and white mixed with an addition of physiological salt
solution.   Probably the addition of some products of acid-fast
bacilli would improve it still further[1].

Griffith uses it without addition of glycerin, since he does
not wish to blunt the sharpness of the distinction between
strains of human and bovine type when tested subsequently
on glycerin-holding media, by allowing opportunity for any
preliminary adaptation of the latter type to glycerin.   But the
precaution is probably unnecessary, and the addition of glycerin
to egg medium undoubtedly improves it for the human type,
while it perhaps makes it a little less favourable for the bovine
type.   It seems therefore best to employ egg both with and
without glycerin for primary cultures, and in this way one will
not only secure the best medium for each type, but obtain preliminary information as to the cultural characters of each strain.

Egg medium is used both with and without glycerin in
America; and on the Continent it has been modified by
Lubenau by the addition of glycerin broth in the place of
saline solution.

*The Choice of a Tuberculous Tissue from which to raise a
Culture.*   It is possible in many cases to raise cultures directly
from human tuberculous tissues at post-mortem examination,
but the attempt will often fail when many hours have elapsed
since the death of the patient.   In such cases it is usual to
inject guinea-pigs with emulsions of the diseased tissues, and
to raise the cultures subsequently from these animals.   The
tissues of the guinea-pig best suited to this purpose are those
which are most likely to be free from other bacteria.   In this
respect the spleen is probably best, though cultures may also
be raised from caseous glands, or, in the case of intraperitoneal

---

[1] A good description of the method of making this medium may be found
in Park and Krumwiede, *loc. cit.* p. 213.

injection, from the caseous omentum, or from the peritoneum covered with miliary tubercles. Lungs are to be avoided as they invariably contain many mould spores and bacteria.

The Antiformin method of obtaining Cultures of Tubercle Bacilli from Tuberculous Sputum. Antiformin which consists of equal parts of Javelle water and a 15 per cent. solution of sodium hydrate, possesses the power of destroying most other bacteria more readily than it does the acid-fast bacilli. Moreover it dissolves mucus. Consequently if sputum be shaken with a suitable proportion of antiformin, not only is there a fair prospect of destroying the contaminating bacteria without injuring the tubercle bacilli, but the sputum is rendered sufficiently fluid to be successfully centrifuged, so that the bacilli from a considerable quantity of the material may be recovered from the deposit. This method, originally introduced by Uhlenhut and Kersten[1], both for microscopical and cultural purposes, has been used with considerable success by Weber and Dieterlen and by Lindemann in the Gesundheitsamt, and by A. S. Griffith in this country. Weber and Dieterlen[2] examined and compared a number of strains isolated both by the antiformin method and from the inoculated guinea-pig and reported that the virulence of the cultures raised by the former method was not impaired by the bactericidal agent.

The amount of antiformin added and the time it is allowed to act differ with different workers. Th. Smith and Brown mixed an equal volume of 30 per cent. antiformin with the sputum, and after thoroughly shaking, allowed the mixture to stand for an hour at the room temperature before centrifuging and washing the deposit. It is probably more usual to add 10 per cent. of antiformin and to allow it to act for a shorter time, say ten or fifteen minutes. Griffith[3], who has had a good deal of experience with the method, employs a 10 per cent. solution of antiformin added to an equal volume of sputum suitably diluted

[1] Uhlenhut and Kersten, "Eine neue Methode zum kulturellen und mikroskopischen Nachweis von Tuberkelbazillen in Sputum und andere tuberkulösem Material," *Zeitschr. f. Experim. Pathol. u. Therap.* 1909, Bd. VI, p. 759.
[2] *Tuber. Arbeiten, etc.* 1912, Heft 12, pp. 7 *et seq.*
[3] *Brit. Med. Journ.* 1914, I, p. 1171.

according to its consistency. The mixture is then stirred up, and after five, ten, or fifteen minutes, according to the speed with which the sputum dissolves, the mixture is centrifuged. The deposit is then washed with salt solution, re-centrifuged and sown upon egg medium. Latterly he has omitted the washing of the deposit, finding the small amount of unreduced formalin which lingers in the deposit insufficient to interfere with the growth of the tubercle bacillus.

He is now experimenting with an even simpler method, which dispenses with the centrifuge, and which, at all events with sputa rich in tubercle bacilli, seems to be practically useful. In this method equal parts of sputum and of a 10 per cent. solution of antiformin are thoroughly mixed, and after the lapse of from 5 to 30 minutes tubes of egg medium are sown directly with the mixture (see App. p. 682).

One or other of these methods of using antiformin can be applied to tissue emulsions also which are contaminated with undesirable organisms, and the emulsions so purified can be used either for sowing cultures or injecting animals.

Prevention of drying. Cultures of tubercle bacilli on solid media should be sealed, since any drying of the medium is very harmful to their growth, which is slow and continues for much longer periods than is the case with most other bacteria. It is best not to wait until the tubes are sown, but to seal them as soon as they are prepared. This may be effected by dipping their ends into melted paraffin. Special tubes with a glass cap containing a small opening for the entrance of air, such as were introduced by Theobald Smith, are not necessary.

The Method of Sowing. It has already been pointed out that it is of considerable advantage when sowing a new culture to transfer a considerable quantity of bacilli from the old to the new tube. And one may often observe in the case of solid cultures that growth takes place freely where one has planted a visible lump of bacilli, while elsewhere, in parts which cannot possibly have escaped being sown, though probably with more or less isolated bacilli, there is no growth.

The explanation of this old observation is supplied by Twort (1910), who has suggested that the tubercle bacillus, having become a strict parasite, has lost, or almost lost, the power to form the substances required for its nutrition out of dead materials, such as coagulated serum, glycerin-potato, etc. ; but that if supplied with dead bacilli (or their extracts) in which the substances required are present ready-formed, the bacilli are enabled successfully to overcome the initial difficulties of adaptation to a saprophytic existence.

In sowing broth cultures of human or bovine tubercle bacilli it is very important that the bacilli introduced should be floated on the fluid, for should they sink no satisfactory growth will occur. This condition is easily satisfied when sowing one broth culture from another, for a little piece of the film may be lifted from the old culture and lightly laid on the surface of the new, but it is not so easy when a strain is sown on broth for the first time. It has long been usual to employ for this purpose the film which spreads over any fluid there may happen to be at the bottom of serum, agar or potato cultures, and, in order to encourage the formation of this film, a few drops of broth are often added to such cultures.

Eastwood improved upon this method in the following manner: into the ordinary 6 or 8 oz. medicine bottle, which was commonly used for broth cultures in the laboratories of the Royal Commission, some serum was introduced, and coagulated while the bottle lay in a nearly horizontal position on its narrow side. The broth was then introduced, and the whole sterilized in the usual way. The culture was sown on the surface of the serum, and the bottle laid in the incubator on its broad side ; growth was therefore free to spread from the serum on to the surface of the broth, just as it spreads from potato or agar on to the surface of the condensation water.

Another simple plan which the author found useful for starting broth cultures is to introduce a little piece of cotton wool into the flask before sterilizing. The wool swells up and extends to the surface, and forms a sufficient support for the bacilli which are planted upon it.

Either of these devices succeeds well, and is quite practical.

The Length of Life of Cultures.

If a strain of tubercle bacilli is to be kept alive, with its powers of growth unimpaired, it is well to transplant it to fresh soil every month or two, if not oftener. Cultures, however, will remain alive for very much longer periods than this, especially if prevented from drying up, as F. Griffith, Weber and others have observed.

Griffith, who kept cultures alive for two or three years, was content to seal his tubes with paraffin. Weber seals his in the flame, and prefers to keep the cultures, after a moderate amount of growth has taken place in the incubator, at the ordinary room temperature.

Griffith thinks they keep better in the incubator, being less likely to become contaminated with moulds, but it is significant that two of his three cultures which lived the longest were kept out of the incubator. He found that primary cultures remained alive longer than subcultures, and he attributed this to the smaller amount of growth in the former, and to the correspondingly lesser demand made upon the food supply.

With regard to the relative endurance of the three types, Weber points out that Jancsó and Elfer had kept avian bacilli alive without any difficulty for one year and hoped that it might be possible to do so for two years. Maffucci found an avian strain alive after two years; and Weber and Bofinger also testify to the long endurance of the vitality of the avian bacillus.

Weber[1] came to the conclusion from his own experiments that the bovine type of mammalian bacillus endures longer than the human. He found the bovine bacillus alive after one year and eight months, but the human type not after one year (serum cultures), and he mentions that Jancsó and Elfer found the bovine tubercle bacillus alive on glycerin-potato after one year and a half, while the human type on this medium, or on glycerin-agar or glycerin-serum, lived scarcely six months.

[1] Weber, 1912, "Zur Tuberculose des Menschen und der Tiere," *Centralb. f. Bakt. u. Parasit.* Abt. 1, Orig. vol. LXIV, p. 260.

Griffith[1] did not venture to draw any conclusion on this point, but his observations are not incompatible with those of Weber. He found the avian bacillus alive after 1067 days, the bovine after 990 days, and the human after 936 days. Again the avian cultures sometimes failed to grow after 180–238 days, the bovine after 181–381 days, and the human after 90–380 days.

The superior endurance of Griffith's cultures over those of other observers may possibly have been due to the fact that the majority tested were grown on coagulated egg[2].

Weber attaches some importance to the greater endurance of bovine as compared with human strains, and he concludes that any strain of mammalian tubercle bacilli which is found alive after one year is in all probability of the bovine type. He relates how Lindemann injected into a guinea-pig a mixture of bacilli of bovine and human types after it had resided eleven months in the test tube, and when the animal was killed, recovered from it bacilli of bovine type only. It may be useful to bear this experiment in mind, for it evidently would not be admissible in a similar case, to conclude from the fact that only bovine bacilli were recovered from the guinea-pig that the original strain contained no bacilli of human type, but the method cannot be relied upon for the separation of a pure bovine strain from a mixture of the two mammalian types.

REFERENCES. VII

(Chapter XI)

The Three Types of Tubercle Bacilli.

Morphological and Cultural Characters.

Burckhardt (1910). Bakteriologische Untersuchungen über chirurgische Tuberkulosen. Ein Beitrag zur Frage der Verschiedenheit der Tuberkulose des Menschen und der Tiere. *Deutsche Zeitschr. f. Chir.* vol. 160.
Cobbett (1907). The Cultural Characters of Tubercle Bacilli obtained from Man. *R.C.T. 2nd Int. Rep.* App. vol. III, p. 1.

[1] F. Griffith, *R.C.T. Fin. Rep.* 1911, App. vol. IV. p. 178.
[2] Numerous observations by other authors will be found in Weber, *loc. cit.* 1912.

Eastwood (1907). The Comparative Study of Tubercle Bacilli from Human and Bovine Sources. *Ibid. Int. Rep.* App. vol. IV, p. 155.

—— (1911). *Ibid. Final Report*, vol. V, p. 211.

A. S. Griffith and F. Griffith (1907). The Cultural Characters of the Bovine Tubercle Bacillus. *Ibid. Int. Rep.* App. vol. III, p. 1.

A. S. Griffith (1914). Further Investigations of the Type of Tubercle Bacilli occurring in the Sputum of Phthisical Persons. *Brit. Med. Journ.* I, p. 1171.

Hutchens (1907). Supplementary Report on the Cultivation of the Tubercle Bacillus. *R.C.T. Int. Rep.* App. vol. III, p. 27.

Jancsó and Elfer (1911). Vergleichende Untersuchungen mit der praktisch wichtigeren säurefesten Bacillen. *Beiträge zur Klinik der Tuberkulose*, vol. XVIII, p. 198.

Kossel, Weber and Heuss (1904). Vergleichende Untersuchungen über Tuberkelbazillen verschiedener Herkunft. *Tub. Arbeit. a. d. Kaiserl. Gesundheitsamte*, Heft 1, p. 1.

Kossel (1912). Der Tuberkelbazillus. Kolle and Wassermann's *Handbuch der Pathogenen Mikro-organismen.*

Krompercher and Zimmermann (1903). *Centralb. f. Bakt. etc.* Abt. 1, Orig. vol. XXXIII, p. 580.

Lindemann (1912). Untersuchungen über den Typus der im Auswurf Lungenkranker verkommenden Tuberkelbazillen. *Tub. Arbeit. a. d. Kaiserl. Gesundheitsamte*, Heft 12, p. 11.

Mohler and Washburn (1907). A Comparative Study of Tubercle Bacilli from Varied Sources. *U.S. Bureau of Animal Industry Bulletin,* No. 96.

Park and Krumwiede (1910). The Relative Importance of Bovine and Human Types of Tubercle Bacilli in the Different Forms of Human Tuberculosis. *Journ. of Med. Res.* vol. XXIII, p. 205.

—— (1911). *Ibid.* vol. XXV, p. 313.

(In vol. XXIII will be found a good review of the whole subject and a bibliography up to date of paper.)

Smith, Th. and Brown. Studies in Mammalian tubercle bacilli. IV. Bacilli resembling the bovine type from four cases in man. *Journ. of Med. Res.* vol. XVI, p. 435.

Twort (1910). A method of isolating and growing the Lepra Bacillus of Man. *Proc. Royal Soc.* B, vol. LXXXIII.

Twort and Ingram (1912). Isolation and Cultivation of Microbacterium Enteritidis, etc. *Ibid.* B, vol. LXXXIV, p. 517.

Ungermann (1912). Untersuchungen über die tuberkulöse Infection der Lymphdrüsen im Kindersalter. *Tub. Arbeit. a. d. Kaiserl. Gesundheitsamte*, Heft 12, p. 109.

Weber (1912). Zur Tuberkulose des Menschen und der Tiere. *Centralb. f. Bakt. u. Parasit.* Abt. 1, Orig. vol. LXIV, p. 243.

Weber and Dieterlen (1912). Untersuchungen über den Typus der im Lungenkranker vorkommenden Tuberkelbazillen. *Tub. Arbeit. a. d. Kaiserl. Gesundheitsamte*, Heft 12, p. 1.

CHAPTER XII

THE MEANS OF DISTINGUISHING THE THREE TYPES OF TUBERCLE BACILLI ONE FROM ANOTHER

Morphological and Cultural Characters.   The Reaction Curve.

I. *Morphological Characters.*

Bovine tubercle bacilli are on the whole shorter than human; but comparison, as we have seen, is valid only when the conditions under which both are growing are the same, and even then there is probably some overlapping.   Difference of size therefore will help us little in deciding to what type a given strain belongs.

Differences in segmentation, and other minute details of structure, also fail us. As evidence of the truth of this statement it may be pointed out that a tendency to stain unevenly has been described by one school (Gesundheitsamt[1]) as characteristic of the bovine type, and by another (Royal Commission[2]) as characteristic of the human type.

Somewhat rarely one sees in sputum bacilli so uniformly short as to suggest that they belong to the bovine type.   This may be misleading.   A specimen was sent to the author for this very reason[3].   But investigation showed that in virulence for calves and rabbits, and in cultural characters, the bacillus was an ordinary representative of the human type.   We have seen that tubercle bacilli are considerably longer when grown in living animal tissues than when cultivated on artificial media (p. 201).   They are usually long in sputum ; but the bacilli present in the sputum in question were quite as short as those which one is accustomed to see in cultures, and they were gathered together into circumscribed groups or colonies, each of some size and containing many bacilli.   This distribution suggested that the bacilli had multiplied in the sputum while it remained undisturbed in some cavity, uninfluenced by the vital processes going on around them, and that the bacilli were short for the same reason—whatever that may be—that they are short when they are growing in artificial culture out of the reach of living tissues and fluids.

[1] At least in broth cultures, see *Tub. Arbeit.* Heft 1, p. 10.
[2] *R.C.T. 2nd Int. Rep.* p. 25.
[3] Strain H 62, *R.C.T. Int. Rep.* App. vol. II.

II. *Cultural Characters.*

The degree of luxuriance and the manner of growth are of much greater importance for determination of type than the so-called morphological characters, and are of considerable value to experienced observers. The cultural characters of the three types of tubercle bacilli have been described already (pp. 202, 209); it will therefore be sufficient to recall the facts (1) that the human type differs from the bovine in superior luxuriance of growth on all media, especially on those which contain glycerin; and (2) that the avian type resembles the human in growing luxuriantly on all media, glycerin-broth excepted, but differs from it and from the bovine type by producing, as a rule, a growth which is moist and glistening, and, especially, in that it lends itself to emulsification more readily than those of the two mammalian types. There now remains to point out the limits of variation in the cultural characters of each type, and the causes which produce such extreme variations as are liable to lead to false conclusions.

Differentiation of the Human and Bovine Types. It is freely admitted that there is often an approximation of the one type to the other; and the slowly increasing luxuriance of growth which accompanies progressive adaptation to the conditions of life on artificial media presents a difficulty which now demands our attention. The question thereby arises at what period of saprophytic life are cultural type characters likely to be most distinct; and to what extent is one justified in comparing strains which have been growing under artificial conditions for different lengths of time.

It might be thought that the most favourable period for bringing out the differences in the cultural characters of different strains of tubercle bacilli would be when they are still freshly isolated from the animal body, and before adaptation to the new conditions of saprophytic life has had time to blunt the points of distinction. But both human and bovine bacilli are equally strict parasites, and both require a certain time to develop their representative capacities for growing on artificial media; moreover, in each type different strains adapt themselves with different degrees of rapidity; so that it is not so much the readiness with which a given strain will grow on artificial media at the start which gives us the desired intimation of the type of the strain, as the character and degree of luxuriance of the growth when once the preliminary difficulties of adaptation to the conditions of saprophytic existence have been got over. For this reason it is probably less easy to judge the type of a strain from very early cultures, than from such as have grown after it has been allowed a reasonable time to settle down to its new kind of life, and to show what it can do.

Now as to the other limit of time : It has already been pointed out that adaptation of tubercle bacilli to the conditions of artificial cultivation is slowly progressive, and may continue for long periods of time. It therefore may reasonably be asked whether this progressive adaptation tends to obscure the distinctive growth-characters of the types, or even in the long run to obliterate them altogether; and whether there is danger, if one does not act promptly, of losing the most favourable opportunity of determining type characters.

An answer to the practical part of this question may be readily given: There is little danger of this happening, and no immediate need to hurry the examination of cultural characters; since adaptation, when once it has overcome the initial difficulties of life on dead and unfamiliar media, proceeds so slowly that many months, during which cultural characters remain practically unchanged, are available for the purpose which we have in view. It is well however to keep the stock strains growing strictly on glycerin-free media, so that when tested from time to time on media which contain this differentiating substance the distinction between the human and bovine strains may be as sharp as possible[1].

[1] Park and Krumwiede, referring particularly to adaptation of bovine strains to glycerin-egg, say that " it is absolutely essential that all comparative observations be made in the first three or four generations if the degree of dysgony is to be estimated " (*Journ. of Med. Res.* XXIII, p. 222). This was at one time the writer's opinion also, and he once ventured to say that if primary cultures could always be used for comparison he believed that strains with intermediate (*i.e.* between the human and bovine types) characters of growth would, to a large extent, disappear, and each group would appear to be more sharply divided from the other. But on maturer reflection he believes that there is no need to restrict the comparison to the early stages

It is not so easy to answer the question whether progressive adaptation tends in the long run to obliterate all difference in the cultural characters of the types. The question really comes to this : Can bovine strains come ultimately to grow so freely on artificial media, and especially on those which contain glycerin, as to become indistinguishable from well-established human strains? They certainly do not do so as a rule when the stock cultures are kept rigidly from glycerin ; but on glycerin media adaptation of bovine strains undoubtedly proceeds far. Some strains would seem more capable of change than others. One that the author possessed, a true bovine strain, came to grow so luxuriantly on the usual glycerin media that it could no longer be used for demonstrating the characters of growth of the bovine type to the students attending the bacteriology class. Grund, whose work will be considered in greater detail later, states that some of her bovine strains grew so vigorously on glycerin-broth (presumably after repeated cultivation on that medium) that the *weight* of the pellicle of bacilli which they formed in a flask of given size " was equal to, or even higher than, that of the average growth of the human type[1]." A. S. Griffith had similar experience[2].

We must therefore conclude that when they are repeatedly cultivated on glycerin media for long periods bacilli of the bovine type tend to approximate closely in the luxuriance of their growth to bacilli of the human type.

Variation of Culture Media. Of far greater practical importance are the accidental variations in the nutritive value of culture media. These are difficult to control, and great care is necessary to select, for the determination of type characters, only such batches of media as have been proved to be of good quality. For, despite every care and attention on the part of bacteriologist and laboratory assistants, it seems impossible

of artificial cultivation if the stock cultures of each strain be grown on glycerin-free media; and that there is much to be gained from a prolonged and oft-repeated study of cultural characters, and moreover he thinks that the true cultural characters of certain human strains do not come out clearly without some opportunity for adaptation.

[1] See page 236.
[2] See page 237.

to prepare successive batches of a given medium, which shall have uniform nutritive value for the cultivation of the tubercle bacillus.

Attention has justly been drawn to this difficulty by Park and Krumwiede[1], who see in it an explanation of the conflicting results of different observers. The difficulty is perhaps most felt with serum, but it is not unknown in the case of potato, agar, broth, or even egg medium.

Even different tubes of the same batch may differ, which may perhaps be explained on the assumption of slight differences of dryness or hardness of surface, due to unequal heating during sterilization, or more probably to some slight defect in the sealing of the tubes.

Ungermann[2] and Lindemann[3] both refer to the difficulty of preparing glycerin-broth of constant quality.

At what age are the Characters of a Culture most clearly marked? Some observers have thought that there is a certain optimum age of cultures when the difference between the strains of human and bovine type is most marked. Park and Krumwiede, who relied mainly on glycerin-egg medium for differentiation of cultural characters, made most of their observations on cultures which were three weeks old. Cultures of one month, however, gave equally good and practically identical results. The continued growth of eugonic strains beyond this time was not marked, but the growth of dysgonic strains continued slowly to increase, and the American observers consequently came to the conclusion that at the age of three weeks to a month the differences are at a maximum[4]. This raises the question whether it is rapidity of growth, or quantity that is important to determine. The present writer is inclined to think that the former is more variable than the

---

[1] These authors write as follows (*loc. cit.* p. 313) : " a point which cannot be too often reiterated is that correct cultural differentiation depends largely on suitable cultural media. Even with long experience one finds irregularities creeping in, namely minimal growth of human viruses on some batches of media, or irregularities of individual tubes planted from the same material."

[2] *Tub. Arbeit. a. d. Kaiserl. Gesundheitsamte*, Heft 12, p. 125.

[3] *Ibid.* p. 17.

[4] *Journ. of Med. Res.* 1910, XXIII, p. 225.

latter, and that it is to the quantity rather than the rapidity of growth that attention should mainly be directed. He therefore is inclined to deprecate laying down any hard and fast rules as to the best age for making comparisons.

It might seem, at first sight, that the best way to judge of the comparative cultural characters of a number of strains of tubercle bacilli would be to sow them all simultaneously on several selected kinds of media, all the tubes of each medium having been prepared at the same time ; and then, after suitable incubation, to sort them out according to the luxuriance and character of the growth. In this way, it might be thought, variations due to accidental differences in the media would best be avoided, and the test made as objective as possible, any unconscious bias on the part of the observer having little opportunity for affecting the judgment.

But this plan does not work well in practice ; for so difficult is it to ensure the most favourable conditions for growth, and so complex are the causes of partial failure, that it is only by repeated subcultivation that the full capacities of any given strain can be brought into view. The author is convinced that a given strain should be judged by *the best growth it produces on each kind of medium after a fairly extended trial*, growths which fall short of the best being passed over as failing, through some accidental cause, to show the full capacities of the strain[1].

The Choice of Differentiating Media. In seeking for a means of clearly determining cultural characters some observers have attached more importance to one culture medium and some to another. Park and Krumwiede trusted mainly to glycerin-egg (Lubenau) supplemented by glycerin-potato. At the Gesundheitsamt, on the other hand, reliance seems to have been placed largely on glycerin-broth[2], though it is admitted that comparison is only to be relied upon in the earlier generations, and (by Ungermann)[3] that broth cultures alone do not suffice.

It is probably a mistake to rely too exclusively on one

[1] Park and Krumwiede take a very similar view when they say : " It is only reasonable to consider that the best tube is an index of the capacity of growth under the most favourable conditions." *Journ. of Med. Res.* XXIII, p. 225.

[2] Weber, *Centralbl. f. Bakt.* etc. 1912, vol. LXIV, p. 263.

[3] *loc. cit.* Heft 12, p. 125.

230 DIFFERENTIATION OF TYPE BY CULTURAL CHARACTERS [CH.

medium, for the determination of cultural characters is not so easy that one can afford to lose any information that might be gained by widening the range of trial media. Ungermann found that strains otherwise conforming to the human type grew unequally on broth. One in particular (No. X), he mentions, grew slowly and formed a smooth translucent thin film upon which fairly numerous nodular thickenings appeared. This type of growth, which is very similar to that produced by the bovine bacillus, was no accidental or transient phenomenon in the case of strain X, but proved constant on repeated cultivation extending over a year (*loc. cit.* p. 125).

Burckhardt also remarks that one of his strains of human type grew on broth exactly as if it were a bovine bacillus, and yet was unlike this type in every other respect.

Differentiation of the Avian from the Mammalian Types. The differentiating value of the cultural characters of the avian type of tubercle bacillus has already been mentioned (p. 209). It will suffice to recall the fact that the growth on various media is moister, and has as a rule a smooth and shining, as opposed to a dull and dry, surface; but that sometimes this characteristic fails one, and growths occur which cannot be distinguished from those of the human type of bacillus.

Perhaps the most constant difference between avian and mammalian cultures is that the former can be readily made to form a fairly homogeneous emulsion when rubbed up with fluid, which is not the case with the latter cultures. This difference impresses itself very strongly on those whose work leads them frequently to prepare emulsions for the injection of animals. Sometimes when one is trying to prepare a uniform emulsion of mammalian bacilli by rubbing a mass of growth between ground glass plates with a drop or two of salt solution it is almost like trying to emulsify soap in an acid fluid, but this difficulty never occurs with the avian bacillus.

Even when sowing subcultures the mere difference in the behaviour of the growth when touched with the platinum needle may be sufficient to reveal the characteristic consistency of the avian culture which is so different from that of the dry crumbling growth of the human tubercle bacillus.

Do Cultural Characters alone suffice for determining the Type of Tubercle Bacilli?

The principal characters of growth, on various artificial media, of the three types of tubercle bacilli have now been described and contrasted, and the limits of their variation pointed out. It has been shown that while the cultural differences which may serve to distinguish the types from one another are sufficiently distinct as a general rule, yet occasionally some uncertainty occurs (see p. 205). We have seen that some observers attach far more importance to these irregularities than others, and we must agree with Rabinowitsch that " the question of the heterogeneity of the various tubercle bacilli and their eventual division into various species, varieties and types will probably not be solved in the near future in a completely satisfactory manner " (*Tuberculosis*, 1907, vol. VI, p. 392). But we have seen that many atypical strains have been resolved into mixtures of two of the types, and that many irregularities may safely be attributed to faults of technique, especially to unavoidable defects in the culture media employed; and while we believe that strains both of bovine and human type vary in their cultural capacities within rather wide limits, we are not prepared to go so far as Eastwood and Rabinowitsch in thinking that they form a continuous series, and would rather hold with Park and Krumwiede, that the more the technique is improved the fewer will be the strains which do not conform to one or other of the types[1].

III. *The Reaction Curve of Human and Bovine Tubercle Bacilli.*

Morphological peculiarities having failed to afford a satisfactory test of type, and the determination of cultural characters being at times attended by considerable difficulty and uncertainty, observers have naturally turned their attention to bio-chemical reactions to see whether one might be found which would serve the purpose of differentiation.

In 1903 Theobald Smith introduced a test of this kind based on a difference in the reaction curves which he had

---

[1] See also App. p. 681.

observed when the two mammalian types of tubercle bacilli were grown on glycerin broth. Such broth, as is commonly used for the cultivation of tubercle bacilli, has an initial acidity to phenol-phthalein, but as the tubercle bacillus of either type grows over its surface the acidity diminishes almost to the point of extinction. From that time onwards, according to Smith, the changes in reaction differ in the two types. With the bovine type the neutral point may be reached or even passed, and there the change ends; while with the human type the reaction, having approached the neutral point, becomes reversed and there is a recovery of acidity. The difference in the two types is thus shown clearly in the final reaction, which is very nearly neutral (slightly acid or slightly alkaline) if the bacillus belongs to the bovine type, and decidedly acid if it belongs to the human type.

This difference in the reaction curves of the two types of mammalian tubercle bacilli Smith regards as the expression of a "fundamental difference of bio-chemical character." But while all observers who have studied the test agree with Smith that the changes which he described commonly occur, they are not all at one with him in thinking that the difference is sufficiently sharp and constant to afford a test of practical value; and it is moreover not yet certain, as we shall see, that the difference in question depends upon any fundamental character, and is not merely a quantitative difference dependent on the luxuriance of growth.

A. S. Griffith (1907)[1] investigated the value of the test for the Tuberculosis Commission, and reported unfavourably. He arrived at the conclusion that his observations had "clearly shown that glycerin-broth culture does not differentiate tubercle bacilli into two classes, and had yielded no evidence that there is an essential difference in the action of different strains of tubercle bacilli on glycerin."

He was "able to confirm Smith in his general statement that the slightly virulent ". (i.e. for calf and rabbit) " bacillus of human origin when grown upon the surface of glycerin-broth causes first a diminution in the acidity of the medium

---

[1] R.C.T. Int. Rep. vol. III, p. 55.

XII]   THE "REACTION CURVE"   233

and then an increase, and that there are strains of bacilli of
bovine origin which steadily diminish the acidity of the broth "
(*loc. cit.* p. 57) but he did not find that such results were constant;
on the contrary there were other strains which produced all
intermediate varieties of reaction ; and, taking all the strains
of tubercle bacilli examined, he says that, if judged by the
difference between " their initial and final reactions, they form
an unbroken series in which there is nowhere a gap that would
justify the conclusion that ‘two essentially different kinds of
organisms were being dealt with"; and he states definitely
that the results of his investigation "do not support the conclusion which Smith draws from his experiments—that the
differences he has observed point to a difference in physiological
properties " (*ibid.*).

Further investigations (*loc. cit.* p. 80) only served to
strengthen this conclusion; additional experiments with
glycerin-litmus-milk (p. 85) gave no better results; and glucose-
broth was found valueless for the purpose[1] (p. 82).

Griffith returned to the subject, and made additional
investigations in 1911. His final conclusions were as follows :

" The bovine tubercle bacillus produces acid as well as alkali
in glycerin-broth when it grows well, the amount of acid produced depending in the main upon the luxuriance of growth."

" The glycerin-broth test does not bring out distinct bio-
chemical differences in the action of the bovine and the human
tubercle bacillus on glycerin-broth[2]."

Meanwhile, abroad, the results obtained were conflicting,
though on the whole they lent but little support to Smith's
position. O. Bang (1907) indeed obtained results which were
identical with those of Smith. But in the United States
Mohler and Washburn (1907) and Lewis (1910), working at

---

[1] It is interesting to note that as a food substance glucose proved a satisfactory substitute for glycerin; all the cultures grew, and the pellicles formed
were the same as those on glycerin-broth, but there was no formation of
acid. " In all cases the acidity of the broth was gradually diminished, the
virulent strain (*i.e.* for calf and rabbit) acting in precisely the same way as
the slightly virulent strains. The greatest diminution of acidity occurred
with those strains which produced the most luxuriant growths " (*loc. cit.*
p. 82).

[2] *R.C.T.* 1911, *Fin. Rep.* vol. 1, p. 26.

Smith's suggestion, got irregular results; sometimes the reaction curve would be that of the type to which the strain in question did not belong, and sometimes different types of reaction would be given by the same virus on repeated tests.

Fibiger and Jensen (1908) investigated the reaction curves of thirty different strains of tubercle bacilli, and concluded that while a difference in the reaction of glycerin-broth cultures of different strains of tubercle bacilli, such as Smith described, undoubtedly occurs, yet this does not support the division of mammalian tubercle bacilli into two types ; for strains were repeatedly met with which in all other particulars corresponded to the human type, and yet gave the reaction of the bovine type[1].

In spite of adverse criticism and want of support Smith (1910) maintained his position, and even went so far as to declare that the reaction test was essential to the complete demonstration of any change of type which was claimed to occur in "passage" experiments[2].

Grund also (1911), working in New York under the general direction of Park and Krumwiede, made an extensive series of investigations of this reaction. The general difference in the reaction curves of the two types which Smith had described were confirmed, but there were too many intermediate types of reaction, and the results, when the test was repeated with a given virus, were too inconstant to have any practical value for the determination of type of a given virus[3].

[1] *Berl. klin. Wochenschr.* 1908, p. 2031.

[2] "Among the criteria for distinguishing the bovine from the human type of bacilli, such as slow or rapid growth, high or low virulence for rabbits, I regard the difference in the reaction curve as the most interesting, and at the same time the most puzzling, phenomenon. It is closely bound up with the vital processes of this species of which we know so little. All claims at transformation by passage of the human into the bovine type, or *vice versa*, must, in my estimation, pass the test of the reaction curve, as well as the others given above, before such a transformation can be accepted as accomplished." (Th. Smith, *Journ. of Med. Res.* vol. XXIII, p. 185.)

[3] Grund's conclusions may be quoted in full, as they appear to form a just and moderate estimate of the value of this test. " Broadly speaking, the reaction curve in glycerin-broth divides tubercle bacilli into two types. The bacilli which possess a low degree of virulence for rabbits, and the power to grow well on glycerin media in the early generations, produce one type of

XII]   THE "REACTION CURVE"   235

Theobald Smith, as we have seen, was of opinion that the difference in the reaction curve of human and bovine tubercle bacilli depended on fundamental bio-chemical differences in the two types, and he quotes in illustration of his meaning the difference between *B. coli* and the hog-cholera bacillus in media containing lactose. "Here one culture acts upon the sugar, the other does not. Some such difference appears to exist between the bovine and human tubercle bacilli" (*Journ. of Med. Res.* vol. XIII, p. 290).

With this view of the case Griffith does not agree. The differences in the reaction curves of the two types are for him "differences in degree and not in kind and are attributable to

reaction curve, while those which are virulent for rabbits and which in the early generations grow slowly and with difficulty on glycerin media, form the other type of curve in glycerin-broth. These two types of glycerin reaction curve are again divisible into groups according to their final reactions. The curves of adjacent groups show much the same general direction and there is a gradation from one group to the next; but the reaction curves of the groups at both extremes are widely divergent. When any large number of viruses is examined there will be found a small percentage of cases, which, by cultural characteristics and virulence, belong to one type of tubercle bacilli, while they would be classed with the opposite type of bacilli if judged by their glycerin reaction curve alone. On repeated tests this reversed glycerin reaction curve may, or may not, be a constant feature of these particular viruses, although the conditions under which they have been cultivated are apparently the same in the several tests. Undetected variations of the culture medium must be taken into consideration. It is not advisable to depend on the reaction curve from one lot of broth only, but several examinations of a virus are desirable. In from thirty to forty per cent. of the viruses retested, the reaction curves belong to different groups, that is, the end reaction may be high in one test, and low or medium in the next. In only three instances was the variation so great as to justify the classification of the reaction curves into different types.

There is also no constant relation between irregularities of culture and virulence on the one hand, and irregularities of the glycerin reaction curve on the other. Some viruses which culturally and in virulence showed nothing unusual have given very atypical curves, while perfectly normal reaction curves were produced by viruses which from cultural and virulence tests could not be called quite typical.

The glycerin reaction curve is undoubtedly a valuable corroborative evidence of a division of tubercle bacilli into two types. Its value is lessened, however, by the number of irregular and atypical reactions encountered, while as a practical aid in determining the types of an individual virus, it is also much handicapped by the length of time required to carry it out" (*Journ. of Med. Res.* 1911, p. 355).

variations in saprophytic power which have been shown to exist on other media " (*loc. cit.* 1907, p. 80).

Smith believed that the chemical activities of the acid-producing group of tubercle bacilli were of two kinds : " during the early growth of the bacilli the acid of the bouillon disappears in part ; later on another process begins, or at least preponderates, which may be associated with the decomposition of the glycerin into acids, and which probably outstrips the alkaline process and masks it " (1904, p. 290).

Now if we may accept this, and bearing in mind how poorly bovine strains of tubercle bacilli grow, as a rule, on broth in comparison with human strains, it seems not improbable that the ultimate state of bovine cultures is usually nearly neutral because their growth stops short of the stage at which acid-production begins to be preponderant. If this be so those bovine strains which have become adapted to the conditions of life in glycerin-broth, so that they grow as freely as strains of human type, should give a human type of reaction, and those human strains which for some reason or other grow but feebly should give a bovine type of reaction. But those who are in the best position to express an opinion on this point agree that it is not so.

Park and Krumwiede (1910, p. 332), probably referring to Grund's experiments which were carried out under their general direction, mention indeed two strains of human type which formed a thin pellicle of growth and gave a bovine type of reaction ; but when they *weighed* the quantity of bacilli produced in different cultures, and compared the results with the final degree of acidity, they failed to find any constant relation. " Seven bovine viruses," they say, " grew vigorously, and the final weight was equal to that of the average growth of human type " and yet their reaction curve was that of the bovine type.

Grund is equally emphatic, and states that she had " not found that the amount of growth, and the degree of acid-production stand in definite and constant relation to one another." She adds that a number of her bovine viruses yielded a weight of dried bacilli equal to, or even higher, than that of the average weight of the human viruses, and yet their reaction curves fell into one of the three groups into which she subdivided those produced by bovine bacilli in general ; while, on the other hand, some of the human viruses which produced a highly acid end reaction were found when dried to have produced only a comparatively small quantity of bacilli[1]. This is strong testimony to the truth of Smith's view.

Fibiger and Jensen also came to the same conclusion, and so indeed did Griffith. The latter found, it is true, that the three strains which caused the greatest reduction of acidity produced much less growth than those which formed most acid ; but beyond this the correlation ceased, and " the remaining estimations " seemed " to show that the majority of the more virulent bacilli were incapable of producing with the same, or even greater, bulk of growth as much acid as the less virulent bacilli " (loc. cit. 1907, p. 80). Here again is support for the fundamental basis of Smith's position if not for the practical value of the test he introduced, and this is hardly consistent with the view, which Griffith expresses on the same page, and which has already been quoted, namely, that " the differences...are differences in degree and not in kind, and are attributable to variations in saprophytic power."

This absence of correlation between the quantity of bacilli grown in the culture and the final degree of acidity, attested as it is by independent observers, all of whom have reported adversely as to the practical value of Smith's test, and who therefore cannot be supposed to be unduly influenced by his undoubtedly great authority on such matters, is of considerable importance, and strongly supports Smith's contention that the difference in end reaction of the two types of bacilli is the result of an essential bio-chemical difference and is not merely dependent on the luxuriance of growth. It suggests too that the irregularities which rob the test of its practical value are due to a want of constancy in the conditions, and that if the technique of the test could be improved it might yet prove to be of considerable utility.

---

[1] 1911, p. 350. Elsewhere Grund states that "in about half the cases the degree of acidity produced has been in direct ratio to the amount of growth."

The question however arises : Can we be sure that there is no correlation between the amount of growth, as measured either by weight or volume of bacilli, and the final degree of acidity ? In other words, can we trust the measurements on which these conclusions are based ? For there are considerable technical difficulties to be overcome in these delicate investigations. Titrations are notoriously difficult when broth cultures are concerned, and even the estimation of the quantity of growth either volumetrically or by the balance, is not easy to carry out with any great accuracy. Every method of measurement, no matter of what kind, has its limits of error, and the question which arises here is: Are the limits in this case so narrow that one can safely trust conclusions founded upon differences of measurement so small as those on which the conclusion in question is based ?

To the mind of the writer the marked difference in the yield of bacilli found by Griffith on comparing the three cultures which produced most acid with the three which produced least acid is of greater significance than the minor departures from strict relation of growth and acidity which was shown by the remainder of his cultures ; he is therefore not yet wholly convinced that the difference of end reaction, which in general is characteristic of the two types of bacilli, is not dependent merely on the fact that as a rule one type grows better than the other.

The question may be put more directly : Does the bovine type of bacillus possess the power of forming acid out of glycerin, or does it not ? Smith apparently believes that it does not, and that in this respect it differs fundamentally from the human type of bacillus. Griffith does not agree with him, for the following reasons. Some of his bovine strains after a preliminary approach toward the neutral point, showed a slight return of acidity, though as a rule this was absent or minimal. He reasoned that if the bovine bacillus could only form alkaline products and no acid the more luxuriant the growth the greater should have been the loss of acidity, but this was not the case, the more luxuriant bovine cultures were often the most acid. After having returned to the question (1911) he finally concluded that " the bovine bacillus produces acid as well as alkali in glycerin broth when it grows well, the amount of acid depending in the main upon the luxuriance of growth." (*R.C.T. Final Report*, vol. I, p. 26.)

During the progress of the researches detailed in the previous pages, the Royal Commission, recognizing the increasing complexity of the question, and the consequent desirability of obtaining help from those trained in the application of the methods of pure chemistry to bio-chemical problems, invited Dr Arthur Harden to undertake an investigation of the subject. Harden consequently carried out a series of investigations at the Lister Institute during 1908–9, on cultures supplied by A. S. Griffith from the Commission's laboratories in Stansted. Harden's report, 1913, gives no support to Theobald Smith's position. He was unable to find " any physiological difference between tubercle bacilli of different origins." And the somewhat unexpected (at least by the present writer) result was reached that " there was no direct production of acid out of glycerol[1]," and no connection between the amount of glycerol used and the change in total acidity, and none was made evident by allowing for the production or disappearance of ammonia, and for the disappearance of acids soluble in ether (*loc. cit.* p. 27).

It seems then that bacteriologists have been misled through failing to understand the complexity of the chemical question. The changes of reaction cannot be explained, apparently, by the ability or disability of the bacilli to feed on glycerin. Alkaline as well as acid products are formed and of each of these some (*e.g.* CO_2 and NH_3) are volatile. The actual reaction of the mixture will depend not only upon the relative activity of formation of each of these products, but also upon the relative activity of their removal. Harden's report is of great interest and should be consulted by those interested. It is impossible to do justice to it in a brief summary[2].

[1] *loc. cit.* p. 21. He adds " that is to say (1) that no definite acid product of such a change has been isolated or detected in the medium after cultivation of the bacillus ; (2) that there is no recognisable relation between the amounts of glycerol used, and the production of acid."

[2] Harden's conclusions may be given in full :

(1) No definite physiological difference has been detected between tubercle bacilli of different origins.

(2) Such differences as exist between the amounts of action exerted

Conclusions as to the Value of the Reaction Curve. From the various investigations which we have considered it seems reasonable to draw the following conclusions :

1. Alkaline as well as acid products are formed by tubercle bacilli and of each of these some (*e.g.* CO_2 and NH_3) are volatile ; rapidity of growth as well as its volume will therefore influence the resulting reaction.

2. The reaction curve produced by the bovine type of bacillus in glycerin broth differs, as a rule, from that produced by the human.

3. These differences have not been shown conclusively to depend upon any fundamental physiological difference in the metabolism of these types, such as a capacity, or a want of capacity, to feed on glycerin, or to form acid out of that substance, as Smith supposed, but seem rather to depend on the differences commonly observed in the rate and vigour of their growth.

4. Such difference of reaction as is observed, only serves in effect to give us information of the same kind as can be obtained far more easily and quickly by observing the quantity and rate of growth on various culture media.

5. As a practical aid to the determination of the type of a given strain of tubercle bacilli the application of the reaction test is difficult and tedious, and has not been shown to add any information beyond what may be gained by more simple means.

on glycerol-beef-broth by different cultures are probably to be attributed to differences between the weights of organism formed, the times of incubation and the individual characteristics of the strains.

(3) When *B. tuberculosis* is cultivated on glycerol-broth, the proteins of the broth undergo hydrolysis to a considerable extent.

(4) Glycerol is partially removed by oxidation. There is no evidence that consumption of glycerol is directly related either to the weight of culture obtained or to the change in acidity.

(5) The initial fall in the acidity of the medium is largely due to the removal of the acids soluble in ether (lactic acid, etc.).

(6) Further important factors in producing changes in acidity are the production and removal of ammonia (free and saline) and the digestion of proteins (*loc. cit.* p. 29).

Summary and Conclusions.

I.   The three types of tubercle bacilli differ morphologically, culturally, chemically and pathogenetically.   The small peculiarities of size and shape, however, which in bacteriology are dignified by the name of morphological characters, differ so little in the three types of bacilli and on the whole are so inconstant that they have little value as differentiating characters.

II.   Cultural differences, on the other hand, are of considerably more importance, and deserve careful study ; but their exact determination is not always an easy matter, and by themselves they are barely sufficient for differentiation.   Of greater value are, as we shall see in the next chapter, differences in the power of producing disease in certain species of animals.

III.   The difference in the growth of the two types of mammalian tubercle bacilli is one of quantity and rapidity, especially on media which contain glycerin.   This in all probability does not depend on any fundamental difference of bio-chemical properties, for bovine bacilli are capable of adapting themselves to glycerin media, and apparently come, in time, to put it to good use.

IV.   Avian tubercle bacilli differ from mammalian in the absence of the tendency to stick obstinately together, which is so marked a character of the latter ; they therefore much more readily lend themselves to the formation of a uniform suspension.

V.   Avian cultures on various media have often a moist glistening appearance not seen in mammalian cultures, but sometimes this character is wanting.

VI.   Avian strains as a rule grow badly on broth, and only with some difficulty, and not in every case can they be induced to form a pellicle.

VII.   The uncertainty which sometimes attends the placing of given strains of tubercle bacilli in their proper class, depends largely on the difficulty of preparing culture media of constant value ; but apparently it also depends partly on differences in the vegetative capacities of different strains in each type, particularly perhaps in those of human type.

c.   16

VIII.   Only media which contain glycerin are of any value for differentiation of type by means of cultural characters.

IX.   Tests should not be confined to any one medium, but should include culture on egg, serum, agar, potato, and broth, to each of which glycerin has been added.

X.   No single tests, however carefully devised and carried out, should be depended on alone.   Cultural characters can only be adequately determined by repeated cultivation on a large variety of media, and carried out over a considerable space of time.

XI.   The earlier in the course of their saprophytic existence cultural characters can be determined the better.   It is, however, impossible to rely on primary cultures, and though a slowly progressing adaptation to the conditions of growth in the test tube gradually tends to obscure the differences in vegetative capacity which are, as a rule, well-marked in strains freshly isolated from the animal body, there is no need to hurry the investigation of cultural characters unduly, for many months at least are available before the distinction in the cultural characters of the types tend to become obscured.

XII.   On the other hand, in order to avoid the tendency which adaptation to a new pabulum has to obscure the sharpness of the distinction, the stock cultures of the various strains of bacilli which are being tested should be kept rigidly from glycerin, and should be grown preferably on plain serum or egg.

REFERENCES.   VIII

(Chapter XII)

The Reaction Curve.

Bang, Olaf (1907).   Einige vergleichende Untersuchungen über die Einwirkung der Säugetier- und Geflügel-Tuberkelbazillen und die Reaction des Substrats in Bouillon-Kulturen.   *Centralb. f. Bakt. etc.* 1. Abt. vol. XLIII, 34.

Beitzke.   Über die Infection des Menschen mit Rindertuberculose. *Virchow's Archiv f. path. Anat.* Beiheft, vol. 190, p. 58.

Duval.   Studies in atypical forms of tubercle bacilli isolated directly from human tissues in cases of primary cervical adenitis.   *Jour. Exp. Med.* 1909, vol. XI, p. 403.

Fibiger and Jensen (1908). Untersuchungen über die Beziehungen zwischen der Tuberkulose und den Tuberkelbazillen des Menschen und der Tuberkulose und den Tuberkelbazillen des Rindes. *Berl. klin. Wochenschr.* 1908, No. 45, p. 2028.

Griffith, A. S. (1907). Report on the Changes in Reaction produced in Broth by Human and Bovine Tubercle Bacilli. *R.C.T. 2nd Int. Rep.* App. 1907, vol. III, p. 53.

—— Additional observations on the changes of Reaction produced in Glycerin-Broth (*ibid.* p. 80), in Glucose-Broth (*ibid.* p. 82) and in Glycerinated Litmus-Milk (*ibid.* p. 85).

—— (1911). The Glycerin-Broth Test. *R.C.T. Final Rep.* App. vol. I, p. 26.

Grund. The Reaction Curve in glycerin-broth as an aid in differentiating the bovine from the human type of tubercle bacillus. Carried out at the suggestion and under the direction of Park and Krumwiede. *Journ. of Med. Res.* 1911, p. 335.

Harden (1913). Report on the Results of a Chemical Investigation. *R.C.T. Final Rep.* App. vol. VI.

Park and Krumwiede (1910). The Relative Importance of Bovine and Human Types of Tubercle Bacilli, etc. See "Smith's Reaction," p. 331.

Lewis (1910). Tuberculous Cervical Adenitis. A study of the Tubercle Bacilli cultivated from fifteen consecutive cases. *Jour. Exp. Med.* vol. XII, p. 82.

Mohler and Washburn, H. J. (1907). A Comparative Study of Tubercle Bacilli from Varied Sources. *Bull.* No. 96. *Bureau of Animal Industry, Dep. of Agriculture, U.S.A.* 1907.

Smith, Th. (1905). Studies in Mammalian Tubercle Bacilli III. A culture test for distinguishing the bovine from the human type of tubercle bacillus. *Journ. of Med. Res.* vol. XIII, p. 286. Also in the *Trans. Amer. Phys.* vol. XVIII, p. 108.

—— (1905). The Reaction Curve of Tubercle Bacilli from Different Sources, etc. *Journ. of Med. Res.* vol. XIII, p. 405.

—— (1910). The Reaction Curve of the Human and the Bovine Type of Tubercle Bacillus in Glycerin-Bouillon. *Journ. of Med. Res.* vol. XXIII, p. 185.

CHAPTER XIII

THE MEANS OF DISTINGUISHING THE THREE TYPES OF TUBERCLE BACILLI ONE FROM ANOTHER (*continued*)

IV. *By Means of Animal Experiment.*

The main distinction between the three types of tubercle bacilli lies in the difference in the power which they possess of producing disease in certain species of animals. It is the existence of such pathogenetic differences that has created the necessity of distinguishing the three types from one another, and it is on them that reliance must in the main be placed when endeavouring to assign a given strain of bacilli to its proper type.

Differentiation of the avian from the mammalian types. It has been said already that domestic fowls and pigeons are insusceptible to infection with either human or bovine tubercle bacilli, while they yield readily to the attack of the avian bacillus. For this reason they afford a ready means of determining whether a given strain of tubercle bacilli belongs to the avian, or to one of the two mammalian types.

In employing these birds for the purpose in question it is best, perhaps, to use intraperitoneal injection, though equally clear and more rapid differentiation may be obtained by intravenous injection, provided that moderate doses only are employed. This precaution is necessary because, as was said before (p. 211), the fowl and pigeon succumb to the toxicity of large doses of mammalian tubercle bacilli injected into the blood stream, although it appears that the bacilli do not get established in the body of the bird, or infect it in the true sense. Subcutaneous or intramuscular injection is better avoided, since, if the bacilli are of the avian type, such procedure is apt to be followed by the formation of an open sore, from which there is risk that the bacilli may become disseminated.

In addition to these birds which are only susceptible to infection with the avian bacillus, it is desirable to employ an

animal which is insusceptible to the avian bacillus and susceptible to the two mammalian bacilli. Such an one is found
in the guinea-pig. It is true that this animal is not entirely
insusceptible to the attack of the avian bacillus, and often
succumbs after intraperitoneal injection of large doses ; but the
type of disease is then so different from that caused by mammalian bacilli, and in particular the absence of the usual caseous
or necrotic lesions is so marked, that no difficulty is presented
on this account to the experienced observer (see p. 437).
However, it is probably better when using the guinea-pig for
this purpose to avoid intraperitoneal injection, and to rely
on subcutaneous injection which is never followed by a fatal
result if the bacilli injected be of the avian type.

If it be desired to differentiate only between the avian and
the human types of bacilli the rabbit may be used ; for, curiously
enough, this animal is much more susceptible to infection with
the avian bacillus than to that with the human type of mammalian bacilli.

Practical details. The strain of bacilli under investigation
should be grown in artificial culture, preferably on serum, and
it should be used for injection after incubation for a definite
number of days. This is desirable, in order that, in comparative experiments, the proportion of living and vigorous bacilli
in the dose injected may be as constant as possible. The
exact number of days assigned for incubation is not very
material, so long as it does not vary. It is obvious that the
younger the cultures are the better, provided that they yield
enough bacilli for the purpose in hand. Those working for
the Royal Commission selected three weeks as the routine
period of incubation for cultures which were to be injected in
test doses ; but a more extended experience has shown that
a somewhat shorter period is practicable, and possibly preferable. These remarks apply equally to comparative investigations with any strains of tubercle bacilli.

Referring now only to the differentiation of the avian
from the mammalian types, the guinea-pig, for reasons given
above, should be injected subcutaneously, and the dose should
be ten milligrammes. The same dose may be given to the fowl

or pigeon intraperitoneally.   If a quicker result is desired the injection into the bird may be intravenous, but if this is done the dose should be reduced to one milligramme.   The vein at the root of the wing will be found a convenient place for such injection.

Animals which do not die within a fixed period of observation may be killed—the guinea-pig six weeks or two months after injection, and the fowl preferably after a longer period.

If the strain which is being tested contains bacilli of one type only, the test may be relied upon to give a clear and decisive result.   Either the guinea-pig develops severe tuberculosis, with the usual characteristic lesions, and the fowl, or pigeon, remains unaffected; or the bird develops tuberculosis, while the guinea-pig remains well, or at most develops some lesions which are not characteristic of tuberculosis.   In the former case the strain may with confidence be pronounced to be mammalian in type, and in the latter avian.

One animal only of each kind has been spoken of, but in practice it is desirable to inject several of each kind, in case of death occurring prematurely from some accidental cause, and in order to have some control in the event of spontaneous tuberculosis (which is not uncommon, at least in the fowl), occurring to confuse the issue.

It is hardly necessary to add that a careful post-mortem examination should be performed in each case, and that the distribution of the lesions in relation to the channels of infection leading from the seat of inoculation should be duly considered. Histological examination of the lesions is hardly necessary, but in no case should a microscopic search for tubercle bacilli in "smear" preparations from the lesions be omitted.   This latter precaution is particularly necessary on account of the frequency with which that confusing disease pseudo-tuberculosis is met with in the guinea-pig (see p. 434).

In earlier days Straus and Gamaléia (1891), following Maffucci, were led to consider the dog as the animal *par excellence* for the differentiation of avian and human tubercle bacilli[1] These observers found that intravenous injection of a dose of

[1] See Straus, *La Tuberculose*, p. 349.

one-quarter of a cubic centimetre or less of "a sufficiently dense emulsion" of human tubercle bacilli provoked a tuberculosis which always proved fatal in a month or two, while an intravenous injection of avian bacilli (except in enormous doses such as 20 or 30 c.c. of a similar emulsion) caused no illness, and when the dogs were killed they presented no lesions. This is undoubtedly the fact[1]; and the injection of the dog may be used with equal success to distinguish avian from bovine bacilli. But one naturally prefers to use other animals for infection experiments, unless the dog is absolutely indispensable; and, fortunately, for the purpose we are now considering the guinea-pig and the fowl provide us with all that is necessary.

Differentiation of the human and bovine types of tubercle bacilli. Various species of animals react very differently to the two mammalian types of tubercle bacilli. Some, such as the common fowl, are, as we have seen, almost totally resistant to infection with either type of bacillus. Others, such as the ox and rabbit, are highly susceptible to the bovine type, and highly resistant to the human type. While others again, such as the guinea-pig and monkey, are almost equally susceptible to either type.

Man alone of all animals is, as we shall see later on, more susceptible to the human than to the bovine type of tubercle bacillus (see p. 659).

A. S. Griffith[2] divides animal species, according to the way they react to tubercle bacilli of human and bovine type respectively, into three groups:

1. The first group consists of animals which are highly susceptible to infection with either type of mammalian tubercle bacilli, and includes the Rhesus and other monkeys, the chimpanzee and the guinea-pig.

2. The second group possesses a comparatively high and approximately equal resistance to both types, and includes the rat, the mouse and the dog.

---

[1] F. Griffith also says " the dog is able to withstand large doses of avian tubercle bacilli inoculated intravenously without suffering any ill effects or developing any tuberculous lesion." *R.C.T. Fin. Rep.* App. vol. IV. p. 173.

[2] *R.C.T. Fin. Rep.* App. vol. I. p. 23.

3. The third is the differentiating group : susceptible to infection with the bovine type, but highly resistant to infection with the human type. This group includes a large number of species, among which the ox, goat, pig, sheep, horse, cat and rabbit may be mentioned.

An attempt is made in the following table to represent the relative degree of susceptibility to infection with the two types of mammalian tubercle bacilli of the various animal species which have been subjected to experimental investigation.

TABLE IX. *Comparative susceptibility of various animals to the two types of mammalian tuberculosis* (as shown by experimental inoculation in all but man).

Animal	1 Human Type	2 Bovine Type	Note
Fowl, pigeon	o	o	Succumb to large intravenous doses.
Rat, mouse	+	+	Succumb slowly to a peculiar form of progressive infection after large intraperitoneal doses of either type of bacillus.
Dog	**+**	**+**	— —
Ox, sheep, goat, cat	+	**++**	Resistant to small doses of bovine bacilli.
Pig	+	**++**	Slightly more susceptible to human tuberculosis than the ox.
Rabbit	++	**+++**	Slightly more susceptible to human tuberculosis than the ox or pig.
Guinea-pig	**+++**	**+++** ⎱ Rather more susceptible to bovine
Monkey, baboon	**+++**	**+++** ⎰ than to human tuberculosis.
Anthropoid ape	**+++**	**+++**	— —
Man	**++**	**+**	— —

o = complete insusceptibility.
+ = a low degree of susceptibility.
++ = a slightly higher but still low degree of susceptibility.
+ = a moderate degree of susceptibility.
++ and **+++** = a high and very high degree of susceptibility respectively.

Among the animals which have been mentioned in the third group as serving to differentiate between the mammalian types of tubercle bacilli some deserve special consideration as being commonly used, or well adapted for use, in laboratory investigation.

The ox, as is natural, has been usually regarded as the most important animal for the differentiation of the two mammalian types of tubercle bacilli, but considering the frequency with

which in all civilized countries it suffers from spontaneous tuberculosis, and the fact that the tuberculin test cannot be absolutely
depended upon to reveal this condition in all cases, the use of
this animal is not entirely free from objection.   It is fortunately
true that spontaneous tuberculosis is very rare in the calf, yet
this animal is expensive both to buy and to keep.   The goat
might reasonably be preferred, since it seldom suffers from
the spontaneous disease, and gives an uncommonly decisive
tuberculin reaction[1].   Moreover, it distinguishes between the
two types of bacilli quite as clearly as the ox.   The rabbit is the
animal which, on account of its cheapness and convenience, is
most commonly used for the purpose now under consideration;
but, as we shall see, it distinguishes between the two types of
bacilli less sharply than the ox and the goat, and on this account its use is sometimes liable to be misleading except in
the hands of the expert in these matters.   The cat differentiates
the two types of bacilli clearly, but is not exempt from spontaneous bovine tuberculosis.

The calf and the rabbit then being the animals most
commonly used for the differentiation of the two types of
mammalian tubercle bacilli, it is desirable to study their reactions to the two types more closely, and to inquire to what
extent, if any, variation in *the method of inoculating*, in *the dose
of bacilli*, and in *the individual susceptibility of the test animal*
may affect the result.

THE CALF AS A MEANS OF DIFFERENTIATING THE TYPES OF
MAMMALIAN TUBERCLE BACILLI.

A.   *Choice of the Method of Injection.*

Of the various ways of causing experimental tuberculosis in
the calf, namely subcutaneous, intraperitoneal and intravenous
injections, inhalation and feeding, subcutaneous injection is the
one usually preferred.   Feeding is too uncertain in its results,
inhalation too difficult and dangerous, and intraperitoneal injection offers no advantages and some disadvantages, as compared
with the subcutaneous method.   Intravenous injection has

[1] See *R.C.T. Fin. Rep.* App. Suppl. vol. 1913, pp. 41 and 73.

in its favour the fact that the bacilli are more completely confined to the body of the animal injected, and that there is, therefore, less risk of the infection spreading to other animals, or to the attendants. On the other hand, this advantage is partly neutralised by the fact that the human type of tubercle bacillus in large doses may cause fatal disease when given by this method, a result which never occurs with subcutaneous injection.

Subcutaneous injection. Subcutaneous injection then, being the method commonly used for the purpose under consideration, must be more fully considered. It is of fundamental importance to bear in mind that no quantity, however large, of tubercle bacilli of human type injected subcutaneously into the calf will produce a fatal or progressive tuberculosis, and that while tubercle bacilli of bovine type cause, in suitable doses, a rapidly progressing general miliary tuberculosis, which proves fatal in almost all cases within a few weeks or months, small doses of this type do not cause more than little local, or if disseminated then minimal and non-progressive, lesions. The dose selected is, therefore, of importance. It must be large enough. To this point we shall return, but it may be said at once that the quantity usually employed is 50 milligrammes.

In the experience of the Royal Commission this quantity of bacilli of bovine type proved fatal in 94·5 per cent. of the calves injected[1].

In the investigations which were carried out at the Gesundheitsamt subcutaneous injections of 50 milligrammes of tubercle bacilli of bovine type were less frequently fatal than in those made by the Royal Commission. The reason for this seems to be two-fold. In the first place the Commission used only Jersey calves (specially imported for the purpose), while this was not the case at the Gesundheitsamt, and there is some reason to suspect that Jerseys are rather more susceptible to tuberculosis than other breeds. In the second place the German investigators employed for injection bacilli grown on the surface of glycerin-broth, while those who worked for the

---

[1] Not including those injected with strains derived from persons suffering from lupus and certain analogous strains from the horse and pig (see chap. xxv).

Commission used bacilli obtained from young cultures on pure serum. The latter method is much to be preferred because growth on serum can be so much more readily induced than growth on broth that it is possible to test the virulence of the strains of bacilli at a much earlier period when serum cultures are used than when glycerin-broth is employed. Moreover, broth cultures have the disadvantage that they grow slowly and at a very variable rate, so that it is not easy to use young cultures for injection, and especially cultures of uniform age, as is easily done in the case of serum.

The method of estimating the dose of bacilli was different in the two institutions. In the Gesundheitsamt the bacilli were weighed on a balance. At the laboratories of the Royal Commission they were measured by volume by a method which is described below[1]. It must clearly be understood,

[1] The method of estimating the doses used in the laboratories of the Royal Commission was as follows : The bacilli were scraped off the surface of the serum and finely emulsified by rubbing between ground glass plates, with a few drops of physiological salt solution. The process was repeated with fresh serum cultures, until sufficient quantity of emulsified bacilli had been collected for the purpose in view. The emulsion was then allowed to stand for some minutes to allow the larger particles to settle, and the rest was pipetted off.

Capillary tubes with a bore of about one or one and a half millimetres and a length of about 10 centimetres were drawn in the blowpipe from ordinary glass tubing, and these were carefully calibrated with a drop of mercury, the length of which was measured in various parts of the tube. Only those tubes which showed a fairly uniform calibre from one end to the other were used, and the rest, the great majority, were rejected. A stock of these calibrated tubes was always kept on hand.

The emulsion having been well shaken to ensure uniformity, one or more of the tubes was filled with a sample of it, and, having had one end sealed in the flame, was put into a centrifuge tube, containing water to give the necessary support, and provided with a small diaphragm of cork with a central aperture to keep the small tube or tubes in an axial position. The tube, or tubes, were then centrifuged for half an hour exactly, and at the end of that time taken out, and, with the aid of a finely-divided scale and a magnifying glass, the length of the little column of bacilli which had been driven to the bottom and the total length of the column of fluid read off. In this way, since the calibre of each tube was uniform throughout its length, was obtained the ratio of the volume of bacilli to that of the emulsion, and consequently when one wanted to give a certain dose of bacilli one only had to multiply the quantity by the inverse of this ratio to obtain the volume of emulsion which contained the dose required.

This method was found to be satisfactory in practice, and sufficiently

therefore, that the doses stated in the Appendices to the Reports of the Commission in terms of milligrammes refer really to cubic millimetres, but, according to A. S. Griffith, this makes no difference, since doses estimated by volume were found by experiment to be "strictly comparable" with doses measured by weight[1].

Lesions produced by the bovine bacillus. The disease produced in the young Jersey calf by the subcutaneous injection of 50 milligrammes of bacilli of bovine type taken from young serum cultures is in nearly all cases a very acute and rapidly fatal miliary tuberculosis, affecting principally the lungs and lymphatic glands, but involving also, more or less severely, almost every other organ in the body. Somewhat rarely a highly resistant individual is met with in which the disease runs a more chronic course, and smaller differences of susceptibility are frequently seen and will be dealt with later. Older animals, so far as experiments have tested the point, prove more resistant to artificial infection than young ones, but it may be questioned whether this is true of cows (see p. 381).

The lungs are often found to be affected with extreme severity. Everywhere may be seen little opaque greyish tubercles scattered as thickly as if showered out of a pepper pot. Around each grey tubercle is a dark translucent zone the colour of plum juice, and often these congested œdematous areas are widely confluent, so that but little lung tissue contains any air. Tubercles are numerous in liver, spleen and kidneys. Every lymphatic and hæmolymph gland may be affected, and the great glands in the thorax are often enormously enlarged, and infiltrated with pinkish white opaque material. In more chronic cases "perlsucht" growths are common on the margins of the lungs and on the serous lining of the thoracic walls, and

---

accurate for the purpose in view, and it remained in use during the whole period of the Commission's labours. It possesses the advantage that it is applicable to small quantities of bacilli and thus facilitates the use of serum cultures at an early age.

In some instances, where emulsions of tuberculous tissues were used for injection the estimation of dose of bacilli was made by counting a sample of known volume (see p. 287).

[1] *R.C.T. Fin. Rep.* App. vol. I, p. 29.

Plate III

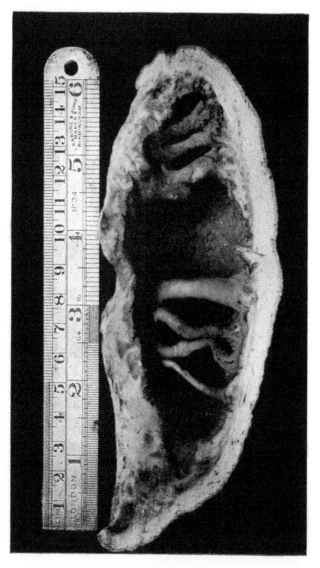

**Section through the Lesion produced in a Calf at the Seat of Injection
of an enormous dose of Human Tubercle Bacilli.**

The softened necrotic tissue has been washed away, leaving a great cavity
with fibrous walls.

Plate IV

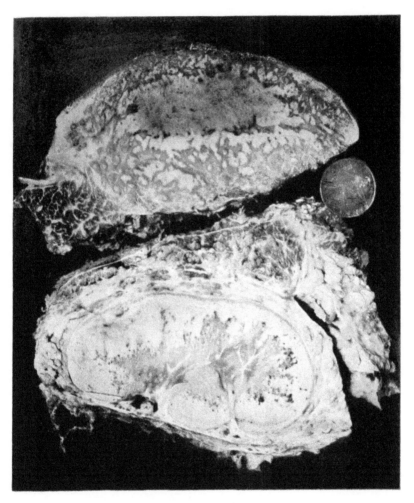

Section through the Lesion at the Seat of Inoculation and the Prescapular Gland of Calf injected with Bovine Bacilli.

Showing the local lesion infiltrating the skin and subjacent muscle, and the gland almost wholly converted into "necrotic" tissue.

tubercles on the surface of the liver may assume a mush-room-like shape, having a wide, flattened, free margin which overhangs a narrower attached base.

At the seat of inoculation an enormous necrotic tumour develops, and infiltrates the skin over it and the subjacent muscles. The nearest lymphatic glands become much enlarged and consist of a firm ivory white, or in some cases slightly pinkish, homogeneous tissue.

It is a curious fact that the local tumours produced by the bovine bacillus do not soften, at least during the usual period of observation, which seldom exceeds three months.

Lesions produced by the human bacillus. The local tumour produced in the calf by the subcutaneous injection of tubercle bacilli of human type, on the other hand, though it may be large when the dose has been 50 milligrammes or more, ceases after a while to grow, and breaks down into a caseo-purulent fluid or semi-fluid substance. Moreover, it never infiltrates the skin or muscle as the lesion caused by bovine bacilli does, but it often ulcerates through the skin and discharges its contents at a comparatively early period. When this has occurred nothing more may be found at the post-mortem examination than a sinus leading to a small fibrous patch containing caseo-calcareous grains situated in the subcutaneous tissue. If ulceration does not occur a very curious tumour with dense thick fibrous walls and semi-liquid contents may result.

Beyond the local lesion very little change is produced in the calf by subcutaneous injection of the human tubercle bacillus. The neighbouring lymphatic glands may contain some small caseo-necrotic nodules, and, in about half the cases, lymphatic glands elsewhere show a few minute foci. These are commonest in the mesenteric glands, and may perhaps in some cases be caused by bacilli which have escaped from the local lesion and have been swallowed and absorbed from the intestine. But this is probably not the usual way, for dissemination undoubtedly occurs by the blood stream, as experiments described in the Appendix have clearly shown (see p. 672). Moreover, these minute lesions are not confined to the mesenteric glands, but occur in other lymph nodes, and in about 50 per cent. of the calves inoculated by the writer, for the Royal Commission, subcutaneously with tubercle bacilli of the human type, one or more, and rarely many, minute submiliary tubercles were found in the lungs or some other organ, evidently due to bacilli disseminated by the blood stream.

As these little submiliary tubercles do not seem to have been noticed by observers other than those who worked for the Royal Commission it may be permissible to describe them in greater detail. The little tubercles in the lung were barely visible, and easily missed. They were best seen when situated on the surface of the organ, and after the latter had been allowed to dry a little by exposure to air. They then looked grey on the paler pink surface, and appeared to be angular; but when picked out on the point of a knife, they shelled out cleanly and were found to be quite spherical; they then appeared slightly opalescent and resembled little seed pearls. They were hard, and could be definitely felt to crack when pressed between glass slides, giving a sensation as though they had a calcareous envelope. Tubercle bacilli were sometimes demonstrated in them. In other organs, such as lymphatic glands, and in the liver where they were seen but rarely, they looked whiter than the surrounding tissue. This appearance was probably only due to the darker colour of the background, for otherwise they were similar to those seen in the lungs.

The most extensive tuberculosis which the present writer has seen produced by the subcutaneous injection of tubercle bacilli of human type into the ox species occurred in Calf 365[1], and may be described as an example of an exceptionally severe infection with that type of bacillus. The virus came from a case of phthisis in a man of 41 years of age, and was proved by the injection of eight calves and five rabbits to be a typical example of the human type, for in none of the animals, with the exception of this calf, was the disease more severe than that usually produced by this type of tubercle bacillus. The calf in question received an injection, under the skin of the side of the neck, of an emulsion of the lung of the phthisical

[1] R.C.T. 1907, Int. Rep. App. vol. II, pp. 555 and 562.

patient, estimated to contain 103 million tubercle bacilli, in 10 c.c. of fairly thick tissue emulsion. This dose of tubercle bacilli cannot be considered excessive[1], but it probably contained many adventitious bacteria, for there was some inflammation at the seat of inoculation shortly after the injection. The calf became somewhat ill, and about a month after inoculation it was suffering from rather high fever, its coat was staring, and it was seen to be shivering. After this it slowly improved in health, but it was still looking a little unwell two months after inoculation. It was killed on the 61st day. At the seat of inoculation there was a large and solid necrotic tumour which showed no signs of infiltrating the surrounding tissues. One of the prepectoral glands on the same side as the tumour was as large as a pigeon's egg and caseous throughout, but the prescapular gland had only two small caseous nodules of the size of cherry stones. In almost all the other lymphatic glands were little yellow foci, and grey tubercles were numerous in lungs, liver and kidneys, and on the peritoneum. The tubercles were small and dark and showed no signs of caseation. One lobule of lung was packed rather densely with these little tubercles which here appeared as whitish spots on a dark background. Over some of the more superficial tubercles were little tufts of villous growth so often seen as the result of chronic inflammation on the serous surfaces of the ox (see p. 548).

This was not a case of spontaneous tuberculosis caused by bacilli of bovine type, for there were no lesions anywhere which were out of harmony with the general pathological picture, and injection of two other calves with an emulsion from the prepectoral gland of this animal produced only the usual minimal lesions. Severe as was the result it was undoubtedly caused by tubercle bacilli of human type, aided, very possibly, by other bacteria contained in the lung emulsion.

A result like this might prove misleading to such as have had but little experience of experimental tuberculosis in these animals, and, as a matter of fact, occurring as it did

---

[1] Cp. Table of injections of tissue emulsions into calves. *R.C.T. Int. Rep.* App. vol. II, pp. 1036, 1038.

comparatively early in the work of the Commission, it proved very puzzling at the time. But further experience showed the true nature of the case, and taught those concerned that the most significant point about the lesions was not so much their widespread distribution and large numbers, as their markedly retrogressive character, as shown by the entire absence of caseation, the local lesion, of course, excepted[1].

We learn from this and other similar instances that the effect of tubercle bacilli of the human type on the calf is to cause a lesion wherever they come to rest. Where the bacilli are very numerous, as for example at the seat of inoculation, the lesion is large, becomes caseous and necrotic, and breaks down and softens ; but where they are few, as for example in the secondary foci produced by distribution by the blood stream, the lesions are minute and become grey and translucent. *The lesions always tend to heal, and the disease is never progressive, and never fatal after subcutaneous injection, no matter how much culture, or tuberculous tissue, swarming with bacilli, is injected.*

Enormous doses of tubercle bacilli of the human type have been injected subcutaneously into very young calves without producing anything more than a transient disturbance of health, a tumour at the seat of inoculation, and minimal lesions elsewhere. For example, on one occasion doses estimated to contain no less than three grammes of tubercle bacilli from broth cultures were injected into each of two calves without producing any disease beyond a large caseo-necrotic softening tumour at the seat of inoculation[2]. Another time 750 milligrammes of bacilli were used with similar results[3], and both A. S. Griffith and the writer have many times injected doses of from 100 to 200 milligrammes of bacilli from young serum cultures with equally little effect. Tissue emulsions also, estimated to contain enormous numbers of bacilli, up to five or ten thousand millions, have been employed, and

[1] Other calves in which similar lesions were seen widely disseminated and in rather large numbers may be compared. These were Nos. 165, 405, and 185. *R.C.T. Int. Rep.* App. vol. II, pp. 458, 460, and 195.

[2] Calves 175 and 177. *R.C.T. Int. Rep.* App. vol. II, pp. 164, 166.

[3] Calves 183 and 185 injected with about 750 mg. *Ibid.* pp. 191, 195. Cp. Calf 741 injected with 275 mg. of young serum culture. (*Ibid.* p. 814.)

none of these injections has produced progressive disease, or indeed anything more, except larger local lesions, than has been described above[1].

Intravenous injection.   When tubercle bacilli of human type are injected intravenously into the calf death may result if the dose is large enough, especially when it is accompanied by finely emulsified tissue in sufficient quantity.   When death occurs it is usually at an early period, and if the animal lives the disease shows very little tendency to spread after the first four or five weeks.   Thus it may be said that as a general rule the animal either dies quickly or recovers altogether.

When death occurs after intravenous injection of tubercle bacilli of this type, either from pure cultures, or contained in emulsified tuberculous tissue, the anatomical type of disease is that of a patchy pneumonia rather than that of a general miliary tuberculosis.   The bacilli, when introduced in this way, come to rest for the most part in the lungs, and around each focus, thus formed by a little clump of bacilli with possibly some emulsified tissue, there arises a little lesion, just as a similar lesion, but on a larger scale, arises around the bacilli when they are injected into the subcutaneous tissue.   The little lesions produced by intravenous injection may then be regarded as so many minute primary or local lesions, each arising around a focus where the bacilli actually introduced have come to rest.

Though there can hardly be any doubt that the bacilli in these lesions multiply somewhat, at least for a time, it is probable that the tubercles are caused mainly by the poisons in the bacilli actually injected, and that, on the whole, the size of these focal lesions is proportionate to the number of bacilli which have come to rest in each.   Here the irritation sets up tissue changes, and a little tubercle is formed, which, as the toxicity of tubercle bacilli of human type for the tissues of the ox is small, has but little tendency to become necrotic or caseous.   Around each tubercle thus produced is apt to appear, temporarily, an œdematous and hyperæmic zone,

---

[1] See list of bovine animals injected with tubercle bacilli from "slightly virulent viruses" (*i.e.* slightly virulent for ox and rabbit, = human type). *Ibid.* pp. 1036 *et seq.*

similar to those one commonly sees around the caseating miliary tubercles in the lungs of calves suffering from an acute infection with tubercle bacilli of bovine type; and if these little areas are sufficiently numerous to become confluent over wide areas of the lung a condition somewhat resembling pneumonia (but studded with minute opaque points) is produced which may destroy life merely by gross mechanical interference with respiration. If, on the other hand, enough functional lung tissue remains to tide over the critical period —which would seem to be about three or four weeks after the injection—the œdema subsides, the consolidation disappears, and there is left behind only a number of very minute fibrous tubercles in a state of retrogression.

The lesions produced by intravenous injection of human bacilli may be not entirely confined to the lungs. Some of the bacilli introduced probably pass at once through the pulmonary capillaries and come to rest in other organs, and it is possible that secondary foci may to a slight extent be developed from those in the lungs.

The disease is characteristically *non-progressive*. But while this is its predominant feature and cannot be too strongly emphasized, the truth of the statement is not absolute. In exceptional cases death has occurred as late as the 57th day; and, as we shall see, little tubercles are liable to persist, if not to progress, in remote situations, such as in the eye, or the carpal and tarsal joints, for a much longer period.

The case of the Calf No. 457[1], which died 57 days after receiving an intravenous injection of tubercle bacilli of human type may be given as an extreme example of the severity of the disease which may be produced in this way. The material injected was not excessive, either in emulsified tissue or tubercle bacilli, for the volume of the emulsion was only 1·5 c.c. and the bacilli it contained were estimated at 20 million; it probably included few if any adventitious bacteria, for it consisted of the emulsified tuberculous thoracic gland of another experimental calf. That the bacilli had no more than the usual virulence of the human type is clearly shown by the fact that two other calves which were subcutaneously injected with the same emulsion, and received doses five times as large as that given to No. 457 developed only minimal or local lesions, while some rabbits also injected with the same material failed to become severely infected. One can therefore only attribute the exceptional severity of the result in Calf 457 to unusual susceptibility on the part of the individual.

[1] *R.C.T. Int. Rep.* App. vol. II, see table 22, p. 431 A.

The disease developed slowly.   At the end of the second week the animal was not so well as usual, " the air of satisfaction and contentment which was very noticeable about this calf had disappeared," and later on respiration became accelerated and the animal grew thin and, gradually becoming worse, died, as we have said already, 57 days after inoculation.

The lungs were found to be in the pneumonic condition described above. Large portions were of a dark purple colour peppered thickly with minute grey points.   A quantity of blood-stained fluid exuded from the cut surface. Samples of the consolidated regions were found to sink in water.   The thoracic glands were moderately enlarged and caseating, but elsewhere there was very little disease[1].

Another exceptional instance of severe infection in which the disease was generalized after intravenous inoculation of tubercle bacilli of human type may be mentioned.   Calf 361 was injected intravenously with 20 c.c., of an emulsion of the tuberculous thoracic gland of another calf, containing 41 million bacilli. The calf remained in good general condition, but after a time respiration became accelerated.   The animal was killed 76 days after injection.   The lungs, as was to be expected, were found to have suffered more severely than other organs.   Everywhere they were thickly peppered with miliary tubercles of uniform size.   A few of the pulmonary lobules were congested and consolidated.   The thoracic glands were enlarged and the cortex of each was almost entirely caseous.

But the disease was not limited to the thorax.   The liver contained numerous little tubercles, the spleen a moderate number of the size of small shot, and about 30 or 40 were counted on the surface of each kidney.   Many of the lymphatic glands in various parts of the body contained tubercles.

The tubercles were not so extensively caseous, as are those seen in equally early cases of infection with bovine bacilli, but had opaque centres surrounded by grey translucent margins.

That this was a pure infection with bacilli of human type is shown by the fact that two calves and a goat injected with an emulsion of the thoracic glands of Calf 361 developed only minimal lesions[2].

Weber and Titze[3] at the Gesundheitsamt also had some experience which makes it necessary to qualify to some slight extent the statement that tubercle bacilli of the human type never produce progressive tuberculosis in the ox.

Three calves which had been given an intravenous injection of tubercle bacilli of the human type[4] for the purpose of immunization became blind soon afterwards.   Two of these came into the possession of the Gesundheitsamt for investigation.   One of them (Ox P) was killed two years and five months after the inoculation.   Behind the cornea was a yellow calcareous nodule as large as a pea ; and an emulsion of this injected into guinea-pigs caused tuberculosis.   From the nodule itself a culture was raised by Weber, which had the characters of growth of the human type and possessed for rabbits and calves the low virulence of that type.

[1] *R.C.T. Int. Rep.* App. vol. II, p. 541.
[2] *Ibid.* p. 175.   See also Table 8, p. 159 A, and a photograph of the calf's lung at the end of the second part of the volume.
[3] *Tub. Arbeit. a. d. Kaiserl. Gesundheitsamte*, Heft 10, p. 184.
[4] Namely of " Tauruman," the virus introduced by Koch and Schütz for the purpose of immunization.

The other animal, known as Cow P, developed a swelling of both carpal joints shortly after an injection of tuberculin given two years and five months after the original intravenous injection of human tubercle bacilli. It was killed six weeks later. In one eye was found a pea-sized yellow nodule, very similar to that present in the former animal and containing many tubercle bacilli.

Three guinea-pigs injected with the nodule from the eye became tuberculous, as also did one of the three injected with fluid from a carpal joint.

Cultures obtained, both from the eye and from one of the joints, grew like bacilli of the human type. That from the eye was tested on rabbits and a calf, the other on rabbits only ; none of the animals developed progressive tuberculosis.

Another calf also had received an intravenous injection of tubercle bacilli of the human type[1] on two occasions for the purpose of immunization. The first vaccine had proved virulent for guinea-pigs, the second avirulent. The first injection only, therefore, concerns us at the present moment. An injection of tuberculin given a year and eight months after this injection of living bacilli was followed by a swelling of one of the carpal joints. Five months later the animal was killed. The inflammation in the joint had in the meantime subsided, but the joint contained 15 c.c. of clear fluid and the synovial membrane was somewhat swollen. Guinea-pigs injected with the fluid remained well, but of eight injected with the synovial membrane two developed tuberculosis. A culture raised from one of these guinea-pigs was of the human type and did not in any way differ from that of the original "bovo-vaccin" culture. Injected into a rabbit it produced only an abscess at the seat of inoculation, and a calf which received an intravenous injection of culture from the joint was found when killed to be free from tuberculosis.

Other instances of swellings of joints after injection of tuberculin into cattle which had some time previously been intravenously injected with tubercle bacilli of human type are mentioned by these authors. From one of these animals tubercle bacilli of human type were obtained from the swollen joint 8½ months after the injection of the bacilli.

The occasional occurrence of small distal lesions, such as those which have just been described, in the calf after intravenous injection of small doses of tubercle bacilli of the human type does not interfere in any way with the value of the intravenous method as a means of determining the type of mammalian tubercle bacilli. The acutely fatal disease which, as we have seen, sometimes occurs is of more practical importance in this connection, but to avoid difficulty which might be caused in this way it is only necessary to employ suitable doses.

---

[1] Namely of "Bovo-vaccin," the virus introduced by Behring for the purpose of immunization.

B.　*The Influence of "Dose" in Experimental Infections*
with Bovine Tubercle Bacilli in the Calf.

It has already been said that the severity of the disease
produced in the ox by inoculating tubercle bacilli of the bovine
type is largely determined by the quantity injected.　It may
be stated generally (1) *that large doses injected subcutaneously
into the Jersey calf produce a very acute form of general miliary
tuberculosis which, with few exceptions, proves rapidly fatal;
in a few weeks, or at most months ;* (2) *that smaller doses produce
variable results, and* (3) *very small doses only minimal or local
lesions.*　The result is, of course, influenced also by the variable
powers of resistance of different individual animals.　It is
worth while examining these factors more closely.

(a)　*As shown by injections of tissue emulsion.*　A few
instances taken from the records of the Tuberculosis Commission will suffice to show that the quantity of bacilli injected is of
great importance.　Three calves each received on one occasion
a subcutaneous injection of a tissue emulsion containing
tubercle bacilli of bovine type.　The tubercle bacilli in the
emulsion were counted, and the quantities of emulsion injected
into each of the calves were estimated to contain 500 million,
3½ million, and 15 thousand bacilli, respectively.　The first
calf, which received 500 million, was killed when dying of
acute general tuberculosis 24 days after the injection.　The
second calf, which received 3½ million, was killed when very ill
63 days after injection, and was found to have severe general
tuberculosis ; while the third calf, which had received the
smallest dose, remained in good condition, and when killed 70
days after injection was apparently quite well, and was found
to have no more than a small calcareous lesion at the seat of
inoculation, and a very few little tuberculous foci of a retrogressive character elsewhere[1].

Several other examples of this kind might be given.

(b)　*As shown by injection of culture.*　A well-grown heifer

---

[1] Calves 315, 321, 325.　*R.C.T. Int. Rep.* 1907, vol. II, p. 279 A.

and a calf each received a subcutaneous injection of 50 milligrammes of tubercle bacilli of bovine type from young serum cultures, and another similar heifer and calf each received the much smaller dose of 1,800,000 bacilli from the same emulsion of bacilli[1]. The two first-mentioned animals developed acute miliary tuberculosis which was rapidly approaching a fatal termination when they were killed, 54 and 34 days respectively after the injections. The other two animals, which received the small doses, remained well, and when killed, after 400 and 200 days respectively, were found to have developed only small calcareous nodules at the seats of injection and a few minute calcareous foci elsewhere[2].

These examples will suffice to show that *small doses do not produce serious lesions in calves and heifers, even when such viruses are used as produce, in large doses, progressive and rapidly fatal tuberculosis.*

The Effect of Injecting Large and Medium Quantities of Bovine Tubercle Bacilli into the Calf compared. In Chapter XVII, opposite page 364, will be found a diagram in which is represented in a graphic manner the severity of the disease which resulted, in each of 146 calves, from the subcutaneous injection of tubercle bacilli of bovine type, in doses of 50 and 10 milligrammes. This table contains most of the subcutaneous injections of culture of bacilli of this type made in the experimental stations of the Royal Commission, only such being omitted as were made with strains derived from cases of lupus, or with others which were considered atypical[3]. The bacilli belonged to 47 different

---

[1] A. Eastwood estimated that 50 milligrammes of tubercle bacilli (or to be more precise 50 cubic millimetres, for the doses were estimated volumetrically), contained 225,000 million tubercle bacilli.

[2] Heifers 249 and 259 and Calves 387 and 385. *R.C.T. Int. Rep.* 1907, vol. II, p. 203. A goat also received the smaller dose at the same time and developed only lesions of moderate severity.

[3] The lupus strains are omitted because many of them were distinctly less virulent than other strains of bovine type, and coming from the surface of the human body it was thought that they might have been subjected to attenuating influences which do not act on bacilli more deeply seated. The other atypical strains were few in number. Most of them were proved to be mixtures, and the others were probably of the same kind.

strains, some derived from the ox, others from man, and a few from the pig and the horse. In Chapter XVII reasons are given for concluding that, excepting three from the horse and one from the pig, these strains did not differ in virulence from one another, or at least that they did not differ sufficiently to make any appreciable difference in the results of the injections; a fact which will be fairly obvious from the diagram. This being the case, it is possible, if we omit these four strains also, to compare the 50 milligramme injections as a whole with the 10 milligramme injections.

The calves were approximately equal in age and weight, and were all of the same breed (Jersey); they were inoculated in precisely the same manner; and as they were nearly all either allowed to die naturally of the disease, or were practically moribund when killed, the duration of life dating from the injection, forms, in each case, a reliable and exact measure of the severity of the disease produced. This duration is expressed by the height of the black column corresponding to each calf. Those which did not die of general tuberculosis within three months of injection were killed at the end of this period, and were found to have tuberculosis of varying degrees of severity. These animals are represented by black columns which reach to the upper limiting line. In three cases where the calves were killed when in fairly good condition before the three months had expired, the black columns are continued upwards by dotted lines to the upper limiting line, to show that, in the opinion of the observer, they would have lived at least to the end of this period.

With 50 milligrammes of bovine bacilli 91 calves were subcutaneously injected (excluding those injected with the three equine and the one porcine virus as already mentioned), and of these all but five died, or were killed when dying, within the period of observation (three months). Thus only 5·5 per cent. survived for 90 days.

Turning now to the 10 milligramme injections we find 47 calves (again excluding those injected with the equine and porcine viruses referred to) and of these no less than 14, or 30 per cent., survived the period of observation. Moreover, those which died, or were killed when moribund, after doses of 10 milligrammes lived, on the average, nearly 10 days longer than those which died, or were killed when moribund, after doses of 50 milligrammes. Lastly, those which survived for three months after 10 milligrammes were found, for the most part, when examined, to have lesions of only moderate severity, while the few which reached this limit after 50 milligrammes were more severely affected.

We find, therefore, that *the results of injecting 50 milligrammes of tubercle bacilli of bovine type from young serum cultures subcutaneously into the calf, are, on the whole, much more severe and much more constantly fatal than those of injecting 10 milligrammes*[1].

Concerning the effect of different doses of tubercle bacilli both human and bovine when intravenously injected into the calf, there exists far less information than is the case with subcutaneous injection. The following experiments have been collected from the writer's own experience[2]:

TABLE X. *Tubercle Bacilli of Bovine Type.*

Intravenous Injections of Emulsions of Tuberculous Tissues.

Animal	Dose expressed in estimated number of bacilli	Fate		Result	
Calf 95	48 thousand T. B.	Died in	40 days	General tuberculosis	
,, 101	48 ,,	,,	41 ,,	,,	,,
,, 59	300 ,,	,,	33 ,,	,,	,,
,, 89	300 ,,	Killed when ill	23 ,,	,,	,,
,, 571	10 million T. B.	Died in	26 ,,	,,	,,
,, 557	49 ,,	Killed when dying	17 ,,	,,	,,
,, 553	99 ,,	,, ,,	18 ,,	,,	,,
,, 539	209 ,,	,, ,,	18 ,,	,,	,,
,, 529	1000 ,,	Died in	13 ,,	,,	,,

[1] A. S. Griffith found that ·02 and ·01 mg. of bovine bacilli injected subcutaneously into calves failed to produce severe or progressive lesions (see Calves 202 and 210, *R.C.T. Int. Rep.* App. vol. I, p. 42).

[2] All these experiments are reported in the Appendices of the *Interim Report of the R.C.T.* vol. II.

TABLE XI. *Tubercle Bacilli of Human Type.*
Intravenous Injections of Emulsions of Tuberculous Tissues.

K = killed.   D = died of tuberculosis.

Animal	Dose expressed in estimated number of bacilli	Fate	Result
Heifer 25	10 c.c.*	K when well 170 days	Normal throughout
,, 27	10 c.c.*	,, ,, 107 ,,	,, ,,
alf 31	10 c.c.*	,, ,, 173 ,,	,, ,,
,, 69	10 c.c.*	,, ,, 144 ,,	Little calcareous focus by the vein
,, 505	11 million T.B.	,, ,, 62 ,,	Minimal lesions
,, 467	11 ,,	,, ,, 62 ,,	,, ,,
,, 441	13 ,,	,, ,, 102 ,,	Generalized tuberculosis, not severe, probably retrogressive
,, 457	20 ,,	D 57 ,,	Miliary tub. lung. Caseation of thoracic glands. Intestines and mesenteric glands not affected. Virus passed on to Calf 505 with minimal results
, 361	41 ,,	K 76 ,,	General miliary tuberculosis
, 812	250 ,,	,, 49 ,,	Minimal (injection partly perivascular)
, 861	346 ,,	,, very ill 30 ,,	Tuberculous pneumonic consolidation
, 399	720 ,,	,, ,, 34 ,,	Tuberculous pneumonic consolidation
, 305	729 ,,	,, ,, 26 ,,	Early general tuberculosis
, 817	891 ,,	,, ,, 31 ,,	Lungs extensively mottled with irregular foci
, 831	1000 ,,	D 17 ,,	Tubercle bacilli in all organs and lymph glands
, 859	2000 ,,	,, 19 ,,	Lungs consolidated

Intravenous Injections of Culture.

Animal	Dose	Fate	Result
alf 685	10 mg.	K in fair condition, 64 days	Moderate number of small tubercles in lungs
, 749	46 ,,	,, very ill 24 ,,	Lungs extensively consolidated. No visible tubercles. Caseation of thoracic glands
, 607	90 ,,	,, in fair condition, 48 ,,	Lungs indurated, no tubercles in them visible to naked eye. A good many small tubercles in the kidneys. Caseous mass outside wall of vein at seat of inoculation. Injection probably partly perivascular
, 551	100 ,,	D in 21 ,,	Lungs consolidated. Thoracic glands enlarged, in early stages of caseation.

* 10 c.c. of emulsion, T.B. not estimated.

From Table X it will be seen that bovine tubercle bacilli injected intravenously have always produced a fatal tuberculosis. But no evidence exists as to the lower limit of the fatal dose of bacilli contained in tissue emulsions, and no evidence at all concerning pure cultures administered in this way.

With the human type of bacillus the smallest number of bacilli contained in a tissue emulsion which proved fatal was 20 millions. Larger doses produced severe results, and doses of 346 millions or over always produced a fatal result, or one which was threatening to prove fatal when the animal was killed.

Pure cultures of tubercle bacilli of the human type have, in the writer's experience, produced a fatal result when injected intravenously into the calf in doses of 46 milligrammes and over, and a dose of 10 milligrammes has failed to cause anything more than a moderate number of small tubercles in the lungs. A. S. Griffith has, however, recorded an injection of five milligrammes which caused a fatal tuberculosis[1].

This experience shows that it would not be safe to use so large a dose as five milligrammes for intravenous injection if the object was to determine whether the bacilli belonged to the human or to the bovine type.

Probably a dose of one milligramme would always be safe when the bacilli were of the human type and could be relied upon to produce severe and fatal tuberculosis if they were of the bovine type. But this cannot be stated with certainty.

C. *The Influence of Differences of Susceptibility in Calves injected with Bovine Tubercle Bacilli.*

We have now to inquire how far individual differences of susceptibility among the animals used for test purposes influence the results and confuse the issue, and whether the part played by such differences is greater with some doses than with others.

---

[1] Calf 1385 inoculated intravenously with culture from virus H 104. The dose was 5 milligrammes, and the calf died in 29 days of acute tuberculosis. Another calf inoculated subcutaneously with 50 milligrammes of the same suspension of bacilli developed slight retrogressive tuberculosis only. The strain of bacilli had been cultivated directly from human lung. *R.C.T. Final Report*, App. vol. I, pp. 31, 470, 472.

It cannot be doubted by any one who has worked much at experimental tuberculosis that differences of individual susceptibility play a very considerable part in determining the severity of the result of injection, both in the calf and rabbit, and, doubtless, in other animals also. One, therefore, cannot measure at all exactly the virulence of a given virus, or make a close comparison of the relative virulence of two or more viruses, without using a considerable number of animals for the investigation of each virus, in order that differences of susceptibility among the animals used may to a great extent neutralize one another.

Let us turn again to the diagram opposite p. 364 for an illustration of this point, and let us take the viruses B xxiv and B ix. With each of these bovine viruses two calves were injected subcutaneously with 10 milligrammes of bacilli. Both calves injected with B xxiv lived for 90 days, and when killed at the end of that period had moderately severe lesions of a chronic type. On the other hand, both calves injected with B ix died of very acute severe miliary tuberculosis in 37 and 34 days respectively after inoculation. Should we be justified in concluding from this evidence that B ix was more virulent for the ox species than B xxiv? Not at all. For we may see results which differ quite as much as these produced in two calves by one and the same virus. Thus for example in the case of B v. With the same dose of the same preparation of bacilli and on the same day two calves, of the same age and then of as nearly as possible the same weight, each received a subcutaneous injection. One of them, No. 352, died 40 days later of acute general tuberculosis, while the other, No. 354, remained in "moderately good health" for three months, and when killed at the end of that period was found to have lesions, generalized indeed, but of a much less severe and more chronic type than those in its companion.

One cannot doubt that this difference in the result was due entirely to a difference in the powers of resistance possessed by the two calves, and one must conclude that if two calves possessing a resistance of the same degree as that of Calf 352 had by accident come together for the test of virus B ix, and two others of the same powers of resistance as those of Calf 354 had chanced to come together for the test of B xxiv, the result would have been just as it actually happened, even though the viruses in question possessed precisely equal virulence.

Again, take the case of virus H 10 B.S. One of the two calves injected with 50 milligrammes of bacilli from this strain was killed when dying of acute tuberculosis 34 days after the inoculation, but the other, No. 667, lived for three months, and when killed was found to have developed tuberculosis of a moderate degree of severity and chronic type. Is this virus to be regarded, therefore, as of lower virulence than others which like H 28 C.L. and many others killed two or more calves with acute tuberculosis? Apparently not; for we find that rabbits injected with the same suspension of bacilli as that injected into Calf 667 died of tuberculosis of the type commonly produced by bovine bacilli, and two other calves inoculated, long afterwards, each with 10 milligrammes of the same strain were both dying of acute tuberculosis 34 days after inoculation— a somewhat exceptionally severe result for doses of this size, as the diagram clearly shows.

The truth is that such irregularities in the results of injection as we have been considering are plainly capable of being accounted for—can indeed, in some cases, only be accounted for—by differences in the susceptibility of the calves used for injection. And from this we learn the important lesson that we must be on our guard against inferring differences of virulence among different strains of tubercle bacilli unless a sufficient number of control animals are inoculated to guard against errors which might arise from the use of an animal or animals with abnormal powers of resistance.

When this condition is fulfilled such an inference may fairly be drawn, as for example in the cases of the viruses P xiv, E ii, and E iv. In each of these cases four calves, each injected with 50 milligrammes, all concur in affirming the comparatively low virulence of the virus; while in the case of two of them, E ii and E iv, this is again confirmed by two calves injected with 10 milligrammes, not to mention numerous experiments made on rabbits. In the case of E iii, on the other hand, the inference is doubtful.   One is tempted to infer from the two calves injected with 50 milligrammes that the virulence of this strain was slightly less than that of the standard bovine type, but then such results might have been obtained with a typical bovine strain, had two calves, with a resisting power similar to that of No. 418 (B XXVI), chanced to have been used.

One point that comes out very clearly from the diagram is that, on the whole, the 50-milligramme injections gave much more constant results than the 10-milligramme injections ; and this is not to be wondered at.   Large doses may be expected to break down the resistance of all but the most highly resistant individuals, and to obscure smaller differences of resisting power ; while with moderate doses where the balance is more even, smaller differences in the powers of resistance will be likely to turn the scale in one direction or the other.

From this analysis of the experiments referred to the following conclusions may be drawn :

I.   That considerable differences of power of resisting infection with tubercle bacilli exist among calves.

II.   That such differences play a more important part when doses of moderate size (10 mg.) are injected than when larger doses (50 mg.) are used.   With the latter dose only very few individuals (of the Jersey breed at least) are able to make sufficient resistance to enable them to survive for three months.

III.   That, consequently, for the practical purpose of determining the type of mammalian tubercle bacilli by injection into the calf, a dose of 50 milligrammes is to be preferred to any smaller dose, and perhaps even a larger one might be better if breeds other than the Jersey are employed[1].

---

[1] Seeing that enormous quantities of tubercle bacilli of human type can be injected into the calf without producing severe or progressive tuberculosis, the test dose might with advantage be greater than 50 mg. were it not that it is inconvenient to have to provide so many cultures as would be required.

The investigators in the Gesundheitsamt also noted considerable variations in susceptibility to tuberculosis among the calves employed by them, and they point out that too much importance must not be attached to the result of injecting a single calf unless this is in complete agreement with the result of inoculating rabbits and with the cultural characters of the virus.   In the

The Goat as a Means of Differentiating the Types of Mammalian Tubercle Bacilli

Experience of experimental infection in the goat is much less extensive than that in the calf, but so far as it goes it shows that the former reacts to the two types of mammalian tubercle bacilli very like the latter ; and there is no reason to think that it is in any way inferior as a means of differentiation. The more uniformly fatal results of 50-milligramme injections of bovine bacilli into this smaller animal is a distinct advantage ; and, on the other hand, there is no reason to think that it is any less uniformly resistant to infection with the human type of bacillus than the calf itself. Its lesser cost, and superior power of reacting to tuberculin when tuberculous[1], the rarity with which it suffers from spontaneous tuberculosis, together

event of any unexpected result being obtained, they say, the experiment should be repeated on another calf.

An example of a calf which possessed great susceptibility is given by Kossel and Weber (*Tub. Arbeit. etc.* Heft 3, pp. 12 and 74). The animal (Calf 18) was about 4 months old when it received a subcutaneous injection of 50 mg. of tubercle bacilli of bovine type from a glycerin-broth culture 37 days old, the strain having been obtained from the mesenteric glands of a child. The calf died of very acute general tuberculosis 40 days later. This was the only instance in their experience up to that time in which such an injection had proved fatal within the period of observation. Control experiments made on other calves, as well as on rabbits, showed that the strain possessed no more than the ordinary virulence of the bovine type ; and they attribute the exceptional result to the peculiarities of the animal and not to those of the strain of bacilli.

An example of the opposite kind was afforded by Calf No. 55 (*ibid.* p. 9). This animal was injected subcutaneously with 50 mg. of bacilli from a strain of bovine type derived from the ox ; yet the tuberculosis which was produced was limited practically to the seat of injection and the nearest lymphatic glands. Other calves injected subsequently with the same strain of bacilli showed that it possessed the usual virulence of the bovine type.

The high resisting power which, as in this case, was sometimes met with among calves the authors are inclined to attribute to an antecedent spontaneous tuberculous infection ; but it must be admitted that the post-mortem notes of this animal (given in Heft 1, p. 50) do not refer to the finding of any calcareous focus or other old or quiescent lesion which would support this explanation.

[1] *R.C.T. Fin. Rep.* App. Supplementary Volume, 1913, " Report on Tuberculin Tests." For those on the goat, see pp. 72 *et seq.*

Plate V

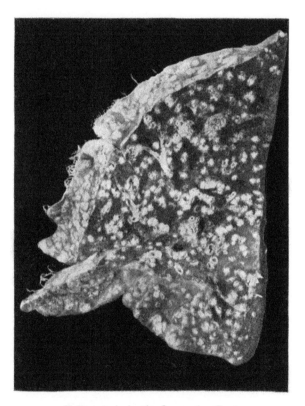

Tuberculosis in the Lung of a Goat.

The animal died 75 days after a subcutaneous injection of bovine tuberculous material, and there were already numerous little cavities in course of formation.

Plate VI

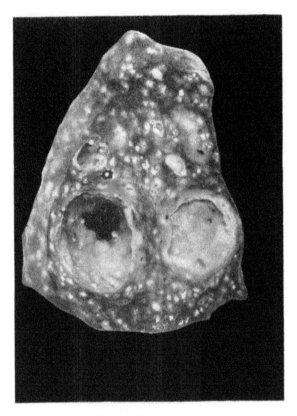

Tuberculosis in the Lung of a Goat.

The animal died 139 days after subcutaneous injection.

From a specimen by A. S. Griffith.

with its moderate size and its hardiness in general, would seem
to combine to make this animal an ideal one for the purpose
of determining the type of tubercle bacilli, and indicate that it
might be used with advantage more frequently than has hitherto
been the case.

On the other hand, it might be urged with some reason
that the tuberculous lesions in the goat are much more liable
to soften and break down than those in the calf ; that the
local lesion at the seat of inoculation becomes an ulcer, and the
lungs filled with little potential or actual cavities ; and that
on this account there is risk of spreading infection among other
experimental animals.

The Rabbit as a Means of differentiating the Types of Mammalian Tubercle Bacilli

The rabbit is very highly susceptible to experimental
infection with the bovine tubercle bacillus, and very fairly
resistant to infection with the human tubercle bacillus.

It is the animal most employed at the present day for
differentiating the two types of mammalian tubercle bacilli.
Weber[1] (1912) said that he regarded it as " the most suitable "
animal for the purpose ; Oehlecker[2] (1907) looked upon the
rabbit as a "complete substitute for the ox"; and Burckhardt[3]
found that rabbit experiments suffice in all cases for the determination of type, provided that enough animals are inoculated.

A. S. Griffith[4] says that "experiments recorded in the Second
Interim Report" of the Royal Commission on Tuberculosis
"showed that the rabbit differentiates between bovine and
human tubercle bacilli in the same way as the calf. Tubercle
bacilli which were highly virulent for the rabbit always proved
highly virulent for the calf, and tubercle bacilli which produced in
the rabbit retrogressive tuberculosis never produced in calves
more than a limited retrogressive tuberculosis. The important
fact was established that with the rabbit alone one is able to

[1] *Centralbl. f. Bakt.* Orig. vol. 64, p. 258.
[2] *Tub. Arbeit. a. d. Kaiserl. Gesundheitsamte,* 1907, Heft 6, p. 103.
[3] *Centralbl. f. Bakt.* Ref. vol. 48, p. 417.
[4] *R.C.T. Fin. Rep.* vol. I, p. 32.

distinguish with certainty the bovine from the human tubercle bacillus."

Park and Krumwiede[1] say that "the rabbit is the best animal to use for testing the virulence for the diagnosis of type "; elsewhere they express the opinion that, except in very unusual instances, rabbit experiments give such clear and even results that the use of calves is no longer necessary. Weber makes a similar reservation. " Calf experiment is only necessary," he says " when the investigation of cultural characters and rabbit virulence has given doubtful results." Jancsó and Elfer, Möller, Rothe, and others give similar testimony. There is, therefore, as Weber says, a very remarkable unanimity concerning the advantages of using the rabbit for determining the types of mammalian tubercle bacilli.

The rabbit has many good points. Above all it is cheap; it is easily housed and fed. It is hardy, and very rarely suffers naturally from tuberculosis[2]. Its cheapness to buy and keep is an immense advantage ; not so much because it saves the pocket of the investigator, though this is something, but because it enables him to use a number of animals in each experiment, and thus to avoid mistakes which might otherwise arise from differences of individual susceptibility. Thus, in other words, it enables a piece of work to be carried out much more extensively and thoroughly than if large and expensive animals alone were to be used.

All these advantages are undoubtedly great. What of the other side of the picture ? It must be admitted that the rabbit is considerably less resistant to infection with the human type of bacillus than the calf or goat. Lungs and kidneys are, by no means unfrequently, affected, and cases of even more generalized and progressive disease have occurred, as we shall see, after injections with this type of bacillus. It is true that these lesions, when they exist, are of a more chronic type than those caused by the bovine bacillus, and that experienced

---

[1] *Journ. of Med. Res.* vol. XXIII, p. 286.

[2] The tuberculin test does not succeed well in the rabbit. Out of 20 tuberculous rabbits tested for the Royal Commission only eight reacted. *R.C.T. Fin. Rep* App. Supplementary Volume, 1913, p. 59.

observers are in little danger of being misled by them, but they undoubtedly present difficulties to the less expert, and it would not be surprising if they had sometimes led to error.

There is also another disadvantage in relying too exclusively on the rabbit. It is too susceptible to the bovine type of bacillus, and gives but little indication of differences of virulence of strains coming within this type.

This is no unreal or fancied objection. Examples may be cited to support it. When the first case of lupus[1] was investigated for the Royal Commission, a strain of tubercle bacilli was isolated which was dysgonic in growth and which produced severe general tuberculosis on injection into rabbits[2]. If this had been all, one would have regarded it as an ordinary bovine strain; but this was not all. Calves were inoculated with measured doses, and showed without doubt that the virulence of the strain was not that of ordinary bovine bacilli, but something considerably below it. This caused further investigation of the viruses concerned in lupus to be made and led to the discovery of some of the most interesting anomalous strains of tubercle bacilli which have yet come to light.

A. *The Susceptibility of the Rabbit to Infection by the Bovine Tubercle Bacillus*

The rabbit is very highly susceptible to infection with the bovine type of tubercle bacillus and succumbs rapidly to an acute and generalized disease if the dose be moderately large. Even exceedingly minute doses prove quickly fatal to young animals; and though older individuals hold out longer against such infections, it is probable that, if they were allowed to live as long as possible, all would succumb to tuberculosis in the end.

[1] See p. 617.

[2] It is true that the rabbits inoculated with this strain lived rather longer than the average of those which received similar doses of typical strains of bovine bacilli. But the difference was so small that it would never have been noticed except for the calf inoculations. The rabbits were injected intraperitoneally; possibly subcutaneous injection of this species would have revealed the low virulence of the virus (see *R.C.T.* 1907, *Int. Rep.* App. vol. II, p. 1128).

The extreme susceptibility of the rabbit to infection with bovine tubercle bacilli is shown by the following experiments. The writer made a series of intraperitoneal injections into half-grown animals with successive ten-fold dilutions of a fine suspension of bacilli, and found that doses down to a millionth of a milligramme proved fatal in about 10 weeks. A. S. Griffith inoculated young rabbits in a similar manner with even smaller doses and found that a quantity of bacilli estimated at one ten-thousand-millionth part of a milligramme produced fatal tuberculosis within three months; while in another series, made with adult animals, a millionth part of a milligramme caused death in 74 days, and a smaller dose produced general tuberculosis, which, however, was not fatal within the period of observation (118 days).

TABLE XII. *Intraperitoneal injection of bovine tubercle bacilli into rabbits.* (*Experiments by L. C.*[1])

G.T. = General tuberculosis.

Dose in milligrammes	Result	Length of Survival
0·00,01	Died	49 days G.T.
0·00,001	,,	34 ,, ,,
0·00,001	,,	53 ,, ,,
0·00,000,1	,,	76 ,, ,,
0·00,000,1	,,	69 ,, ,,

(*Experiments by A. S. G.*[2])

Dose in milligrammes	Young rabbits		Adult rabbits	
	Result	Length of Survival	Result	Length of Survival
0·1	Died	15 days G.T.		
0·01	,,	22 ,, ,,	Died	63 days G.T.
0·00,1	,,	27 ,, ,,		
0·00,01	,·	47 ,, ,,	Died	118 days ,,
0·00,001	,,	40 ,, ,,		
0·00,000,1	,,	30 ,, ,,	Died	74 days ,,
0·00,000,01	,,	68 ,, ,,	Killed	118 ,, ,,
0·00,000,001	,,	29 ,, ,,	Killed	118 ,, No T.
0·00,000,000,1	,,	89 ,, ,,		
0·00,000,000,01	,,	82 ,, ,,		

[1] See *R.C.T.* 1907, *Int. Rep.* vol. II, p. 1127.
[2] *Ibid.* vol. I, pp. 468, 469.

Plate VII

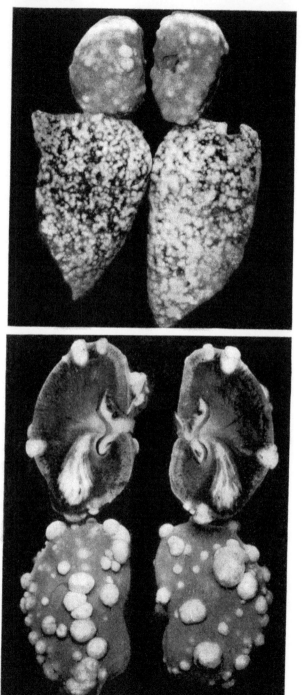

Tuberculosis in the Lungs and Kidneys of the Rabbit produced by injection of the Bovine Type of Tubercle Bacillus.

The animals died 103 and 171 days respectively after subcutaneous injection.

Intravenous injections of culture or emulsion of tuberculous tissue prove rapidly fatal, doses of 0·1 or 0·01 milligramme of the former killing in about three or four weeks.
Intraperitoneal injections of 1·0 milligramme of culture are
fatal after an average period of 26 days[1].

Subcutaneous injections cause tuberculosis with equal certainty, and the disease is severe and progresses towards a fatal
termination, even in adult animals and when doses so small
as 0·1 mg. or even less are used; but the disease induced by
this method runs a less rapid course than that caused by
intraperitoneal, and still less than that caused by intravenous
injection, and, as a rule, after the subcutaneous injection of
1·0 milligramme of bacilli the average duration of life is between
two and three months.

Feeding with bovine bacilli causes tuberculosis with a
considerable degree of certainty, doses of 10 milligrammes and
1·0 milligramme having proved sufficient. But the disease
runs a rather chronic course, and often does not prove fatal
within three months[2].

The lesions produced by bovine tubercle bacilli in the rabbit.
At the seat of inoculation, wherever this may be, lesions are
developed. Thus if the injection be subcutaneous a caseo-
necrotic tumour appears and usually ulcerates, and the nearest
lymphatic glands become enlarged and caseous. If it be intraperitoneal, tubercles are freely developed on the omentum and
diaphragmatic and somatic peritoneum. If intravenous, the
brunt of the attack falls on the lungs. But, apart from the
changes produced in the tissues into which the bacilli are
directly introduced, the lungs, as in nearly all other animals
the guinea-pig excepted, are the organs most severely affected.
The kidneys, however, which in other species, especially the
guinea-pig, are not usually so severely affected as are other
organs, in the rabbit come only second to the lungs in susceptibility. The spleen and liver are never the seat of such marked
changes as one sees in the guinea-pig.

The lungs in acute cases are beset with innumerable little

---

[1] 10 mg. intrap. proves fatal in about 19 days, and 0·1 mg. in about 35 days.
[2] *R.C.T.* 1907, App. vol. II, pp. 1130, 1131.

grey tubercles with caseating centres. In others there may be irregular nodules, evidently made by the coalescence of smaller tubercles ; and some of these may be ¼ or ⅓ of an inch in diameter or even more. By their outstretching processes they tend to run into one another, and so to form an irregular network. The nodules are largest in the more chronic cases, and in such they are extensively caseous, showing yellow centres and translucent margins. After the lapse of many months they may break down into cavities. In other cases again large areas of lung may consist of a uniform cream-coloured, firm, necrotic tissue.

The kidneys are usually studded with hemispherical ivory-white nodules which on section are found to extend wedge-wise into the cortex, but not, as a rule, into the medulla. Sometimes these are numerous and small, but it is not uncommon for them to be as big as large peas.

The spleen often contains numerous tubercles, and some may usually be found in the liver, but the yellowish-white necrotic areas so characteristic of tuberculosis in the guinea-pig are not seen in the rabbit. Occasionally other parts such as the testes, mammary glands or joints may be affected. In acute infections miliary tubercles are seen in the rib marrow[1].

B. *The Susceptibility of the Rabbit to Infection by the Human Tubercle Bacillus.*

Intravenous Injection. The result of intravenous injection of human tubercle bacilli into the rabbit depends largely on the quantity of bacilli employed, and unless this is small a fatal result may ensue. One milligramme of bacilli, indeed, injected into the veins usually causes death ; even 0·1 milligramme proves fatal in more than a third of the cases, and the fact that death may occur after three months shows that the disease is in such cases progressive. Only when doses so small as 0·01 milligramme are used can the human type of bacillus introduced into the veins be trusted not to cause a fatal infection[2].

---

[1] See also p. 429.

[2] A. S. Griffith injected 105 rabbits intravenously with various strains of tubercle bacilli of human type. 33 received 1 mg.; of these 27 died—9 within 4 weeks, 12 within 3 months, and 6 after a longer period. 40 rabbits received 0·1 mg.; of these 15 died—6 within 4 weeks, 3 within 3 months,

Plate VIII

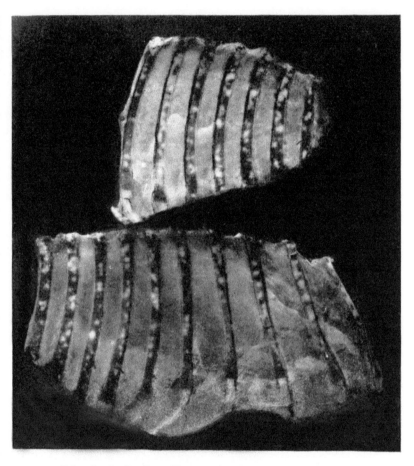

Tubercles in the Bone-Marrow of a Rabbit seen through the semi-transparent ribs.

In an animal injected 80 days previously with bovine bacilli.

From a specimen by A. S. Griffith.

In the rabbits which died in the laboratories of the Royal Commission of an acute form of the disease after intravenous injection of tubercle bacilli of human type the lesions were not unlike those produced by bovine bacilli. In the more chronic cases, whatever the dose, and whether fatal or not, the disease when severe was of a slowly progressive character, and lesions were found not only in the great organs and lymphatic glands but occasionally in many other parts of the body also, joints, bones, eyes, brain, testes, mammary glands, muscles, and areolar tissue having in one case or another been found affected. The lungs and kidneys, however, did not show the massive caseous nodules so characteristic of an infection with bovine bacilli[1].

The view that progressive tuberculosis may occasionally be induced in the rabbit by human tubercle bacilli is also supported by Continental experience. Some rabbits which had been intravenously injected with human tubercle bacilli by Heymans[2] were kept under observation for as long as two years, and from the result of their post-mortem examination and their clinical histories he was led to believe that old and quiescent lesions may become again active, or as he himself says " an old focus may after several months flare up, and the bacilli may, in a manner, seek out new fields to colonise, and so it may result in a chronic infection of the joints, testes or iris."

From this description it will be seen that the interpretation of the results of intravenous injection into the rabbit is not unattended with difficulty, and can only be undertaken without risk of error by experienced observers. If this method is used for diagnosis of type it is imperative to employ a means of accurately measuring the quantity of bacilli injected, and this latter should not exceed 0·01 milligramme.

Intraperitoneal injection. Injected into the peritoneal cavity of the rabbit tubercle bacilli of the human type

and 6 after a longer period. In the majority of the fatal cases, " death was undoubtedly due to tuberculosis." Thus intravenous injection of tubercle bacilli of human type in doses of 1·0 and 0·1 mg. proved fatal in more than half the rabbits. *R.C.T. Fin. Rep.* App. vol. I, pp. 34 *et seq.*

[1] *Ibid.*
[2] Quoted by Oehlecker, 1907, *Tub. Arbeit. a. d. Kaiserl. Gesundheitsamte,* Heft 6, p. 106.

sometimes produce no visible lesions of any kind, and, as a rule, if the dose be not excessive, only a limited amount of chronic disease which shows but little tendency to progress to a fatal termination. It is a marked feature that the rabbits continue in good health and grow fat. On the other hand, it is necessary to recognize that rather extensive lesions may sometimes be produced in this way in unusually susceptible individuals, especially in the lungs and kidneys, and after large doses. Excessive quantities of bacilli, such as 50 milligrammes, not unfrequently prove fatal, and evidence of progressive disease is not wanting in exceptional cases.

After the injection of large quantities of emulsified tuberculous tissue the material is often found, more or less softened and converted into a pultaceous mass, contained in one or more thin-walled cysts loosely attached to the omentum, or to one of the abdominal viscera. In other cases there may be irregular caseous patches in a thickened omentum, and long sinuous yellow lines of similar material are often seen in its dorsal layer, evidently following the lymphatic vessels. Sometimes there are fibrous patches on the mesentery. The mesenteric glands escape.

The lungs are quite commonly the seat of tuberculous changes, especially along their thin margins, and the disease is not unfrequently rather extensive. The lesions usually consist of well-defined grey fibrous patches. They may be more or less confluent, and sometimes they have small caseous centres. These lesions, however extensive they may be, differ considerably in their distribution from the evenly scattered miliary tubercles which occur in acute tuberculosis set up by the bovine type of bacillus, and caseation is far less marked.

Lesions are present in the kidneys nearly as commonly as in the lungs. They take the form of inconspicuous grey tubercles, or of whitish or yellowish streaks or wedges running right through the cortex and medulla, and sometimes forming a little prominence on the surface. They may resemble those caused by the bovine type of bacillus, but they do not form such large and prominent hemispherical white nodules on the surface of the organ. Very often when a kidney is thus affected

Plate IX

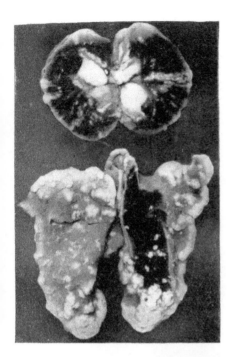
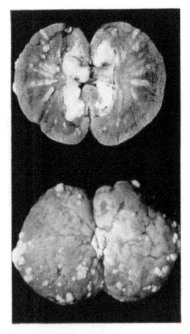
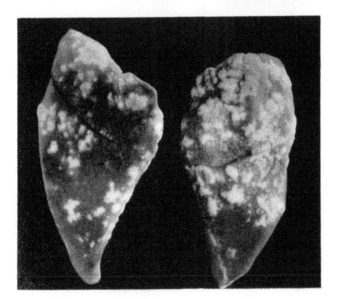

Kidneys and Lungs of Rabbits injected with Tubercle Bacilli of Human Type.
Selected to show unusually severe results.
No. 3 is from a preparation by A. S. Griffith.

Plate X

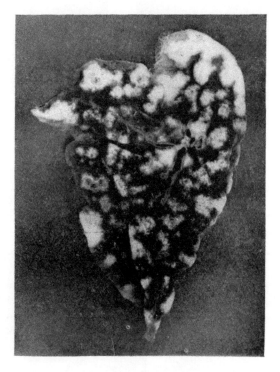

Lung of Rabbit injected with Tubercle Bacilli of Human Type.

Exceptionally severe result.

From a preparation by A. S. Griffith.

Subcutaneous injection of 50 mg. of eugonic cult. from human cervical glands. A culture obtained from these lungs also was eugonic, and, injected subcutaneously in a dose of 10 mg. into a rabbit, produced minimal lesions. *Lancet*, 1915, I, p. 1280. R. 320.

XIII]   RESULTS PRODUCED BY THE HUMAN BACILLUS   279

its pelvis is distended with a muco-purulent material, which may be swarming with tubercle bacilli. Another lesion, seen not unfrequently in the female rabbit, is distension of the uterus with a creamy fluid resembling the pus of a psoas abscess in man (R 261, 382, and 376). This, too, has been found swarming with tubercle bacilli (R 416).

In rarer cases small tubercles may be seen in the liver (R 665) and spleen (R 665), and tubercle bacilli without visible lesions have not unfrequently been found in the latter organ (*e.g.* in R. 332, 326, 350, and 615). Tuberculosis has been seen in the vas deferens, the vesiculæ seminales (R 631), in the epididymis and testes (R 62, 228, and 912), in the empty uterus (R 261) and in the pregnant uterus (R 212). Acute and fatal tuberculosis may sometimes be caused in the rabbit by the intraperitoneal injection of human tubercle bacilli if the dose be so large as 10 or 50 milligrammes, and in such instances tubercle bacilli have repeatedly been found in the bone-marrow in the ribs (R 326, 332, 350, and 365). In rare instances a slowly progressing tuberculosis is set up and may prove fatal after many months. In such cases bones, joints, testes, or eyes may become involved—as Heymans found after intravenous injection. Tuberculous joints have only been seen when the animals were allowed to live two or three hundred days (R 263, 271, and 539), and in one animal which had been injected 205 days previously cavities were found in the lungs (R 260)[1].

A few exceptionally severe results may be given. R 332, a very young rabbit, received an intraperitoneal injection of 50 milligrammes of tubercle bacilli of human type. It died 13 days later, when innumerable scarcely-visible tubercles were present in the mesentery, numerous small yellow collections were seen in the omentum which was not thickened and no definite tubercles were found in the organs, but tubercle bacilli were numerous in liver, spleen, and rib marrow.

---

[1] Unfortunately the full post-mortem notes of these cases have not been preserved. But abstracts may be found in the Reports of the Commission. *Int. Rep.* App. vol. II, pp. 1068 *et seq.*
For particulars of R 260, 263, 271, see *R.C.T. Fin. Rep.* App. vol. III, p. 331.

R 615 received an intraperitoneal injection of 10 milli-grammes of bacilli. It died 18 days later. Very early acute peritonitis was found. The omentum was a solid mass of tissue with caseating foci. The lungs contained many small ill-defined tubercles. Tubercle bacilli were found in spleen, kidneys, liver, and rib marrow.

R 219 was injected intraperitoneally with 50 milligrammes of bacilli, and died 69 days later. There was a good deal of caseous deposit in the omentum; numerous small tubercles were found in the kidneys; and the lungs were extensively consolidated with irregular grey patches largely confluent.

R 638 received an intraperitoneal injection of 0·1 milli-gramme of bacilli. It died 100 days later. At the post-mortem examination there was seen chronic tuberculous peritonitis and numerous grey yellow-centred tubercles in kidneys and lungs, in the latter often confluent.

One other instance of progressive tuberculosis caused in a rabbit by tubercle bacilli of human type may be quoted. It occurred in an animal injected intraperitoneally with a tissue emulsion, but it is selected because the possi-bility of the animal being infected with a spontaneous bovine disease is absolutely excluded. The animal was one of a series used in a passage experiment and had been injected intraperitoneally with an enormous dose of tissue emulsion (30 c.c.) made from the tuberculous lesions of the pre-ceding animal of the series. The reason for giving so large a dose was that it was feared the strain might be lost, the tissue being so poor in bacilli that none could be found on microscopic examination of the emulsion. It is probable, therefore, that the dose of bacilli received by the animal was small, but they were provided with a large amount of dead tissue to serve them as a preliminary culture medium. This rabbit died after 145 days, of "chronic progressive tuberculosis," especially severe in lungs and peritoneum. That this result was caused by a bacillus of human type, and was not the result of a spontaneous infection with bovine bacilli, was placed beyond all doubt by the fact that the injection of an emulsion of the tuberculous lungs of this animal into another rabbit produced only the usual minimal lesions[1].

Subcutaneous injection. It may be stated with con-fidence that tubercle bacilli of the human type do not cause fatal tuberculosis in the rabbit when injected subcutaneously. A. S. Griffith[2] injected 125 animals in this way, with doses varying from 1 to 100 milligrammes of bacilli, the majority

[1] *R.C.T.* 1911, App. vol. III, Rabbit 640, pp. 331 and 133. See also *postea*, p. 347.   [2] *R.C.T. Fin. Rep.* vol. I, p. 36.

receiving 10 milligrammes, and none of them died of tuberculosis[1]. A caseous or necrotic lesion developed at the seat of inoculation, and the lungs usually suffered to some extent, the kidneys also in many cases being slightly affected.

The lesions have been described by A. S. Griffith as follows : " The organs of rabbits after a subcutaneous inoculation of slightly virulent tubercle bacilli[2] are generally only slightly affected. Sometimes they are free from tuberculous lesions. In other cases one organ only is affected, usually the lungs, occasionally the kidneys.

" The lungs usually contain sparsely scattered lesions only, in the form of minute grey tubercles, caseous or calcareous tubercles (sometimes aggregated together), grey nodules containing caseous foci, or caseous and softened nodules gritty from calcification, the latter situated chiefly towards the posterior tips or in the thin margins of the lungs ; together with the above lesions there may be irregular grey caseating patches of varying size and extent in the thin margins or on the dorsal surfaces of the caudal lobes. The kidneys are in the large majority of cases normal, or show in the cortices sparsely scattered miliary tubercles ; sometimes they contain in the cortices grey nodules which project from the surface and extend deeply into the substance, and in the medulla caseous streaks ; rarely caseo-pus has been found in the pelvis ; small pits are frequently seen on the surfaces of the kidneys and occasionally a few small scars.

" Lesions are not generally found anywhere else in the body ; in a few cases there have been a few miliary tubercles on the pleura.

" In six out of the 125 rabbits, a more severe tuberculosis was produced than is described above. The lungs of all these animals were more severely affected than any other organ ; in five instances they contained large caseating nodules which

[1] One of them " died after 89 days, apparently from a secondary infection of the local lesion."

[2] An expression designedly used during the earlier stages of the investigations of the Commission, because it did not commit the user to any theory of types, but which may now be interpreted to mean tubercle bacilli of the human type.

sometimes by coalescence replaced the greater part of a lobe. In the sixth the lungs were even more extensively tuberculous ; they were large and did not collapse, and appeared from the surface to be composed throughout of tuberculous tissue ; the cephalic lobes were solid and caseating almost throughout ; the caudal lobes were tuberculous for a varying depth from the surface and were crepitant in the centre, the crepitant tissue containing caseating nodules. The severe disease in this case was possibly due to the immediate dissemination of a larger number of tubercle bacilli than usual, since a very similar result has occasionally been produced by the intravenous inoculation of slightly virulent cultures.

" The kidneys of five of the six rabbits showed either no lesions at all, or one or two miliary tubercles. The kidneys of the remaining rabbit contained scattered, grey, slightly caseous nodules, some projecting from the surface.

" In four of the six rabbits the tuberculosis within the body was confined to the lungs and kidneys. In one there were 'perlsucht' growths on the pleura, and in the other a number of miliary tubercles in the liver[1]." After describing these severe and exceptional results Griffith points out that " The important points in regard to the results are (1) that though the tuberculosis produced in the rabbits was severe, it was not so severe as that which follows the inoculation of bovine tubercle bacilli; (2) that death from tuberculosis did not ensue in any of the rabbits within the period of observation (from three to five months) ; and (3) that the number of severely infected rabbits bears but a small proportion to the total number inoculated (6 out of 125 or 4·8 per cent.)[2]."

Thus we see that even with subcutaneous injection rather

[1] Griffith adds : "Whether these more severe results are to be attributed to greater susceptibility of the individual rabbits, or to higher virulence of the particular cultures, cannot be definitely determined. On the one hand, each culture produced in two other rabbits inoculated subcutaneously, as well as in calves, slight tuberculosis such as is often produced by the human tubercle bacillus. On the other hand, each of the two viruses (H 124 and H 129) produced severe tuberculosis in more than one of the rabbits inoculated subcutaneously, and a third (H 78) produced unusually severe results by intravenous and intraperitoneal inoculation."

[2] A. S. Griffith, *R.C.T. Fin. Rep.* App. vol. i, p. 37.

severe tuberculosis is sometimes produced in the rabbit by tubercle bacilli of human type, and that the results of such injection may occasionally be misleading to those who are not aware of this fact.   Doubtless the most important point is the entire absence, after injections of bacilli of this type, of the rapidly fatal miliary tuberculosis which is produced by the bovine bacillus.

Oehlecker[1] has attached some diagnostic importance to the alleged immunity of the lymphatic glands near the seat of inoculation in the rabbit when the tubercle bacilli belong to the human type.   His injections were made in the abdominal wall, and ulceration occurred and led to the escape of the tuberculous products.   It may be for this reason that the glands were free from lesions in his animals.   A. S. Griffith, who inoculated his rabbits under the skin of the back, between the shoulders, with the definite object of avoiding, if possible, an open ulcer, found the lymphatic glands tuberculous in nearly half his cases.

The method of inoculation adopted by Griffith usually resulted in the formation of a cyst, but sometimes the skin gave way and caseo-purulent material was discharged.   The tendency to the formation of an open sore with the attendant risk of the infection spreading to other animals, is undoubtedly a grave objection to the subcutaneous method of inoculating rabbits as ordinarily used, and Griffith's plan is an undoubted improvement.

The dose of bacilli recommended to be employed in rabbit experiments made with the object of determining the type of mammalian tubercle bacilli.   As we have seen, the human type of tubercle bacillus is by no means entirely devoid of virulence for the rabbit, and may cause a fatal result, or (rarely) progressive tuberculosis when large doses are used, especially when the injection is intravenous, and sometimes even when it is intra-peritoneal or even subcutaneous.

This is a strong reason for employing small doses only for the determination of type.   As Oehlecker has said: "The smaller

---

[1] *Tub. Arbeit. a. d. Kaiserl. Gesundheitsamte*, 1907, Heft 6, p. 109, § Sub-cutane Impfung Kaninchen mit Reincultur.

the dose, the clearer is the difference in the result." But even with small doses rather severe results sometimes follow the injection of human tubercle bacilli, due apparently to an unusually high degree of susceptibility in an individual rabbit. It has been truly said that "the rabbit is a capricious animal." This, however, is not an insuperable obstacle to its use. We must be prepared for exceptional results, and must inoculate several animals in each experiment, so that we may not be misled by an exceptional individual.

The method of inoculating. It may be said that the best method will be that which gives the clearest difference in the effect produced by the two types of bacilli. Other things being equal a quick result is to be preferred. And lastly, it is desirable to avoid such methods as lead to a discharging tuberculous lesion, and the consequent escape of tubercle bacilli which may open the door to spontaneous infection in other research animals.

Oehlecker prefers intravenous inoculation, and this is supported by Park and Krumwiede, and to some extent by A. S. Griffith. If this method be adopted the dose, as we have seen, should not exceed 0·01 milligramme.

Kossel, Weber and Heuss mainly used the subcutaneous method, and this was largely employed (together with the intravenous) by A. S. Griffith also. With this method 10 milligrammes may be injected, and the result is certainly quite as sharp, though not so quick, as when 0·01 milligramme is injected intravenously.

The intraperitoneal method of inoculation has few supporters, but in the opinion of the writer it is preferable to the other methods, and for the following reasons. Intravenous inoculation requires a careful estimation of dose, a process in which it is possible mistakes may occur. Too large a dose may give very misleading results. The results of such experiments, therefore, when published do not carry quite the same conviction to the reader as those obtained by other methods.

Subcutaneous injection is open to objection, as mentioned already, on account of the open ulcer which usually results; for in such investigations as we are considering it is of paramount importance to open no door to the possible transmission of infection accidentally to other animals used in the research. It is this danger which, in the writer's opinion, has resulted in such inextricable confusion in attempts to modify the type of tubercle bacilli by passage.

Intraperitoneal injection is free from these objections. It gives a very sharp and decided result in the immense majority of cases, especially if 1·0 milligramme be the dose employed. In the rare case of an indecisive result in one of the animals used in a given experiment the doubt can always be dispelled by the injection of a second rabbit with material taken from the one which gave the doubtful result. Why then is not this method generally chosen ? It is, I believe, because of the fear of accidentally wounding the cæcum, or some other part of the intestine. This fear is unfounded. Such wounds, in an experience extending over more than a thousand injections of this kind, have seldom occurred, and when they have done so have led to no confusion[1].

Summary. It may be said that the rabbit is one of the most susceptible of all animals to infection with the bovine type of tubercle bacillus, however injected ; that it shows as a rule a high, but somewhat variable, resistance to the human type of tubercle bacillus, lesions of a chronic type being not unfrequently seen in the lungs, and sometimes in the kidneys. Some considerable experience, therefore, is necessary in the use of this animal to avoid being misled by exceptional results, unless a number of animals are used in each experiment.

Subcutaneous or intraperitoneal injection, of 10 or 1 milli-grammes respectively, is the method least likely to mislead. But equally good results may be obtained in skilled hands by intravenous injections, provided that the doses are accurately measured and do not exceed 0·01 milligramme of bacilli.

[1] The writer prefers to use for intraperitoneal injection in the place of the ordinary hypodermic syringe an extemporized glass pipette. In order to regulate exactly the depth to which the pipette penetrates the end of the pipette is drawn out abruptly into a fine capillary tube about $\frac{1}{4}$ inch long. The sudden alteration of diameter thus produced forms a shoulder which arrests the further progress of the pipette when it penetrates, as it often does, with a jerk through the abdominal wall. For this beautiful method the writer is indebted to Dr Haffkine who demonstrated it many years ago in the Cambridge Laboratory.

CHAPTER XIV

THE STABILITY OF TYPE OF TUBERCLE BACILLI IN ARTIFICIAL CULTURE

A. *The Stability of Cultural Characters.*

This part of the subject has been dealt with already. We have seen that tubercle bacilli exhibit a capacity for slowly adapting themselves to the conditions of artificial cultivation, and come gradually to grow in the test tube more and more luxuriantly, the dysgonic bovine strains thus tending to approximate to the eugonic human strains and the distinctive cultural characters of the types to become at length obscured. At the same time it may be doubted whether bovine strains ever, or at least during the course of observations even when extended as long as is reasonably possible, assume to the full the eugonic characters which distinguish the human type.

B. *The Stability of Virulence during Artificial Cultivation.*

It is natural to suppose that step by step with this slowly progressing adaptation to the conditions of saprophytic existence some loss of correspondence to the conditions of parasitic life must occur, and some degree of attenuation of virulence consequently ensue. How far this is the case we must attempt to ascertain by an examination of the available evidence. But, in order to avoid being tedious, the verdict may be anticipated, and it may be said at once, *that attenuation under artificial cultivation is as a rule very slight, and often imperceptible after one or more years. That when it occurs it does so capriciously, and would seem to be determined by causes about which at present little is known.* Tubercle bacilli indeed, we shall find, are, as to their virulence, amongst the most stable of all bacteria.

Do tubercle bacilli, on transference from the animal body to artificial culture media, lose immediately some of their virulence? In the laboratories of the Royal Commission in the earlier period of their investigations tuberculous tissues were frequently employed for inoculation. In these cases the number of bacilli injected were estimated by counting. At a later period injections of pure culture were almost exclusively used. It was found on comparing the results of the two methods that a given number of tubercle bacilli taken from artificial cultures and suspended in a small quantity of salt solution, produced a far less severe disease than the same number of bacilli from the lesions of a tuberculous animal injected together with an emulsion of animal tissue[1]. It was, as a matter of fact, estimated from actual experiments that to produce in the calf by injection of culture results as severe as those caused by the injection of tuberculous tissue emulsions containing bacilli belonging to the same original strain several hundred times as many bacilli were required[2]; and this held good of cultures quite recently isolated from the animal body. The question, therefore, arose—do tubercle bacilli lose some of their virulence almost immediately on changing from a parasitic to a saprophytic existence? Or is the difference in the results mentioned above due to the adjuvant action of the emulsified animal tissue injected along with the bacilli in one case but not in the other? The question might, of course, have been settled by a direct experiment. One had only to take some culture and inject equal doses into two series of animals, suspending the bacilli in the one case in physiological salt solution, and in the other in an emulsion of animal tissue. But there was so much more important work going on that this was not done. In the absence of direct experiment of this kind one can only consider probabilities, and it may at least be said that no immediate loss of virulence on the change of the conditions of life which we are considering has been *proved* by the experiments referred to above, and that,

---

[1] For examples see Calves 385 and 199, Heifers 259 and 237, and Goats 3 and 17. *R.C.T. Int. Rep.* App. vol. ii, pp. 202 and 203.

[2] *R.C.T. Int. Rep.* App. vol. iii, p. 187.

on the contrary, it appeared likely that the difference in the severity of the disease which was observed was due to the adjuvant action of the dead tissue injected along with the bacilli in the one part of the experiments. For dead and emulsified tissue may reasonably be thought to afford the microbes at once a suitable and accustomed culture medium, and a mechanical protection against the bactericidal forces which the new host would otherwise be able to bring against them unimpeded, and thus to allow them to multiply in comparative security. Possibly also the difference may be due, in part at least, to preformed toxins present in the tuberculous tissues injected along with the bacteria.

Does progressive attenuation occur in artificial cultures? Koch, Schütz, Neufeld and Miessner have recorded the attenuation of a strain of bovine tubercle bacilli which originally was highly virulent, but which, after long-continued cultivation on broth, suffered such a loss of virulence that even large doses could be injected intravenously for the immunization of cattle.

Trudeau also mentioned a strain which after more than 14 years of artificial cultivation was capable only, when injected into guinea-pigs, of producing an enlargement of glands and spleen which never led to a fatal termination. De Schweinitz described an attenuated strain of tubercle bacilli, obtained from Trudeau, which is possibly identical with that mentioned above. Vallée has described the attenuation of a strain of tubercle bacilli, isolated by Nocard from a horse. This strain was said to have been very virulent originally, but to have lost its virulence little by little, so that, at length, the subcutaneous injection of 1·0 milligramme into guinea-pigs caused only a transient retrogressive disease of the neighbouring glands, while eight or ten milligrammes were required to produce severer lesions. Lindemann, who also worked with the strain, confirmed this statement.

Arloing and Courmont produced an attenuated strain of tubercle bacilli, which grew as a homogeneous suspension in fluid culture media by means of cultivation in glycerin-broth which was frequently shaken.

Park and Krumwiede speak of loss of virulence of two of

the bovine strains which they examined[1]. On the other hand, Kossel, Weber and Heuss[2] found that the bovine tubercle bacillus retained its virulence during two years' artificial cultivation on serum.

Very little evidence of loss of virulence was observed by those who worked for the Royal Commission, although certain strains were kept under observation for considerable periods of time, and their virulence tested after long intervals. Such evidence as bears on the question has now been gathered together from the Appendices to the Reports of the Commission, and is set out here for the first time. The following table contains experiments made on the calf with accurately measured doses of bacilli of bovine type, the mode of injection in each case being subcutaneous, and the dose of bacilli the same. The experiments are arranged in the order of the total duration of artificial cultivation to which each strain had been subjected at the time the test was made, with the object of seeing whether the results become any less severe as one passes from the beginning to the end of the table. Such a comparison can only be justified if we have good grounds for assuming that all the strains possessed originally the same degree of virulence. We believe that this was the case for reasons which have been discussed at length in the previous chapter (pp. 267 *et seq.*)[3].

The number of strains of tubercle bacilli of bovine type available for this comparison are forty. They include 19 of human, 16 of bovine, and 5 of porcine origin.

The conditions, apart from the point under consideration, were as nearly as possible the same in the various experiments. The strains had never been grown on glycerin media, nor indeed on anything but plain serum, unless perhaps in primary culture, on plain egg. The cultures actually used for injection were grown on serum for 21 days.

---

[1] These authors think it is important to use early generations for measuring the virulence of strains of tubercle bacilli; and they add—"Although our work as well as that of others has shown that there is a marked degree of stability in this characteristic, still where one is using this characteristic for differentiation no reliance should be put on such stability in individual cultures." *Journ. of Med. Res.* 1910, vol. XXIII, p. 283.

[2] *Tub. Arbeit. a. d. Kaiserl. Gesundheitsamte*, Heft 3, p. 11.

[3] See also footnote on page 291.

TABLE XIII. *Relation of virulence to duration of artificial cultivation,* as shown by 40 strains of bovine type. Tested by subcutaneous injection into 87 calves, the virulence being measured by the duration of the disease. Dose 50 milligrammes of bacilli.

H = Human origin.   D = Died of uncomplicated tuberculosis.
B = Bovine   ,,   K = Killed when dying, or; in a few cases, when
P = Porcine   ,,   apparently about to die in a day or two.
K Well = Killed when capable of living some considerable time longer.

Strain of Bacilli	Duration of Artificial Cultivation	No. of Calf	Duration of Disease	Strain of Bacilli	Duration of Artificial Cultivation	No. of Calf	Duration of Disease
H 31	1¼ months	519	D 21 days	B IX	8 months	244	K 19 days
H 31	1¼ ,,	521	D 31 ,,	H 29	8 ,,	693	D 63 ,,
B I	1½ ,,	228	K 43 ,,	H 29	8 ,,	697	K 35 ,,
H 59	1½ ,,	965	K 60 ,,	H 10	8 ,,	387	D 34 ,,
H 59	2 ,,	1063	D 28 ,,	H 20	8 ,,	547	D 36 ,,
H 64	2 ,,	1115	D 38 ,,	H 20	8 ,,	561	D 33 ,,
H 64	2 ,,	1091	D 37 ,,	B VI	8¼ ,,	240	K 54 ,, Well
H 69	2 ,,	1249	K 101 ,, Well	B VII	8¼ ,,	236	K 32 days
H 128	2½ ,,	1579	K 41 days	B VII	8¼ ,,	238	D 22 ,,
H 128	2½ ,,	1567	K 42 ,,	B XII	9 ,,	274	D 39 ,,
B XVIII	3 ,,	258	D 18 ,,	B XII	9 ,,	276	D 24 ,,
H 32	3 ,,	587	D 35 ,,	P XII	9½ ,,	444	K 48 ,,
H 32	3 ,,	589	D 40 ,,	P XII	9½ ,,	450	D 41 ,,
H 88	3 ,,	1271	D 45 ,,	B X	10 ,,	260	D 33 ,,
H 127	3 ,,	1585	K 48 ,,	H 19	10 ,,	577	D 37 ,,
H 128	3 ,,	587	D 46 ,,	B XXVI	10¼ ,,	418	D 76 ,,
H 128	3 ,,	1589	K 37 ,,	B XXVI	10¼ ,,	422	D 44 ,,
P XI	3¼ ,,	338	D 37 ,,	B V	11 ,,	224	D 42 ,,
P XI	3¼ ,,	376	K 19 ,,	B VIII	11 ,,	254	D 19 ,,
H 65	3¾ ,,	1093	D 30 ,,	B VIII	11 ,,	256	D 37 ,,
P VIII	4 ,,	328	D 28 ,,	H 29	11 ,,	841	D 23 ,,
H 28	4 ,,	489	D 28 ,,	H 29	11 ,,	847	K 31 ,,
H 28	4 ,,	464	K 29 ,,	B I	12 ,,	230	D 34 ,,
H 89	4 ,,	1275	K 105 ,, Well	B II	12 ,,	212	D 25 ,,
H 127	4 ,,	1569	K 105 ,, Well	H 77	12 ,,	1349	D 19 ,,
H 127	4 ,,	1593	K 34 days	B III	14 ,,	214	K 45 ,,
H 127	4 ,,	1595	K 45 ,,	B V	14 ,,	246	K 47 ,,
P VI	4¼ ,,	326	K 29 ,,	H 38	14 ,,	643	D 28 ,,
P IX	4¼ ,,	334	D 45 ,,	H 38	14 ,,	647	D 32 ,,
P V	4½ ,,	336	D 29 ,,	B IV	15 ,,	218	K 32 ,,
B III	5 ,,	248	D 46 ,,	B IV	15 ,,	220	D 36 ,,
B XVI	5 ,,	296	D 32 ,,	B VI	15 ,,	330	D 32 ,,
H 69	5 ,,	1267	K 56 ,,	H 14	15½ ,,	545	D 45 ,,
B X	5½ ,,	332	K 35 ,,	H 10	16½ ,,	667	K 90 ,, Well
B X	5½ ,,	334	D 38 ,,	H 19	18 ,,	597	K 45 days
H 32	6 ,,	837	D 33 ,,	H 19	18 ,,	885	D 25 ,,
H 32	6 ,,	849	D 23 ,,	H 14	19 ,,	671	D 33 ,,
B XV	6½ ,,	250	D 41 ,,	H 7	20 ,,	563	K 32 ,,
B XV	6½ ,,	262	K 47 ,,	B I	21 ,,	222	D 35 ,,
H 89	7 ,,	1351	K 44 ,,	H 38	22 ,,	887*	K 33 ,,
B XIII	7¼ ,,	268	D 27 ,,	H 7	25 ,,	773	K 40 ,,
B XIII	7¼ ,,	272	K 46 ,,	H 7	25 ,,	775	K 47 ,,
B II	7½ ,,	226	K 25 ,,	H 14	27 ,,	899	D 44 ,,
B IX	8 ,,	242	K 43 ,,				

* Dose 23 mg.

The figures in Columns 1 and 3 are for reference to further particulars given in the Appendices to the Reports of the Royal Commission.

The calves were as nearly as possible of the same age and size, and all of the same breed (Jersey). The disease caused by the bacilli injected was either allowed to terminate naturally, or the animals were killed only when obviously dying, except in five cases where the animals were killed when they were apparently capable of living some considerable time longer ; when this was the case it is indicated by the word " well " in the table. In no case included in this comparison was any serious complication present. Consequently, the rapidity with which the disease reached a fatal termination in each case may fairly be accepted as a measure of the severity of the results attributable to the inoculation, and, therefore, with reserve, of the virulence of the bacilli injected. The only disturbing factor is the variation in the susceptibility of individual calves. This is admittedly considerable, but calves of high and low virulence may be expected to be distributed fairly evenly over so long a list, and thus to a great extent these variations will neutralize one another[1].

Table XIII contains the results of the subcutaneous inoculation of 87 calves each with 50 milligrammes of bacilli of bovine type grown under the conditions of artificial cultivation on plain serum for periods which varied from five weeks to $2\frac{1}{4}$ years.

The first point which comes out clearly from the table is that in almost every case (five only excepted) the disease terminated fatally (or threatened to do so in a few hours or at most a day or two) within a period of a month or two of the injection ; and this was the case whether the virus had been freshly isolated from the animal body, or had been a year or two under artificial cultivation.

Thus the five animals which suffered least severely are not among those inoculated with the oldest strains, but are scattered impartially about the table. And, conversely, the

[1] In cases such as H 69, H 89, B vi, H 10, where only one animal appears as having been injected with each strain, it might be thought that the strain in question was of lower virulence than the standard. But in each of these cases the results of inoculation of other calves with 10-milligramme doses or with tissue emulsions, as well as those of inoculating rabbits and other animals with these strains lends no support to this supposition.

severest results, as shown by a termination, actually fatal or immediately threatened, in three weeks or less, occurred with viruses which had been grown for very different periods of time, namely, for 5 weeks, 3, 3¼, 8, 8¼, 11, and 12 months.

If the experiments are arranged according to the number of months during which the viruses had been cultivated artificially and the average duration of life of the calves of each group calculated the results are as follows:

Duration of artificial cultivation in months	No. of calves in each group	Average duration of disease	Duration of artificial cultivation in months	No. of calves in each group	Average duration of disease
1–2	4	38·75 days	10–11	4	47·5 days
2–3	5*	37·2 ,,	11–12	5	30 ,,
3–4	10	35·5 ,,	12–13	3	26 ,,
4–5	8†	33·4 ,,	14–15	4	38 ,,
5–6	5	41 ,,	15–16	3	36·25 ,,
6–7	4	38 ,,	16–20	4§	34·3 ,,
7–8	4	35·5 ,,	20–22	3	33 ,,
8–9	9‡	35 ,,	25–27	3	44 ,,
9–10	4	38 ,,			

* Excluding one which was killed in fairly good condition more than three months after inoculation.
† Excluding two which were killed in fairly good condition more than three months after inoculation.
‡ Excluding one which was killed in fairly good condition fifty-four days after inoculation.
§ Excluding one which was killed in fairly good condition three months after inoculation.

These results are rendered irregular by the fact that there are not enough calves in each group to neutralize the effect of differences in the resisting power of different individuals. It is, therefore, better to arrange them in larger groups, as follows:

Duration of artificial cultivation	No. of calves in each group	Average duration of disease
Under six months	32*	36·5 days
Six to eleven months	30†	36·6 ,,
One to two-and-a-quarter years	20‡	35·4 ,,

* Excluding three which were killed in fairly good condition.
† Excluding one which was killed in fairly good condition.
‡ Excluding one which was killed in fairly good condition.

From this analysis, then, we find no evidence whatever of progressive attenuation[1].

[1] The experiments included in the tables above were made partly by A. S. Griffith and partly by the present writer, and it is noticeable (if we select the calves injected with strains of human origin, which form the

Experiments made with single strains of bacilli tested when freshly isolated from the animal, and again from time to time after long intervals of cultivation, would probably be considered only class which contains enough animals injected by each of us for satisfactory comparison) that those injected by Griffith lived, on the whole, a little longer than those injected by the writer. Possibly this is due merely to chance, for both authors used identical methods, but lest it should be thought that the results obtained independently by two observers are not so strictly comparable as those obtained by one only, the results of the writer's inoculations are given separately below.

The author's own inoculations alone.

Duration of artificial cultivation	No. of calves in each group	Average duration of disease
Under 6 months	17	33·6 days
6–11 ,,	11	35·7 ,,
12–20 ,,	9	37·7 ,,
25–27 ,,	3	43·7 ,,

Here, indeed, would appear to be some trace of evidence of progressive attenuation, but it is very slight, amounting only to a prolongation of the disease by a few days after more than two years' cultivation. Moreover, the number of animals in each class is too small to afford a basis for any definite conclusions.

From the records of the Commission another series of calves, injected with doses of 10 milligrammes might be examined to see whether they afford any evidence of attenuation occurring in the course of artificial cultivation. But the results are so irregular as to be of little value for this purpose. This irregularity is no doubt due, as we have seen already, to differences in the individual susceptibility of different calves, for sometimes of two calves injected at the same time and with the same suspension of bacilli, one would develop disease of very different degree of severity from that developed by the other. Irregularities due to this cause were, as was to be expected, much greater with the smaller dose (10 mg.) than with the larger dose (50 mg.) of bacilli.

There were 47 calves injected with 10 milligrammes and while most of them died of acute miliary tuberculosis a few weeks after inoculation, 14 were less severely affected, and when killed at the end of three months were found to have developed a tuberculosis of a more or less chronic type. It may be interesting to see how these less severely affected calves were distributed among the strains of different ages. Seven of them had been inoculated with strains which had been under cultivation less than a year, and the same number with strains which had been under cultivation for one to three years.

One of the viruses which produced these comparatively mild results had been grown under artificial conditions for three years, and two others for two years and three months. On the other hand, one had been cultivated for six weeks only, another for two months, and two others for four and a half and seven months respectively. The low degree of severity of the disease in these cases, therefore, cannot be attributed in any degree to attenuation of the strains by long continued cultivation. Indeed, in many of the cases the production of disease of typical severity in other calves injected at the same time and with the same doses of these strains, served to show that there was nothing

more satisfactory evidence than that brought forward above. Unfortunately evidence of this kind is very scanty. Such as is contained in the Reports of the Royal Commission is almost all included in Table XIII.

B I after six weeks' artificial cultivation, injected in a dose of 50 mg. brought a calf to the point of death in 43 days. After 12 months' artificial cultivation it killed, with the same dose, another calf in 34 days. Tested again after 21 months' cultivation it killed a third calf in 35 days.

B II after 7½ months' cultivation brought a calf to the point of death in 25 days. Cultivated for 12 months it was tested again and killed a calf in 25 days.

B III was first tested after 5 months' cultivation and killed in 46 days. Tested again after 14 months it killed in 45 days.

H 14 was tested on three occasions but not before it had been already 15½ months under artificial cultivation. It then killed a calf in a dose of 50 mg. in 45 days. Three and a half months later it killed another calf in 33 days, and after a further interval of 10½ months, it killed a third calf in 44 days.

H 38 was first tested after 14 months' cultivation. It then killed two calves injected subcutaneously with 50 mg. doses in 28 and 32 days respectively. Five and a half months later it was injected subcutaneously in 10 mg. doses into two calves. One of these animals died of general tuberculosis in 36 days ; the other was killed after 108 days, and found to have developed tuberculosis of moderate severity only. When the strain had been cultivated for 22 months—that is to say 8 months after the first test—it was again injected into a calf, this time in a dose of 23 mg., and killed in 33 days.

These experiments afford no evidence of progressive attenuation during artificial cultivation within the comparatively short period (up to 2¼ years) under observation[1].

unusual about the virulence of the strains, but that the lesser degree of severity of the disease produced in certain calves was due to their possessing higher powers of resistance than the average.

Further particulars of these calves may be found in the Appendices to the Reports of the Commission. See *Int. Rep.* App. vol. I, p. 41, and vol. II, p. 1057.

[1] In another case, however, where the interval was longer, some attenuation would seem to have occurred (unless, indeed, this was an additional instance of separation of the more eugonic element from an originally mixed virus). This strain was known as H 19 S.W. and came originally from the mesenteric glands of a child. It appeared to possess when first tested the virulence of the bovine type, but the tests are not entirely convincing owing to the small doses of bacilli given. According to its cultural characters it was classed by Eastwood in Grade III, among the more easily growing bovine viruses. However this may be, it is quite certain that a sub-strain isolated from a goat after the virus had already passed through two calves was fully virulent. It killed calves in doses of 10 and 50 mg. and rabbits after the usual intervals of time (*R.C.T. Int. Rep.* App. vol. II, p. 471). This strain was retested on rabbits by A. S. Griffith after it had been growing for four years in the incubator and

Evidence of stability of virulence derived from rabbit experiments. Let us now examine the rabbit experiments and see whether they confirm or correct the inferences which have been drawn from the calves. Over 100 rabbits received intraperitoneal injections of tubercle bacilli of bovine type in doses of 10, 1·0, 0·1 and 0·01 milligrammes. The results of these injections are arranged according to the duration of artificial cultivations of the strains of bacilli used for inoculation, set out in the following table.

TABLE XIV. *Average duration of disease of rabbits after intraperitoneal injection of strains of tubercle bacilli of bovine type which had been grown in artificial culture for various periods.*

Duration of artificial cultivation	Duration of disease in days			
	10 mg.	1·0 mg.	0·1 mg.	0·01 mg.
Under 1 year	18·5 (9)	23·2 (14)	35·7 (15)	43·8 (3)
1–2 years	19·2 (14)	27·1 (18)	33·7 (12)	40·2 (4)
Over 2 years	16·2 (2)	36·7 (3)	40·2 (4)	39 (1)

(The figures in brackets indicate the number of animals in each group.)

These results are not of much value, since in many of the groups, especially those in which strains more than two years in cultivation were employed, the numbers of the animals are not large enough to neutralize the disturbing effect of differences of individual powers of resistance, which differences are probably as great in the rabbit as in any other animal. But they serve at least to support the evidence given by the calves to the effect that if any attenuation occurs in the course of two years' artificial cultivation it is so slight as not to be easily put in evidence.

Rabbit experiments were made by F. Griffith with three bovine strains which had been over three, and in one case over four, years under artificial cultivation, in order to see whether any attenuation had taken place, but he was unable to obtain any evidence that this had occurred[1].

Whatever one may think of the evidence of attenuation of

was " found to be much less virulent than the original culture" (*Ibid. Fin. Rep.* App. vol. I, p. 26). This strain gave a reaction curve similar to that commonly shown by tubercle bacilli of human type (*loc. cit.*).

[1] *R.C.T. Fin. Rep.* App. vol. IV, pp. 391 and 434.

tubercle bacilli under the conditions of artificial culture, the existence of strains of true tubercle bacilli which possess a low degree of virulence for animals cannot be denied. Such, as we shall see, have been found by A. S. Griffith to constitute a large proportion of the viruses which have been obtained from cases of lupus in man, as well as some of those which were found in cases of tuberculosis in the horse. Instances of strains of low virulence have also been recorded by Kleine, and one by those who have worked in the Gesundheitsamt, from cases of human surgical tuberculosis (see p. 645).

The cause of attenuation under artificial cultivation. As to the cause of the attenuation which occasionally occurs under artificial cultivation but little is known. It would seem reasonable to believe that as a strain of pathogenic tubercle bacilli adapts itself to the conditions of a saprophytic existence in our artificial cultures it loses to some extent its adaptation to the conditions of parasitic life, but, as we have seen, but little evidence of the truth of this can be gathered from the experience of the Royal Commission.

Beck has suggested that glycerin in culture media causes a loss of virulence. The present writer investigated this suggestion but was unable to confirm it[1]. He found, indeed, that strains of bovine type produced in animals a somewhat more severe disease when the bacilli actually injected had been grown on pure serum than that which was caused when the bacilli had been grown on serum to which glycerin had been added. But if in each case the bacilli actually injected were grown on pure serum it made no difference whether their previous growth had been on pure serum or glycerin-serum. Glycerin then does not really attenuate, though it may weaken temporarily the action of tubercle bacilli actually grown in its presence. Possibly the slight difference which is then seen may be due to a difference in the products of the bacilli grown under the two conditions.

The evidence of the truth of this statement is as follows :
Eighty-two rabbits were injected intraperitoneally with various strains of bovine tubercle bacilli, all presumably of approximately the same degree of

---

[1] Stability of tubercle bacilli in artificial culture. The influence of glycerin. *R.C.T. 2nd Int. Rep.* App. vol. III, p. 191.

virulence originally. The effect of injecting cultures grown on pure serum and glycerin-serum respectively is shown in the following table.

Average duration of disease in rabbits (82 in number) after intraperitoneal injection of cultures grown on pure serum and on glycerin-serum respectively.

Dose	On pure serum	On glycerin-serum
10 mg.	14 days	20 days
1·0 ,,	21·7 ,,	28 ,,
0·1 ,,	26 ,,	37·6 ,,

The following experiment was carried out on similar lines with a single virus of bovine type:

Average duration of disease after intraperitoneal injection of cultures (29 rabbits).

Dose	On pure serum	On glycerin-serum
10 mg.	13·8 days (5)	23·2 days (5)
1 mg.	30·5 ,, (2)	27·6 ,, (5)
0·1 mg.	50·7 ,, (3)	52·7 ,, (4)
0·01 mg.	60·5 ,, (2)	79·7 ,, (3)

(The figures in brackets indicate the number of animals in each group.)

From these experiments it is quite clear that glycerin-serum cultures produce in corresponding doses somewhat less severe disease in the rabbit than do pure serum cultures. But, from the second experiment, particularly, in which a stricter comparison is possible owing to the fact that only one strain of bacilli was used throughout, it will be seen that the difference is greater with large doses than it is with small. This supports the suggestion that the difference in the severity of the disease caused by pure serum and glycerin-serum cultures respectively may be due to a difference in the chemical products rather than to any essential difference in the virulence of the bacilli themselves·

The effect of continued cultivation on glycerin-serum was tested in the following experiment. A strain of tubercle bacilli of bovine type was grown in parallel series on (1) pure serum, and (2) glycerin-serum for a whole year. At the end of that time cultures were made on pure serum from the last tube of each series and injected intraperitoneally into rabbits, with the following results:

Effect of continued and repeated cultivation of a strain of tubercle bacilli on pure serum and glycerin-serum respectively shown by injection into rabbits.

Dose	Duration of disease	
	Pure serum series	Glycerin-serum series
10 mg.	16 days	12 days
1 ,,	23 ,,	24 ,,
1 ,,	23 ,,	20 ,,
0·1 ,,	31 ,,	29 ,,

From this experiment it is evident that growth on glycerin serum continued for one year had produced no attenuation.

F. Griffith[1] also compared the comparative virulence of tubercle bacilli

[1] *R.C.T. Fin. Rep.* vol. IV, p. 434.

of bovine type after growing in parallel series on pure serum and glycerin-serum respectively. Three strains were used and the cultivation on these media was extended to three and four years (1487, 1224 and 1189 days respectively). No attenuation of the strains grown on glycerin media as compared with those grown in the absence of glycerin was observed.

Summary and Conclusions.

An examination of the records of the Royal Commission has failed to yield any good evidence of attenuation of tubercle bacilli when grown in artificial cultures prolonged in some cases for two, three, or even four years. On the contrary, the general impression gained has been one of unusual stability. Some very slight falling off in virulence is visible in some of the series of results examined however, and it cannot be affirmed that this might not proceed much further if longer periods of time were allowed.

On the other hand, it would appear from the evidence of foreign observers already alluded to, that tubercle bacilli may undergo a considerable loss of virulence[1]. If this is so the experience of the Commission would seem to suggest that this loss does not depend simply on adaptation to the conditions of saprophytic existence and a parallel loss of correspondence with a parasitic environment, but rather on some adventitious or accidental condition; for attenuation when it takes place seems to be irregular and capricious; and the suggestion naturally occurs that it may perhaps be caused by some such circumstance as unintentional exposure to diffuse daylight—or possibly even to the direct rays of the sun—on the laboratory bench when the cultures are being examined or

---

[1] Although the existence of attenuated strains of tubercle bacilli is often spoken of as a matter of common knowledge, the evidence that such have really descended genetically from true tubercle bacilli is not always conclusive. The question is beset with the same kind of difficulties which surround the kindred question of the stability of type of tubercle bacilli in the animal body and which will presently be discussed. Before finally accepting instances of apparent attenuation one would have to be convinced that no acid-fast bacillus belonging to one of the non-pathogenic or slightly pathogenic species were present originally in, or had obtained access subsequently to, the strain of tubercle bacilli in question.

resown, or to partial drying of the media, to resowing at too long intervals, or to some imperfection of the culture medium.

The question of the attenuation of tubercle bacilli is of some importance. The conditions which produce it are, as we have seen, imperfectly known, and the very occurrence of attenuation, and the degree to which it may be carried seem worthy of further study.

P.S. The evidence cited in this chapter from the records of the Royal Commission relates only to cultivation on serum. The possibility of attenuation on other media has not been considered and is therefore not excluded.

CHAPTER XV

THE STABILITY OF TYPE OF TUBERCLE BACILLI IN THE ANIMAL BODY

INTRODUCTORY: DIFFICULTIES AND PITFALLS OF THE EXPERIMENTAL INVESTIGATION OF THE QUESTION OF MODIFICATION OF TYPE.

THE ALLEGED ATTENUATION OF MAMMALIAN TUBERCLE BACILLI IN THE BODIES OF COLD-BLOODED ANIMALS.

THE QUESTION OF TRANSFORMATION OF MAMMALIAN INTO AVIAN TUBERCLE BACILLI AND VICE VERSA.

Introductory : The Difficulties and Pitfalls of Experimental Investigation of the Question of Modification of Type.

All three types of tubercle bacilli possess, as we have seen, many characters in common, including the capacity to produce in appropriate animals disease which, though it shows minor variations in different species, is nevertheless so uniform that it has been universally regarded as one and the same. The three types of bacilli are, therefore, regarded by all as closely allied, and are held to have descended at no very remote period from a common ancestor ; and each type is thought to owe its peculiarities to adaptation to its particular host. But here agreement ceases, for while some observers hold that this special adaptation has been carried so far that three entirely distinct and stable sub-species have been formed, others see in them only subordinate and temporary varieties, and think that a change of environment to a new species of host is capable of readily reversing the adaptation, and of causing the conversion of one variety into another.

The question thus raised is not merely of academic interest, but of great practical importance ; for if tubercle bacilli can readily change their type, it follows that our views concerning the etiology of tuberculosis will be modified greatly ; for we shall no longer be able to infer the source of infection in any given case of the disease from the type of bacillus found in it. If, for example, the bovine tubercle bacillus can become so changed by residence in the human body as to take on the characteristics of the human type of bacillus, we shall not be justified in inferring a bovine origin for the infection in those cases only in which bacilli of the bovine type are found, but we shall have to admit that many more cases of human tuberculosis may be derived from infection from the cow than can actually be proved to have been so caused.

We have, therefore, now to consider the question of the stability or instability of type of tubercle bacilli when transferred to a new species of host. This question has been keenly contested in recent years and is by no means settled yet.

The experimental investigation of this problem is beset with peculiar difficulties, and surrounded by hidden sources of error. For all attempts at its solution involve the passage of a given strain of bacilli into a new species of host, with the object of seeing whether in its new environment the strain will, by adaptation, acquire the special characters which distinguish that type of bacillus which is commonly found in the new host. The experiments necessarily extend over a considerable period of time, and may involve the passage of the strain through not one only but a whole series of animals ; consequently, it is difficult to exclude completely the possibility of spontaneous infection with the very type of bacillus into which one is attempting to convert the strain under investigation, a type to infection with which, by the necessities of the case, the new species of host is liable. Such an infection may occur without exciting any notice. It may either be latent at the time of the experimental inoculation and escape detection for one reason or other, even with the help of the tuberculin test, or it may by some accident creep in insidiously after the experimental inoculation.

Moreover, the very slightest contamination of a strain of tubercle bacilli of one type with tubercle bacilli of another type will lead in time, during passage through a species of animal which is a more favourable host to the contaminating organism than to the one under investigation, to the complete substitution of the latter for the former type of bacillus. Such a sequence of events has been actually demonstrated by direct experiments with purposely mixed cultures; and it is possible that, in certain of the experiments where a change of type has apparently taken place, the cultures selected for testing the possibility of modification may have contained the two types of bacilli from the start. Mixed infections with two types of tubercle bacilli have repeatedly been met with both in man and in the lower animals.

Let us take a concrete case as an example. Suppose there were to occur in a tuberculous focus in some human being a very small number of tubercle bacilli of the bovine type along with a large number of bacilli of the human type, and suppose the investigator were first to determine the type of the virus, and then to proceed to try to modify it by passing it through cattle. In the experiments made for the preliminary determination of type it is possible that the bovine bacilli might not be detected. The cultures would, of course, grow like those of the human type, and the small number of bovine bacilli injected into the calves might make little or no appreciable difference in the extent or distribution of the lesions within the few months usually allowed in these experiments. The injection of rabbits, it is true, would almost certainly reveal to an experienced observer a virulence superior to that of the human type[1]; but even this

[1] Strains of tubercle bacilli with cultural characters of the human type and low virulence for the ox, together with high virulence for the rabbit have frequently been described (as for example by Schroeder and Mietsch, *Deutsch. med. Wochenschr.* 1910). They are often described as atypical or transitional in type, but in the hands of some observers strains of this kind have been, as we shall see, resolved into mixtures of human and bovine bacilli.

might be overlooked, or the injection of rabbits might be omitted, as in some of the earlier modification experiments of the Royal Commission.   Thus it is quite possible that such a strain might pass for an ordinary example of the human type and might be selected for the purpose of testing the possibilities of modification by passage through the calf.   If that were done, the bovine element of the virus, which owing to its numerical inferiority was powerless to produce serious disease in the calf injected with the original strain, would soon increase at the expense of the human bacilli during repeated passages through bovine animals and in the end a pure bovine strain would be obtained.

Spontaneous tuberculosis then, especially of a minimal or latent kind, in the animals used for passage, and the existence of two types of bacilli in very unequal proportions in the lesions which provide the strain to be investigated, are the two chief pitfalls which beset the path of one who sets out to investigate experimentally the possibility of transmutation of type.

Having examined the difficulties which are associated with the experimental investigation of the question of the stability of type of tubercle bacilli in the animal body, we may now pass on to consider critically the work of various researchers which bear upon this question.

The Alleged Attenuation of Mammalian Tubercle Bacilli in the Bodies of Cold-blooded Animals.

An acid-fast bacillus which grows freely at ordinary temperatures, but otherwise somewhat after the manner of a tubercle bacillus, was discovered in 1887 by Bataillon, Dubard and Terre in a carp believed to be suffering from tuberculosis. Since that time very similar bacilli have been found in many kinds of cold-blooded animals, for example by Friedmann in turtles, by Möller in the blind worm, by Hansemann in a python, and by Rupprecht, as well as by Küster, and more recently by Weber and Taute, in the frog.   These various strains of acid-fast bacilli are probably not all of them identical, but at least they represent closely allied varieties, and they are usually grouped together under the convenient name of fish-tubercle bacillus, because the first known strain was derived from a carp. By German writers they are frequently called Kaltblütertuberkelbazilli. But neither name is altogether free from objection, for the pathogenicity of these bacilli, even for cold-blooded animals, seems to be low ; and it is by no means certain that they cause tuberculosis in them, or that the lesions with which they have sometimes been found associated have not been set up by some other parasite. It would appear that they are not uncommonly present in cold-blooded animals, unassociated with any lesions whatever, for Weber and Taute (in the Gesundheitsamt) have isolated no less than 38 strains of these bacilli from apparently healthy frogs, and also from the mud of the aquarium in which they were living. It is, therefore, questionable whether they should be called *tubercle* bacilli at all[1]. But however this may be, these names have become established by usage, and appropriate or inappropriate they will probably continue to be employed.

Certain observers have regarded these organisms simply as tubercle bacilli modified by residence in a cold-blooded host ; and some have believed that they were successful in attempts to attenuate mammalian tubercle bacilli by placing them in the bodies of such animals, and that these organisms by gradual adaptation to their new hosts had become so altered in their virulence and cultural characters as to be more or less identical with the fish-tubercle bacillus (Bataillon, Dubard and Terre, Möller, Dieudonné, Friedmann, Küster, Bertarelli, and more recently Klimmer, of the Veterinary School in Dresden). But the discovery of the frequent presence of fish-tubercle bacilli in frogs by Weber and Taute, and the recognition of the fact that mammalian tubercle bacilli slowly die in the bodies of cold-blooded animals has thrown quite a new light on these experiments.

Klimmer himself injected human tubercle bacilli into carp,

[1] It is true that they may be made to cause a certain amount of disease associated with some sort of tubercles by injecting the tissues of a frog harbouring them into another frog, but so may other kinds of acid-fast bacilli which are ordinarily regarded as harmless, if they are injected along with cream or milk (Möller), and the latter are not considered to be tubercle bacilli on this account.

and found that the injection of the emulsified organs of these fish into guinea-pigs caused tuberculosis if not more than 160 days had elapsed since the injection, but that after 260 days no disease was caused by such injections.

If then some acid-fast bacilli, not pathogenic for guinea-pigs, were discovered in the organs of some of the fish injected with tubercle bacilli, it does not follow that they were the descendants of the bacilli which had been injected. It is much more probable that the mammalian tubercle bacilli had died out in the unaccustomed environment, and that fish-tubercle bacilli happened to be present in these particular fish, just as they did in so many of Weber and Taute's apparently normal frogs.

Such is the state of the question to-day. It is hard to believe that bacteria so different as mammalian tubercle bacilli and the so-called fish-tubercle bacillus can be readily converted the one into another by simply changing the environment for a short time. The real battle of metamorphosis must be fought over the alleged conversion of human into bovine bacilli and vice versa. And until the interconvertibility of such closely related forms has been placed beyond doubt, one cannot accept the alleged conversion of these others which are far more widely separated.

The Question of Transformation of Mammalian into Avian Tubercle Bacilli and vice versa.

I. *The alleged transformation of mammalian into avian tubercle bacilli in the bodies of birds.* In earlier and less critical days than the present Nocard (1898) believed that he had succeeded in converting mammalian tubercle bacilli into avian by passage through fowls. These experiments were at one time accepted by many as conclusive evidence of the possibility of such metamorphosis, and it is unfortunate that they have got into some of our text books ; for, as we shall see, there is good reason to doubt whether they ought not to be interpreted in quite another manner.

In Nocard's experiments human, or sometimes bovine, tubercle bacilli obtained from cultures were placed, enclosed in collodion capsules, in the peritoneal cavities of fowls, in order that the bacilli might become accustomed to growing in the fluids of the bird while they were protected from the attack of its leucocytes. After remaining in this position for varying intervals of time the capsules were taken out, and their contents were tested by injection into various animals, and by sowing cultures from them.

Avian tubercle bacilli, we have seen, possess but slight virulence for the guinea-pig, but are capable of causing fatal tuberculosis in the rabbit. Like these, the bacilli recovered by Nocard from the capsules produced, as a rule, but slight effect on the guinea-pig, and more severe disease when injected (intravenously) into rabbits. But this is but slender proof that they belonged to the avian type, and it seems more probable that they produced but slight disease in the guinea-pig because they were dead or dying (for it must be understood that it was the actual contents of the capsules after they were recovered from the fowls, and not bacilli from recent cultures raised from them, that were injected), and that the severe disease in the rabbit was due to the injections being intravenous—a method which is capable of causing severe pulmonary disease when bacilli which have only slight virulence for the animal employed are injected (e.g. human tubercle bacilli into the calf) or even when dead bacilli are used in sufficient quantity. The crucial proof of conversion into the avian type, namely acquisition of virulence for the fowl, was in most of the experiments wanting.

In two of the experiments, however, tuberculosis occurred in fowls which were injected with the contents of the collodion capsules ; and it is necessary to examine these more closely. In the first of these experiments the bacilli came originally from human sputum, and after passing, in collodion capsules, through three fowls in succession, were injected directly into other fowls to test their virulence for this species. One of these birds, injected intravenously, died nine weeks later of intense miliary tuberculosis affecting the liver, spleen and bone marrow. Another, injected intraperitoneally, remained well, and when killed had no tuberculous lesions. From yet another

C.   20

fowl, also of the third passage, a capsule was taken, and two more of these birds were injected with the bacilli which it contained. One of these, injected intravenously, died two months later with considerable enlargement of liver and spleen without visible tubercles, and numerous tubercle bacilli were found in these organs and in the bone marrow; the other, injected intraperitoneally, was found to be suffering from intense miliary tuberculosis of liver and spleen " identical with that of the natural malady." There does not seem to be any doubt then that Nocard, at this stage of the experiment, was dealing with a bacillus virulent for domestic fowls. But whether this bacillus of avian type had really descended from human tubercle bacilli with which the *passage* was started, or had, by some unknown means, crept into the virus—possibly from a spontaneous infection of one of the birds used for the passage—is not so certain.

The other experiment which resulted in the ultimate production of a strain of bacilli virulent for the fowl was commenced with a culture obtained from the mammary gland of a cow. This culture, enclosed in collodion capsules, was placed in the peritoneal cavities of three fowls. The bacilli recovered some time later from two of these capsules were injected directly into other fowls and found to possess no virulence for these birds. They grew however in artificial culture, in Nocard's opinion, like avian tubercle bacilli. They had, it seems, acquired the cultural characters, but not the pathogenic properties of the avian type of bacillus. The third bird, a cock, into whose peritoneal cavity a collodion capsule had been inserted, was killed nine months later when ill and wasted. Post-mortem examination showed that the capsule had ruptured. In the region of the left testis there was an irregular tumour of sarcomatous appearance, as large as a pigeon's egg, containing multiple caseous foci full of tubercle bacilli, and in its midst was the torn capsule. In addition there was fibrous ascites, a confluent eruption of small grey tubercles on the peritoneum, and the liver and spleen were infiltrated with miliary tubercles, with caseous centres surrounded by thick greyish margins.

This bird had remained well for some long time before it

began to fail, and Nocard believed that the capsule had only ruptured after the bacilli had grown accustomed to live and multiply in the fluids of the fowl, and so, when the time came that they were no longer sheltered from the attack of the leucocytes by the protective capsule, they were able to hold their own, and to invade the tissues of the bird. Other students, however, impressed by the negative results of almost all the modern attempts to convert mammalian into avian tubercle bacilli, will see in this occurrence only an instance of spontaneous tuberculosis arising naturally in a bird which by chance had been chosen to receive an injection of tubercle bacilli of a type incapable of infecting it.

More recently Olaf Bang (1908) has made a series of experiments like those of Nocard and has obtained similar results, and he also believes that he has succeeded in converting mammalian into avian tubercle bacilli[1].

On the other hand, only negative results were obtained by Shattock, Seligmann, Dudgeon and Panton (1907), who injected pigeons subcutaneously with tuberculous sputum, and investigated the properties of the bacilli which were ultimately obtained from them. Tubercle bacilli were found in the apparently unaltered spleens of the birds. These organs, and in some cases also the local lesions caused at the seat of inoculation, were emulsified and injected into guinea-pigs. The latter developed tuberculosis of the usual mammalian type, showing that the bacilli had not acquired the low virulence for this species, or the power of producing a kind of septicæmia rather than a condition marked by anatomical tubercles, which is characteristic of the disease sometimes produced in the guinea-pig by tubercle bacilli of avian type (see p. 437).

These experiments, however, convincing enough as far as they go, do not carry us very far, for the length of sojourn of

[1] Prof. Delépine of Manchester is also among those who believe that tubercle bacilli are unstable in type. His views are based on his own experimental investigations which now extend over many years, but the evidence on which they rest has never been fully published. At the International Medical Congress 1913, however, he exhibited a series of specimens showing progressive changes in the character of the lesions produced in guinea-pigs by inoculating these animals in series with avian tubercle bacilli.

the bacilli in the avian tissues was short, varying only from seven days to eight weeks ; and it is of course open to the supporters of the modification hypothesis to maintain that no particular change of characters could be expected to take place in so short a time.

Far more convincing are the very numerous and lengthy experiments carried out for the Royal Commission by A. S. Griffith and F. Griffith.

A. S. Griffith (1911)[1] investigated the cultural and pathogenetic characters of mammalian tubercle bacilli after more or less prolonged residence in the fowl and pigeon.

In the first series of experiments the cultures were injected directly into fowls. Eight different strains of tubercle bacilli were used, one an ordinary example of the human type, others, both of human and bovine type, being strains of attenuated virulence derived from cases of lupus. The total duration of residence of the bacilli in the body of the fowl varied from 28 to 239 days. These strains were recovered from the fowls, their cultural characters re-determined, and their virulence tested for rabbits and guinea-pigs, and (in three cases) fowls. Except in one experiment no change whatever was observed in the bacilli.

In the exceptional case the culture grown from the bird (No. 81) was quite a typical example of the avian type. It was obtained from the spleen of a fowl inoculated intravenously 239 days previously with a culture derived from a case of lupus. Post-mortem examination showed early tuberculosis of intestines, spleen and liver. " The distribution of the disease," Griffith remarks, "leaves little room for doubt that the bird was suffering from spontaneous tuberculosis."

Another series of experiments was made with cultures enclosed in collodion capsules. The strains used were either of human type, or attenuated bovine strains from cases of lupus; in one a mixture of the two standard types was employed. The capsules after being filled with culture, were inserted into the peritoneal cavities of fowls or pigeons.

Altogether 41 capsules were inserted, and 12 different

---

[1] *R.C.T. Fin. Rep.* 1911, App. vol. I, p. 59.

strains of tubercle bacilli were investigated by this method. In some cases the bacilli were passed in capsules through a series of birds. When this was done a culture always intervened between the successive passages.

The total period of residence in the peritoneal cavity of birds varied in the case of the different experiments from 59 to 685 days.

In many cases the bacilli were found at the end of the experiment to be dead. But from 13 capsules, representing five different original strains of bacilli, cultures were obtained. These grew on artificial media precisely like the original cultures, and inoculation tests of the bacilli taken from the capsules on guinea-pigs, rabbits, and fowls or pigeons, showed that the organisms had not undergone any change of virulence. These negative results will be found to be very impressive if we reflect that in two cases the virus was kept resident in the bodies of fowls or pigeons for no less than 643 and 685 days respectively without undergoing the slightest modification of character in the direction of the avian type. The experiments, Griffith justly concludes, do not lend any support to the view that mammalian tubercle bacilli can acquire the characteristic properties of avian tubercle bacilli by residence in the body of the fowl.

F. Griffith[1] also made similar collodion capsule experiments with mammalian tubercle bacilli in fowls and pigeons. In this series 36 collodion capsules were inserted into 16 fowls and 20 pigeons. Ten different strains of bacilli were used. When passage was made from one bird to another a culture always intervened. The capsules remained in the bodies of the individual birds for periods varying from 55 to 186 days, but when passage was made from bird to bird the total length of residence in the avian body was much longer, and in one case amounted to 475 days. In ten of the experiments with fowls and in ten with pigeons cultures were ultimately obtained, and were found to be unchanged in characters. In the 16 remaining cases the bacilli were dead[2].

---

[1] *R.C.T. Fin. Rep.* App. vol. IV, p. 388.

[2] Two other *direct* passage experiments through a series of fowls, each lasting two years and a half, were made with negative results. See *R.C.T. Fin. Rep.* App. vol. IV, p. 389.

II. *Attempts to convert avian into mammalian tubercle bacilli in the bodies of mammals.* F. Griffith[1] attempted also to modify avian tubercle bacilli by passage through the calf. Two experiments of this kind were made, each lasting one year. In each the virus was passed intravenously[2] through five calves in succession, emulsions of the spleen or liver of the preceding animal being used for injection at each step of the passage. Finally the virus was tested by injecting tissue emulsions subcutaneously into calves and guinea-pigs.

Numerous cultures were isolated from animals of various species in the course of these experiments, and, except for a single instance, none showed any change in cultural characters, or increased virulence for guinea-pigs.

The exception was one of two cultures obtained from the final calf of passage No. 2, which showed, when killed in good health after 109 days, a local tuberculosis at the seat of inoculation and some small lesions in the neighbouring lymph nodes, together with a caseous nodule in a bronchial gland. From the latter situation a culture was isolated which grew like a bovine bacillus and was virulent for rabbits and guinea-pigs, while from the prescapular gland another culture with typical avian characters and identical in every respect with that inoculated was obtained.

Some perhaps might be found who would claim this as a proof of modification. The bacilli in the gland next to the seat of inoculation, they might argue, remained there because they underwent no change, but such as acquired virulence for the ox made a further invasion and reached the bronchial gland, where, being more adaptable than those left behind, they acquired all the characters of the bovine type, while their less progressive brethren remained behind unaltered. The author however would point out that the facts of this case would have been to him more convincing evidence of modification had the change of type been less complete in the sub-strain from the bronchial gland, and if some signs of commencing modification

[1] *Loc. cit.* p. 385.
[2] Avian tubercle bacilli when injected *intravenously* into calves multiply and cause rapidly fatal tuberculosis, but injected *subcutaneously* into these animals they produce little more than local lesions. See. p. 392.

at least had been seen in the sub-strain from the prescapular gland. The simple suggestion that the bronchial lesion was caused by an independent spontaneous infection with bovine tubercle bacilli seems more easily acceptable.

In addition to the experiments already described, F. Griffith[1] investigated cultures obtained from a large number of animals each of which had been injected with avian tubercle bacilli, and in fairness to those who hold the view that modification is possible these must also be mentioned, for several instances occurred in which bacilli of bovine type were isolated from the animals.

From 169 animals injected with avian tubercle bacilli, including 1 horse, 22 calves, 6 goats, 12 pigs, 9 monkeys, 3 cats, 1 dog, 4 rats, 3 mice, 34 rabbits and 74 guinea-pigs, cultures were recovered which showed no change of character.

On the other hand, the cultures obtained from seven animals differed from those used for injection.

A. From the prescapular gland of Calf 456, inoculated subcutaneously with avian tubercle bacilli, a culture was obtained which was typically mammalian in its characters of growth, and highly virulent for guinea-pigs and rabbits; but it also produced general tuberculosis in three out of four fowls injected with it, and from two of these typical avian cultures were ultimately obtained. This culture was probably a mixture of mammalian and avian bacilli.

B. Calf 390, inoculated subcutaneously with a bacillus of avian type obtained from a pig, and killed after 90 days, was found to have a chronic general tuberculosis. Typical avian cultures were isolated from the prepectoral gland, the portal gland, and the suprarenal bodies. But from the lung a mammalian culture which grew like a bovine tubercle bacillus was obtained, and from the bronchial gland both avian and bovine types were obtained.

C. Goat 36 was inoculated with a culture of avian type obtained from a pig; killed 131 days later, it was found to have, besides local lesions, a little cavity and two small nodules in the lungs, caseous nodules in the thoracic glands, and a calcareous tubercle in the mesenteric glands.

"From the lung a culture was obtained typically mammalian in character, resembling a bovine tubercle bacillus."

Griffith remarks that in his opinion there can be little doubt that Calf 390 and Goat 36 became accidentally infected with mammalian tubercle bacilli.

D. Rabbit 777 was inoculated subcutaneously with a culture of avian type obtained from a pig, and when killed 91 days later showed a cystic local lesion, and a caseating nodule in the lung from which a typical bovine tubercle bacillus was obtained in culture.

[1] *R.C.T.* 1911, vol. IV, pp. 385, 398 and 402.

E. Two guinea-pigs, 1856 and 1857, were inoculated, one subcutaneously the other intraperitoneally, with an emulsion of the inguinal gland of Pig 106, inoculated with a strain of avian type of porcine origin.

The animal subcutaneously inoculated developed slight tuberculosis of the usual avian type. The other, No. 1857, died after 119 days of general tuberculosis, and a culture of bovine character, virulent for rabbits and guinea-pigs, was obtained from its bronchial gland.

Griffith believes that both Rabbit 777 and Guinea-pig 1857 became infected accidentally with bovine tubercle bacilli.

F. Guinea-pig 1612 was injected subcutaneously with an emulsion of the spleen of a calf, which had been injected with a culture of avian type derived from a pig, and died 150 days later. From the bronchial gland a culture was obtained which grew like a tubercle bacillus of human type, and which was virulent for guinea-pigs, slightly virulent for calves and rabbits, and produced no effect on a fowl fed with it.

G. Monkey 118 was inoculated subcutaneously with a culture of avian type derived from a pig, and when killed after 98 days had general tuberculosis, severe in the lungs. A culture obtained from the lungs grew like a bovine tubercle bacillus and was virulent for guinea-pigs and rabbits. A fowl fed with 20 milligrammes remained healthy. A culture made directly from the local lesion was avian in type, while one obtained from a guinea-pig injected with an emulsion of the local lesion was mammalian in type like that obtained from the lung.

These seven instances will be interpreted differently according as the reader is inclined to believe in instability of type, or the reverse. But in judging of their significance the far larger number of experiments which gave negative results, and the great length of some of these passage experiments, must be kept in mind.

A remarkable point, which the reader may have noticed, is that in six of these seven cases in which the final culture differed from the original, the virus used, while belonging to the avian type, was obtained originally from the pig, an animal which, of course, is far more susceptible to infection with bovine than with avian tubercle bacilli[1]. Although Griffith is probably right when he attributes the changes of type of the bacilli in these exceptional cases to spontaneous tuberculosis, it appears to the writer that the evidence of the pure avian

[1] These viruses were P 27 (for Experiments B and D), P 2 (for Experiments C, E and G), and P 3 (for Experiment F). For a complete account of the various experiments made with them, and especially for those which were held to establish their original avian character, the report on "the investigation of avian tubercle bacilli obtained from birds and swine" should be consulted R.C.T. 1911, App. vol. IV. pp. 167 et seq., and especially the tables on pp. 343–346, 358–360, and on p. 376 A.

character of some of the original viruses is not absolutely conclusive.

M. Koch and L. Rabinowitsch (1907)[1] investigated the effect of passing avian tubercle bacilli through guinea-pigs. In all experiments but one no increase of virulence for the guinea-pig occurred, but the strains after passing through three or four of these animals in succession died out, as indeed had occurred in a much earlier investigation of the same kind made by Straus and Gamaléia. In some of Koch and Rabinowitsch's experiments, residence in the mammalian body was continued for a long time, and in one, passage was made through ten animals in succession during a period of 18 months, but with no alteration of the virulence of the bacilli. In another, however, passage through 20 guinea-pigs during the space of two years and eight months led to the obtaining of a strain of bacilli of mammalian type. The success of this experiment can, however, scarcely be attributed to the great length of time afforded to the bacilli for adapting themselves to their new hosts, for the virulence of the strain for the guinea-pig was already high at the third passage, and it does not appear that it increased notably after this.

The importance of this result as evidence of change of type is diminished by the fact that the original tuberculous material was obtained from the liver of a parrot, a bird which is more commonly infected with human than with avian tuberculosis. It is, therefore, possible that the strain of bacilli may have been a mixed one from the start. The authors themselves recognized this and made several attempts to separate human and avian bacilli by cultivating from single colonies on plate cultures. In this they did not succeed ; but negative evidence of this kind is of little value in the case of so difficult a procedure[2].

These authors found also, as Courmont and Dor had done before them, that passage of avian tubercle bacilli through rabbits did not cause any increase of virulence for mammals,

---

[1] *Virchow's Archiv*, Beiheft zum Bande 190, etc.   See pp. 337, 358, 402 (Table of Experiments), and 473 (conclusions).

[2] For this experiment see *loc. cit.* p. 409, Leber Papagei 300.

as measured by guinea-pig inoculations ; and in another series of experiments they demonstrated that mammalian tubercle bacilli were not in any way altered by being grown in fowl's eggs (*loc. cit.* p. 428).

Weber and Bofinger[1] report, very briefly, the result of modification experiments with avian tubercle bacilli in mammals. They state that after even one or two years' residence in the guinea-pig, rabbit, or mouse, they were unable to detect any increase of virulence for the guinea-pig, or loss of virulence for the fowl.

Kleine mentions in a foot-note that he himself obtained results similar to those of Weber and Bofinger (*loc. cit.* p. 507).

Summary.

Attempts have been made to attenuate mammalian tubercle bacilli, or to transform them into so-called fish-tubercle bacilli, by growing them in the bodies of cold-blooded animals. The possibility of such a transformation has not been proved ; though in some cases fish-tubercle bacilli have been obtained from animals previously injected with mammalian tubercle bacilli. In such cases it seems probable that the mammalian tubercle bacilli which were injected had died out, and that the fish-tubercle bacilli were present as the result of an independent infection, since they are known to be quite common in cold-blooded animals which have not been injected, at least in frogs.

The relationship between mammalian tubercle bacilli and the so called fish-tubercle bacillus appears much more distant than that between avian and mammalian bacilli, or between the human and the bovine types of the latter. The real battle of stability of type must, therefore, be fought over these more nearly related forms, and until this is decided in favour of instability of type the alleged instances of transformation of more distantly related forms cannot be accepted.

With respect to the relationship of avian and mammalian tubercle bacilli numerous experiments have been carried out by many observers with the object of determining whether

[1] *Tub. Arbeit. a. d. Kaiserl. Gesundheitsamte*, 1904, Heft 1, p. 15.

mammalian tubercle bacilli are able to adapt themselves to the conditions of life within the body of the fowl, and in so doing to lose the special characters of growth and of virulence which distinguish the mammalian type and to acquire those of the avian type. Many other experiments also have been undertaken to try whether avian tubercle bacilli can be transformed into bacilli of one or other of the two mammalian types, by being made to grow in the body of some mammal.

These experiments have shown that mammalian tubercle bacilli can be grown in the bodies of fowls for considerable periods of time and passed from bird to bird without necessarily undergoing any change of type (A. S. Griffith). They have also shown that mammalian bacilli, enclosed in collodion capsules, may be kept alive in the bodies of fowls and the process repeated in a series of these birds, so that the total duration of residence of the bacilli in the avian body has amounted in some cases to considerably more than a year and in one case to nearly two years, without the bacilli losing any of the characters which mark the mammalian type, or taking on any of those of the avian type (A. S. Griffith, F. Griffith).

These experiments have shown also that avian tubercle bacilli can be grown in the bodies of various mammals for long periods, and passed from one animal to another, without necessarily becoming altered in type—the residence in the mammal having in some cases been prolonged to 18 months or two years (M. Koch and Rabinowitsch, Weber and Bofinger, F. Griffith).

On the other hand in some of these experiments a strain of bacilli, differing in type from that of the strain with which the experiment was commenced, and identical with that of the bacilli which naturally attacks the species of animal used in the experiment, was recovered. Such an experience seems to have occurred in the work of nearly all investigators, both those who concluded in favour of the possibility of modification (Nocard, O. Bang, M. Koch and Rabinowitsch), and those who did not (A. S. Griffith and F. Griffith). When this has occurred the change from one type to the other has usually been complete, but in a few instances bacilli with the combined characters of the two types have been obtained. These latter may possibly have been mixtures.

Such results will be interpreted differently by different observers. By some they will be regarded as examples of transformation, by others as the consequence of spontaneous tuberculosis occurring in certain of the animals used in the experiments, and due to accidents which are difficult to avoid in such investigations.

Whichever view be taken we may safely say that neither change of type, nor indeed any modification whatever of cultural characters or virulence *necessarily* occurs when a mammalian tubercle bacillus is made to live in a bird, or an avian bacillus in a mammal, at least within a period of one or two years.

This transformation or substitution—call it which you will —has occurred irregularly and capriciously, and though it has sometimes taken place in some of the longest passage experiments this has been by no means generally the case ; and it may be said quite fairly *that changes of type have not been in proportion to the length of time allowed the bacilli to adapt themselves to the new environment.*

Such changes of type when they have occurred have been abrupt, and strains of bacilli with characters intermediate between the types in question have rarely been met with.

It may, of course, be argued that changes of type when they occur in other regions of biology are apt to be abrupt, and without assignable reason, and that the changes which are alleged to have occurred in tubercle bacilli are not exceptional in this respect. Alteration of type, so the argument might run, does not occur every time a tubercle bacillus changes its host, but it has been shown to have done so in several instances, and we ought to recognize the possibility of there being certain conditions which bring about this change, although these conditions, as in other regions of botany where saltation occurs, are not yet known.

But the plain fact is that many of the instances of apparent change of type which we have been considering took place at an experimental station where spontaneous tuberculosis was not uncommon among the animals used for experiment, and it would seem surprising to anyone who has made practical acquaintance with the difficulties of excluding completely such infections in the course of researches into tuberculosis, if, under these circumstances, some instances of spontaneous infection among the animals which now concern us had *not* occurred during the progress of so many modification and *passage* experiments as we have been considering.

Conclusion.

We must therefore conclude (1) *that transformation of type from avian to mammalian, or vice versa, or indeed any modification of cultural characters or virulence, does not necessarily occur whenever a tubercle bacillus of the one type is made to reside for a year or two in the body of a new host in which tuberculosis, when it occurs naturally, is caused by the other type ; and* (2) *that transformation of type, or modification of characters, occurring apparently capriciously, that is to say, under special and as yet unknown conditions, and by no means regularly, has not yet been proved to take place.*

CHAPTER XVI

THE STABILITY OF TYPE OF TUBERCLE BACILLI IN THE ANIMAL BODY (*continued*)

THE QUESTION OF TRANSFORMATION OF HUMAN INTO BOVINE TUBERCLE BACILLI IN THE BODIES OF VARIOUS ANIMALS.

I. *The Alleged Transformation of Type of Human Tubercle Bacilli by Passage through Goats and Calves.*

In 1902 Behring, Römer and Ruppel reported a successful *passage* experiment in which a strain of bacilli highly virulent for calves was obtained from a goat inoculated ten months previously with tubercle bacilli of the human type. The announcement attracted considerable attention at the time ; and the experiment has proved to be the prototype of many a similar attempt to change the characters of the human tubercle bacillus.

The details of this investigation were submitted to a critical examination by Kossel, Weber and Heuss, who abstracted from the various papers in which they appeared the particulars relevant to the case. The following abbreviated summary is taken from their report[1]. The original strain of bacilli was obtained in artificial culture indirectly from human sputum, after several guinea-pigs had been inoculated with it. From one of these the culture was raised. The goat, referred to above, was injected intravenously five times with this culture. When killed ten months after the first injection it was found to have general tuberculosis. The original strain of culture, when injected into calves intravenously, in doses of 2·5 to 10 mg. of bacilli, had produced no illness, or at most a temporary disturbance of health ; but a subculture derived from the goat, similarly injected in a dose of 10 mg. into another calf, caused tuberculosis which was rapidly fatal.

The authors say " it is worthy of emphasis that in all our experiments on cattle with tubercle bacilli of human origin disseminated miliary tuberculosis of lungs, running an acute course and ending in death, has only occurred after previous passage through the goat[2]"; thus implying that a similar alteration of virulence had occurred in other instances also. Yet, as Kossel, Weber and Heuss point out, this seems to be the only instance of change of type which occurred. Moreover, Römer in a further paper admits that passage through the goat does not always raise the virulence of human tubercle bacilli[3].

The critics of the Gesundheitsamt suspected that in the experiment described above an accidental introduction of bovine tubercle bacilli might have occurred in the course of the *passage* of the virus, arising possibly as the result of spontaneous

---

[1] *Tub. Arbeit. a. d. Kaiserl. Gesundheitsamte,* Heft 3, p. 41.

[2] *Beiträge zur Experimentellen Therapie,* Heft 5, p. 36.

[3] " Wir verfügen selbst über mehrere derartige Erfahrungen, auf die ich weiter unter bei der Besprechung der Kulturen 5 und 6 zurückkommen werde, und die uns zeigten, dass die Erhöhung der Virulenz der Msch. Tb durch den Ziegenkörper durchaus nicht eine gesetzmässige Erscheinung ist." *Beiträge zur Experimentellen Therapie,* Heft 6, p. 31.

tuberculosis in one of the guinea-pigs; and they point out that it was not so much an example of gradual increase of virulence for the ox as a complete change of type.

Investigations at the Gesundheitsamt. In addition to criticizing Behring's results Kossel, Weber and Heuss, 1905 (*loc. cit.*) repeated the experiment. A strain of human tubercle bacilli (H 1) was passed through four goats in direct succession, and another strain (H 2) was passed also through four goats, but with a culture intervening at each *passage.* The total length of time that the strains remained in the goats was 188 and 202 days respectively; but no modification occurred. Cultures obtained from the last goat of each series grew even more luxuriantly than the originals, and showed on inoculation no increase of virulence either for goats themselves or for rabbits. Injected subcutaneously into calves they caused only minimal lesions.

Meanwhile certain experiments which were held by their authors to prove the transformation of the human into the bovine type of bacillus having been reported both by de Jong and by Dammann and Müssemeier, the investigations undertaken at the Gesundheitsamt were continued by Weber in 1907[1]. Accordingly the passage of the strain H 1 was carried through yet another goat; but no change in the character of the bacilli was observed. A culture obtained from this animal, the fifth of the series, was injected subcutaneously into a calf without producing anything more than the local changes which occur in that species of animal when the human type of bacillus is similarly employed; and another calf, which was injected intravenously, was found when killed to be free from tuberculosis. The strain H 2 was passed through three more goats (making eight in all), and the total duration of residence of the strain in the bodies of these animals carried to 515 days. Yet not the least change of virulence was observed when the bacilli were recovered from the last goat and finally tested.

In another series of experiments Weber passed a strain of tubercle bacilli of human type through a series of four calves, the total duration of residence in their bodies amounting

[1] *Tub. Arbeit. a. d. Kaiserl. Gesundheitsamte,* Heft 6, p. 77.

thereby to nearly two years (685 days), but again no change
of virulence took place.   In still another experiment fifteen
strains of human type were injected into a pig, and after 300
days there was obtained from this animal a substrain of bacilli
which possessed all the characters of the human type.

Weber and Titze (1910[1]) who also worked in the Gesundheitsamt, mention three instances in which calves, injected
intravenously with bacilli of human type (for the purpose of
immunization) developed tubercles in the eye (two cases), or
swellings of the joints (three cases), some long time afterwards.
From these lesions the tubercle bacilli were ultimately recovered
in culture ; and when finally tested showed no deviation from
the human type, although the bacilli had been living for considerably more than two years in bovine tissues.

Another instance of the same kind is related by these
authors.   A heifer received several injections, both intravenous and subcutaneous, of tubercle bacilli of human type,
and from its milk tubercle bacilli were recovered a year and
seven months after the last injection.   Cultures of these bacilli
were thoroughly investigated, and were found to possess the
characters of growth, and the low virulence for calves and
rabbits, of the human type[2].

By these experiments the authors demonstrated that
tubercle bacilli of human type might remain for a long time
(one or two years) in the tissues of the living ox without
undergoing any change.   And the conclusions which they
drew from their experience is uncompromisingly opposed to
the hypothesis of instability of type.

The Experiments of Dammann and Müssemeier (1906).
These experiments, mentioned above as having been put
forward in support of the doctrine of instability of type,
must now be considered more closely.   The observers passed
through a series of goats a strain of tubercle bacilli of human
type, and ultimately obtained from one of these animals a
strain of bovine type.

[1] *Tub. Arbeit. a. d. Kaiserl. Gesundheitsamte*, Heft 10, pp. 188, 189.
[2] *Ibid.* 1907, Heft 7, p. 11.   These observations have already been referred
to in Chapter XIII (p. 259).

The original strain was cultivated from the sputum of a phthisical patient, and at first produced on injection only slight tuberculosis in calves and swine. It was then injected into a goat and caused minimal lesions.

A second goat, which seems to have escaped the usual preliminary tuberculin test applied by these authors to their other animals[1], was injected subcutaneously with an emulsion of the tuberculous prescapular gland of goat No. 1. This animal developed a swelling at the seat of inoculation, which increased for a time, but afterwards subsided, shrinking to the size of a bean. It was killed nine months after inoculation. At the autopsy the prescapular gland on the side of the inoculation was found enlarged but not tuberculous ; in a tracheal gland was found a small greyish translucent nodule the size of a pea ; and in the middle of one lung was a tuberculous focus the size of a hazel nut, which was greyish yellow in colour, partly caseous and partly hard and crumbly.

The third goat was injected with the contents of this pulmonary nodule, and died 15 weeks later of general tuberculosis, and, after this, further *passage* consistently produced the bovine type of disease.

On the other hand, a culture derived from the tracheal gland of Goat No. 2 injected into a calf and into a pig produced only minimal lesions.

The nodule in the lung of Goat 2 is an important landmark in the history of this passage experiment. It was, as we have seen, hard and crumbly, and therefore probably of some long standing. The injection of this animal had produced only the most trivial lesion locally, and, though it apparently caused a focus in a tracheal gland, it seems to have failed to render the nearest lymphatic glands tuberculous ; it is difficult therefore to believe that it was the cause of this pulmonary nodule.

The description of the lesion reminds the writer of one which he found in a calf (No. 447) in the course of one of his own passage experiments (H 21, G.B. described fully later, p. 339), a lesion which, he did not hesitate to suggest at the time, might

[1] *loc. cit.* p. 116 (see *postea*, p. 370.)

be the result of a spontaneous infection.   If this was the case also with the pulmonary nodule in Goat 2 the transformation of type which occurred in this passage experiment of Dammann and Müssemeier is capable of a simple explanation.

The Experiments of Professor Eber of Leipzig.   Among the foremost of those who maintain that the human tubercle bacillus can, in certain circumstances, be converted into the bovine tubercle bacillus is Prof. Eber, who has carried out numerous *passage* and other experiments in the Veterinary School of Leipzig since 1893.

Since Eber attaches special importance to the particular methods which he uses, and attributes largely to them the difference between his results and those obtained in the Gesundheitsamt, it is necessary to describe them.   In all but his very early experiments he employed a combination of subcutaneous and intraperitoneal injection for his cattle ;   the subcutaneous being originally intended to test the virulence of the bacilli, and the intraperitoneal to afford the bacilli, accustomed to live in human tissues, the most favourable conditions possible for getting a hold on the tissues of the ox and of adapting themselves to their new host.   For the sake of economy both kinds of injection were usually performed in the same animal.

As material for injecting the calves he employed as a rule the coarsely divided tuberculous glands and other organs of guinea-pigs injected with human tuberculous tissues ;   and this formed the starting point of each *passage* experiment.   In some of the researches, however, a parallel series of inoculations was made with culture ;   but it was not in these that the majority of the alleged instances of modification occurred.

Eber, since 1903, has investigated 31 cases of human tuberculosis, and in seven instances has observed a change of type after passage of the strain of bacilli through the ox.   In these seven instances the bacilli are stated to have been, either not virulent, or not fully virulent, for the ox at the start.   Three of them came originally from children and four from adults.   In six of these seven instances of alleged modification the change of type occurred after direct inoculation of the original material

XVI] EBER'S EXPERIMENTS

into the animal, and only in one (No. XIX) by the passage of a culture obtained from the original material.

Three of the experiments may be described briefly as examples of the work now under consideration. The first is selected because Eber evidently considered it of considerable importance as being the earliest instance of a successful modification experiment, and regarded it as the starting point of all the experiments which he undertook later The second is chosen as an example of one of the more recent experiments. The third because it is the only instance in which passage of a culture resulted in an increase of virulence.

Case XI[1]. A youth died of phthisis at the age of 17. A portion of the lung was injected into guinea-pigs, and the tuberculous organs of these animals were emulsified and injected subcutaneously into a goat, and, both subcutaneously and intra-peritoneally, into a calf.

The fact that the goat, when killed $6\frac{1}{2}$ months after injection, was free from tuberculous lesions showed that the virus at that time was devoid of virulence for these animals. Moreover, a culture obtained from the original material of this case grew well and proved itself almost avirulent for the rabbit when injected subcutaneously in a dose of 10 mg., and only slightly virulent when 1 and 2 mg. were injected intravenously.

The calf was killed six months after injection. Its general health was slightly impaired. There was tuberculosis of some cervical glands, and of those in the prescapular region, the thoracic opening and the axilla on the side of the subcutaneous injection. The abdominal cavity showed, in the neighbour-hood of the intraperitoneal injection, a chronic tuberculous peritonitis which had extended to the omentum and the diaphragm. There was also some tuberculosis commencing on the posterior part of the costal pleura, and on the visceral pleura covering the diaphragmatic surface of one of the lungs.

Guinea-pigs were injected with the peritoneal tubercles of this calf, and subsequently their tuberculous organs were emulsified and injected into a second goat and a second calf. The result of these latter injections was that both the animals

[1] See *Centralbl. f. Bakt.* etc., 1. Abt. Orig. Bd. 70, pp. 234, 238 and 252.

died of acute general tuberculosis, in 60 and 83 days respectively.

Case XXVI[1].   A woman, aged 37, died of phthisis, and was found to have, in addition to caseous disease of the lungs, tuberculosis of the tonsils, the larynx, and the mediastinal glands, ulceration of the intestines, and tuberculosis of the mesenteric glands.

Guinea-pigs were injected with a portion of the woman's lung ; and after a due interval one of these animals was killed and an emulsion of its organs injected subcutaneously and intraperitoneally into a calf.   The calf remained in good condition, and was killed 122 days after injection.   In the neck the tuberculous infiltration about the seat of the subcutaneous inoculation was localized, and there was the usual slight tuberculosis of the prescapular gland on that side.   In the abdomen, on the other hand, there was widespread chronic tuberculous peritonitis which is said to have been of the " perlsucht " type.

The virus contained in the peritoneal nodules of this calf was, after further direct passage through a rabbit and several guinea-pigs, injected subcutaneously and intraperitoneally into a second calf.   It then produced acute general miliary tuberculosis and death from disseminated tuberculous peritonitis in 35 days.   A culture obtained from the peritoneal tubercles of this calf grew sparsely on various media, like a bovine bacillus, and was found to possess that degree of virulence for rabbits which is typical of the bovine type.   Injected into a calf, subcutaneously in a dose of 50 mg. of broth culture, it caused general miliary tuberculosis and death in 32 days.

The virus from the second calf, therefore, was a typical bovine bacillus.   Moreover, cultures obtained from the first calf of the series, both those grown directly and others obtained indirectly through rabbits, grew feebly on artificial media, and produced severe tuberculosis when injected into calves and rabbits.

On the other hand, cultures obtained directly from the human lesions grew well, and when injected into calves both subcutaneously and intraperitoneally produced so little disease,

[1] *Centralbl. f. Bakt.* etc., 1. Abt. Orig. Bd. 70, p. 264.   Also see Table of Experiment, opposite p. 244.

and that of so transient a nature, that injection of the emulsified peritoneal lesions into guinea-pigs failed, on two occasions, to cause any tuberculosis.

Case XIX. The original material which formed the starting point of this investigation was some tuberculous granulation tissue removed by operation from the knee joint of a child nine years of age. The injection of a calf, both subcutaneously and intraperitoneally, with the emulsified organs of a guinea-pig infected with this material, failed to provoke any tuberculosis.

On the other hand a culture raised directly from the original material injected into another calf, in doses of 50 mg. subcutaneously and 50 mg. intraperitoneally, caused a lesion at the seat of inoculation in the neck and chronic tuberculosis of the peritoneum. From each of these lesions a culture was obtained.

Now the culture obtained from the local lesion in the neck was exactly like that grown from the original material; that is to say it grew freely, had low virulence for the rabbit, and produced in the calf, injected both subcutaneously and intraperitoneally with 50 mg. doses, a localized tuberculosis of chronic type. It belonged, clearly, to the human type.

On the other hand the culture from the peritoneum of the calf was unlike the original culture. It grew sparsely and was virulent for the ox, and after further passage the strain took on all the characters of the bovine type.

If this is an instance of modification (rather than substitution) then modification failed to occur in the tissues of the neck, but succeeded in the peritoneal cavity of the same animal.

Experiments of Neufeld, Dold and Lindemann (1912). In the Gesundheitsamt Neufeld, Dold and Lindemann[1] repeated Eber's experiments as closely as possible, but were unable to obtain any evidence of modification.

Tuberculous material was obtained by them from 12 cases of human tuberculosis, and 13 calves were injected by the combined subcutaneous and intraperitoneal method to which Eber had largely attributed his success. Eleven of the calves were injected with emulsions of the organs of guinea-pigs infected with the human tuberculous tissues, and two with cultures

---

[1] *Centralbl. f. Bakt.* etc., 1. Abt. Orig. Bd. 65, p. 467.

derived from this material.   In no single instance, the authors
say, did modification occur, nor was there any suggestion of
transformation of type.   None of the calves developed peritoneal tuberculosis, or any progressive disease in connection
with the seat of inoculation.

Two of the calves were, indeed, found to be tuberculous,
but the authors hold that these were instances of spontaneous
tuberculosis.   In one of them there was found tuberculosis of
the mesenteric glands ; in the other tuberculosis of bronchial
glands, lungs, and liver.   Rabbits inoculated with emulsions of
lesions from each of these calves developed progressive tuberculosis.

The authors point out that some of Eber's results are like
those which Lindemann had previously obtained by *passage* of
an artificial mixture of bovine and human tubercle bacilli
through animals ; and they would explain the change of type
which occurred in some of the Leipzig experiments on the
hypothesis that the strains in question originally contained
both types of tubercle bacilli, the bovine being probably present
in very small numbers ; or, failing that, they would attribute
it to some chance contamination with bovine bacilli occurring
during the progress of the experiment.   " The principal source
of error in researches of this kind lies " they say " in the
possibility of some small quantity of tubercle bacilli of a foreign
type being present in the original material, or slipping in during
the course of the experiment " (*loc. cit.* p. 475).

Further they point out that nearly all Eber's instances of
alleged modification occurred in strains of bacilli which came
originally from pulmonary lesions obtained at autopsy, and
that concerning the collection of the material no special precautions are stated to have been taken ; while, on the other
hand in the case of experiments made with tissue removed by
surgical operation during life, and which were therefore necessarily collected with every possible care to guard against
accidental contamination, very little evidence of modification
was forthcoming[1].

[1] The original material used in the seven successful experiments was as
follows: No. vi, mesenteric glands from a child which died of primary intestinal

To the present writer also, but for another reason, it appears significant that in no less than five of Eber's seven experiments in which a change of type of bacillus occurred on passage the original material came from pulmonary tissue, and in one only from a case of surgical tuberculosis (knee joint), although eight cases of this latter class were investigated. Pulmonary lesions (caused by human tubercle bacilli) would seem to be more exposed to contamination with bovine tubercle bacilli than are lesions in any other part of the body, the alimentary canal and its lymphatic glands alone excepted; for, as we have seen, there is reason to think that milk containing bovine tubercle bacilli may occasionally slip past the glottis in minute amounts, and that in this way bacilli of this type may sometimes find entrance into the cavities and other lesions caused by human tubercle bacilli[1].

The evidence of the frequent escape of bacteria from the mouth or pharynx into the bronchial tubes and lung has already been discussed in Chapter IX, and the author's own feeding experiments with *B. prodigiosus*, in which, in spite of all precautions, these micro-organisms were found almost constantly in the lungs shortly after introduction into the mouth, have been described. From this and other evidence it appears that the direct passage of finely divided material in minute quantities from the mouth to the lungs is not uncommon; and it therefore seems not improbable that an admixture of bovine tubercle bacilli from milk, or other food, would occasionally be found in the products of a lung rendered tuberculous by the human tubercle bacillus, in spite of all precautions taken in removing the organ.

As a matter of fact mixed cultures of bovine and human tubercle bacilli have been obtained several times from lungs or bronchial glands. One such mixture was found on two occasions by Kossel[2] in the sputum of a woman aged 27, who was

tuberculosis; Nos. XI, XXVI, XXVII and XXX, lungs from cases of phthisis; No. XIX, tuberculous tissue from the knee of a nine-year-old child; and No. XXV, lung from a case of subacute miliary tuberculosis.

[1] A similar argument was advanced by Koch in explanation of a case brought forward by Arloing in 1908. (See p. 559, also footnote p. 361.)

[2] Kossel, *Deutsch. med. Wochenschr.* 1911, No. 43.

suffering from phthisis, and another was obtained by Lindemann[1] from the sputum of a man of 20 years.   The well known
de Jong-Sturmann strain, described elsewhere, which is believed
by some to have been a mixture, came from a similar source,
and an " atypical " strain was obtained from sputum by Mohler
and Washburn[2].   In one instance (or perhaps two) investigated by the Royal Commission both types of bacilli were
obtained from bronchial glands[3] and recently another strain
from a bronchial gland investigated by A. S. Griffith has
been found to be a mixture[4].

Eber himself admits that in two of his successful modification experiments which started from pulmonary lesions (Nos.
VI and XXV), it is conceivable that the original material may
have contained a mixture of human and bovine tubercle bacilli,
though he does not favour this interpretation.   But he thinks
that it is just possible because the experiments made with the
strains before they became modified give grounds for the
suspicion that the virulence for the ox was, even then, not
entirely of the low order of the human type[5].

He is himself, however, inclined to regard the cases of human
tuberculosis which provided the original material for these experiments as instances of bovine infection, in which in consequence
of long residence in man the bacilli had lost, more or less, their
virulence for the ox.   In the other successful modification
experiments he holds that there are no grounds whatever for
the assumption that " other than so-called tubercle bacilli of
human type were present in the original material."   But he
admits that in such cases exact proof is scarcely possible, and
he tacitly allows that he did not give sufficient attention to

---

[1] Lindemann, *Tub. Arbeit. a. d. Kaiserl. Gesundheitsamte*, Heft 12, p. 68.

[2] U.S. Bureau of Animal Industry, 1907, *Bulletin* No. 96.

[3] H 13, A.D. and H 60, W.B. *R.C.T. Fin. Rep.* App. vol. III, pp. 17 and 19.

[4] *Reports to the Local Government Board*, 1914, N.S. No. 88, p. 115.

[5] For example the first calves which were inoculated in each of these experiments developed a tuberculosis which, although it ran at the start a favourable
course, proved ultimately to be progressive; and he might have added as
additional evidence (in the case of xxv) the fact that the original material
proved moderately virulent for rabbits. *Tub. Arbeiten. a. d. Kaiserl. Gesundheitsamte*, 1912, Heft 12, p. 68.

this important point, when he adds that in future experiments, as for example in a new series which he is now undertaking in collaboration with the Gesundheitsamt, the original cultures will be investigated with especial care to test the possibility of both types being present.

As to the possibility of spontaneous tuberculosis occurring in one or other of the experimental calves, either before or after inoculation, Eber rejects it altogether. He admits that tuberculous foci may sometimes be present in animals which pass a successful tuberculin test. But he points out that tuberculosis in young calves is in any case very rare, and when it does exist is found to be limited to the bronchial, portal or mesenteric glands. Moreover, he says that, in the opinion of veterinary inspectors of great experience to whom he showed his animals, the presence of tuberculosis limited to part of the peritoneum and omentum, and not involving any of the inner organs, cannot be explained by spontaneous infection, and such were the lesions which in his experiments were used for further passage.

Experiments of the Royal Commission. During the earlier work of the Commission several instances of apparent conversion, on *passage* through animals, of a bacillus of human into one of bovine type occurred. But on repetition of these experiments (which for one reason or another were not considered entirely satisfactory), and on the carrying out of new ones under improved conditions, no evidence of modification came to light ; and the Commission finally arrived at the conclusion that no real change of type had occurred, and that the apparent modification which had taken place in some of the earlier experiments " were due, certainly in most, if not in all, cases, to the presence of two types of bacilli, the human and the bovine, in the original material, and that during the course of the passage the human type, not developing in the calf, had died out, leaving the bovine type which multiplied and exerted its virulence on that animal[1]."

The experiments in which a change of type occurred must

[1] *R.C.T. Fin Rep.* 1911, " The Question of Modification," p. 32. See also pp. 14 *et seq.*

however be examined.   They concern seven strains of bacilli ;
namely H 49, T.C., H 13, A.D., H 17, Sp.B., H 21, G.B., H 60,
W.B. and H 90, I.P.

H. 49, T.C.[1]   From a young man who died of pulmonary
tuberculosis a strain of tubercle bacilli was obtained in culture
from a mesenteric gland. This strain grew on artificial media like
a bacillus of human type, but for rabbits it was virulent, and
when injected into calves in measured doses it produced disease
far more severe than that which is caused by bacilli of human
type, though distinctly less severe than that caused by equal
doses of bacilli of bovine type. On closely examining the
rabbit experiments also, a failure to attain quite to the standard of virulence of the bovine type becomes apparent; for
the disease caused in these animals, though generalized and
fatal, is stated to have been " protracted beyond the usual
limits."

A sub-strain of bacilli, obtained from the prescapular gland
of one of the calves injected with the original culture, was found
to possess the full virulence of the bovine type.

On the other hand the original strain of culture after
it had been grown in artificial culture for some months was
found to have lost its virulence for calves and rabbits, and
to behave now towards these animals exactly like a strain
of human type.

Thus the original strain, atypical, and in regard to its
virulence for ox and rabbit intermediate between the human
and bovine types, was found to be capable of modification in
two directions.   On the one hand, passage through a single
calf converted it into a typical strain of bovine type, and on
the other, growth on artificial media resolved it into a typical
strain of human type.

The readiness with which these conversions occurred
was in strong contrast with the repeated failure to modify
other strains by similar means, and caused this experience to
be regarded as the consequence of a separation of two pure
strains from an original mixture, rather than as one of true

[1] R.C.T. Int. Rep. App. vol. II, p. 836, and Fin. Rep. App. vol. III, pp. 12
and 317.

modification of a strain occupying at the outset of the investigation an intermediate position between the two types.

To test the truth of this view experiments were undertaken with artificial mixtures of bacilli of well-determined human and bovine character respectively, with the result that it was found possible, in some cases at least, to eliminate the less-readily growing bovine type from such a mixture by cultivating on glycerin media, and so to obtain the human type in pure culture, and, on the other hand, in all cases, to isolate the bovine type by passage through an animal susceptible to infection with that type but not with the other[1].

After these experiments with purposely mixed strains A. S. Griffith (who continued the investigation of virus H 49 which was begun by the present writer) succeeded in obtaining, from another branch of the original strain which had not lost its virulence for the ox, one of pure human type by growing on glycerin-agar.

Finally, the existence of two distinct types of bacilli in this strain was proved conclusively by Griffith by the isolation from single colonies of two sub-strains, one of pure human type and the other of pure bovine type[2].

H 13, A.D.[3] This strain of tubercle bacillus was obtained from a child aged four, who died of tuberculous meningitis with miliary tubercles in lungs, spleen and liver. The bronchial glands contained caseous nodules which seemed to be older than the lesions elsewhere.

An emulsion (not very rich in bacilli) was made from the bronchial glands and a portion of the spleen, and two calves

[1] Cobbett, "Experiments with Mixed Viruses," *R.C.T. Fin. Rep.* App. vol. III, p. 141. It has been shown in an earlier chapter that the addition of glycerin to culture media greatly favours the human type of tubercle bacillus, while it seldom helps the bovine type, and then but slightly, and is often distinctly detrimental to its growth. Bovine bacilli, however, become less dysgonic after being cultivated for some time, and grow accustomed to glycerin and able to make use of it. This method of separation therefore is not always successful, and indeed can only be expected to succeed with strains recently removed from the animal.

[2] A. S. Griffith, *R.C.T. Fin. Rep.* App. vol. III, p. 116.

[3] *R.C.T. Int. Rep.* App. vol. II, p. 279, and *Fin. Rep.* vol. III, pp. 14 and 314.

were injected subcutaneously with it.   These animals developed local tuberculosis only.

Direct passage of the virus from the prescapular gland of one of these calves was made into Calf 225, but without producing anything more than a local lesion.

On the other hand, an increase of virulence occurred in a parallel passage experiment.   In this case the virus was passed from one of the original calves through three guinea-pigs in succession, and from the last of these an emulsion, rich in bacilli, was made from the tuberculous lesions, and injected in large doses into two new calves.   In the case of one of these calves the injection was intraperitoneal, and caused a tuberculous peritonitis of chronic type, which had spread through the diaphragm to the thoracic glands after 87 days, but had not affected any of the great organs.   The other calf, No. 301, was injected subcutaneously with a similar dose; it became very ill; and when killed 33 days after the inoculation, was found to have developed severe general tuberculosis[1].

The virus was then passed into other calves, an emulsion of the thoracic glands of Calf 301 being injected in various doses into three more of these animals.   They developed general tuberculosis of a severity proportional to the numbers of bacilli injected in each case, and equal to that produced by comparable injections with viruses of the bovine type.   One of these, Calf 325, which received a dose estimated to contain the same numbers of tubercle bacilli as that given to Calf 301, died of acute tuberculosis in 24 days.

The virus had evidently increased in virulence by passage

[1] The contrast between these two calves is striking; both received the same dose (a rather large one containing 541 million tubercle bacilli) of the same emulsion at the same time, and if there were to be any difference in the severity of the disease in the two animals due to the difference in the mode of inoculation one would have supposed that the calf which received the intraperitoneal injection would have been the one to suffer more severely, but it was not so.   The difference in the severity of the disease in this case can only be attributed to a difference in the powers of resistance of the two calves, or to an extraordinary inequality in the distribution of the bacilli in the emulsion.

A peculiar feature in the lesions of Calf 301 was the unusually large number of bacilli present, especially in those of the peripheral lymph glands.

through the ox. For at the stage when it was injected into Calf 301, its virulence for this species fell short of the standard of the bovine type (as was shown by the fate of the animal injected intraperitoneally), but after residence in this animal it had all the virulence for the ox of the bovine type of tubercle bacillus.

A culture derived from the emulsion of the lesions of Calf 301, which had proved so exceedingly virulent for Calf 325, grew like the human type, and when again tested after it had been growing for 15 months on artificial media, was found to possess only slight virulence for the calf and moderate virulence for the rabbit. Virulence for these species must therefore have been lost during artificial cultivation, for it was undoubtedly present in the material from which the cultures were made.

On the other hand, a culture derived after further passage, namely from Calf 321, grew like bacilli of bovine type, and when tested, after $15\frac{1}{2}$ months' artificial cultivation, in measured doses, was found to possess for calves and rabbits the virulence normal to that type. The strain was then not only virulent, but its virulence was stable under artificial cultivation.

The sub-strain of bacilli from Calf 301 was, we have seen, unstable; but its virulence for the ox did not entirely disappear on artificial cultivation. It was retested by A. S. Griffith after it had been artificially cultivated for over three years. It was then still capable of causing chronic general tuberculosis in rabbits, and general, but not severe, tuberculosis in the ox; and again further passage through the calf produced a fully virulent strain of bacilli of bovine type, thus repeating the experience obtained when the original strain was passed through Calf 301 to 321.

Griffith then proceeded to investigate separate colonies grown from the sub-strain obtained from Calf 301. In order to get the bacilli well separated from one another, so as to reduce as much as possible the risk of individual colonies springing up from two kinds of bacilli if such should be present, the strain was first injected into a guinea-pig, and cultures were subsequently sown with an emulsion of the caseous sternal gland of this animal, the emulsion being spread over the surface of glycerin-serum plates with a camel's hair brush. These plates, after several weeks' incubation were "found to be covered with growth which in the main consisted of two quite distinct kinds of colonies. One kind was small and grey and not pigmented, and the other was large, yellow and wrinkled, spreading in some cases up the sides of the plate."

Strains of bacilli raised from two of the smaller colonies were found to be fully virulent for calf and rabbit; while others, raised from the larger colonies, possessed only the low degree of virulence for the rabbit characteristic of the human type.

It is then perfectly clear that in this virus at the stage when it was obtained from Calf 301, two distinct types of tubercle bacilli were present—one a perfectly typical example of the human type, and the other an equally typical example of the bovine type. And it is equally clear that the change which took place in the virus on further passage through the calf was caused by the elimination of the human type, leaving only the bovine type of bacillus present. A marked diminution in the proportion of bovine bacilli in the mixed strain seems to have taken place under artificial cultivation.

The only possible conclusion to be drawn from this investigation is that we were dealing, at a certain stage if not from the very beginning, with a mixture of the two types of bacilli.

So much is certain. But exactly when the bovine bacillus got into the virus remains obscure. Was it present in the bronchial glands of the child? did it creep in through some accident during the course of the experiment? or did it develop out of the bacilli of human type?

As to the first possibility: unfortunately, at the start no rabbits were injected, and by this omission there was lost the only chance of detecting small quantities of bovine bacilli. The calves originally injected give us no help, because the doses were too small, and we know that very small doses of bovine bacilli produce no more disease in these animals than do larger doses of human bacilli. Of slightly more significance is the small amount of disease produced in Calf 225. This animal was injected with an emulsion (containing a considerably larger number of bacilli) of the prescapular glands of one of the calves which received the original emulsion of human tissues. But, even allowing for the proportion of bovine bacilli having considerably increased by passage through a calf, the dose in this case also is small. The possibility of spontaneous tuberculosis in the guinea-pigs which intervened between Calf 129 and Calf 301 must also be considered, but the question thus raised cannot be settled.

And so we are left undecided whether there were bovine bacilli present along with human tubercle bacilli in the lesions of the child A.D. or whether they gained admission to the virus by some accidental infection.

H 16, J.H.[1] This virus was obtained from synovial membrane removed by operation from the knee joint of a man aged 38 years. The investigation of the virus was long, and involved the inoculation of a large number of animals. It would be tedious to describe it in full detail here; it may perhaps be sufficient to say that a strain of tubercle bacilli was obtained from this case which at the commencement had all the characters, both cultural and pathogenetic, of the human type, but which, after passing through a series of calves, gradually acquired high virulence for the rabbit and ox and the dysgonic characters of growth peculiar to the bovine type of tubercle bacilli.

In its transitional stage the virus (like the one already considered) was unstable in both directions; for not only did it afterwards increase further in virulence, as already mentioned, but it lost, after growing for some time on artificial media, the partial bovine virulence which it had then acquired. This loss of virulence occurred in the following manner: a culture derived from the first calf which developed general tuberculosis (Calf 273) grew like a bacillus of human type, and after cultivation for ten months on pig's serum had no longer the power to produce progressive tuberculosis in calf and rabbit. On the other hand three additional sub-strains obtained in culture after further passage through the calf grew like bovine bacilli, and retained their bovine virulence after continued cultivation.

In this series of experiments there is no absolute proof that the virus was at one time a mixture of the two types of mammalian tubercle bacilli, since no sub-strains were isolated from single colonies. But the double instability of the virus in its transitional stage was so like that which occurred in the cases of A.D. and T.C., where the presence of a mixture of bacilli was

[1] *R.C.T. Int. Rep.* App. vol. II, p. 349, and *Fin. Rep.* App. vol. III, pp. 9 and 299.

demonstrated, that it is almost certain that this was the case with J.H. also.

H 17, Sp.B.[1]   The next series of experiments in which a change of type of the bacilli occurred had for its starting point the sputum, collected during four months, from many patients in a large hospital.   This experiment was even longer and more complicated than the last; a brief summary must therefore suffice.   Four calves were repeatedly fed with this sputum, and when at length they were killed some small calcareous tuberculous foci of a retrogressive character were found in their abdominal lymph glands.   From each of these animals a separate passage experiment was started.   In three of these parallel series of inoculations no change whatever took place in the characters of the virus, though in one of them it passed through three calves in succession, in another through two calves, and in the third through two calves and two goats.

Quite otherwise was the result of the fourth passage experiment with this virus.   An emulsion made from tubercles taken from the abdominal glands of one of the calves fed with the sputum was injected into guinea-pigs, and from these other guinea-pigs were infected.   An emulsion made from the tuberculous organs of one of these latter animals was injected subcutaneously into a second calf and produced only tuberculosis at the seat of inoculation and in the neighbouring glands.

A third calf, No. 475, inoculated intravenously with an emulsion of the organs of guinea-pigs injected with the prescapular gland of the second calf, developed tuberculosis of lungs and a few tubercles elsewhere.   After this further passage through calves by means of intravenous injection consistently caused general tuberculosis.

Four cultures were obtained from different animals in this series and tested for their virulence for ox and rabbit.   The first of these, obtained from the second calf of the series, was eugonic and produced only minimal lesions in these animals. The second was obtained from a rabbit infected from the fourth calf, which it will be remembered died of general tuberculosis.   It was,

---

[1] R.C.T. Int. Rep. App. vol. II, p. 397, and Fin. Rep. App. vol. III, pp. 10 and 305.

on the whole, eugenic.   When first tested for virulence, after
ten months' artificial cultivation, it was highly virulent for
calves and rabbits ; but when again tested after 19½ months'
artificial cultivation it was found incapable of producing
progressive tuberculosis in these animals.   Thus it possessed
bovine virulence at the start ; but this was unstable, and was
lost during prolonged artificial culture.   The third and fourth
cultures, derived respectively from the sixth and eighth calves
of the series, were in every respect typical examples of the
bovine type.   Here again, as in the other passage experiments previously reviewed, the strain of bacilli when first
obtained from man had the cultural characters and low virulence for the ox which is characteristic of the human type, but
after passing through various animals including several calves
it acquired the cultural characters and virulence for the ox
which are characteristic of the bovine type.   Somewhere in the
course of this transition was obtained a sub-strain which
possessed along with the cultural characters of the human type
the virulence (more or less) of the bovine type.   This sub-
strain, like certain sub-strains in all the preceding experiments
which we have been considering, was unstable in both directions:
it lost what virulence it had for calf and rabbit after prolonged
cultivation on artificial media, and, on the other hand, increased
in virulence for these animals and lost its eugenic cultural
characters by further passage through a calf.

It can hardly be doubted that we were dealing with a
mixture, although in this case no efforts were made to cultivate strains of pure human and bovine type from single
colonies, as was done in the case of T.C. and A.D.

The question then arises where did the bovine bacillus get
in ?   Now, in attempting to answer this question, the lesions
in Calf 475 are important, inasmuch as they offer a possible
explanation.   It will be remembered that this animal was
injected intravenously with the emulsified organs of a guinea-
pig which had been infected with the virus before the latter
had shown any signs of bovine virulence.   The calf became
ill, but improved slightly towards the end, when it was killed,
88 days after inoculation.   The dose had been very large

namely 20 c.c. of emulsion estimated to contain over 100 million tubercle bacilli.

The disease was found to be confined chiefly to the lungs, where there were some interesting lesions, for "the posterior corners were found to be riddled with cavities for the last two or three inches. The larger of these were about the size of peas though somewhat irregular in shape. They had thin walls to which calcareous grains were adherent, and were filled with thick cream-coloured pus[1]." "The softening" (thus indicated) "of the caseous nodules in the lungs was unusual, not having been seen before in our experimental animals; and this raised the question whether so advanced a lesion could have been produced within the 88 days which elapsed between injection and death, and whether it might not have been a spontaneous antecedent lesion[2]." This suspicion was supported by the fact that rabbits injected at the same time and with the same emulsion as this calf developed only minimal lesions. It only remains to be said that previous to inoculation this calf had passed a tuberculin test without exciting any suspicion. In spite of this the author, who was personally responsible for all these inoculations, feels convinced that this calf was suffering from a spontaneous infection with bovine tubercle bacilli affecting the lungs, and that the increase of virulence for ox and rabbit, which occurred at this point and was shown by all animals afterwards injected with this strain, was due to the presence of bovine bacilli derived from this lesion mixed with the original strain of pure human type.

H 21, G.B.[3] This virus was obtained from a girl, aged 16, who died in hospital of heart disease. No suspicion of tuberculosis existed during life, but at the post-mortem examination a number of small tubercles were found in the bronchial glands.

An emulsion of these glands injected, necessarily in small doses, into calves and rabbits produced only minimal lesions.

From one of these calves the virus was next passed through guinea-pigs, to increase the number of bacilli, and an emulsion,

---

[1] *Loc. cit.* App. to *Int. Rep.* vol. II, p. 418.
[2] *Loc. cit.* App. to *Fin. Rep.* vol. III, p. 306.
[3] *R.C.T. Int. Rep.* vol. II, p. 515, and *Fin. Rep.* vol. III, p. 322.

rich in bacilli, made from the organs of one of these animals, was injected subcutaneously, in large doses, into two calves. One of these latter developed minimal lesions only, but the other, No. 447, was found when killed to have, in addition to small retrogressive lesions near the seat of inoculation, some tubercles in the lungs and thoracic glands, which will be described more minutely in the sequel.

Three strains of bacilli were obtained in culture, directly or indirectly, from this calf. One, obtained from a rabbit inoculated with the prescapular gland of the calf, caused, when tested in measured doses in rabbits, minimal lesions only. Another obtained from the same prescapular gland through a guinea-pig produced severe general tuberculosis in rabbits and one calf and general tuberculosis of moderate severity in another, while the third strain, derived directly from the posterior thoracic gland of the calf itself possessed the full virulence, for calves and rabbits, of the bovine type. Thus the virus present in this calf seems to have been of unequal virulence in different parts of the body, as in one of Eber's cases already considered (Case XIX, see p. 325).

Now the lesions found in Calf 447 are important, inasmuch as they offer a possible clue to the virulence manifested subsequently by this virus ; they therefore demand a closer examination.

At the seat of inoculation and in the prescapular gland nearest thereto the lesions were of the chronic type which is produced in the calf by viruses of human type. But elsewhere there was another lesion which pointed to an older and more severe infection. This was found in the posterior lobe of the right lung, and consisted of a hard calcareous nodule about as large as a blackbird's egg.

There were besides several small tubercles in each lung, and in the posterior thoracic glands, in addition to some small calcareous foci which might well have been caused by tubercle bacilli of human type, was a hard nodule, as large as a gooseberry, and full of calcareous grains, very unlike any lesion known to be produced by bacilli of that type. It was from this nodule that the fully virulent culture was obtained and there can hardly be any doubt that both it and the nodule in the lung were the result of an accidental infection[1].

Thus in each of the two investigations which we have just been considering (namely Sp.B. and G.B.) the change of type seems to have been due to spontaneous infection with tubercle bacilli of bovine type. In this way the virus came to consist of two types of bacilli—human and bovine ; and the former became eliminated by further *passage* through the calf.

The facts are no doubt open to another interpretation : an originally pure strain may have undergone a gradual modification. In so doing it is natural to suppose that it would have passed through an unstable stage, during which the transformation towards the bovine type was capable of being carried to a conclusion by further *passage* through the ox, or of being reversed by conditions such as artificial culture, which tend to encourage the eugonic rather than the dysgonic elements. Even the cultivation from single colonies of pure strains corresponding to the standard types, which was successfully carried out with the strains A.D. and T.C., might be made to fit in with this hypothesis : for it might plausibly be argued that during the transitional period certain individual bacilli would have changed their type, while others would still have remained in their original condition. This hypothesis then

---

[1] In view of the importance of these lesions it may be of interest to show the impression produced at the time of their discovery, that is to say before any hint had been received that the virus was about to manifest bovine virulence. In describing the post-mortem examination the following words were written. " The larger lesion in the lung of Calf 447 was obviously an old one, it was quite unexpected, and unlike anything found in a similar case before. It might be thought possibly due to an independent infection, but the original tuberculin test was satisfactory" (*loc. cit. Fin. Rep.*). Further experience, however, has since led the writer of the above to think that a negative tuberculin test is not invariably to be relied upon*.

The contrast in virulence of the two sub-strains obtained in culture indirectly from the prescapular gland of this calf is difficult to interpret. It is possible however that bovine tubercle bacilli from the (spontaneous) pulmonary lesion wandered in small numbers through the blood stream and reached the lesion in the prescapular gland caused by the human bacilli injected; and that of the two cultures raised indirectly from this gland (through a rabbit and a guinea-pig respectively) the one lost the trace of bovine bacilli in culture while the other retained it.

* Report on Tuberculin Tests, *R.C.T. Fin. Rep.* App. Supplementary Volume, p. 17.

appears to be tenable. But, to the writer at least, the balance of probability seems to lean the other way ; and, as we shall see, repetition of the experiments with the same original viruses as well as with others, under more rigorous conditions, failed to produce any modification.

Two further cases which yielded atypical viruses demand attention. In these there was definite evidence of the co-existence of bacilli of different virulence in the lesions of the human subject. From each of these viruses a perfectly typical strain of bovine bacilli was readily obtained by passage through animals.

These viruses came from cases known as H 60, W.B.[1] and H 90, I.P.[2] W.B., aged four years and seven months, died of general miliary tuberculosis and meningitis. " Cultures from the meninges, lungs and mesenteric glands of the child were only slightly virulent for calves and rabbits, and grew luxuriantly on artificial media." They were, therefore, typical examples of the human type. But a culture derived from a bronchial gland was atypical, for, while it grew luxuriantly on artificial media its virulence for calves and rabbits corresponded to that of a bovine tubercle bacillus

I.P. was a man aged 70, who died of pneumonia, and in whose body a tuberculous retroperitoneal gland was found after death. A culture derived from this gland " grew luxuriantly on artificial media, like the human tubercle bacillus ; and produced, when inoculated into calves, slowly progressing tuberculosis not severe and not fatal within the period of observation, and in rabbits progressive tuberculosis not so quickly fatal as after the inoculation of equivalent doses of bovine tubercle bacilli."

These two atypical strains, then, possessed the cultural characters of the human type. One possessed practically the full virulence of the bovine type, and the other a virulence for calves and rabbits which fell a little short of this, but was clearly above that of the human type. Both acquired the cultural characters of the bovine type, and the latter recovered the full virulence of that type, on passage through the ox.

From single colonies of the original strain, in each case, several sub-strains were cultivated by A. S. Griffith. Some of

---

[1] R.C.T. Fin. Rep. App. vol. I, p. 109.   [2] Ibid. p. 134, and vol. III, p. 18.

these proved to be typical bovine, and others typical human bacilli.

It might be argued that these two strains were originally bovine, and were caught in process of transition as they were about to acquire the characters of the human type in consequence of residence in man ; and that they had arrived at a stage when their newly acquired human characters were still unstable, and their old bovine characters still capable of being restored by a return to the old (bovine) environment. If so it must be admitted that some individual bacilli had become completely changed while others had remained entirely unaltered by residence in man, for, as we have seen, Griffith again succeeded in each of these cases, as he had done before in the cases of T.C. and A.D. in cultivating from single colonies two sub-strains, one exactly resembling the human type, and the other equally representative of the bovine type[1]. It cannot be doubted then that the atypical character of the original strains was caused by a mixture of bacilli of two types ; but here our certitude

[1] The following experiments are quoted from Griffith's Report as examples of his method of analysis by single colonies.

Culture derived from the bronchial gland of the child W.B.
(through a guinea-pig).

Sub-strain from colony No. 1

Animal	Method	Dose	Result
Calf 1481	Subcut.	50 mg.	Well when killed 90 days later. Local and minimal lesions
Rabbit 1947	,,	10 mg.	Killed after 161 days. Local lesion, slight tuberculosis of lungs and kidneys
Rabbit 1947	Intrav.	0·1 mg.	Killed after 128 days. Tuberculosis of lungs and kidneys (slight)

Inference : Virulence for calf and rabbit low, like that of the human type.

Sub-strain from colony No. 5

Animal	Method	Dose	Result
Calf 1425	Subcut.	50 mg.	Dying when killed 45 days later. General tuberculosis
Rabbit 1948	,,	10 mg.	Died 49 days. General tuberculosis (not severe)
Rabbit 1606	Intrav.	0·01 mg.	Died 67 days. General tuberculosis

Inference : Virulence for calf and rabbit high, like that of the bovine type.
(*R.C.T. Fin. Rep.* App. vol. III, p 44.)

ends, for we have no means of knowing whether this was due
to a double infection of the patient in each case, or to the
transformation in an originally pure strain of certain bacilli
only, while other bacilli remained unaltered.

If this latter hypothesis be accepted it will have to be
admitted that in the case of W.B. the transition from bovine
to human had been complete in the lungs, meninges, and mesenteric glands, while in the bronchial glands alone—possibly the
primary seat of the disease—some of the bacilli still retained
their bovine characters unaltered.

In consequence of the suspicious nature of certain of the
lesions found in Calves 475 (Sp.B) and 447 (G.B.) it was felt
that none of the modification experiments of the Commission
hitherto recorded could be entirely trusted as revealing a transformation of type, and it was thought that fresh experiments
ought to be undertaken under more rigorous conditions.

It must now be explained in what way the conditions under
which the experiments which we have been considering were
made were capable of improvement. The investigations were
carried out in the experimental station at Blythwood Farm,
Stansted, Essex, generously lent to the Commission (along with
Walpole Farm, where viruses of animal origin were investigated)
by Sir James, now Lord, Blyth. It must be understood that the
general conditions were extremely good, that no expense or care
was spared in providing and caring for the animals, and that at
Blythwood only viruses of human origin were allowed to be
investigated. But, inasmuch as some cases of human tuberculosis proved to be caused by the bovine type of bacillus,
there were, necessarily, always present on the premises many
animals infected with this type of micro-organism. If in all
cases cultures had first been grown, and the character of their
growth ascertained before any animals had been injected it
might perhaps have been possible to have separated entirely the
animals injected with bacilli of human from those injected with
bacilli of bovine type ; but at the time when these investigations
were begun much had to be learnt ; and as a matter of fact
during the earlier period of the work, including the time when
most of the modification experiments which we have been

considering were begun, viruses of human origin were injected *directly* into calves and other animals without preliminary cultivation, and no segregation was then possible, because at the time when the primary injections were made not the slightest indication of the nature of the viruses had as yet been revealed. Apart from this every possible precaution was taken. The calves and other of the larger animals infected with each virus were kept in separate houses, each with its own entrance, though a number were under a common roof. The guinea-pigs and rabbits had their separate cages. But it was impossible to secure complete isolation, because the men had to go from house to house and from cage to cage to feed the animals and to clean out their stalls, etc. Moreover, temperatures had to be taken and other observations made ; nor was it possible to exclude flies (stomoxys) of which there were many in summer.

Now these conditions, excellent though they were on the whole, and sufficiently rigorous for the determination of the primary virulence of viruses, were, as we now think, not nearly strict enough for experiments whose object was to settle the vexed question of stability of type of tubercle bacilli in the animal body.

A little consideration will show that the risk that spontaneous infection will interfere with the *primary determination* of the type of a given virus in a well-regulated experimental station is small. For neither calf, goat, guinea-pig or rabbit is particularly liable to spontaneous tuberculosis, and in the case of the calf, at least, we know that infections with small quantities of bacilli do not lead to progressive tuberculosis within the time during which it is usual to keep the animals under observation.

Quite otherwise, however, is it with passage experiments which necessarily extend over considerable periods of time, and involve the inoculation of a large number of animals each with the tuberculous tissues of another, or with cultures derived from them. There is *then* good reason to think that a spontaneous infection with bovine bacilli occurring in one of the calves in a series through which a virus of human type is being passed will (even if it be of a minimal kind, and one which might never have caused any trouble in the animal which received it) lead nevertheless, on further passage through these animals being made, to an entire replacement in the virus of the human type of bacillus with one of bovine type. This, as was said before, has actually been borne out by direct experiments with mixtures of human and bovine bacilli.

With these considerations in mind a new series of experiments was undertaken. There was in an outlying meadow, a quarter of a mile from the buildings which housed the experimental animals, a new animal house which had been reserved as an isolation hospital for such beasts as might develop some intercurrent disorder possibly of an infectious nature, but which had never been used for this or, indeed, for any other purpose. It was in this house that the new series of passage experiments was carried out, and a special staff of farm servants was told off, whose sole duty was to look after the animals involved in them ; and all communication between this building and the rest of the experimental station was reduced to a minimum.

The New Series of Passage Experiments carried out by the Royal Commission. In the meantime one had learnt that tubercle bacilli of human type might cause severe and even fatal disease in the calf if injected intravenously and in large doses, and might in this way be got even to multiply in the body of this animal. The intravenous method (previously used in the passage experiments with Sp.B.) seemed therefore to offer very favourable conditions for giving human tubercle bacilli an opportunity of adapting themselves to the conditions of life in the body of the calf, and of transforming themselves, if they were able, into bacilli of bovine type.

Several experiments[1] were now made in this way and under the improved conditions, some with new viruses, others with the original strains of some of the viruses which in the older experiments had undergone a change of type. Great difficulty however was experienced in keeping up the passage by direct inoculation through a series of calves.

Eight passage experiments in all were attempted by the present writer, using the method described above, but in several it proved to be impossible to carry the virus through more than one calf, owing to paucity of tuberculous material ; and it was found necessary to use very large doses capable of killing rapidly (in a few weeks), or run the risk of losing the virus altogether.

Nevertheless, one virus was successfully passed through four calves in direct succession, during a period of 87 days ; two others were passed, each through three calves, in 153 and 104 days respectively; while a fourth was passed through two

[1] "Further Passage Experiments." *R.C.T. Fin. Rep.* App. vol. III, p. 327.

calves in 102 days. No modification of virulence occurred in any of them. In still another experiment subcutaneous inoculation was used, and the virus passed through three calves in direct succession in 293 days. Again there was no change in the characters of the bacilli.

After this the work was continued by A. S. Griffith on a more extensive scale[1]. Realizing the risk of the strain dying out when passed directly from calf to calf, and with the object of giving a sufficiently large dose of bacilli to each calf to ensure the production of tuberculous lesions, Griffith adopted the expedient of inoculating a guinea-pig whenever the bacilli in the calf were so scanty that there appeared to be danger of losing the strain; and in such cases it was with the tuberculous organs of this guinea-pig that the next calf in the series was injected. These experiments were carried out, for the most part, under the improved conditions described above.

Six different strains of tubercle bacilli of human type were passed each through a series of calves ; and in the majority of experiments two parallel lines of experiments were carried out with each strain in order to have a control should any modification of type occur in one of the lines.

The number of calves used in each line varied from two to seven, and the total duration of residence of the bacilli in bovine tissues from 247 to 512 days.

A culture was raised from the last calf of each series, and its properties were compared with those of the original culture. *In no case was there any alteration in the cultural characters of the bacillus or of its virulence for calves and rabbits.*

II. *Passage of Tubercle Bacilli of Human Type through the Rabbit and other small Animals.*

The passage of tubercle bacilli of human type through the rabbit was tried in the Gesundheitsamt without any increase of virulence for this animal being observed. L. Rabinowitsch[2]

---

[1] " Modification Experiments with Human Tubercle Bacilli." *R.C.T.* *Fin. Rep.* App. vol. I, p. 55.

[2] *Tuberkulose des Menschen und der Tiere : Arbeiten aus dem Pathologischen Institut zu Berlin,* 1906. A. Hirschwald, Berlin Sonderabdruck, p. 24.

also made similar experiments without change of character, as Vagedes and Th. Smith had done before.

Some similar experiments were made by the writer in 1904–6 for the Royal Commission[1]. The transference was made directly from rabbit to rabbit by means of emulsions of tuberculous organs. Twelve different viruses were used. In one case the virus passed through five rabbits and the experiment lasted 21 months. In others it passed through two to four rabbits, the total duration of residence in the rabbit in several of the experiments varying from one to two years. In one case (H 22, F.W.) the experiment ended with the production of "chronic progressive tuberculosis with cavities in the lungs" 205 days after injection of the rabbit (R 260). The death of this animal occurred unfortunately in the absence of the investigator, and the virus could not be tested further.

In another experiment one (R 640) of two rabbits injected with the same material developed "chronic progressive tuberculosis," and died 145 days after injection. Thus a presumption of an increase of virulence for the species was raised; but the sequel proved that this indicated no increase in virulence, but was only an abnormally severe result in a susceptible individual; for the injection of the emulsified pulmonary lesions of this animal into another produced only the chronic trivial disease which is characteristic of infection of this species with the human type of bacillus. In no other instance was severe tuberculosis produced.

A. S. Griffith also made a similar passage experiment in the rabbit extending over a year and four months without any change occurring in the virus[2]. And he made also a very extended passage in the rat[3] extending over four years, in the course of which a virus of human type passed through no less than eight of these animals in direct succession without change.

Finally he reported on several strains of human type recovered after long residence each in a single animal. In one case the bacilli had lived for 529 days in a cow, in another for 378 days in a pig, while in a third they had lived for 413 days

---

[1] R.C.T. Fin. Rep. App. vol. III, pp. 329, 331.
[2] Ibid. vol. I, p. 71.   [3] Ibid. vol. I, p. 72.

in a dog, and in a fourth for 454 days in a rat. In each of these cases the strain of bacilli ultimately recovered in culture was adequately tested and found to have maintained the characters of the human type entirely unaltered[1].

Conclusions.

The large array of " passage " experiments by various authors in which no alteration of type occurred, extending as some of them did over considerable periods of time (two or more years) and involving often a number of animals in succession, show quite conclusively that tubercle bacilli of human type do not necessarily become changed into bacilli of bovine type merely because of a change of host from man to ox or some other animal. Some changes of type have occurred in other experiments, but they have been exceptional.

It may be, however, that every strain of human type is not to be thus converted, but only those whose special characters have been recently acquired by residence in man. But on the other hand we have to remember the special dangers and pitfalls of such investigations, especially the possibility of the occurrence of spontaneous tuberculosis in some of the animals employed, or of two types of bacilli in the original virus investigated.

When one recalls the fact that changes of type have occurred not only in the investigations of those who believe in mutability of type, such as Eber, and Dammann and Müssemeier, but equally in the experiments of those who believe in stability, such as the Germans who worked in the Gesundheitsamt, and Griffith and the writer who were responsible for the investigations of the Royal Commission, it must be obvious that if some of the changes of type which have occurred are here attributed to spontaneous infections in experimental animals the writer is not imputing carelessness to others or casting blame which he does not himself equally share. He is convinced that in some of his own experiments change of type was due to spontaneous infection, and he is naturally inclined to believe that some of the results of other investigators which seem to be similar to his own were due to the same cause.

[1] *R.C.T. Fin. Rep.* App. vol. III, p. 72.

It seems indeed very improbable that accidental infections should not sometimes occur among the experimental animals, kept as they almost necessarily are not far removed from others suffering from bovine tuberculosis.   Some of the results then, we hold, have been due to spontaneous infections.

Other changes of type which have occurred in passage experiments may reasonably be attributed to an admixture of bovine bacilli with the strain of bacilli of human type primarily responsible for disease in the human patient from which the experiment started.   As we have seen, mixed infections with human and bovine tubercle bacilli undoubtedly occur in man, and not very unfrequently, and it seems not unlikely that mixed infections with a relatively minute proportion of bovine bacilli—so small as to easily escape notice in primary investigations of virulence—may be commoner than is usually supposed.

That such admixture would satisfactorily account for all the phenomena of a successful passage experiment has been shown by similar experiments carried out with purposely mixed viruses.

CHAPTER XVII

THE STABILITY OF TYPE OF TUBERCLE BACILLI IN THE ANIMAL BODY (continued)

THE QUESTION OF MODIFICATION OF BOVINE TUBERCLE BACILLI IN MAN, THE CHIMPANZEE AND OTHER ANIMALS.

Modification Experiments with Tubercle Bacilli of Bovine Type.
Are Tubercle Bacilli of Bovine Type derived from Man Identical in every respect with those derived from the Ox?
Comparison of Strains of Bovine Type derived from the Pig and the Horse with those derived from the Ox.

The question under consideration in the preceding chapter was whether it is possible to convert the *human* type of tubercle bacillus into the *bovine* by causing it to live in the ox or other animals; in the present chapter we have to consider the

possibility of a change in the opposite direction taking place—
namely from the *bovine* to the *human* type—when a bacillus of
the former type is passed through the chimpanzee or other
animals, or takes up its residence in man.

Modification Experiments with Tubercle Bacilli of Bovine Type.

Many passage experiments with bovine tubercle bacilli were
made for the Royal Commission by A. S. and F. Griffith (1907)[1]
in various species of monkey (including *Macacus rhesus*) several
kinds of baboon and the chimpanzee.   Some experiments were
made also in dogs, one of the very few animals, besides the
monkey, which is known to suffer naturally from tuberculosis
caused by tubercle bacilli of human type.   The results of these
experiments were, on the whole, negative.   In the very great
majority there was no change either in the cultural or pathogenic characters of the various strains of bacilli after residence
more or less prolonged in these animals.   But there were some
exceptions which will be described in detail presently.

The experiments with the chimpanzee are of special interest,
because it seems that, if the bovine tubercle bacillus is capable
of being transformed into the human bacillus by living in man,
a change in the same direction is more likely to occur in one of
the higher apes than in any other species of animal.

In one of these experiments a bovine virus passed through
five chimpanzees in succession, during a period of 542 days,
without showing the slightest tendency to approximate to the
human type ; and in another experiment a similar virus passed
through two chimpanzees in 198 days without undergoing any
change[2].

In the experiments with baboons and smaller monkeys the
period of residence of each strain in the bodies of these
animals varied from 198 to 375 days.   In all these experiments the bacilli when ultimately recovered were tested for

---

[1] A. S. Griffith and F. Griffith.   *R.C.T. Int. Rep.* App. vol. III, p. 87 (for
summary and conclusions see p. 92), continued by F. Griffith in the *Fin. Rep.*
App. vol. IV, p. 383.

[2] *Ibid. Int. Rep.* App. vol. III, p. 94.   *Fin. Rep.* vol. IV, pp. 390 and
424 *et seq.*

virulence on the rabbit and their cultural characters carefully re-determined. Again the results were negative, with the exception that in one instance there was some increase in the luxuriance of growth.

This exception occurred in an experiment with baboons. The strain of bacilli had passed through two of these animals in 198 days; originally it was one of the most dysgonic of the bovine type, but after the passage it grew more luxuriantly "like a bovine culture which had been modified by repeated subcultivation on glycerin media"; the virulence for rabbits however remained unaltered[1].

More important exceptions to the rule stated above occurred in the experiments made on the dog[2]. These were five in number. In two there was no change in the characters of the bacilli after passage; in one there was an increase in luxuriance of growth without change of virulence for the rabbit; and in two there was a decided change both in character of growth and in virulence. The details of these two latter experiments were as follows :

Dog No. 18[3] was fed with an emulsion made from the organs of two guinea-pigs infected with tubercle bacilli of bovine type. It was killed 135 days later, when it was found to have tuberculosis of two mesenteric glands, and a few doubtful tubercles in the lungs. A culture derived from one of the glands grew "more luxuriantly than any bovine virus" and "was not virulent for rabbits."

Dog No. 50[4] was fed with 1 mg. of bacilli from a culture of bovine tubercle bacilli. Killed 111 days later, it showed no disease of the alimentary tract or glands connected with it, but there was consolidation and a small cavity in the cephalic lobe of one lung.

A strain derived from a guinea-pig injected with this lung grew "like slightly virulent bacilli of human origin" and, injected subcutaneously into a calf in a dose of 50 mg., produced minimal lesions. A second calf, inoculated subcutaneously with an emulsion of the prescapular glands of the first calf, developed only a local lesion.

Here then, in each of these instances the change—if indeed there had been a change and not a substitution—was complete. The new virus had all the characters of the human type, and, in the second of these experiments the human characters were stable, that is to say they were not changed by passage through the calf.

[1] R.C.T. Int. Rep. App. vol. III, p. 90. Baboon passage Virus B 1.
[2] Ibid. p. 91.
[3] Ibid. vol. III, p. 104.
[4] Ibid. pp. 106 and 142.

The results of these two experiments, as A. S. and F. Griffith themselves remark, may be explained on one or other of two hypotheses : either the strain of bacilli used became modified, or the lesions from which the eugonic cultures without virulence for calves were obtained were not caused by the bacilli introduced into the animals.

In order to determine which of these explanations was the correct one new experiments were carried out, the original virus previously used for Dog 18 being passed through two new series of dogs, and that previously used for Dog 50 through one series.

The period of residence in the dog in these latter experiments amounted to 206, 237 and 185 days respectively, while in the earlier experiments in which a change of type occurred it was only 135 and 111 days. " The results of these newer experiments were negative "; no change of type occurred, " the cultures isolated from the last animal in each series showing not the least change in cultural characters or virulence."

The authors provisionally concluded that "the bovine tubercle bacillus is very retentive of its special cultural characters and high virulence[1]." But they were not entirely satisfied until another and more conclusive series of experiments had been carried out.

For the report dealing with these latter experiments F. Griffith was alone responsible, his brother meanwhile having been transferred to Blythwood farm, where only viruses of human origin were investigated. Five new passage experiments through dogs were made with viruses of bovine type. The number of animals used in each series varied from three to ten, and the total period of residence in the canine body in each series lasted from 320 to 1222 days. In spite of this long period of residence, amounting in one case to nearly three and a half years, these experiments yielded no further evidence of modification, the final culture in each case being exactly like the original, both in character of growth and in virulence[2].

It may, therefore, fairly be concluded that bovine tubercle bacilli do not become converted into human tubercle bacilli in

[1] loc. cit. Int. Rep. vol. III, p. 92.
[2] loc. cit. Fin. Rep. vol. IV, p. 389.

the body of the dog. Indeed it would be a very remarkable and surprising thing if they did so[1]. Perhaps the chief interest of these experiments lies in the fact that they show that the same kind of evidence for a change of type on *passage* can be obtained when the bovine bacillus is passed through the dog, where the conversion (into the human type) would seem very improbable, as occurs in the much more probable case where the human bacillus is passed through the ox.

Are Tubercle Bacilli of Bovine Type which are derived from Man Identical in every respect with those derived from the Ox?

If the characters of tubercle bacilli which distinguish the types from one another are unstable, and if a transformation of type tends to occur when bacilli of one type are transferred to a new species of host such as is commonly infected by another type of bacillus, then one might reasonably expect that some at least of the strains of bovine type which are recovered from cases of human tuberculosis would show a departure from the standard characters of that type, and would be somewhat more luxuriant in growth on artificial media, and slightly less virulent for calf and rabbit when injected than strains of bovine type derived from the ox itself. We have seen hitherto that the balance of experimental evidence is distinctly against a *complete* change of type occurring with a change of host, such as is defined above, within the period of the few years which can be covered by laboratory experiments; but it is conceivable that modification of type may take place slowly—so slowly indeed that it is difficult to produce even in the most prolonged passage experiments of the laboratory. Some human cases of tuberculosis are however of much longer duration than any of the laboratory experiments which we have been considering, and we might reasonably expect to find in such of these as were caused originally by bovine bacilli some strains which, while exhibiting in the main the characters of the bovine type, show some departure from the standard of that type and some degree of approximation to the human

---

[1] The dog is susceptible to spontaneous infection with bovine as well as with human tubercle bacilli (see pp. 486 *et seq.*).

type. The question then arises : Do such transitional strains in man occur ?

Let us assume that transformation of type from bovine to human takes place in man ; it is conceivable that the characters which serve to distinguish the bovine type, namely (*a*) dysgonic growth and (*b*) high virulence for ox and rabbit, might disappear *pari passu,* or again it is possible that one of these characters might prove less stable than the other, and be the first to change. We have already considered the cases of atypical strains of human origin which are at once eugonic, like the human type, but show a virulence for ox and rabbit which is only somewhat less than that of the bovine type (such as T.C. and W.B. pp. 330 and 341), and we have seen reason for believing that these are mixtures of the two types. We have now to consider certain strains which possess the dysgonic characters of the bovine type together with low virulence for those animals which are resistant to the human type.

A. *Strains of tubercle bacilli from man, of bovine type, the virulence of which, however, is more or less decidedly below the standard of that type.* It has already been mentioned that strains of tubercle bacilli obviously in the main of bovine type but possessing a low degree of virulence for animals have been discovered, not only among such strains as have been grown in artificial cultivation for long periods, but among others also which have recently been isolated from the bodies of men and animals. These latter must now be discussed more fully.

In 1906 Kleine[1] published an investigation of seven strains of tubercle bacilli obtained from five cases of *Tuberculosis verrucosa cutis* in butchers. The material, taken from warts on the hands, was inoculated into guinea-pigs, and from these animals cultures were obtained and tested on calves. The cultures all grew feebly and with extraordinary slowness, and were very difficult to establish on glycerin-broth. Microscopically examined, the bacilli appeared short and thick. Four of the cultures injected subcutaneously in 50 milligramme doses caused general tuberculosis in calves and were considered by

[1] Kleine, *Zeitschf. f. Hygiene*, vol. LII, p. 495.

XVII] DYSGONIC BACILLI OF LOW VIRULENCE 355

Kleine to be typical members of the bovine type. Another caused general tuberculosis indeed, but of a sub-acute type. The other two produced in these animals lesions which did not extend beyond the glands nearest to the seat of inoculation, and were therefore considered to be attenuated. The falling off of the virulence of these strains below the standard of the bovine type showed no relation to the duration of the disease in the patients, and from one case in which the warts had existed for eight years a culture was raised which was as virulent as any of the others.

The experiments are not very satisfactory, one calf only having been used for each culture, and no rabbits inoculated. Moreover, the age of the cultures actually used for inoculation is not given, and it is probable that they were not very young ones, for it is stated that they grew extraordinarily slowly, and were used " as soon as a sufficient quantity of bacilli was present."

The existence of attenuated strains of bovine bacilli was confirmed and greatly extended by A. S. Griffith. This observer obtained from man many dysgonic, and therefore presumably bovine, strains of tubercle bacilli, the virulence of which for ox and rabbit fell short, and often considerably short, of the standard of virulence of the bovine type. All these strains came from cases of lupus, that is (as in Kleine's cases also) from situations on the surface of the body more or less exposed to light. These strains have already been mentioned (p. 214), and we shall have to consider them again at greater length in Chapter XXV when we are dealing with the types of bacilli found in lupus. In the present connection, therefore, their description must be brief, and it must suffice to say that they cannot be regarded as transitional—that is to say as strains, originally bovine, which were gradually becoming converted into human strains by residence in the human body—for the following reasons : 1. Unlike tubercle bacilli of human type they had low virulence, not for the ox and rabbit only, but for guinea-pig and monkey also. Now bacilli of human type are highly virulent for these animals; these strains therefore must be regarded as attenuated, rather than transformed. 2. Other

strains also were obtained from cases of lupus equally attenuated with these but possessing the eugonic characters of the
human type, the evidence of their attenuation being that they
possessed less than the normal virulence for monkeys and
guinea-pigs, animals very susceptible of infection with bacilli of
that type. It would seem therefore that residence in the
human skin is capable of attenuating tubercle bacilli no matter
to which type they belong.

Weber and Steffenhagen (1912) obtained a strain of bovine
type showing some evidence of slight attenuation from the
metacarpal bone of a child who was suffering from tuberculosis
which had existed some years in that situation and which had
undergone various kinds of treatment[1] (see p. 629).

Eastwood and F. Griffith[2] reported two strains of tubercle
bacilli which were distinctly dysgonic in their cultural characters,
but which possessed only low virulence for the rabbit. One of
them seems to have been not fully virulent for the guinea-pig
also.

These authors have quite recently described ten additional
strains of this kind from human cases of bone and joint
tuberculosis. A. S. Griffith also has met with ten strains of
a similar kind. Whether these should be regarded as dysgonic
varieties of the human type or attenuated representatives of
the bovine type is as yet uncertain; but the fact that their
peculiar low virulence is a stable feature and unalterable on
passage through rabbits is against the possibility of regarding
them as in a state of transition from the bovine to the
human type; moreover their nearest analogues seem to be
certain strains derived from the horse and pig (see pp. 403,
404 and 470).

B. *Strains of tubercle bacilli from man, of bovine type, and
possessing approximately the virulence of that type.* Having now
dealt with those strains of bacilli of human origin which belong
apparently to the bovine type and are dysgonic, but show a
more or less decided departure from the normal standard of

---

[1] *Tub. Arbeit. a. d. Kaiserl. Gesundheitsamte,* Heft 11, p. 1.
[2] *Rep. to the Loc. Govt. Board,* 1914, N.S. No. 88, pp. 74, 76. See *postea,*
p. 604.

virulence of that type, let us turn to the examination of those human strains of bovine type—the vast majority—which are generally considered to be ordinary examples of the type, and let us see whether when examined closely they exhibit precisely those cultural characters and that degree of virulence for ox and rabbit which are to be found in strains of bovine type derived from the ox itself.

As to the first point it may be stated at once that no difference in cultural characters was detected between these strains and those of bovine origin by any of the various observers who worked for the Royal Commission. Eastwood[1] who made a comparison of the cultural characters of a large number of strains of all kinds derived from man and the ox arranged them, according to their luxuriance of growth, into five grades. Into the first three of these grades fell all those of bovine origin and all those of human origin which were virulent for calves and rabbits; that is to say all the strains of bovine type irrespective of origin. In each of these three grades strains derived from man may be found alongside those derived from the ox itself. In other words strains which possessed bovine virulence were equally dysgonic whether they came from their true host, the ox, or their new and unaccustomed host, man[2].

For the purpose of close comparison of the virulence for the ox of strains of tubercle bacilli of bovine type derived from man with those of the same type from the ox itself, we possess among the records of the Royal Commission a large number of results of injecting calves with carefully measured doses of tubercle bacilli. These have already been utilized in treating of the influence of individual susceptibility and of dosage on the results of experimental infection in Chapter XIII and the way in which the following diagram is compiled is there

---

[1] *R.C.T. Int. Rep.* App. vol. IV, p. 234.

[2] It ought perhaps in fairness to be pointed out that into Eastwood's most dysgonic grade No. 1 fell ten human and 17 bovine strains; in grade No. 2 there were four human and eight bovine strains; while in his least dysgonic grade No. 3 there were eight human and four bovine strains. This increased proportion of viruses of human origin in the third grade is pointed out for what it is worth. It may perhaps show a slight tendency to increasing eugony when bovine bacilli take to living in man.

described.   But it may perhaps be permissible to redirect attention here to the following points :

Every care was taken at the time the experiments were made to render them as strictly comparable with one another as possible. The cultures injected were all of the same age, and grown on the same medium (plain ox serum). The calves were all of one breed (Jersey), and as nearly as possible of the same age and weight.

The disease was for the most part allowed to run its natural course, or the animals were killed only when moribund. For this reason, as we have argued before, the duration of the disease in these animals is a fair measure of its severity, and, if we take a sufficient number of animals to neutralize differences of individual susceptibility, a measure also of the virulence of the strains of bacilli which caused the fatal issues.

In a minority of cases the disease was less severe, and had not commenced to threaten life within a period of three months from the injection, at the end of which time the animal was killed.

In compiling the following diagram (p. 364) experiments with certain viruses, as was stated before, have been omitted. These include the atypical viruses, already considered fully, namely those which underwent modification and concerning which evidence has been given that they were probably mixtures of the two types, and all those derived from lupus because many of them showed a more or less definite attenuation of virulence.

There remain experiments on 156 calves subcutaneously injected with strains of tubercle bacilli of clearly recognized bovine type.   105 of these animals received doses of 50 milligrammes, and 51 received doses of 10 milligrammes of bacilli.

Of the 48 strains of tubercle bacilli tested in this way 19 came from man and 18 from the ox.   The remainder came from the pig and from the horse, and will be considered in a subsequent section.

Comparison of the Virulence for Calves of Strains of Tubercle Bacilli of Bovine Type derived from Man with others of the same Type derived from the Ox.

Let us first consider the 50 milligramme injections, and compare the severity of the result caused by viruses of bovine type and human origin with those of the same type but of bovine origin. Very little difference is apparent. The subcutaneous injection of tubercle bacilli of this type obtained from young cultures in this dose is almost invariably fatal to young Jersey calves within three months, whether the bacilli are derived from man or the ox.

TABLE XV.   *Analysis of* 128 *subcutaneous injections.*

Dose	Origin of strains	No. of strains tested	No. of calves inoculated	No. of calves which died	Range of duration of disease when fatal	Average duration of disease	No. of calves which survived	Percentage which survived
50 mg.	Man	19	47	43	19–63 days	37·0	4	8·5
	Ox	18	34	33	18–76 ,,	35·9	1	2·9
10 mg.	Man	13	35	25	31–72 ,,	45·6	10	28·6
	Ox	5	12	8	33–53 ,,	41·3	4	33·3

Forty-seven calves were injected with this dose of bacilli of human origin. Of these four survived for three months. Thirty-four calves were injected with the same dose of bacilli of bovine origin, and of these only one[1] failed to develop a rapidly fatal tuberculosis. These five calves which failed to succumb to acute tuberculosis undoubtedly owed their escape to the possession of abnormal powers of resistance, for other calves injected with the same strains of bacilli died in the usual time. They were therefore exceptional individuals. It would not be surprising if such were found to be unequally distributed between the two groups of animals injected with viruses of bovine and human origin respectively, therefore one must be cautious in drawing conclusions as to the comparative virulence of the two groups of viruses from the larger proportion of survivals in the one group (8·5 %) than in the other (2·9 %).

Let us see whether this is supported by other evidence. Among the 43 calves which died after receiving subcutaneous injections of 50 mg. of bacilli of bovine type derived from man the duration of the disease varied from 19 to 63 days, while among the 33 calves which died after receiving similar injections of bacilli of bovine type derived from the ox the duration of the disease varied from 18 to 76 days. The average duration of disease was in the case of the human group 37 days, and in

---

[1] This animal was actually killed two months after inoculation; but it was then in good general condition, and on post-mortem examination was found to have tuberculous lesions of a sub-acute type. A. S. Griffith who made the examination had no doubt that it would have survived for at least three months if it had been allowed to do so. (*R.C.T. Int. Rep.* App. vol. I, p. 222.)

the case of the bovine group nearly 36 days.   This difference
is exceedingly small, and taken by itself negligible.

Turning to the smaller number of 10 milligramme injections
we find the proportion of surviving calves actually higher in
the group of viruses of bovine origin (namely 4 out of 12 =
33·3 %) than in the group of viruses of human origin (namely
10 out of 35 = 28·6 %).   But of those which died the average
duration of disease was, in the human group 45·6 days, and in
the bovine group 41·3 days[1].

On the whole then the evidence is very strong that strains
of tubercle bacilli of bovine type but of human origin (certain
lupus strains, and a few others which seem to have been mixtures
of the two types excepted) possess very nearly the same
virulence for the calf as that found in strains of bovine origin.

Some difference does indeed seem to exist, if the number
of observations is sufficient to justify a conclusion, but it is so
small that it requires delicate analysis of a carefully prepared
series of experiments to put it in evidence.

Such difference as has come to light then is in favour of
the view that bovine tubercle bacilli when they live in human
tissues slowly lose a little of their virulence for the ox.   Small
as is this loss within the period of the infections which came
to examination[2], it may nevertheless point to an adaptation to
the new host, but it lends no support whatever to the alleged

[1] Compare also similar experiments in the guinea-pig, p. 437 f.

[2] It cannot be stated precisely what the duration of infection in these
cases was; but it could not have been long seeing that, with two exceptions,
they were all children aged from thirteen months to eight years.   The two were
cases of phthisis, aged 21 and 31 years respectively (H 127 and H 128).   The
bacilli obtained from the latter of these produced the average effect on four
calves inoculated with it; while that from the former killed three calves out
of four in the usual time, but failed to produce a fatal effect on another within
three months.   In addition to this one the strains which produced least effect
on the calves were as follows: H 10, tuberculous peritonitis in a child of one
year and nine months; H 69, tuberculous meningitis in a child of two; and
H 89, general tuberculosis in a child of four.   Cases are on record in which
disease caused by the bovine tubercle bacillus has existed for several years
in the human body without the microbe losing the special characters which
mark the bovine type.   At the Gesundheitsamt a case (already referred to)
of tuberculosis in a metacarpal bone has been under investigation for some
years, and five separate strains of bacilli obtained from this case on different
occasions have been studied.   Small fluctuations in virulence did indeed

instances of experimental modification, for, as we have seen, in many of them a complete change of type (in this case from human to bovine) is claimed to have occurred within a few months. Such change as we find a mere hint of in the series of injections which we are now considering, and in those which have been considered in the footnote to p. 292, must be immeasurably slower than that which is alleged to have occurred in modification experiments, and it seems probable that it would take very many years for change at this rate to effect anything like a complete change of type[1].

occur of which more will be said in another place (p. 629). But the point which concerns us now is that the culture last obtained, at a time when the disease had been in existence for over ten years, showed all the cultural characters of the bovine type unaltered and its virulence undiminished.

[1] The reader will naturally ask whether among the strains of bacilli of *human type** any difference of virulence has been observed when one strain was compared with another. As the evidence on this point is scanty, and somewhat inconclusive it is relegated to a footnote. The calf inoculations, as might be expected, reveal no difference, the resistance of the species to this kind of infection being too great. For the opposite reason the guinea-pig injections are of no greater value. There remain the rabbits. The writer has looked through the post-mortem abstracts of 250 of these animals inoculated by him with various viruses of the human type. The great majority were injected intraperitoneally ; more than half received injections of culture the rest of tissue emulsions; various doses were used. Striking differences in the severity of the disease which resulted occasionally occurred ; and these could by no means always be explained by differences of dose, or mode of inoculation. But in no instances were *all* the rabbits injected with a single virus affected with unusual severity. On the contrary severe and mild results occur side by side in a series of animals injected with the same material. The conclusion was obvious; the differences in the severity of the results could not be attributed to differences in the virulence of the viruses, but, so far as they could not be accounted for by differences of dose and mode of inoculation, they could only be explained on the assumption that the individual rabbits differed much in susceptibility to tuberculous infection.

A. S. Griffith, on the other hand, who also noted the occasional occurrence of severe results after injections of bacilli of human type, was unable to explain them all on this hypothesis. He says in a passage already quoted (p. 282 footnote). "Whether these more severe results are to be attributed to greater susceptibility of the individual rabbits, or to higher virulence of particular cultures cannot be definitely determined." In some cases the former explanation seems to have been valid, but this can hardly have been the case with the sputum viruses 124, 129, and 143 (*R.C.T. Fin. Rep.* App. vol. I. pp. 9, 485, 503 and 516), where in certain experiments a number of rabbits developed " a more severe form of tuberculosis than had been produced by human

* Other than those from lupus.

*Comparison of the Virulence for Calves of Strains of Tubercle
    Bacilli of Bovine Type derived from the Pig with others of
    the same Type derived from the Ox*[1].

Six strains of bacilli of bovine type derived from the pig
produced disease of the usual severity in the calf.   One strain
(P XIV) differed from the rest.   Four calves received 50 mg.
of bacilli from this strain.   One indeed died of general tuberculosis in 76 days, but in the others the injections " gave rise
to general tuberculosis much less severe than that ordinarily
produced by 50 mg. of bovine tubercle bacilli."   This strain
became fully virulent on passage through the ox; for a culture
from one of these calves, inoculated in the same doses into
two other calves, "caused fatal tuberculosis within the usual
period[2]."   The cultural characters of the original strain seem
to have been those of the bovine type, otherwise one would
suspect that this was a mixture of bovine and human bacilli
—for human tubercle bacilli have not unfrequently been found
in the submaxillary glands of the pig, and the strain in question
came from this source.

The exceptional character of this virus has made it desirable
to give it separate consideration, just as for similar reasons

tubercle bacilli."   Further experiments were made to determine whether these
results were due to the presence in the cultures of a small proportion of bovine
tubercle bacilli introduced accidentally into the sputum (possibly by milk
or some other food).   It would take too long to discuss these experiments
fully, for the results are anomalous and difficult of explanation.   It must
suffice to state here that in the case of the two viruses first mentioned passage
did not produce an increase of virulence, and Griffith came to the conclusion
that there was no admixture of bovine tubercle bacilli.   In the third case
he admitted there was such a mixture, but thought it more probable that it
came from a spontaneously affected rabbit, rather than from bovine bacilli
present in the original culture.

Those who believe in instability of type may perhaps see in these strains
the last flicker of bovine virulence in strains originally bovine, but whose
transformation into strains of human type was almost complete.   It is difficult
to say what was the duration of the disease in the three patients from whom
these strains were derived (for such information as is available, see *loc. cit.*
pp. 147, 161 and 164).   The question whether there are intrinsic differences
of virulence between different strains of bacilli of human type has recently
been discussed by Eastwood and F. Griffith (*Journ. of Hyg.* vol. xv, p. 269).

[1] *R.C.T. Int. Rep.* App. vol. III, p. 145.

[2] *R.C.T. Fin. Rep.* vol. III, p. 149, see also table on pp. 240–241.

when considering strains of human origin the attenuated (lupus) viruses were treated apart from the others.

The other strains of tubercle bacilli of bovine type derived from swine, six in number, did not differ at all from strains derived from the ox. Injected into eight calves in 50 mg. doses they produced rapidly fatal general tuberculosis. The average duration of disease was even slightly less than that of the disease produced by strains of bovine origin, but this probably is merely accidental.

TABLE XVI. *Analysis of 42 subcutaneous injections.*

Dose	Origin of virus	No. of viruses tested	No. of calves inoculated	No. of calves which died	Range of duration of disease when fatal	Average duration of disease	No. of calves which survived	Percentage which survived
50 mg.	Pig	6	8	8	19–48 days	34·5	0	0
	Ox	18	34	33	18–76 ,,	35·9	1	2·9

If then the pig derives its tuberculosis from the ox, as seems probable, either directly, or indirectly through other pigs, the transference of the bacilli from the one species of animal to the other does not seem to produce any modification of its specific virulence—unless indeed the exceptional virus P XIV be taken as evidence of modification caused by such a change. It is just conceivable that in this particular case the virus, originally bovine, had passed from pig to pig and had become modified in time by adaptation to its new host ; while in the other six cases of swine tuberculosis the infection had been contracted directly from the ox, and there had therefore been insufficient time for adaptation to proceed far enough to be demonstrable. But the evidence is quite insufficient to support so far-reaching a conclusion. One must therefore not attempt to build a house with a single stone. And it would seem that the more reasonable conclusion to draw from the evidence, so far as it goes, is that generalized tuberculosis in swine yields, as a rule, the ordinary (unmodified) bovine tubercle bacillus[1].

---

[1] Eastwood and F. Griffith have more recently obtained two more strains like P XIV from the pig (see *postea*, p. 406).

Comparison of the Virulence for Calves of Strains of Tubercle Bacilli of Bovine Type derived from the Horse with others of the same Type derived from the Ox[1].

The tubercle bacilli derived from the horse would, so far as it is possible to judge from the limited number of viruses investigated, seem to possess, in a considerable proportion of cases, a virulence for the calf which is distinctly less than that shown by viruses derived from the ox.

Four strains were examined. These were, apparently, in the main of bovine type, growing like bovine bacilli and virulent, or moderately virulent, for rabbits. Two of these (E II and E IV) possessed a distinctly lower degree of virulence for the calf than viruses of bovine origin, and moreover were of lower virulence than the latter for other animals also (rabbit, monkey, pig, guinea-pig). A third strain (E III) was *possibly* a little below the standard of virulence of viruses of bovine origin, while one (E I) appeared in every way to be a typical example of the bovine type. (See also p. 470.)

E II was tested on seven calves in doses of 100, 50 (three calves), 20 and 10 milligrammes (two calves). All the animals remained in good health and developed merely retrogressive tuberculosis, slight in extent, and similar to that produced in this species by tubercle bacilli of human type. For rabbits the virus was moderately virulent.

E IV was tested on six calves in doses of 50 mg. (four calves) and 10 mg. (two calves); five of these remained in good health and showed when killed, after about three months, slight non-progressive tuberculosis; the other died of a peculiar tuberculous pneumonia after 89 days. For rabbits the virulence of this strain was "moderate[2]."

Several passage experiments were made with these strains. The results, which were very irregular, were as follows: With each strain, passage through calves produced, in one series no change whatever, in another a slight increase of virulence, and in still another a complete change of virulence to that of the full standard of the bovine type.

[1] See F. Griffith, *R.C.T. Fin. Rep.* 1911, vol. IV, p. 7.

[2] The tests of the original virulence of these strains were made as follows: E I after 482 days, E II after 405 and 841 days, E III after 188 and 410 days, and E IV after 390 and 795 days of artificial cultivation (*loc. cit.* pp. 40, 49, 52, 67, 68, 74 and 76). The long duration of artificial culture opens the question whether attenuation may not have occurred after the bacilli left the horse. This explanation however is hardly consistent with the degree of uniformity shown by the injection of several sub-strains of each original virus.

It is generally admitted that equine tuberculosis is derived, either immediately or remotely, from the ox. Nocard believed that the infection was direct from the one species to the other, but it may be that in this he was mistaken. If we may assume that equine tuberculosis is derived sometimes directly from the ox, and sometimes from another horse, it would go far to explain the unequal virulence for the ox of strains of bacilli derived from the horse. For in the former case there would be but little time for the bacilli to adapt themselves to the new (equine) environment and lose their adaptation to their old (bovine) environment, while in the latter, especially if the virus had passed through many horses since it came from the ox, progressive adaptation to the new host might possibly have proceeded so far that some of the virulence for the ox had become lost.

Unfortunately for this rather attractive hypothesis the viruses E II and E IV which had low virulence for the ox had also somewhat lower virulence for the horse itself than that of bovine viruses of bovine origin, or of the virus E I which was fully virulent for the ox. Intravenous injection indeed, in 10 mg. doses, produced a fatal result in two horses, but the illness lasted 40 and 90 days respectively, while similar injections of E I produced a fatal result in 17 days, and one with a strain of bovine origin killed in 20 days[1].

Passage through the horse of a typical bovine strain of bovine origin was tried in two instances, but in neither case was the strain after recovery from the horse altered in virulence for calf or rabbit ; the duration of residence of the bacilli in the horse was 124 and 132 days respectively[2].

The plain fact is this, the question of equine tuberculosis is difficult and presents many interesting problems which still await solution. Their further discussion cannot profitably be attempted at this stage of our inquiry, but the subject will be resumed when we come to deal at length with equine tuberculosis (p. 461)[3].

---

[1] *R.C.T. Fin. Rep.* App. vol. IV, p. 19.

[2] *loc. cit.* pp. 8 and 137.

[3] The question whether there is an equine type of bacillus is discussed more fully in Chapter XXI.

Summary and Conclusions.

A review of the numerous experimental investigations dealt with in this and the preceding chapter shows that many instances of apparent modification, and even of complete transformation of type have been recorded during the course of passage experiments, both with human and bovine tubercle bacilli. Such changes of type have occurred not only in the work of those who have concluded that true modification takes place, but also in that of those who have become convinced that none of the proofs of modification will stand critical examination.

On the other hand the great majority of passage experiments have had negative results; that is to say the strains of bacilli employed have emerged, after a more or less prolonged residence in the new species of host completely unaltered.

It is quite certain therefore, whatever we may think of the general merits of the question of modification, that alteration of type does not *necessarily* and *constantly* occur whenever a strain of tubercle bacilli of one of the two mammalian types is made to reside for a time in a new species of host such as is liable to be infected under natural conditions with the other type of bacillus. Such changes as have occurred in experiments of this kind have been exceptional.

As to the changes of type which have undoubtedly occurred in some of these experiments, three explanations may be put forward for consideration:—

(1) that they represent true transformations of type;

(2) that they have been caused by substitution of one type of bacillus for the other, owing to accidental spontaneous infection of some of the animals employed; and

(3) that the original virus in these cases contained a mixture of the two types of bacilli, perhaps in very unequal proportions, and that the change of type was due to the elimination of one type and the establishment in sole possession of the other.

Now as to No. 1 we have seen that transformation of type

is not the rule when a change of host takes place, and there are no explanations put forward to explain why it should occur in one case and not in another. When a change of type has occurred it has been by no means always in the course of the longest experiments; moreover it has never been a gradual one.

With respect to No. 2 it must be admitted that the danger of spontaneous infections among the research animals is by no means imaginary, even in the most carefully managed establishments. As we have seen cause to believe certain lesions found in some of the animals employed by the Royal Commission were probably caused in this way, and there is no reason to think that the Commission's experiments were conducted less carefully than, or under conditions inferior to, those of other authors.

Moreover experience has shown that the more the conditions for carrying out such researches are made to approach the ideal the rarer become the instances of apparent modification of type. Specially instructive in this direction has been the work of the Royal Commission. In their earlier modification experiments, conducted under the same conditions as all their other researches and on premises where bacilli both of human and bovine type were being freely employed for the inoculation of animals, several instances of change of type occurred. But when the experiments were transferred to a new site, where accidental contamination by spontaneous infection with bovine bacilli was excluded as far as was humanly possible, no instance of modification took place.

Now as to explanation No. 3, it does not seem, on due consideration, at all improbable that in man traces of bovine tubercle bacilli should sometimes become mixed with the human tubercle bacilli living in pulmonary or intestinal lesions or in the lymph glands which receive the drainage from the lung or alimentary canal. The way is open, and bovine bacilli are common in milk and other food. Indeed several instances of tuberculosis in these regions have been investigated in which it is practically certain that both types were present. It is therefore quite possible that some of the alleged instances of modification of strains of bacilli of human type have arisen in consequence of the use of viruses which contained originally a small admixture of bovine tubercle bacilli. In some of the passage experiments, we have seen, the possibility that bovine bacilli were present at the commencement was not excluded in the only way practicable, namely by the injection of the extremely sensitive rabbit.

Direct experiments with mixtures of the two types of bacilli have shown that all the changes of virulence and cultural character which have been observed in passage experiments with single viruses may be imitated in similar passage experiments with mixtures.

Thus we see that there are good grounds for suspecting that the alleged instances of modification have been due, either to an admixture of two kinds of bacilli in the original virus, or to a bovine bacillus creeping in through some accident during the course of the experiments.

Of great interest in this connection has been the work of A. S. Griffith who by a most painstaking investigation of plate cultures, and the successful isolation of sub-strains from single colonies has in several instances of apparent transformation of type been able to show that both typical human and typical bovine bacilli were present. Of course it is open to anyone to argue that such a mixture is the natural result of an incomplete transformation, for it is probable that certain individual bacilli will be more easily modified than others, and that the descendants of the more stable ones will retain their type, while those of the less stable will be transformed. On the whole, however, the simpler explanation of Griffith's result would seem to be that two originally different kinds of bacilli were present.

It may be said then in conclusion that direct experiment has not succeeded in proving that a tubercle bacillus of given type can be transformed into one of another type by being made to reside in the body of a new host in which tuberculosis when it occurs naturally is caused by the latter type of bacillus.

One must not lose sight of the very numerous and often prolonged passage experiments in which no change of type has occurred. They are apt to be forgotten, owing to the larger amount of attention demanded by the more interesting experiments in which a change has resulted. But in reality they are of great importance, and demonstrate the extraordinary stability of tubercle bacilli in general; a stability of virulence which presents so great a contrast to the instability of certain other kinds of bacteria [1].

The existence of true transitional strains of tubercle bacilli which stand midway between the bovine and the human types has not been established.   Atypical strains indeed have been found, and not unfrequently; but some of these have, in our opinion, been resolved into mixtures of the two types of bacilli (e.g. H49, T.C., H13, A.D., H60, W.B. and H90, I.P.), while others, obtained from cases of lupus, and from other sources, have been shown to be attenuated rather than intermediate forms; and it seems highly probable that many other atypical strains concerning which no conclusions have as yet been arrived at belong to one or other of these categories [2].   Some of the attenuated strains have shown themselves capable of being readily transformed into typical examples of the type from which they seemed to have been derived; but in others restoration of virulence proved difficult to accomplish and in many attempts to bring it about failed altogether.   The restoration of virulence to some of these attenuated strains constitute, in our opinion, the only certain instances of experimental modification which so far have come to light.

But if transformation of type does not occur in our laboratory experiments which, prolong them how we will, are necessarily limited in time, it does not follow that an exceedingly slow modification of type does not take place when a suitable change of host occurs, as for example when bovine tubercle bacilli take up their residence for several generations in man, pig or horse. Such a change is perhaps dimly indicated in the analysis which in the previous pages has been made of experiments with viruses of bovine type taken from these species.   This slow alteration which appears probable (though the actual evidence for its existence is very slender) is, if it occurs at all, of a magnitude altogether different from that of the more or less sudden and complete changes of type which have appeared in some of the passage experiments.

[1] E.g. streptococci.   [2] For evidence of a new sub-type see Appendix, p. 681.

Such slow changes as are hinted at here are of little more than theoretical importance. They cannot interfere with the identification of the type of bacillus which has caused a given case of tuberculosis, since during the course of the disease in a single individual, however it may be prolonged, there would seem to be no time for such changes to occur. This is of great practical importance, because we may thereby feel assured that it is possible to recognize—of course after systematic investigation—the bovine source of infection in every case of human tuberculosis which may occur as the result of infection from the ox, and that the magnitude of the danger of bovine tuberculosis to mankind may be measured accurately by the frequency with which bacilli of bovine type are to be found in cases of human tuberculosis.

REFERENCES. IX

(Chapters xiii–xvii)

The Stability of Type of Tubercle Bacilli.

Arloing (1906). Production expérimentale de variétés transmissibles du bacille de la tuberculose et des vaccines antituberculeux. *Acad. d. Sciences.* June 18th.

Bang, O. (1908). Geflügeltuberkulose und Säugetiertuberkulose. *Centralbl. f. Bakt.* etc., 1. Abt. Orig. Bd. xlvi, p. 461.

Behring, Römer and Ruppel (1902). Betreffend die Abstammung und Gewinnung von Modifikationen des Tuberkulosevirus und des Tuberkulosegiftes. *Beiträge zur Experimentellen Therapie.* Heft 5.

Cobbett (1907). The Pathogenic Effects of Human Viruses. *Roy. Comm. on Tuberculosis, 2nd Int. Rep.* App. vol. ii.

—— (1907). The Stability of Virulence of Tubercle Bacilli in Artificial Culture ; and the Influence of Glycerin in Culture Media. *Ibid.* vol. iii, p. 185.

—— (1911). The Stability of Virulence of Tubercle Bacilli in the Living Animal. *Ibid. Fin. Rep.* App. vol. iii, p. 297.

—— (1911). The Fate of Mixed Viruses. *Ibid.* p. 342.

Dammann and Müssemeier (1905). *Untersuchungen über die Beziehungen der Tuberkulose des Menschen und der Tiere.* M. and H. Schaper. Hanover.

Eber (1906). Experimentelle Uebertragung der Tuberkulose vom Menschen auf das Rind, nebst Bemerkungen über die Beziehungen zwischen Menschen- und Rinder-tuberkulose. Berlin, *Tierärztliche Wochenschr.* No. 28, p. 527.

Eber (1908). Einige weitere Fälle erfolgreicher Uebertragung von menschen stammenden tuberkulösen Materiales auf das Rind. *Ibid.* No. 42, p. 601.

—— (1909). *Münch. med. Wochenschr.* No. 43, p. 2215.

—— (1910). Die Umwandlung vom menschen stammenden tuberkelbazillen des Typus Humanus in solche des Typus Bovinus. *Ibid.* Nos. 57, 115.

—— (1910). *Centralbl. f. Bakt.* I. Abt. Orig. vol. 59, pp. 193–364.

—— (1913). "Was lehren die in Veterinärininstitut der Universität Leipzig bisher durchgeführten Untersuchungen über die Beziehung zwischen Menschen- und Rinder-tuberkulose." Kritische und antikritische Bemerkungen zur Arteinheit der Säugetiertuberkelbazillen. *Centralbl. f. Bakt.* I. Abt. Orig. vol. 70, p. 229.
(This article contains a useful summary of all Eber's experiments on the subject.)

Griffith, A. S. (1911). Modification Experiments with Human Tubercle Bacilli. *R.C.T. Fin. Rep.* App. vol. I, p. 54.

—— (1911). Investigation of viruses derived from Sputum. *Ibid.* p. 8.

—— (1911). Investigation of Viruses obtained from Cases of Lupus. *Ibid.* vol. II.

Griffith, A. S. and Griffith, F. (1907). Modification Experiments with Tubercle Bacilli of Bovine Origin.
(a) Modification by Culture. *R.C.T. Int. Rep.* App. vol. III, p. 89.
(b) Modification by Animal Passage. *Ibid.* p. 89.
(c) Influence of Glycerin on Virulence. *Ibid.* p. 179.

—— (1911). Certain Human Viruses of Irregular Type. *R.C.T. Fin. Rep.* App. vol. III, pp. 5 and 18.

—— (1911). Swine Tuberculosis. *Ibid.* vol. III, p. 145.

Griffith, F. (1911). Investigation of Tubercle Bacilli from Tuberculosis occurring naturally in the Horse. *Ibid.* vol. IV, p. 4.

—— (1911). Modification Experiments with Tubercle Bacilli derived from Animals other than Man. *Ibid.* vol. IV, p. 383.

—— (1911). An Investigation of Artificially Mixed Cultures. *Ibid.* vol. III, p. 145.

Hamilton and Young (1903). An Investigation into the Relationship of Human Tuberculosis to that of Bovines. Univ. of Aberdeen, Department of Agriculture. *Trans. of the Highland and Agricultural Society of Scotland.*

Jancsó and Elfer (1910–11). Vergleichende Untersuchungen mit den praktisch wichtigeren Säurefesten Bazillen. *Beitr. z. Kl. der Tuberkulose,* vol. XVIII, p. 183.

De Jong (1902). Expériences comparatives sur l'action pathogène pour les animaux, notamment pour ceux de l'espèce bovine, des bacilles tuberculeux provenant du bœuf et de l'homme. *La semaine médicale,* No. 3.

De Jong (1902). *De éénheed der Zoogdiertuberculose.* Leiden.

Kleine (1906). Impftuberkulose durch Perlsuchtbazillen. *Zeitschf. f. Hygiene,* vol. LII, p. 495.

Koch, Schütz, Neufeld and Miessner (1905). Über die Immunisierung von Rindern gegen Tuberkulose. *Archiv f. wissensch. u. praktische Tierheilkunde,* vol. 31, p. 545.

Koch, M. and Rabinowitsch, L. (1907). Die Tuberkulose der Vögel und ihre Beziehungen zur Säugetiertuberkulose. *Virchow's Archives,* vol. 190, Beiheft, p. 246.

Kossel, Weber and Heuss (1905). Vergleichende Untersuchungen über Tuberkelbazillen verschiedener Herkunft. Anpassungsversuche mit Bazillen des Typus Humanus. *Tub. Arbeit. a. d. kaiserl. Gesundheitsamte,* Heft 3, p. 40.

Lindemann (1912). Ueber die Veränderung der biologischen Eigenschaften des Tuberkelbazillus ausserhalb und innerhalb des Organismus. *Berlin. klin. Wochenschr.,* p. 1185.

Malm (1912). On the so-called Types of the Tubercle Bacillus. *Journ. of Comp. Pathol. and Therap.* vol. XXV, p. 202. (See also *Official Report of Tuberculous Conference,* Rome, 1912, p. 87.)

Mohler and Washburn (1906). The Susceptibility of Tubercle Bacilli to Modification. *23rd Ann. Rep. U.S. Bureau of Animal Industry,* Washington, p. 113.

Neufeld, Dold and Lindemann (1912). Über Passageversuche mit menschlichen Tuberkulosematerial nach Methode von Eber. *Centralbl. f. Bakt.* I. Abt. Orig. vol. 65, p. 467.

Nocard (1898). Sur les Relations qui existent entre la Tuberculose Humaine et la Tuberculose Aviaire. *Ann. de l'Inst. Pasteur,* vol. XII, p. 561.

Park and Krumwiede (1910). The Relative Importance of the Bovine and Human Types of Tubercle Bacilli in the Different Forms of Tuberculosis. *Journ. of Med. Res.* vol. XXIII, p. 205. See § on Passage Experiments, p. 321.

Rabinowitsch (1906). Tuberkulose des Menschen und der Tiere. *Arbeiten aus dem Pathologischen Institut zu Berlin.*

Römer (1903). Beiträge zur Experimentellen Therapie. Heft 6.

Royal Commission on Tuberculosis (1907). *Interim Report.*

—— (1911). *Final Report.*

Salmon (1903). Some Observations on the Tuberculosis of Animals. *20th Ann. Rep. U.S. Bureau of Animal Industry,* p. 69. § Modification of the Morphology and Virulence of Tubercle Bacilli by Culture and Passing through Various Species of Animals.

Shattock, Seligmann, Dudgeon and Panton (1907). Relationship between Avian and Human Tuberculosis. *Proc. Roy. Soc. of Med.*

De Schweinitz (1898). The Attenuated Bacillus Tuberculosis, etc. *15th Ann. Rep. U.S. Bureau of Animal Industry.*

Trudeau (1890).   An Experimental Study of Preventive Inoculation in Tuberculosis. *Med. Record*, 1890, p. 565.

Vallée (1906).   Sur les Vaccinations Antituberculeuses. *Bull. de la Société centrale de Médec. Vétér.* p. 407.

Weber and Bofinger (1904).   Die Hühnetuberkulose. *Tub. Arbeit. a. d. Kaiserl. Gesundheitsamte,* Heft 1, p. 83.

Weber (1907).   Weitere Passagenversuche mit Bazillen der Typus Humanus. *Tub. Arbeit. a. d. Kaiserl. Gesundheitsamte,* Heft 6, p. 77.

Weber and Steffenhagen (1912).   Was wird aus den mit Perlsuchtbazillen inficierten Kindern, und welche Veränderungen erleiden Perlsuchtbazillen bei jahrelangem Aufenthalt im menschlichen Körper. *Tub. Arbeit. a. d. Kaiserl. Gesundheitsamte,* Heft 11, p. 1.

CHAPTER XVIII

THE SUSCEPTIBILITY TO TUBERCULOSIS OF VARIOUS ANIMAL SPECIES

Tuberculosis in the Ox.

Frequency of Infection.   It is difficult to ascertain with any degree of exactness the frequency with which tuberculosis occurs among the cattle of our own and other countries.   This much is certain however: it is exceedingly common both in Europe and America; and it may be said, on the authority of Sir John McFadyean, that it is "immensely more frequent among cattle than among any other farm animals," "and that bovine tuberculosis is the fountain head of the disease in these other species[1]."

One point must be kept clearly in mind when examining in detail the evidence of the frequency of bovine tuberculosis: the disease is far commoner among older animals than among younger ones.   It is very common among cows, especially old cows, it is comparatively rare among calves; while among bullocks and heifers of one or two years of age the frequency of the disease is intermediate between these extremes.   Hence

[1] *Journ. of Comp. Pathol. and Therap.* 1914, vol. XXVII, p. 218.

statistics are useless for comparative purposes unless the age composition of the groups of animals concerned is taken into account.

For the same reason too there is usually wide discrepancy between statistics based on slaughter-house inspection and those founded on the tuberculin test; for the former are necessarily concerned with animals killed for food, and therefore in the main young ones, while tuberculin tests are often made on herds consisting largely of cows.

There is, of course, another weighty reason why figures based upon tuberculin tests should show a far higher incidence of tuberculosis than those founded on slaughter-house inspection. Tuberculin reveals even the smallest traces of incipient tuberculosis, while inspection at the slaughter-house cannot be anything more than a somewhat rough and ready test, calculated to detect gross lesions, but liable to miss many smaller ones hidden in one or more of the numerous lymphatic glands or in the voluminous organs[1].

Thus while figures based upon slaughter-house returns must be held to under-estimate greatly the real frequency of tuberculosis among cattle, those based upon tuberculin tests are probably more reliable. But here again caution is necessary, for one must remember that tuberculin tests are usually made on selected material, and not unfrequently on individuals or herds concerning which a suspicion of tuberculosis has already arisen.

Bearing in mind these sources of error let us proceed to

---

[1] The exhaustive examination of the whole of the carcass of an ox is a long and tedious business. The number and size of the lymphatic glands alone would astonish anyone who had not worked systematically through them; while the length of the intestine is calculated to fill the conscientious pathologist with despair. In the well equipped laboratories of the Royal Commission, with numerous skilled assistants each trained by almost daily practice to do his appointed part, the post-mortem examination of even a calf was the work of a morning. Such systematic examination, or anything approaching it even remotely, is, of course, out of the question in the slaughter-house; it is certain then that many small lesions must there be overlooked. Hence the wide disparity of the returns from different slaughter-houses is easily explained if, as seems reasonable, we may assume that the inspection is carried out more carefully in some centres than in others.

examine the evidence of the frequency of bovine tuberculosis in different lands.

It will not do to take the statistics of any one country as representative of another, for the distribution of the disease is very unequal. In some countries it is rare. In Japan, as we learn from Kitasato, the disease is almost unknown among the native cattle, and, according to de Haan, a similar state of things prevails in Java. In the Island of Jersey also tuberculosis among the cattle is said to be rare[1]. In other countries the disease is exceedingly common; and, in some of them, at least in certain districts, probably half the cows are tuberculous.

In one and the same country there may be great disparity in different localities. Nocard, speaking in 1894 of bovine tuberculosis in France, said: "there are some districts where one estimates it at 10, 15 or 25 per cent., or more; there are others where it is unknown[2]." In the United States of America in 1908 the percentage of animals which reacted to tuberculin varied from 46·67 in Nebraska and 40·33 in Missouri, to 0·51 in New Jersey and 1·04 in Oklahoma[3].

. Let us now look more closely into the statistics of various countries.

The amount of tuberculosis among the cattle of the United Kingdom may be judged from some statistics published in 1900 by the editor of the *Journal of Comparative Pathology and Therapeutics*, Sir John McFadyean. The Royal Veterinary College had issued tuberculin to veterinary surgeons who applied for it, and the following figures are based on reports received from them If the reports received during the three

[1] Eighty-one animals, the majority probably being milch cows, were tested with tuberculin in 1899 without any reacting. This result is said to have been entirely in keeping with the results of the two previous years. (Editor of the *Journ of Comp. Pathol. and Therap.* vol. XIII, p. 69.)

Over 2000 calves, as well as a small number of cows and heifers, specially imported from Jersey, were tested by the Royal Commission, and all animals whose temperature reactions were considered in any degree doubtful or unsatisfactory were killed and examined, but no instance of tuberculosis came to light.

[2] *Les tuberculoses animales*, p. 8.

[3] Melvin, 25*th Ann. Rep. U.S. Bureau of Animal Industry*, p. 100.

years 1897–8–9 are taken together we find that somewhat over 15,000 animals were tested, and that of these 26 per cent. reacted. The animals tested comprised cattle of various breeds[1] and ages, but it is definitely stated that the majority were milch cows[2].

The proportion of reacting animals varied very much in different parts of the country: thus of 1175 animals tested in Cornwall, Devon, Dorset and Somerset in 1899 only 7 per cent. reacted. In some other counties unnamed, out of 2090 animals 33 per cent. reacted. Two veterinary surgeons tested 1238 cattle in the counties of Sussex and Hampshire and of these 50 per cent. reacted. In the neighbourhood of the South Coast 264 animals were tested and of them 62 per cent. reacted.

The local disparity being such as is shown here these figures clearly cannot be accepted unconditionally as representative of the whole of England; moreover it is possible that in some, or perhaps many, cases the test was applied because there was reason to suspect tuberculosis in the herd in question. This is not stated definitely to have been the case, but the possibility cannot be overlooked. These figures however may be controlled by comparing them with others elicited by the very careful investigations of MacLaughlan Young and Walker in Aberdeen and by Delépine in Manchester.

Young and Walker's investigation, 1899, was based both upon tuberculin tests and post-mortem examination, and was carried out on a limited number of animals, but the care with which the post-mortem examinations were conducted makes them more valuable than slaughter-house statistics based on far greater numbers. These observers found, out of 240 cattle, 77 (or 32 per cent.) tuberculous.

Delépine, in 1910, by the same methods examined 128

[1] It is very generally supposed that susceptibility to tuberculosis varies in different breeds of cattle. In this country tuberculosis is much more prevalent among shorthorns, Jerseys and Ayrshires than among West Highlanders, Galloways or Herefords; but McFadyean is of opinion that this is mainly, if not entirely, ascribable to the different circumstances in which those breeds are usually kept. As to the general question whether constitutional susceptibility varies in different breeds he says he would prefer to leave the matter doubtful: probably, he adds, it does so, but at least in this country the circumstances seldom if ever furnish a fair test. (*Journ. of Comp. Pathol. and Therap.* 1896, vol. IX, p. 279.) Experimental evidence however is slowly accumulating which shows that the shorthorn calf is more resistant than the Jersey (see p. 250).

[2] *Ibid.* vol. XIII, p. 68.

animals more than one year old, derived from the neighbourhood of Manchester. Of these 27 per cent. were tuberculous.
As to the composition of this group of animals it may be said
at once that many of them were cows, but we shall have to
return to this investigation in a moment when the question of
the age incidence of tuberculosis in cattle comes up for discussion.

If these investigations can be accepted as representative,
and great caution is necessary in drawing conclusions from
such small numbers, it would seem that from one-quarter to
one-third of our cows are infected in some degree (in many
cases probably not very severely)[1] with tuberculosis.

Turning once again to foreign countries we see that, at
the International Congress held at Budapest in 1905, Bang
declared that out of over 40,000 cattle of all ages (including
a large proportion of cows) examined in December by means of
the tuberculin test 35 per cent. reacted.

Malm, 1914, stated that, in the course of the campaign
against bovine tuberculosis which was being carried out in
Norway, over 39,000 herds of cattle, including more than
324,000 (or, as one may say in round numbers, nearly
a third of a million) animals were tested with tuberculin
between 1895 and 1913. In 1897 the proportion of reacting
beasts was 8·3 per cent.; by 1912 it had fallen to 4·8 per cent.

The extent of tuberculosis among the cattle of the United
States may be judged by the following figures published in
1908 by the Bureau of Animal Industry at Washington. Out
of 400,000 animals tested with tuberculin, the majority being
dairy cattle, 9·25 per cent. reacted[2].

[1] Tuberculosis as it occurs naturally in the bovine species is usually a
chronic disease; and, though it may be extensive, often causes remarkably
little constitutional disturbance or deterioration of condition. Schroeder
and Cotton were so impressed with this fact that they went so far as to speak
of the existence of advanced tuberculosis with extreme and voluminous lesions
in cows that presented no visible sign of disease during life. (1904, 21st
Ann. Rep. U.S. Bureau of Animal Industry, p. 64.)

McFadyean also says that "a stock owner may find when he tests his animals
(with tuberculin) that he has 20 or 30 per cent. of them affected, and yet he
may not have lost a single animal from tuberculosis, or noticed any deterioration of their health in previous years." (Journ. of Comp. Path. and Therap.
1899, vol. XII, p 269.)

[2] 25th Ann. Rep. U.S. Bureau of Animal Industry, p. 99.

The difference between these figures is remarkable enough, but if now we look at the statistics of the slaughter-house there will be seen such extraordinary discrepancy as will go far to undermine any confidence which we might otherwise place in such returns. Thus, to take a rather ancient example from Straus's work, we find that, though bovine tuberculosis was notorious in Saxony, so much so that Straus calls it "celle terre classique de la tuberculose bovine[1]," the returns for that country for the age periods when bovine tuberculosis is commonest (over 3 years) are given by Siedamgrotsky as only about one-third as high as those for the whole of Germany as collected by Röckl. The figures may be seen on the opposite page. It may be added that Straus himself did not call attention to the discrepancy.

Again the frequency of tuberculosis among the cattle of France was estimated in 1889 by Arloing[2] at only 0·5 per cent., while among those over two years old slaughtered in Berlin it was put by Ostertag, who for six years was one of the chief inspectors there, at 33 per cent.[3] Such extreme differences in neighbouring countries are beyond belief, and only show the unreliability of estimates based upon slaughter-house inspection.

In the United States the following report was made by Melvin, Chief of the Bureau of Animal Industry. Out of 7,000,000 cattle (not including calves) slaughtered under Federal inspection in 1908, 0·961 per cent. were found to be tuberculous. Melvin adds that a larger proportion of the animals privately slaughtered are tuberculous, and he arrives at the estimate that "more than 1 per cent. of the beef cattle in the United States are affected with tuberculosis in some degree[4]"; and, he adds, 10 per cent. of the dairy cattle are tuberculous[5].

[1] Straus, *La tuberculose*, p. 320.
[2] Arloing, "Tuberculosis considered from the point of view of Sanitary police." Translation of a paper communicated to the International Veterinary Congress in Paris in 1889, *Journ. of Comp. Pathol. and Therap.* vol. II, p. 199.
[3] Cited in an Editorial Article, *Journ. of Comp. Pathol.* etc., 1892, vol. V, p. 56.
[4] *25th Ann. Rep.* p. 98. This may be compared with the 9·25 per cent. of dairy cattle which reacted to tuberculin.
[5] *loc. cit.* p. 101.

The Age Incidence of Tuberculosis among Cattle. Whatever we may think of the *absolute* value of slaughter-house figures, relatively, as to the comparative frequency of gross lesions in animals of different ages in any one locality, they may doubtless be accepted. They all show an immensely greater frequency in the older animals, that is to say in the cow (for there are few bulls of comparable age), than in young ones.

Take for example the old figures already mentioned as quoted by Straus from Siedamgrotsky and Röckl. Though they differ greatly in absolute magnitude they agree fairly well in showing a remarkable increase of tuberculosis as age advances.

Tuberculosis among Cattle in Saxony (Siedamgrotsky) and Germany (Röckl)[1]. (Showing Increase with Age.)

Age	0—6 weeks	6 weeks— 1 year	1—3 years	3—6 years	6 years and over
Saxony 1889	0·006	0·3	7·0	9·3	16
Germany 1888–89	0·4	0·6	11·4	33·1	43·4

These figures may be supported by others based on the tuberculin test. The following were communicated by Bang to the International Tuberculosis Congress held at Washington in 1906.

Results of 40,000 Tuberculin Tests on Cattle in Denmark (Bang)[2]. (Showing Increase of Infection with Age.)

Age	0—6 months	6 months— 1½ years	1½—2½ years	2½—5 years	Over 5 years
Number Examined	5559	7744	5047	10,350	11,924
Percentage Reacted	12·1	27·5	38·6	44·9	48

---

[1] *La tuberculose*, pp. 321 *et seq.*
[2] "Bekämpfung der Tuberkulose der Haustiere." *Rep. VIth Internat. Cong. on Tuberculosis*, Washington 1895, vol. IV, pt. 2, p. 855.

With these results some statistics collected in this country by Delépine in 1912 may be compared. These are based not only on tuberculin tests, but are controlled by careful post-mortem examination. They refer to 379 animals from the neighbourhood of Manchester and Cheshire, and in some cases from Scotland. Over one-third of the examinations were made by Delépine himself, and the rest by Prof. Hamilton or by veterinary surgeons.

Tuberculosis of Cattle in Manchester and Elsewhere (Delépine)[1]. *(Showing Increase of Infection with Age.)*

Age in years	0—1	1—2	2—3	3—5	5—9	9—13	Total
Number Examined	29	68	112	51	94	25	375
Percentage Tuberculous	3·4	13·2	24·1	23·5	48·9	76·0	30

All these figures combine to show that tuberculosis is extraordinarily frequent among cows[2]. In young cattle it is less common; McFadyean in 1894 stated that the proportion of tuberculosis among bovine animals between six and eighteen months of age is quite insignificant[3].

[1] " Bovine tuberculosis," *Proc. Nat. Vet. Ass.* 1912.

[2] Young and Walker, already referred to, found among 76 cows no less than 42 tuberculous—that is to say 55 per cent. The increase in the frequency of infection with age is shown in the following analysis of their results.

Tuberculosis in Cattle in Aberdeen (Young and Walker). Showing Increase with Age.

	Heifers, Bulls, Bullocks	Cows		
Age in years............	2—3	4—6	7—10	11—13
Number Examined	158	33	30	13
Percentage Tuberculous	19	45	57	77

The above is a modified arrangement of Delépine's analysis of the Aberdeen figures. See *Ann. Rep. Med. Off. Loc. Gov. Bd.* 1908–9: fig. opposite p. 408.

[3] Editorial Article. *Journ of Comp. Pathol. and Therap.* 1894; vol. VII, p. 269.

In the calf tuberculosis is probably unfrequent, though here there is a good deal of discrepancy in the figures. Delépine referring to abattoir returns published chiefly in Germany, Denmark and France stated that only one out of 3300 calves was reported to have been found tuberculous. Small as this figure is it agrees fairly well with that given for the United States by Melvin, who stated that, while about 1 per cent. of all the cattle slaughtered were tuberculous, among nearly 2,000,000 calves killed during the same period only 0·026 per cent. were similarly affected. These figures however are not borne out by tuberculin tests, and as we have already seen Bang found that about 12 per cent. of the calves in Denmark reacted[1].

Perhaps we can best judge of the frequency of tuberculosis in the calf, at least in the neighbourhood of London, by some figures published annually by Blaxall, who is responsible under the Local Government Board for the production of vaccine lymph. A number of calves are purchased each year for the purpose of inoculation; and when the lymph has been obtained the animals are killed and subjected to a searching examination by the veterinary inspectors of the Board. From time to time a tuberculous animal is detected, and the lymph which it has supplied is destroyed. Now the proportion of tuberculous calves found each year has been published since 1903; and if we add together the figures for the eleven years 1892–93 to 1912–13 we find that, in all, 5092 calves were slaughtered and examined and that of these 54 were found to exhibit evidence of tuberculous disease. This gives an incidence of 1·05 per cent.[2]

The Age at which Infection Occurs. Predisposing Causes. The Influence of Lactation. The statistics which we have just been reviewing show clearly the increasing frequency with which tuberculosis is recognized in cattle as age advances; and more particularly they show that the cow is very often affected and the calf comparatively rarely. But since the figures are compiled mainly from the returns of slaughter-houses, and are therefore based to a large extent on gross

---

[1] Cp. Bang's post-mortem results at Aarhus (see p. 125).

[2] *Ann. Rep. Med. Off. Loc. Gov. Bd.* Reports, Nos. 32 to 42.

anatomical lesions, it may be objected that after all the calf may very probably be affected much more frequently than these figures imply, since, if the disease progresses very slowly as is probably the case, lesions at the age in question may not, as a rule, have attained such a size as to attract notice in the slaughter-house. Probably this objection is not without foundation, and it is supported by the fact that Bang found so considerable a proportion of his calves reacted to tuberculin. But even Bang's figures show a remarkable increase in the frequency of infection as one passes from the lower to the higher age periods. Consequently, unless we are prepared to maintain that animals with early or latent tuberculosis do not react to tuberculin, we cannot uphold the view that the majority of infections take place early in life: on the contrary it would appear that they occur with increasing frequency as age advances.

If this is the case it follows: (1) either that the *external* conditions predisposing to tuberculous infection are more frequent among the older than among the younger animals—which is improbable—or (2) that the *internal* forces of the body, whose object it is to resist infection, become weaker as age advances, either continuously and gradually, or irregularly, at certain critical periods of life. A third possibility also there is, namely that by their cumulative effect repeated invasions of tubercle bacilli are particularly liable to produce progressive disease, and that consequently the longer the animal lives the more chance there is that such repeated invasions shall have occurred in sufficient quantity and sufficiently often to produce disease. But experimental investigation lends no support to any such view, and on the contrary shows that doses of bacilli individually too small to cause progressive disease have, when repeated, an immunizing effect. We therefore seem driven to conclude that *the reason why the frequency of infection increases as age advances is to be sought in physiological changes which tend to increase susceptibility.*

This conclusion however seems, at first sight at least, to be sharply opposed to experience derived from experimental infection. For the latter shows, with no uncertainty, that young

XVIII] CAUSE OF THE GREAT SUSCEPTIBILITY 383

calves may be infected much more easily and more severely than animals several months older. But we do not know that the power of resisting tuberculous infection, which is thus shown to increase greatly during the first year or two of life, continues to do so afterwards, or indeed remains at the high level which it attains about the end of that period, for experiments on adult bovine animals have, owing to the expense which they entail, been limited in number. Judging however from such facts as have come to light from experimental research, as well as from common experience of the natural disease, it seems probable that the power of resistance reaches a maximum about the end of the period of growth, and remains after that at a fairly constant level, but subject to depressions brought about by various disturbing causes.

What then are the causes which produce depressions in the resisting power of the bovine species? Doubtless they are many; but there is one which seems to be of more importance than all the rest. We must remember that it is the cow with which we are mainly concerned. We know little or nothing about the prevalence of tuberculosis in the males of equal age, since they are seldom permitted to live so long; but it may be doubted whether, if they were allowed to attain the same age, it would be anything like so great in them as in the cow; and we shall probably not be wrong if we look for the predisposing causes of tuberculosis in the latter among the physiological crises which are peculiar to the life of the female.

It will not be forgotten that it is only by artificial selection, practised on countless generations, that the cow has been brought to yield such unnatural[1] quantities of milk as it commonly does; and it would not be surprising if an

---

[1] It was found by the writer when working at Stansted for the Royal Commission that the richness and quantity of the Jersey cow's milk was such that if calves was allowed freely to suck their mothers and to take as much milk as they could get they usually died of diarrhœa and their intestines were found filled with decomposing curd. The writer, who was responsible for this method of feeding, obstinately persevered in it for some time, insisting, against expert advice, that it was absurd to think one could improve upon Nature's method of allowing the young to feed from their own mothers. But after losing a good many calves, and always finding in their intestines

accomplishment of so exacting a nature had been acquired at
the expense of some other capacity, such as the power of
resisting tuberculous infection[1].   It seems probable then that
it is because of the excessive demands made by the processes
of lactation, which have been developed far beyond the bounds
of what is natural, that the cow is so much more frequently
infected with tuberculosis than the younger members of its
own race, and it is probably also because these demands fall
largely on the mammary gland that this organ is so often
implicated[2].

the conditions described above, he gave way, and allowed the calves afterwards
born on the place to be brought up by hand on a *portion* of the mother's milk,
suitably diluted; and after this there were no further losses.

[1] The reader will note that in the vegetable kingdom a similar law seems
to hold, and that many a plant which has been brought artificially to yield
particularly beautiful flowers is highly susceptible to infective disease.   One
might point, for example, to the prevalence of disease in the hollyhock and the
mallow, and the liability of the choicer kinds of cineraria to be attacked by
black fly.

[2] This argument may be supported by negative evidence derived from
other species of animals.   Mammary tuberculosis is uncommon in many animals
which frequently suffer from tuberculosis in other organs, for example in the
guinea-pig, in which species, among his experimental animals, the author has
never seen this gland affected.   Tuberculosis no doubt occurs in the human
breast; but the disease is far from common, and it is possible that many
cases so diagnosed are due to another cause.   The latest review of the subject
is that published by Deaver in 1914 (*Am. Journ. of Med. Sciences*, vol. CXLVII,
p. 157).   This author, after rejecting all cases unsupported by microscopic
examination, was able to collect from the records of the previous decade
only 74 cases (including five of his own).   But if we were to insist, as we
have surely a right to do in these days, not on histological evidence only,
but on demonstration of the tubercle bacillus, few cases would remain in
the list.   The following instances are gathered from Deaver's paper.   Fuller,
Bransburg and Stromberg demonstrated tubercle bacilli in stained sections;
and Ingier, Schley, Duvergey and Davis found them in smear preparations.
Only two instances of transmission of tuberculosis to animals by inoculation
(by far the most satisfactory test) are recorded.   Both Zvioni and von Eberts
are said to have grown tubercle bacilli from lesions of the human breast.
The author has not seen the former's paper, but in the latter (*Am. Journ.
Med. Scien.* 1909, vol. CXXXVIII, p. 70) it is merely stated that cultures were
sown on egg media and soon died out; even the fact that they grew at all
is left to be inferred.   Among English cases there are but few in which the
diagnosis is based upon the presence of the tubercle bacillus.   No mention
of them occurs in the description of the case recorded by Shattock (1889),
and in those of Hebb (1888) and Lane (1890) they were looked for in
vain.   In Scott's collection of 27 cases (1904), 21 of which were verified

Portals of Infection. Susceptibility of Various Tissues. The organs most frequently affected in the ox in cases of naturally acquired disease are the lungs, pleuræ and thoracic lymphatic glands. Less frequently the principal lesions are found in the glands or organs of the abdominal cavity. For this reason it

by microscopic examination, the finding of tubercle bacilli in the breast itself is only recorded in two cases, and in another these micro-organisms were found in the axillary glands. In the rest diagnosis depended on "foci of granulation tissue and endothelial cells" sometimes with and sometimes without giant cells, and on other similar and, as I think, not quite convincing histological evidence (*St Bart. Hosp. Rep.* vol. XL, p. 97).

In Germany (1891) Mandry reported seven cases of human mammary tuberculosis which he had himself observed in the Surgical Clinic at Tübingen. But he says that tubercle bacilli were rare; he only found them in two cases; and in one of these it was only a single bacillus that was seen. The diagnosis, then, depended mainly on anatomical structure; and no animals seem to have been injected. Soon after this Beuder added three more cases from Heidelberg. In these tubercle bacilli were found, but they were relatively scarce, and again no animals seem to have been inoculated.

The writer has examined two supposed instances of tuberculosis of the human breast, and injected emulsions of the diseased tissues into guinea-pigs; but he did not succeed in producing tuberculosis on either occasion.

We may, I think, conclude from the evidence just considered that tuberculosis of the human breast is not a common condition; one might venture even to describe it as rare. On the other hand mammary tuberculosis would seem to be frequent not only in the cow but in other animals also on whose milk-supply a large demand is made.

A case of mammary tuberculosis has been reported in the goat. (*Recueil de méd. vét.* 1900, abst. in the *Veterinary Journal*, vol. II, N.S. p. 109.)

In female animals which produce a large number of young at a birth a corresponding strain must be imposed upon the milk-producing system. In such animals mammary tuberculosis would seem to be particularly common. Thus it occurs frequently in the prolific pig, though probably less commonly than in the dairy-supplying cow (Mohler and Washburn). Among the 59 swine examined by A. S. Griffith and F. Griffith, although these included but few adult animals, tuberculosis was twice seen in the mammary gland, and in another case in the supra-mammary lymphatic gland (*R.C.T. Fin. Rep.* App. vol. III, pp. 154 et seq.). In the rabbit, which not only produces many young at a birth, but those too in a very immature condition, so that they have to remain for a long time dependent on their mother's milk for sustenance, the writer has more than once seen mammary tuberculosis; and A. S. Griffith remarks of this species that even the human tubercle bacillus, which has in general very little virulence for it, may cause tuberculosis in the functional mammary gland (*R.C.T. Fin. Rep.* App. vol. I, p. 36).

From these examples it seems permissible to conclude that susceptibility to tuberculosis in any given organ is greatly increased by excessive functional activity (compare also the dog's heart, p. 491 footnote).

is believed that the disease is more often contracted by inhalation than by deglutition.   (Nocard, Straus, McFadyean.)

The muscles are very seldom affected[1], but the mammary gland in the cow is often the seat of tuberculosis; and it is this fact and the consequent contamination of the milk with tubercle bacilli that gives to bovine tuberculosis most of its importance in relation to human pathology.

Whether the milk may become infected by bacilli carried by the blood stream to the mammary gland, and in the absence of tuberculous changes in that organ itself has been much debated.   Recent researches[2] clearly show that it may sometimes become contaminated in this way.   But it is probable that in such cases the number of bacilli is seldom large; and it can hardly be doubted that whenever these organisms are present in dangerous quantities in the milk almost invariably the udder itself is tuberculous.   Of more practical importance is the fact that early tuberculosis of the udder is difficult to detect, and that even advanced disease of this organ cannot easily be distinguished from induration due to other causes.

A curious point well worthy of consideration is the immunity shown by certain organs and tissues which remain unaffected even in the severest cases of generalized tuberculosis.   We have seen that the muscles almost always escape; but this is not all; certain glandular organs seem to be equally immune.   Even in the most acute forms of experimental tuberculosis, when dissemination has occurred by the blood stream, and after intravenous injection, although all the great organs and the

[1] Ostertag says that tuberculous lesions are very rarely present in the muscular system, or flesh proper; nor does the muscle juice often contain bacilli even in cases of generalized tuberculosis.   He goes on to say that Nocard injected muscle juice from 21 cows affected in this way into guinea-pigs.   Only in a single case did one of the guinea-pigs (out of four used in the experiment) develop tuberculosis.   Gaultier repeated the experiment in the case of 15 cows and caused tuberculosis, twice.   Perroncito injected 200 rabbits and as many guinea-pigs with the muscle juice of tuberculous animals without obtaining a single positive result.   (Ostertag, *Journ. of Comp. Pathol. and Therap.* 1899, vol. XII, pp. 243–245.)

[2] A. S. Griffith and F. Griffith, "The Excretion of Tubercle Bacilli into the milk of Cows and Goats," *R.C.T. Fin. Rep.* App. vol. III, p. 81.

Plate XI

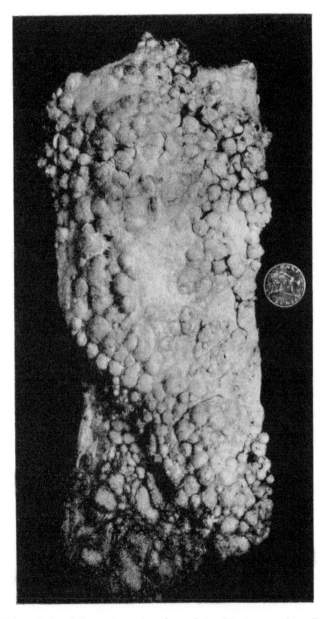

Tuberculosis of the peritoneal surface of the Diaphragm of an Ox.
Natural disease.

intestinal mucosa may be crowded with minute tubercles, and when no single lymph or hæmolymph gland is free from obvious lesions, yet the muscles and salivary glands escape, and generally too the pancreas and thymus.

These facts raise the question: Do the organs in question owe their immunity to superior powers of resistance (being either able to destroy tubercle bacilli, or indifferent to them) or to absence, on the part of the endothelium of their capillaries, of power to arrest tubercle bacilli which are brought there by the blood? We know that this power of arrest varies in different organs in relation to the taking up of indifferent substances such as carbon or carmine, and it seems probable that it varies also in relation to tubercle bacilli; but the question cannot yet be answered, and it seems to invite direct investigation[1].

The Comparative Susceptibility of the Ox to Infection with the Three Types of Tubercle Bacilli.

Natural Tuberculosis. Practically in the ox tuberculosis is always caused by the bovine type of bacillus. The human

---

[1] The organs immune to tuberculosis are not always the same in different species of mammals. The kidneys, for example, are very susceptible in the rabbit, and seldom affected in the guinea-pig. The skeletal muscles it is true seem to be insusceptible in most mammals, but the writer has twice seen them severely affected in the monkey.

In some species a special weakness would seem to be associated with certain organs or structures, which makes them liable to disease caused not by the tubercle bacillus only but by other pests also. Thus in the rabbit a specially weak point would seem to be the joints; for not only are they sometimes the seat of tuberculosis, but, in the writer's experience, are not unfrequently attacked by pyogenic cocci, when these have been experimentally injected into the blood-stream and a rapidly fatal result has not ensued.

The guinea-pig too would seem to have a weak spot in its structure, namely in the system which deals with the drainage of the pleural cavities. Those who have worked at the standardization of diphtheria antitoxin will have observed that the great majority of guinea-pigs which die within a few days of an injection of diphtheria toxin, succumb to effusion into the pleuræ and consequent collapse of the lungs. This result is not peculiar to diphtheria toxin, but may be seen with equal frequency in guinea-pigs which have perished from acute tuberculosis. Neither with diphtheria nor tubercle is a similar result produced in the rabbit, or, so far as the writer is aware, in any species other than the guinea-pig.

type of bacillus has never been found[1]; the avian rarely, and
then probably only in unimportant lesions, or in association
with the bovine bacillus.

Thirteen instances of natural tuberculosis in the ox were examined by
the Committee of the Gesundheitsamt[2]; thirty were examined by the Royal
Commission[3]; in each series only the bovine type of bacillus was found.

It is possible however that the avian type of bacillus may at times cause
trivial lesions in the ox, as it does, as we shall see, in the pig; or that it may
be present in open tuberculous lesions caused by the bovine bacillus. Kruse[4],
in 1893, mentioned a strain, isolated by San Felice from the tuberculous lung
of an ox, which was presumably a pure strain of avian bacilli, for it caused
tuberculosis in the hen and rabbit but not in the guinea-pig. Pansini[5] appears
to have obtained a mixture of avian and bovine strains from the lung juice
of an ox, for the virus caused tuberculosis, not in the hen only, but also in the
guinea-pig. These are ancient examples. More recently A. S. Griffith[6] found
an avian bacillus in a pea-sized gritty caseous nodule in the mesenteric glands
of a calf which had previously been injected under the skin with human
tubercle bacilli. Review of the literature however shows that instances in which
avian tubercle bacilli are reported to have been found in the ox are few in
number, and they require support before any conclusions can be based on them.

Johne's Disease. The avian tubercle bacillus has been
suspected, by some investigators, to be the cause of a peculiar
form of chronic enteritis which occurs in the ox, and is
characterized usually by immense numbers of acid-fast bacilli
in the affected mucosa. It was first described by Johne and
Frothingham, and has been named, after the first of these
observers, Johne's disease. A similar disease has been observed
in the sheep by Stockman. It was suggested by Markus and
de Jong that the disease might be caused by the avian tubercle
bacillus, and indeed a strain of·tubercle bacilli, obtained from
a case of this kind by Stuurmann, was investigated by M. Koch
and L. Rabinowitsch and pronounced to be of this type[7]. But
more recently a bacillus which is certainly not an avian tubercle

---

[1] Certain exceptions are mentioned in the Appendix (p. 675).

[2] Weber, *Tub. Arbeit. a. d. Kaiserl. Gesundheitsamte*, Heft 6, p. 9.

[3] *R.C.T. Fin. Rep.* p. 9.

[4] Kruse, "Ueber das Vorkommen der sogennanten Hühnertuberkulose
beim Menschen und bei Säugetieren," *Zieglers Beiträge zur path. Anat. u.
allgem. Pathol.* vol. XII, p. 544.

[5] Pansini, "Einige neue Fälle von Geflügeltuberkulose beim Menschen und
Säugetieren," *Deutsch. med. Wochenschr.* 1894, p. 694.

[6] *R.C.T. Fin. Rep.* App. vol. I, pp. 374 B and 386 (Calf 1225).

[7] "Die Tuberkulose der Vögel," *loc. cit.* p. 475. Cp. also Goat 48, p. 419,
small type.

bacillus has been repeatedly cultivated from cases of the disease in question. This was first successfully accomplished by Twort and Ingram (1912) by use of a special culture medium, which they introduced, containing dead acid-fast bacilli or extracts made from them. It was repeated by Holth, then by McFadyean, Sheather and Edwards (1912), and afterwards by Meyer (1913). The bacillus belongs to the acid-fast group, as do the tubercle bacilli, but it grows with difficulty in artificial media. It defied cultivation for a long time, and so far has only been grown on the special media already mentioned. McFadyean, Sheather and Edwards give a detailed description of the cultures. These do not at all resemble those of the avian tubercle bacillus which as is well known grows readily on various kinds of media. Moreover, O. Bang and others have found that material taken from cases of Johne's disease and containing the bacilli in question is not infective for fowls and rabbits[1]; and Twort and Ingram have obtained negative results on injecting their cultures into these animals. Holth also states that the injection of cultures into rabbits produced only small suppurative lesions. In the face of these facts it is clear that Johne's disease is not caused by the avian tubercle bacillus.

Experimental Infection. This subject has already been considered fully in a former chapter in which the question of the differentiation of the various types of tubercle bacilli was discussed; it will therefore be sufficient to recall here the following facts and conclusions. The ox possesses a considerable power of resisting tuberculous infection, even when the bacillus belongs to the bovine type. Small doses (see p. 261) of this type of bacillus injected subcutaneously into the calf produce only a minimal amount of disease which shows no tendency to progress beyond the initial stages, at least during the period which is usually allowed to elapse before the animal is killed and its body examined (3–6 months). Larger doses (50 mg.) however produce in the (Jersey) calf acute, and generally fatal, miliary tuberculosis which affects almost every great organ, and every lymphatic and hæmolymph gland, almost without exception.

[1] Rabbits are susceptible to experimental infection with avian bacilli (see p. 428).

Intravenous injection, as may well be imagined, is a more certain method of infection, and causes fatal disease even when the doses are much smaller than those required to produce this result by subcutaneous injection.

Serious disease is easily produced also by inhalation of bovine tubercle bacilli; but attempts to infect by feeding are not always successful, and rapidly progressing disease, such as is caused by subcutaneous injection in suitable doses, has not been produced in this way.

Intra-mammary injection, on the other hand, practised on the cow during lactation, produces, at least when the dose is a large one, an extraordinarily severe form of tuberculosis which may be rapidly fatal (in a few weeks). The disease is peculiar; and there is some reason to think that death may be due to toxæmia, for the animals may die at an early period, before visible lesions have extended beyond the mamma itself and its lymphatic glands. The severity of this toxæmia would seem to be accounted for by the very large mass of tissue which becomes primarily tuberculous, and by the absorption of the products from so large a lesion at an early stage before tolerance or immunity to those poisons has been acquired.

In this method of injection no tissues are wounded, the material containing the bacilli being introduced into the milk sinuses through the duct of the teat by means of a cannula. The injection is followed by a little massage which distributes the material along the tubules. It is very remarkable how completely the bacilli penetrate into every part of the affected quarter, and how even may be the distribution of the miliary tuberculosis which arises therein. The udder swells enormously, and, in severe cases, in a short time a very large quantity of tissue indeed is swarming with tubercle bacilli. The tissues around the udder become œdematous; and petechial hæmorrhages may occur in liver or lungs. The animal sometimes assumes an extraordinary attitude with arched back and feet close together as if suffering from pain in the udder, and convulsions and rigidity with retraction of head may occur towards the end.

During the progress of the work of the Royal Commission 13 cows received intra-mammary injections of bovine tubercle bacilli. All but one were injected with emulsions of tuberculous tissues, the other was injected with culture. No less than nine of these cows died, or were killed in a moribund condition, within 32 to 48 days of the inoculations. The rest, which probably received smaller doses[1] developed a more chronic form of tuberculosis. In three of the cows which died from the tuberculous infection (Nos. 44, 64 and

[1] The numbers of bacilli injected were not estimated in these cases.

Plate XII

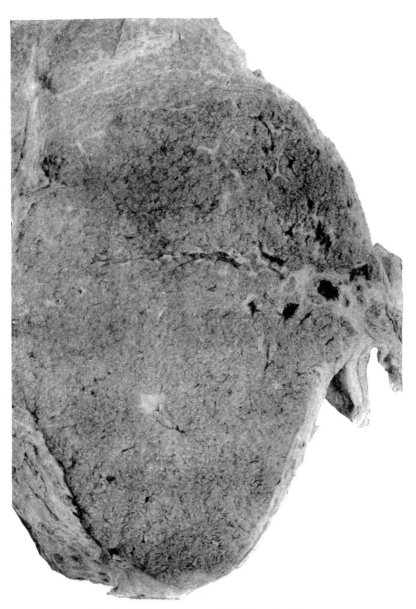

Result of intra-mammary injection of a Cow.
Killed when dying 34 days after injection.

500) there were no macroscopic lesions beyond those in the mamma itself and the lymph glands nearest to it; and in another (No. 75) the visible lesions had extended only as far as the iliac glands. In three others (Nos. 18, 4 and 43) there were lesions in the great organs, but these for the most part were very small and early ones[1].

To infection with the human type of bacillus (except when intravenously injected) the ox is extremely refractory. A necrotic lesion occurs at the seat of injection, and the neighbouring lymphatic glands develop tuberculous changes. The tubercle bacilli probably multiply to some extent in the local lesion, and dissemination undoubtedly occurs, for semi-microscopic lesions may often be found in small numbers in various organs (see p. 253). But the disease never develops a progressive character, no matter how large the dose may have been; and the animals, after a transient disturbance of health, recover their condition, and continue to put on flesh at a normal rate. The lesions however do not necessarily become quickly cured, nor the bacilli killed, outright; for in some cases animals which had been given small doses intravenously, for the purpose of protective inoculation, have developed lesions in the iris or in one of the joints after a year or more[2].

Intravenous injection of human bacilli, however, when the dose is large, and especially when the bacilli are contained in an emulsion of tuberculous tissue, may produce an acute infiltration and œdema of the lungs which proves rapidly fatal; and in some instances of the kind the lesions may even extend to other organs[3]. It seems almost certain that in such cases the bacilli multiply after injection, but they do not continue to do so indefinitely, for in the great majority of cases the disease so produced, if it does not cause death in a few weeks, quickly subsides (see p. 257). This type of fatal disease is not to be regarded as a true infection, but rather as a local intoxication; for the bacilli seem incapable, so to speak, of taking root. Wherever groups of them of sufficient size come to rest, there, owing to the toxin which they contain, little tubercles arise; and these become surrounded by a zone of hyperæmia and œdema.

---

[1] *R.C.T. Int. Rep.* App. vol. I, p. 38, and vol. II. p. 1033.

[2] See pp. 259 and 676.

[3] *E.g.* Calf 361. *R.C.T. Int. Rep.* App. vol. II, p. 175.

If such tubercles occur in the lungs in sufficient number, as they may do after large intravenous injections, they become confluent over considerable regions and produce consolidation sufficiently extensive to cause death by mechanical interference with the respiratory function.

The ox then may be said to be entirely refractory to true infection with the human type of bacillus. If further evidence of this is necessary it may be found in the fact that even direct injection into the functional mammary gland of the cow—a procedure which, when practised with the bovine bacillus, produces such extraordinarily acute results—fails to produce any notable effect if the bacillus is of the human type[1].

Experiments with avian tubercle bacilli on the ox species are not numerous. The most extensive series was made by F. Griffith for the Royal Commission[2]. Fifteen calves were injected subcutaneously with this type of tubercle bacillus derived either from birds or from swine, the doses varying from 10 to 500 mg. In no case was there any disturbance of general health; and when the animals came to be killed they were in good condition, and showed on post-mortem examination little beyond a local lesion, and a caseous or calcareous nodule in the nearest lymphatic gland. There were indeed, in some cases, a few little disseminated lesions, but these were of small size and non-progressive in character. Intravenous injection usually proved fatal; but feeding with an enormous dose of avian bacilli, in the only instance in which this method of infection was tried, resulted only in producing a few small yellowish foci in three of the rectal lymphatic glands.

[1] During the work of the Royal Commission six cows were injected in this manner, five with emulsions of tuberculous tissue containing tubercle bacilli of human type and one with culture. In one of the five (Cow 3) some miliary tubercles appeared in the gland, but the infection did not develop or spread further; in two others (Cows 33 and 43) slight induration of the inoculated quarters was the only result produced; and in the remaining animal (Cow 1) there was no change whatever. (See *R.C.T. Int. Rep.* App. vol. II. See also *postea*, pp. 673 and 674 footnote.)

[2] *R.C.T. Fin. Rep.* App. vol. IV, p. 186.

REFERENCES. X

(Chapter XVIII)

TUBERCULOSIS IN VARIOUS ANIMAL SPECIES.

General.

Friedberger and Fröhner. *Pathologie und Therapie der Haustiere,* vol. II, pl 446.

Gesundheitsamt, Berlin, 1904–1912. *Tuberculose Arbeiten,* Hefte I, III, VI, VII, IX, X, XI, XII.

Koch, R. (1884). *Die Aetiologie der Tuberculose.* Eng. Trans. in *Micro-organisms in Disease.* New Sydenham Soc. 1886.

Nocard (1894). *Les Tuberculoses Animales.* Masson, Paris.

Nocard and Leclainche (1903). *Les Maladies Microbiennes des Animaux.* Masson, Paris.

Report on Tuberculosis in Saxony in the year 1895 (cattle, goats, sheep, and pigs). Abstract in the *Journ. of Comp. Pathol. and Therap.* vol. IX, p. 233.

Royal Commission on Tuberculosis (1907–1911). Reports and Appendices.

Straus (1895). *La Tuberculose.* Rueff, Paris.

United States. *Reports of the Bureau of Animal Industry,* Washington.

Tuberculosis in the Ox.

Bang (1899). Measures to be taken against Tuberculosis of the Domesticated Animals. *Journ. of Comp. Pathol. and Therap.* vol. XII, p. 189.

—— (1905). Bekämpfung der Tuberkulose der Haustiere. *Report VII. Internat. Veterin. Cong. Budapest.*

—— (1908). Measures against Animal Tuberculosis in Denmark. *Report VIth Internat. Cong. on Tuberculosis, Washington,* vol. IV, pt. 2, p. 850.

Cobbett (1907). The Virulence of Tubercle Bacilli of Human Origin for the Ox Species. *R.C.T. Int. Rep.* App. vol. II, p. 1028.

De Haan (1903). Experimentelle Tuberkulose. Java. *Virchows Archiv,* vol. 174, p. 2.

Delépine (1901). The Control of Milk Supplies. *Trans. Brit. Cong. on Tuberc. London,* vol. II, p. 235.

—— (1910). Investigations on the Prevalence and Sources of Tubercle Bacilli in Cow's Milk. *Ann. Rep. Med. Off. Loc. Gov. Bd.* for 1908–9.

—— (1912). Bovine Tuberculosis. *Proc. Nat. Vet. Ass.* 13th Ann. Meeting, Manchester.

De Schweinitz, Dorset and Schroeder (1904). The Comparative Virulence of Human and Bovine Tubercle Bacilli for some large Animals. *21st Ann. Rep. U.S. Bureau of Animal Industry*, Washington, p. 169.

Dorset, M. (1904). Experiments concerning Tuberculosis. *Ibid.* p. 159.

Editorial Article (1892). The Prevalence of Tuberculosis among the Cattle of Great Britain. *Journ of Comp. Pathol. and Therap.* vol. v, p. 56.

—— (1894). Tuberculosis in Young Cattle. *Ibid.* vol. vii, p. 269.

—— (1898). The Relationship between Human and Bovine Tuberculosis. *Ibid.* vol. xi, p. 344.

—— (1900). The Frequency of Tuberculosis among British Cattle. *Ibid.* vol. xiii, p. 68.

Griffith, A. S. (1907). *R.C.T. Int. Rep.* App. vol. i.

—— (1911). The effects produced in Different Species of Animals by the Inoculation of Human Tubercle Bacilli of Bovine and Human Origin. *Ibid. Fin. Rep.* vol. i, p. 28.

Griffith, A. S. and Griffith, F. (1911). The Excretion of Tubercle Bacilli in the Milk of Animals. *Ibid. Fin. Rep.* vol. iii, p. 81.

Griffith, F. (1911). *Ibid. Fin. Rep.* vol. iv.

Kitasato (1904). Ueber das Verhalten der einheimischen Japanischen Rinder zur Tuberculose. *Zeitschf. f. Hygiene*, vol. 48, p. 471.

Koch and Schütz (1902). Menschliche Tuberkulose und Rindertuberkulose. *Archiv f. wissensch. u. prakt. Tierheilkunde*, Nr. 1 and 2.

Kossel, Weber and Heuss (1904). Vergleichende Untersuchungen über Tuberkelbazillen verschiedener Herkunft. I. *Tub. Arbeit. a. d. Kaiserl. Gesundheitsamte*, Heft 1, p. 1.

—— (1905). Pt. ii. *Ibid.* Heft 3, p. 1.

Kruse (1893). Ueber das Vorkommen der sogennanten Hühnertuberkulose beim Menschen und bei Säugetieren. *Zieglers Beiträge zur path. Anat. und allgem. Pathologie*, vol. xii, p. 544.

McFadyean (1889). Tubercular Mastitis in the Cow. *Journ. of Comp. Pathol. and Therap.* vol. ii, p. 119.

—— (1896). Tuberculosis of Cattle. *Ibid.* vol. ix, p. 277

—— (1896). The Infectivity of the Blood, Muscular Tissue and Lymphatic Glands in Generalised Tuberculosis in the Ox. *Ibid.* vol. xi, p. 298.

—— (1898). The Situation and Order of Development of the Lesions in Bovine Tuberculosis. *Ibid.* vol. xi, p. 226.

—— (1914). Tuberculosis. *Ibid.* vol. xxvii, p. 218.

Malm, O. (1914). Tuberculosis. *Ibid.* vol. xxvii, p. 234.

Melvin (1908). The Economic Importance of Tuberculosis of Food-producing animals. *25th Rep. U.S. Bureau of Animal Industry*, p. 97.

Mitchell (1914). The Milk Question in Edinburgh. *The Edinburgh Medical Journal*, April, 1914.

Ostertag (1899). The Use of the Flesh and the Milk of Tuberculous Animals. *Journ. of Comp. Pathol. and Therap*, vol. XII, p. 240.

Pansini (1894). Einige neue Fälle von Geflügeltuberkulose beim Menschen und Säugetieren. *Deutsch. med. Wochenschr.* p. 694.

Ravenel (1902). The Intercommunicability of Human and Bovine Tuberculosis. *Journ. of Comp. Pathol. and Therap.* vol. XV, p. 112.

Royal Commissions on Tuberculosis (1911). *Final Report*, p. 9.

Schroeder and Cotton (1904). Danger of Infection with Tuberculosis by different kinds of exposure. *21st Ann. Rep. U.S. Bureau of Animal Industry*, p. 44.

Schroeder (1908). The Tuberculous Cow and Public Health. *Ibid. 25th Ann. Rep.* p. 109.

Siedamgrotsky (1892). *Das Vorkommen der Tuberkulose bei Schlachttieren i. Kgr. Sachsen.* Abst. in *Baumgarten's Jahresbericht* (1893), vol. IX, p. 767.

Weber (1907). Vergleichende Untersuchungen über Tuberkelbazillen verschiedener Herkunft. *Tub. Arbeit. a. d. Kaiserl. Gesundheitsamte*, Heft 6, p. 1.

Johne's Disease.

De Jong (1905). Das Verhältniss der Tuberkulose des Menschen, des Rindes, des Geflügels, etc. *VIII. Internat. tierärztliche Kongress, Budapest.*

Holth (1912). *Zeitschr. f. Infekt. parasit. Krankh. u. Hyg. d. Haustiere,* vol. XI, p. 378. Abstract in the *Journ. of Comp. Pathol. and Therap.* vol. XXV, p. 148.

Johne and Frothingham (1895). Ein eigentümlichen Fall der Tuberkulose beim Rind. *Deutsch. Zeitschf. f. Tiermedizin,* vol. XXI, p. 138.

McFadyean, Sheather and Edwards (1912). Johne's Disease. *Journ. of Comp. Pathol. and Therap.* vol. XXV, p. 217.

Markus (1904). Eine specifische Darmentzündung des Rindes wahrscheinlich tuberkulose Natur. *Zeitschf. f. Tiermedizin,* vol. VIII, p. 68.

Meyer (1913). The Specific Paratuberculosis of Cattle in America. *Journ. of Med. Res.* vol. XXIX, p. 147.

Twort and Ingram (1912). Myobacterium enteritidis chronicae pseudotuberculosae bovis Jöhne, etc. *Proc. Roy. Soc.* Series B, vol. LXXXIV, p. 517.

Tuberculosis in the Human Breast.

See p. 612.

CHAPTER XIX

THE SUSCEPTIBILITY TO TUBERCULOSIS OF VARIOUS
ANIMAL SPECIES (*continued*)

TUBERCULOSIS IN SWINE, GOATS AND SHEEP.

Tuberculosis in Swine.

Next to the ox, among the domesticated mammals which
suffer from tuberculosis, the pig takes the second place. In
the former species, as we have seen, it is the milch cow which
is the chief sufferer, and young animals are less often affected.
The pig probably suffers from tuberculosis almost as often as
these latter, and, in some countries at least, among the animals
slaughtered for food is more commonly found affected with
the disease than the ox itself[1].

Tuberculosis in pigs is believed to be contracted, as a rule,
from the ox, either in consequence of their being fed on
separated milk, or of consuming the fæces· of tuberculous
cattle. It is very common in certain districts and on particular
farms, and especially rife in localities and countries where the
dairy industry is largely developed, as in Denmark[2]; while
in other parts, such as the states of Arkansas, Oklahoma and
Texas in the United States where the hogs are allowed to
roam over large areas of pasture and shift for themselves,
and in the forest regions of Hungary where they run in the
woods, swine tuberculosis is said to be rare[3].

[1] In U.S.A., in 1908, nearly 750,000 pigs slaughtered under Federal
inspection were found to be tuberculous; and the proportion of animals
recognized as thus infected was 2 per cent. At the same time the proportion
of slaughtered cattle found to be similarly affected was, as we have seen
already, not quite 1 per cent. (Melvin, 25th Rep. U.S. Bureau of Animal
Industry, p. 98.)

The statistics of the Federal slaughter-houses in the Argentine Republic
show that the percentage of tuberculous swine is greater than that of tuberculous cattle. This is however not the case in most European countries.
(Mohler and Washburn, 24th Rep. U.S. Bureau of Animal Industry, p. 218.)

[2] See footnote No. 2 on p. 399.

[3] Mohler and Washburn, loc. cit. p. 217.

The prevalence of tuberculosis in pigs, as revealed by slaughter-house statistics, varies greatly in different countries; being low in France, moderate in England and the United States, and high, for the most part, in Germany, Denmark, New Zealand and Argentina. The older returns as a rule are much lower than modern ones; and for this reason swine tuberculosis is believed to be on the increase; but it is by no means certain that the increase in the number of cases reported is not due to more thorough inspection, and especially to an increasing recognition of local tuberculosis[1]; nevertheless it is probable that where the dairy industry has developed there tuberculosis among pigs has been increasing.

Among the older figures we may take those of Lydtin, who collected the statistics of Baden Baden for the years 1874–82. Though about 8000 pigs were slaughtered there each year, only 22 were reported in these nine years as tuberculous; at Rouen, among 38,164 pigs slaughtered in four years, Veyssière found only 15, or 0·04 per cent., tuberculous. At Berlin, however, in 1883–4 the proportion at different abattoirs varied from 0·5 to 0·9 per cent.[2]

More recent statistics give considerably higher figures. As examples of these we may conveniently take those quoted by Buchanan in a Report to the Local Government Board in 1906[3]. In Prussia during the three years 1900–1–2 the proportion of pigs regarded as tuberculous was 2·49, 2·72 and 2·91 respectively. In Berlin alone in each of the four years ending March, 1902, the corresponding figures were 3·9, 4·0, 5·79 and

[1] Deetz, who examined the statistics of the slaughter-houses of Berlin extending over a series of years, came to the conclusion that tuberculosis was increasing, not only among hogs, but also among cattle. In Buenos Ayres the percentage of hogs recognized as tuberculous among those slaughtered at the abattoirs rose steadily from 6·5 in 1898 to 10·23 in 1904. But it may well be questioned whether this indicates a real increase in the frequency of the disease; for an analysis of the figures for Liniers, one of the districts of the city (as given by Mohler and Washburn) shows that the increase in the returns was due entirely to an increase in localized tuberculosis (from 3·32 to 9·33 per cent.), while the proportion of hogs reported as affected with general tuberculosis actually fell, during the same period, from 3·21 to 0·9 per cent. (Mohler and Washburn, *loc. cit.* p. 218.)

[2] Straus, *loc. cit.* p. 341.

[3] *Reports of the Medical Inspectors of the L.G.B.* No. 225.

5·13 respectively. These percentages are based on large figures, between 650,000 and 850,000 pigs being annually slaughtered in Berlin.

In 17 German towns, in 1901–2, the proportion of swine recognized as tuberculous at the public slaughter-houses exceeded 4 per cent. For the whole Kingdom of Saxony the corresponding percentages for the five years ending with 1903 were 3·03, 3·5, 3·79, 4·81 and 4·81. In the Kingdom of Bavaria, on the other hand, the proportion of swine recognized as tuberculous in the years 1895–1903 did not exceed 1 per cent.[1]

In the Netherlands, out of 368,428 pigs slaughtered in 1903–4, under official supervision, for export to Great Britain, 5516, or 1·5 per cent., were found to be tuberculous (Buchanan).

In New Zealand, in 1907, out of 100,731 pigs examined 5·89 per cent. were found to be affected with tuberculosis of one degree or another (Mohler and Washburn).

In the Argentine Republic tuberculosis of swine seems to be exceedingly common; the proportion of these animals found to be tuberculous in the abattoirs of Buenos Ayres having been 6·5 per cent. in 1898, and 10·86 per cent. in 1903.

In the United States the proportion of tuberculous hogs among all those slaughtered under Federal inspection was stated by Mohler and Washburn in 1907 to be 1·5 per cent.[2] In 1908, however, it was 2·0 per cent.[3]

In the London Corporation slaughter-houses at Islington, Buchanan tells us, the veterinary inspector found tuberculosis in 75 out of 15,225 pigs examined in 1904, that is to say in 0·5 per cent. On the other hand in the same year in Glasgow, where there are no private slaughter-houses, and

---

[1] Most of these German figures seem very high in comparison with those of other countries, and Buchanan remarks concerning them that doubtless the diagnosis was based on naked-eye appearances without microscopical examination, and there is a possibility therefore that certain non-tuberculous affections were classed from time to time as tuberculous. But one would suppose that this source of error would apply equally to the statistics of other countries also; and, on the other hand, it is possible that in Germany inspection was stricter than elsewhere.

[2] *loc. cit.* p. 215.　　　　　　　　[3] Melvin, *ibid.* 25*th Rep.* p. 98.

where consequently all pigs killed come under official inspection, no less than 4·24 per cent. were found to be tuberculous in one degree or another, a proportion which corresponds closely enough with those recorded in Berlin.

Quite recently in this country the Local Government Board has conducted a laboratory investigation of swine tuberculosis[1] in which great care was taken to seek for minimal and localized, as well as more severe, lesions. For the purpose of this investigation over 24,000 pigs slaughtered in the borough abattoir at Brighton were specially examined, with the result that 2·74 per cent. were found to have tuberculous lesions of some kind. These cases are classified according to the distribution of the lesions as follows:

Tuberculosis in 24,000 swine at Brighton.

General Tuberculosis	0·87 per cent.
Slightly Disseminated Tuberculosis .	1·63 per cent.
Localized Tuberculosis . . .	0·24 per cent.

This large proportion of cases of localized and slightly disseminated disease strongly suggests that stricter inspection in one locality than in another may go far to explain differences in the frequency with which tuberculosis is reported in different places; for easy-going inspectors are not likely to take cognizance of local or minimal disease. Nevertheless there can be no doubt at all that a very real difference of this kind actually exists, however much it may be obscured or exaggerated by the source of error referred to.

The Sources of Tuberculous Infection in Swine. The tuberculosis of swine is, as was said before, commonly believed to be contracted from cattle, either by feeding on the separated milk of tuberculous cows, or by consuming the droppings of tuberculous cattle[2]. For evidence of this we must refer to

[1] Eastwood and F. Griffith, 1914, *Reps. of the L.G.B. on Public Health and Medical Subjects*, N.S. No. 91, p. 184.

[2] The importance of the kind of food given to the pigs is shown by the following example cited by Mohler and Washburn. "A great many hogs in Texas are raised on alfalfa (lucerne) supplemented with corn, and the result is clearly shown in the Bureau statistics, which indicate that from Jan. 1 to June 30, 1907, only 0·1 per cent. of several thousand hogs slaughtered at Fort Worth showed tuberculous lesions. In striking contrast to this are the

Mohler and Washburn's paper, already quoted more than once. Swine tuberculosis is undoubtedly very prevalent in states and countries where the dairy industry is important, and probably too much importance in this connection cannot be attributed to separated milk. Nevertheless it is by no means certain that tuberculosis does not also spread from pig to pig; and, as we shall see, some of the localized and less severe forms of tuberculosis in swine are probably caused by eating the bodies of tuberculous fowls or their droppings, or even tuberculous sputum from man.

Distribution of the Lesions. Tuberculosis in the pig may be more or less widely generalized, or limited to one or several lymphatic glands, especially to the submaxillary. Localized tuberculosis is probably rather common. In the Brighton series, as we have already seen, the disease was localized in about one-eleventh of the infected animals; and localized or only slightly disseminated in more than two-thirds.

When the disease is generalized the lungs as a rule are affected more or less severely; liver and spleen too are very liable to be attacked; but the kidneys are said usually to escape. When the lesions are disseminated widely tuberculous foci are not uncommon in the bones[1]. Tuberculosis in the muscles has been recorded both by Straus[2] and by Koch[3].

In the series of cases examined by A. S. and F. Griffith the joints were affected in three cases out of 63[4], and the shaft

percentages, for the same period, of three cities in one of the leading dairy States which show a frequency of infection of 3·1, 3·4 and 6·4 respectively." (*Loc. cit.* p. 217.) In Denmark too, where the dairy industry is of great importance, tuberculosis is very common in pigs. In 1895 no less than 11·38 per cent. of 8569 swine slaughtered in Copenhagen were found by Bang to be tuberculous. (Straus, *La tuberculose*, p. 342.) (Mohler and Washburn, *loc. cit.* p. 220.)

For evidence of the presence of tubercle bacilli in the fæces of tuberculous cattle, and the part played by them in the propagation of swine tuberculosis see Mohler and Washburn, 24*th Rep. Bureau of Animal Industry*, pp. 220 and 224, and also Bulletin No. 99 of the same Bureau. Melvin's opinion on this point may be found in the 25*th Report*, p. 50.

[1] Kersten and Ungermann, 1912, *Tub. Arbeit. a. d. Kaiserl. Gesundheitsamte*, Heft 11, p. 184.   [2] *La tuberculose*, p. 343.
[3] *The Etiology of Tuberculosis*, Eng. trans. p. 127.
[4] *R.C.T. Fin. Rep.* App. vol. III, pp. 154–166. See p. lvi, p. lix, and p. lxiii.

of a rib in another[1]. The mammary glands of the sow are said by Mohler and Washburn to be less often affected than that of the cow. In two cases recorded by the Griffiths, however, these glands were tuberculous[2], and in another case there was tuberculosis of the supramammary lymphatic gland[3]. These facts, seeing that the great majority of pigs in this series were young ones, and that there do not seem to have been more than five adult sows among the tuberculous, are suggestive, and seem to point to a rather high incidence of tuberculosis in the functional mammæ of the sow.

The pig may continue to fatten in spite of the advance of tuberculous disease; and several observers, including Mohler and Washburn, have remarked how good may be the apparent condition of these animals even when severely affected. The writer also, while he was working for the Royal Commission, was very much struck by the apparently healthy appearance of pigs suffering from rather advanced experimental tuberculosis.

Portals of Entry. On the question of the portals through which tubercle bacilli most commonly reach the living tissues of the pig, opinions differ. Koch, in 1884, seems to have believed that these micro-organisms usually enter with the air directly into the lungs; and he described five cases where there was a peculiar caseous pneumonia which appeared to him to have arisen from the inhalation of large masses of bacilli. Kersten and Ungermann, 1912, supported this view. They examined seventeen cases of natural tuberculosis in the pig, and found the lungs and thoracic glands affected in every one.

On the other hand Straus thought that primary tuberculosis of the lungs was uncommon in the pig; and in one of Koch's cases the disease, which looked as if it was recent in the lungs, appeared to have originated in the tonsils; for in the situation where these should have been were deep tuberculous ulcers[4].

---

[1] *Ibid.* p. lxiii.   [2] *Ibid.* p. vi, p. lviii.
[3] *Ibid.* p. lxiii. The mammary glands in this case were not sent for examination.
[4] *The Etiology of Tuberculosis*, Eng. trans. p. 126.

In many instances of natural tuberculosis in swine the disease is limited to the lymphatic glands which receive the lymph from one part or another of the alimentary canal. Sometimes it is the mesenteric glands which are thus affected; but far more often it is the glands of the neck, and especially the submaxillary. Mohler and Washburn, 1907, referring to slaughter-house statistics, state that these glands are affected in 93 per cent. of the tuberculous animals; and they believed that infection takes place usually through some part of the alimentary canal.

A. S. Griffith and F. Griffith, 1911, who examined 63 cases of natural tuberculosis in pigs for the Royal Commission, found the submaxillary glands affected in 90 per cent. In many the only lesion seemed to be in this situation. In every one of their animals with two exceptions, they say, the disease appeared to be of alimentary origin[1].

The close association of swine tuberculosis with the dairy industry to which reference has already been made, and the fact that in districts where this industry prevails separated milk, which, as we know, frequently contains tubercle bacilli, is largely used for feeding pigs, are also greatly in favour of the view that tuberculous infection in this species occurs commonly through the walls of some part of the alimentary canal.

Again, experimental investigation has shown that pigs are very easily infected by feeding with substances which contain tubercle bacilli; especially young pigs, in which the disease so caused may spread rapidly to the various great organs. In older animals it is apt to remain limited to the glands in the neck or mesentery. The intestinal mucous membrane in such cases often escapes infection, but the tonsils and the pharyngeal mucous membrane are more commonly the seat of macroscopic lesions[2].

On the whole then it seems that pigs when they contract tuberculosis do so commonly by taking in tubercle bacilli with

[1] R. C. T. Fin. Rep. App. vol. III, p. 151. In the two cases excepted the condition of the glands of the alimentary canal were not ascertained.

[2] A. S. Griffith, R.C.T. Int. Rep. App. vol. I, pp. 591, 631, 696 and 707. See also p. 408 of this volume.

their food; and that the bacilli enter the tissues through some part of the pharyngeal or, less frequently, the intestinal mucous membrane. At the same time it is not impossible that in some instances infection arises in consequence of bacilli suspended in the air entering the bronchi.

The Comparative Susceptibility of Swine to Infection with the Three Types of Tubercle Bacilli.

Natural Infection. The tubercle bacillus which is found in the great majority of cases of tuberculosis in swine conforms, as might be supposed, to the bovine type. As a rule it does not depart from that type in any particular, but sometimes, in rare cases, attenuated strains are met with. On the other hand in no inconsiderable minority of cases the bacillus belongs to the avian, and in a few even to the human type. Such however are, almost without exception, cases of localized disease. It is scarcely too much to say that in generalized tuberculosis in swine the bacillus is always of the bovine type.

A. S. Griffith and F. Griffith, working for the Royal Commission[1], made a careful investigation of the types of tubercle bacilli present in swine tuberculosis. For this purpose tuberculous organs of pigs were sent to them from the Metropolitan Meat Market. Cases of localized disease were specially sought for, but instances of tuberculosis of all degrees of severity were included. From these sources 59 strains of tubercle bacilli were isolated in culture and their properties thoroughly investigated, many different kinds of animals being used for the purpose.

Forty-nine of the strains resembled in every particular strains of bovine bacilli derived from the ox itself. In addition there was one strain which conformed to the bovine type except that its virulence for various animals was not up to the bovine standard. There was also one mixture of bovine and avian bacilli, and there were five pure avian strains, and three pure human strains.

Thus bovine tubercle bacilli either alone or mixed with others were found in 86 per cent. of the cases, and pure bovine strains,

---

[1] *R.C.T. Fin. Rep.* App. vol. III, p. 145.

typical in every particular, in 85 per cent. The proportion of bovine strains would doubtless have been considerably higher if the material had been unselected; for all the strains other than those of bovine type came from cases of localized tuberculosis, and, as was said above, such were specially sought out for the investigation.

The bovine type of bacillus alone was found in every case of generalized disease, and in nine out of the 17 or 18 cases of localized tuberculosis, as well as in nine cases in which the extent of the disease was not recorded.

More recently Eastwood and F. Griffith, 1914, have conducted for the Local Government Board a somewhat similar investigation to which we have already referred. We have now to consider what types of bacilli were found by these authors.

The tuberculous material was obtained from pigs slaughtered in Birmingham and Brighton, and was selected from cases in which the disease, so far as could be ascertained by careful inspection, was limited to certain glands. A few cases of slightly disseminated tuberculosis were added for comparison. Strains of tubercle bacilli were isolated from this material, and their cultural and pathogenetic properties determined by suitable experiments. The results were as follows:

Of five cases of disseminated tuberculosis all yielded the bovine type of bacillus.

Of 73 cases of apparently localized tuberculosis 44 yielded only bovine bacilli. In two of these the virulence was less than the standard of the type. No less than 26 yielded avian bacilli. In only one case was the human type of bacillus alone. In addition one case yielded both bovine and avian, and another both bovine and human bacilli.

Two of the 26 cases from which the only *tubercle* bacillus isolated was of the avian type yielded in addition some other acid-fast bacilli.

The avian bacillus was thus the only tubercle bacillus found in nearly 36 per cent. of the cases of localized tuberculosis. But the proportions were very different in the Birmingham and Brighton series; in the former it was 29 per cent.; in the latter it was 40 per cent. This is perhaps no more than might be expected,

for the ratio of avian to bovine infections in any given place
will doubtless depend largely upon the extent to which the pigs
associate with fowls and with cows respectively, and this will
be likely to differ a good deal in different localities[1].

Types of Tubercle Bacilli found in Tuberculous Swine
(Eastwood and F. Griffith).

Type of Bacillus	Local Tuberculosis			Disseminated Tuberculosis
	Birmingham	Brighton	Total	Brighton
Bovine ..	20	22	42	5
,, attenuated	1	1	2	0
Avian ..	9	17	26	0
Human ..	0	1	1	0
Bov. + Av. ..	1	0	1	0
Bov. + Hu. ..	0	1	1	0
Total ..	31	42	73	5

The avian bacillus alone was found only in cases of localized
tuberculosis. But it must be understood that this term is
used in the sense in which it would be commonly employed
in the slaughter-house, and is not strictly accurate. As a
matter of fact more careful search in the laboratory revealed,
in about one-third of these "localized" cases, minute tubercles
in lungs and liver, and in bronchial or portal lymphatic glands.
In the remainder, 18 in number, the submaxillary or mesenteric glands alone were visibly tuberculous, even on minute
inspection in the laboratory, but it must be added that in about
one-third even of these more strictly limited cases inoculation
of guinea-pigs with emulsions of one or more apparently
normal organs (lungs, liver, spleen and, in one case, muscle)
revealed the presence of tubercle bacilli in one or other of
these situations[2].

[1] In the Royal Commission investigation the proportion of cases of localized
tuberculosis which yielded only avian tubercle bacilli seems to have been
about 29 per cent. as in Birmingham.
[2] *loc. cit.* p. 129.

The two atypical, or attenuated, strains of bovine bacilli deserve special mention. In cultural characters they were quite typical, one being "highly dysgonic," and the other "producing no more than a thin, translucent, somewhat moist, finely wrinkled or warty layer on glycerin-agar[1]." In virulence for the rabbit however, and in one case for the guinea-pig also, they fell below the standard of the bovine type. Passage through the rabbit did not increase the virulence of either strain for this species.

The two cases which yielded more than one type of bacillus were as follows: In one the submaxillary glands yielded a pure strain of bovine bacilli, and the mesenteric a pure strain of avian bacilli. In the other the submaxillary glands yielded a pure culture of bovine bacilli, while from the apparently normal liver there was obtained through a guinea-pig inoculated with an emulsion of the organ a culture which was "eugonic in growth, and, like the common eugonic bacillus of human origin, of low virulence for rabbits[2]."

In the meantime, in the Gesundheitsamt, investigation of tuberculosis as it occurs naturally in the pig had, with one exception, resulted only in the discovery of the bovine type of bacillus. This is easily explained on the ground that the investigators did not specially study local tuberculosis.

Kossel, Weber and Heuss, 1904[3], investigated seven cases of tuberculosis in swine. All yielded cultures of the bovine type.

Zwick, 1908[4], likewise investigated four cases and found only bacilli of bovine type.

Kersten and Ungermann, 1912[5], investigated 19 cases (17 unselected, and 2 selected because there was a suspicion that they might be caused by bacilli of human type[6]). All 19 yielded cultures which corresponded exactly in cultural characters and pathogenicity for the rabbit with the bovine type of tubercle bacillus.

Weber and Bofinger, 1904, briefly reported the isolation of a strain of tubercle bacilli of avian type from the mesenteric glands of a young pig which showed no signs of tuberculosis elsewhere[7].

The conclusion to be drawn from all these investigations is obvious. Tubercle bacilli of avian and even of human type

---

[1] *loc. cit.* p. 82. [2] *loc. cit.* p. 127.

[3] *Tub. Arbeit. a. d. Kaiserl. Gesundheitsamte*, Heft 1, p. 24, and Heft 3, p. 52.

[4] 1908, *Zeitsch. f. Hygiene u. Infect.* vol. IV, p. 161.

[5] 1912, *Tub. Arbeit. a. d. Kaiserl. Gesundheitsamte*, Heft 11, p. 171.

[6] Two of Kersten and Ungermann's cases were investigated because there was a suspicion that the infection might have spread to the pigs from a tuberculous attendant. The owner of one of the animals in question had a tuberculous fistula in his leg, and the pig had never been given cow's milk. In the case of the other animal the tuberculosis seemed to have spread from a castration wound. But the suspicion in neither case was confirmed, both the strains of bacilli isolated from these animals being typical examples of the bovine type.

[7] *Ibid.* 1904, Heft 1, p. 95.

do occasionally cause tuberculous lesions in the pig under natural conditions. But their virulence for this species of animal is low, and the disease which they cause does not spread appreciably, but remains as a rule limited, at least so far as gross lesions are concerned, to one or more of the lymphatic glands nearest the portal of entry. Practically all cases of generalized, or at least of obviously generalized, tuberculosis in the pig seem to be caused by the bovine type of tubercle bacillus.

At the same time it has been shown that the apparently normal organs of pigs in which foci of dissemination, however minute in size, are to be discovered may contain tubercle bacilli; and in one case avian tubercle bacilli have been demonstrated (by guinea-pig inoculation) in the apparently normal muscle of a pig infected with "localized" tuberculosis[1].

But the danger to man arising out of this source of infection in his food cannot be great, for in such cases as we are now considering the bacilli present in apparently normal tissues are few in number, and it must be seldom that they escape death by cooking.

These investigations which we have been considering, together with the inoculation and feeding experiments which will presently be described, dispose once and for all of the legends of epidemics of swine tuberculosis derived from infected fowls or tuberculous human attendants[2].

Experimental Infection.

(A) *The Bovine Tubercle Bacillus.* It is easy to cause tuberculosis experimentally in the pig by any of the ordinary processes of artificial infection, provided only that the bovine type of bacillus is employed. The avian and the human types have, as we shall see, much less effect.

Subcutaneously injected in doses of 10 or 50 mg., the bovine bacillus produces rapidly fatal miliary tuberculosis. Doses of 1·0, or even 0·1 mg., of bacilli have caused general

---

[1] Eastwood and F. Griffith, *loc. cit.* pp. 129 and 131.

[2] For one such legend see Mohler and Washburn, 1908, *25th Rep. Bureau of Animal Industry,* p. 166.

tuberculosis of a severe and progressive type. But the pig is not incapable of resistance, and, according to A. S. Griffith, the disease after such small doses may sometimes become arrested[1].

By feeding with bovine bacilli contained in milk it is quite easy to infect the pig. In experiments made by the Royal Commission 10, 1·0, and even 0·1 mg. thus administered produced general tuberculosis. The disease after 10 mg. was severe, but that caused by the smaller doses was, at the end of three months, only of moderate severity[2].

Eastwood and Griffith[3] fed 16 pigs, when about four months old, with much smaller doses of bovine bacilli. Quantities of ·001–·005 mg. given to eight pigs caused local tuberculosis in two, and nothing at all in the other six. Larger amounts— ·01–0·1 mg.—given to eight pigs caused disease in all but one, and in six there was more or less dissemination.

A. S. Griffith was struck by the difference in susceptibility of young and old pigs. He says that tuberculosis is readily set up in either by feeding. But while in the young it is usually of the progressive type, in the adult, which is much more resistant, the disease does not spread so readily, and may even become arrested at the glands nearest the portal of entry[4].

To sum up then it may be said that experiment has shown that the pig reacts to infection with the bovine type of tubercle bacillus very much like the ox, but that its powers of resistance are distinctly inferior[5].

(B) The Human Tubercle Bacillus. There has been some confusion in the past concerning the susceptibility of swine to infection with the human tubercle bacillus, largely owing to some early experiments in America; and an erroneous belief grew

[1] R.C.T. Int. Rep. App. vol. I, p. 47.
[2] Ibid. p. 632 and vol. II, p. 1156.
[3] L.G.B. Reports on Public Health, etc. N.S. No. 91, part 2, p. 130.
[4] R.C.T. Int. Rep. App. vol. I, pp. 706 and 592.
[5] A. S. Griffith says "the calf is much less susceptible (to experimental infection with the bovine bacillus) than the pig, and a larger dose of bacilli is necessary to produce generalized disease." Ibid. vol. I, p. 707.

Schroeder and Mohler, 1907, believed that swine are more easily affected by feeding than guinea-pigs, and this is certainly the case.

up that "pigs are susceptible to infection with both bovine and human tubercle, and bovine tubercle is no more active for these animals than human sputum[1]." That this is not the case has been proved conclusively by more recent experiments, the work of the Royal Commission and of the Gesundheitsamt having made it clear that the pig is highly resistant to human tuberculosis, though not quite to the same extent as the ox.

In the laboratories of the Commission 50 mg. of bacilli of human type have produced definite lesions at the seat of inoculation together with some slight dissemination, very like what is sometimes seen in the calf. But the disseminated lesions in the pig are more constant, more numerous, and more severe. Some of them may have caseous centres. Nevertheless the human bacillus seems to be just as incapable in the pig as in the ox of producing a progressive type of disease[2].

Administered by the mouth the human tubercle bacillus is even less capable of causing progressive tuberculosis in swine than when injected under the skin. Lesions indeed of some sort commonly occur in the lymphatic glands which receive the lymph from the alimentary canal, and occasionally some small disseminated foci may arise in one or other of the internal organs. But the severity of the disease is minimal, and its character non-progressive. It makes no appreciable difference to the animal's condition[3].

As evidence of this the following example may be given. Two young pigs were fed, for five and eight months respectively,

---

[1] Dinwiddie. Quoted from Mohler and Washburn, 24th Rep. Bureau of Animal Industry, 1907, p. 230.

[2] R.C.T. Int. Rep. App. vol. II, p. 1156. A. S. Griffith says on this point: "The pig, like the calf and the goat, is very resistant to the human tubercle bacillus. It appears however to be slightly more susceptible than the calf, since disseminated lesions were" (in his experiments) "numerous and more frequently present." (R.C.T. Fin. Rep. App. vol. I, p. 44.)

[3] With this opinion the German investigators are in substantial agreement. Kossel, Weber and Heuss say indeed that their experiments show that the human type of bacillus is more virulent for pigs than for cattle: in the former the lesions caused by feeding are not confined to the mucous membrane and the regional lymphatic glands, but may extend to the (deep) cervical glands, and to the thoracic organs. "Nevertheless," they add, "the virulence of the human type of bacillus for swine stands far behind that of the bovine bacillus." (Tub. Arbeit. a. d. Kaiserl. Gesundheitsamte, Heft 3, p. 30.)

almost daily, with enormous quantities of human sputum containing innumerable tubercle bacilli. They throve and grew fat, and when killed no lesions were found except a few small calcareous tubercles in the mesenteric and submaxillary glands, and, in one animal, a little group of doubtful tubercles contained in a pea-sized nodule in one of the lungs[1].

A. S. Griffith, who fed five pigs with tubercle bacilli of human type, remarked that even when the glands were affected the mucous membrane never showed any lesion which might indicate the point at which the bacilli had penetrated[2].

Eastwood and F. Griffith fed two pigs with cultures of tubercle bacilli of human type, the doses being 10 and 50 mg.[3] of bacilli respectively. Both animals developed tuberculosis of the submaxillary and mesenteric glands and also exhibited a slight amount of visible dissemination in the organs.

(C) *The Avian Tubercle Bacillus.* After what has been said in another chapter concerning the serious effects of injecting intravenously tubercle bacilli of a type which is incapable, when administered in any other way, of causing fatal or progressive disease in the species of animal in question, the statement will not appear surprising that injected in this manner, in sufficient quantity, avian bacilli prove fatal to the pig. Introduced by any other channel they show themselves incapable of setting up progressive disease, though they may multiply at the outset and become disseminated about the body, where they remain alive in the organs for considerable periods of time.

That they are not entirely harmless the experiments which are about to be related will show; but on the whole it is rather surprising than otherwise, when one remembers that naturally

---

[1] *R.C.T. Int. Rep.* App. vol. II, pp. 68 and 71, Pigs 1 and 3.

[2] *Ibid. Fin. Rep.* App. vol. I, p. 49. Griffith, summing up the results of his experiments, says that "they prove conclusively that the human tubercle bacillus is unable when ingested to set up anything more than a limited retrogressive tuberculosis in swine," and he adds that "repeated doses continued during long periods are not more effective than a single dose." (*Ibid.*)

[3] It will be noticed that these doses were several hundred times as large as the doses which they employed in the case of bovine bacilli. See Pigs 13, 14, *loc. cit.* pp. 117–118.

acquired tuberculosis in the pig is sometimes caused by the avian bacillus (although the disease is then, as we have seen, always more or less limited in extent) to find that the results of experimental inoculation of this type of bacillus into the species in question are not more considerable.

Mohler and Washburn[1], 1908, investigated an outbreak of swine tuberculosis in Oregon which appeared to have spread to these animals from poultry. Owing to the distance of Oregon from Washington where the investigations were carried out and to the consequent condition of the organs on arrival at the laboratory, it was not possible to study the type of bacillus present in the lesions of the pigs; but the organs of some of the infected birds were used for feeding experiments. Two pigs were infected in this way. One developed tuberculosis in mesenteric and submaxillary glands and liver, and tubercle bacilli were found in the apparently normal spleen. The second pig developed tuberculosis in submaxillary and mesenteric glands. From the affected animals cultures were obtained which conformed in morphological and cultural characters with the avian type.

The authors seem to have been greatly impressed with these results, but subsequent investigations have shown that their importance was exaggerated.

Titze[2], working at the Gesundheitsamt, fed during 58 days four young pigs with 40 glycerin-serum cultures of avian tubercle bacilli. The results were local or minimal.

One pig, killed about six months after the commencement of the experimental feeding, was found to have some dry yellow tubercles, varying in size from a pin's head to a hazel nut, in the portal and mesenteric glands; another, killed after a year, had numerous pin-head yellow foci in all the mesenteric glands; a third, also killed after a year, was found to be sound throughout. The fourth animal is interesting. It died much wasted with a severe infection of the intestines with nematoid worms. In the mucous membrane of the small intestine, and in the cæcum, were numerous yellow dry crumbly nodules, many of them ulcerated, and others with a central pin-sized opening. The mesenteric and portal glands were much swollen and the spleen greatly enlarged. There were no tuberculous lesions, but in the spleen, liver, and abdominal lymphatic glands there were numerous acid-fast bacilli. In the

---

[1] "Transmission of Avian Tuberculosis to Mammals," 25th Rep. U.S. Bureau of Animal Industry, 1908, p. 165.

[2] Tub. Arbeit. a. d. Kaiserl. Gesundheitsamte, Heft 6, p. 216, Pig No. 2.

bronchial glands and lungs these could not be found. Titze thinks that the extensive ulceration of the intestine caused by the worms afforded an opportunity for the avian tubercle bacilli to penetrate in large numbers into the organs.

Numerous experiments with the avian tubercle bacillus were made for the Royal Commission, 1911, by F. Griffith[1]. Referring to the pig and to some other animals he says: "after subcutaneous inoculation and feeding these animals never developed a progressive tuberculosis, and have rarely shown more than disease localized to the seat of inoculation and to the nearest lymphatic glands[2]." But he goes on to point out that there may be a remarkable dissemination and multiplication of avian bacilli in the organs of the pig, just as occurs in the guinea-pig[3]. "After intravenous inoculations with moderately large doses, they succumb almost invariably to the toxic effects of the bacilli multiplying in their tissues."

Tuberculosis in the Goat.

The goat was at one time believed to be immune to tuberculosis; but this supposed immunity, like that ascribed to several other species, proved to be a myth. Several investigators, Bollinger, 1873, Colin, 1891, and Cadiot, Gilbert and Roger, 1893, succeeded in producing tuberculosis experimentally in this species; and during the last part of the century many cases of naturally acquired disease came to light[4].

[1] R.C.T. Fin. Rep. App. vol. IV, pp. 167, 245 et seq.

[2] Ibid. p. 172. In respect to its reaction to infection with the avian tubercle bacillus F. Griffith classes the pig along with the calf, horse, monkey, cat and guinea-pig.

[3] "In the case of three pigs, inoculated intraperitoneally, subcutaneously, and by feeding, respectively, with culture of the same virus, there was dissemination and great multiplication of tubercle bacilli in the organs, and though the animals had not apparently suffered in general health up to the time when they were killed they nevertheless did not increase in weight at the usual rate." (Loc. cit. p. 172.) Titze also observed a very similar dissemination in the pig fed with these bacilli. (Tub. Arbeit. a. d. Kaiserl. Gesundheitsamte, Heft 6, p. 218.)

[4] Frosch and Hertha, 1901, thought that among the domesticated animals, classed according to their liability to suffer from tuberculosis, the goat took the third place, after the ox and the pig. But it is only a bad third at the best, and it may be doubted whether the dog is not as frequently a victim, and possibly the cat and the horse are not a very long way behind.

In 1884 Koch described a single case, and noted the existence of cavities in the lungs (which are now known to be rather characteristic of tuberculosis in this species) and the presence of tubercle bacilli. Lydtin in 1884 described three cases, Nocard in 1890 another. At the Congress for the Study of Tuberculosis held in Paris in 1892 Thomassen reported a case from the abattoir at Amsterdam, and Moulé and Weber another, while Siegen stated that he had seen no less than 10 cases.

Mr Alston Edgar in 1892 reported an instance which was confirmed by McFadyean who found tubercle bacilli in the lesions. McFadyean considered that this was probably the first authentic case described in this country.

A. S. Griffith has met with a case quite recently.

An outbreak of tuberculosis in a herd of 28 goats in Saxony was mentioned by Thompson (1904) as having been related by Eichhorn[1]. One of the animals was brought to the veterinary school because it was ill; and having died there, was found to be tuberculous. The rest of the herd was then tested with tuberculin, with the result that no less than 18 animals reacted. The owner would only allow three of them to be slaughtered. This accordingly was done, two animals which had reacted and one which had not reacted being selected. The latter was found free from disease, but the other two were proved to be tuberculous.

In the Report of the United States Bureau of Animal Industry, 1904, some interesting slaughter-house statistics are quoted by Thompson[2]. In Saxony in 1894 10 goats out of 1562 slaughtered were pronounced to be tuberculous, or 0·64 per cent.[3] In Prussia in 1899 tuberculosis was detected in 148 out of 47,705, or 0·3 per cent. of the goats slaughtered.

In the United States tuberculosis would seem to be extremely rare in the goat, for Melvin[4], Chief of the Bureau

[1] Quoted by Thompson, 1904, in the *21st Rep. of the U.S. Bureau of Animal Industry* from the *Deutsche landwirtschaftliche Presse*.

[2] *Ibid.* p. 342.

[3] In the following year (1895) out of 3007 goats slaughtered in Saxony 13, or 0·4 per cent., were found to be tuberculous (see article in the *Journ. of Pathol. and Therap.* vol. IX, p. 233).

[4] *25th Ann. Rep. U.S. Bureau of Animal Industry*, p. 98.

of Animal Industry, states that out of 46,000 goats slaughtered under Government inspection in that country one only was reported to be affected with tuberculosis.

Whether we accept as representative the American figures, or the much higher ones quoted by Thompson for Prussia, it is evident that goats enjoy a comparative freedom from tuberculosis which is in marked contrast to the frequency of the disease in the ox. And this is the more remarkable because, as we shall see, the goat is not a whit behind the ox in its susceptibility to tuberculosis artificially induced, either by inoculation or by feeding.

Petersen, referring to the figures for Prussia mentioned above, remarks with astonishment on the small amount of tuberculosis among the goats, for they were kept, he says, under conditions very favourable to the spread of tuberculosis, running freely among the cattle[1]. But, after all, the amount of tuberculosis found in them, namely 0·3 per cent., though of no great magnitude, is not nearly so small as that shown by the abattoir statistics of the United States where the conditions presumably are better.

G. F. Thompson is inclined to attribute the comparative rarity of tuberculosis in the goat "to the feed and climate where the animals are found, and to the exercise obtained in roaming over the mountain side...in other words to environment rather than to a physiological immunity."

Tuberculosis in the goat, when it does occur, is commonly supposed to be derived from cattle; and in some of the recorded instances close association with bovine animals has been noted. Thus in Edgar's case, mentioned above, "the goat had the run of the farmyard and mixed freely with the cattle"; but he adds that "the latter were all healthy, except for an attack of husk." In Griffith's case the evidence is stronger, since the tuberculous goat was known to have been brought

---

[1] Quoted by Thompson (*loc. cit.* p. 342) from the *Deutsche landwirtschaftliche Presse*. He adds that they "ate out of the same racks with tuberculous cows and, owing to their well-known proclivities for mischief, took hay out of the mouths of cattle whereby they exposed themselves to the greatest possible (risk of) infection." But we may perhaps doubt whether this description applied to all the goats included in the statistics.

XIX]   REASON FOR COMPARATIVE IMMUNITY OF GOAT   415

up on cow's milk[1].   Frosch and Hertha, 1901, thought they
saw evidence in Germany that the amount of tuberculosis
among the goats in different districts was proportional to
the tuberculosis among the cattle.   But one would suppose
that it would depend rather on the closeness of association
which prevails in different places between the goats and the
cattle.

If we conclude that tuberculosis in the goat is commonly
derived from cattle, we have yet to ask why, when the goat
is so susceptible as experimental research has shown it to be,
the disease does not spread from goat to goat.   One would
like to have more information from such countries as Spain,
where the goats go about in flocks instead of leading isolated
lives as they so often do in other countries; possibly the disease
does, under such circumstances, spread through the flock; at all
events the experience related by Eichhorn and mentioned just
now points in this direction.

In England at least tuberculosis seldom spreads from
goat to goat because these animals are not brought very much
together.   They often are kept by poor country people, who
cannot afford a cow; and they live an isolated life, feeding on
the margins of the road before the cottage.   For this reason
goats do not often meet the chance of catching tuberculosis
from one another or from the cow.   When they are brought
into contact with the latter they are liable, as we have seen,
to become affected.   What it may be in other countries one
cannot say, but one thing is certain, the goat is decidedly
susceptible constitutionally to tuberculosis, as the following
experimental investigations will show.

[1] This animal was one of twins bought for the purpose of research.   Both
kids were accordingly tested with tuberculin; and when one reacted it was killed
and examined.   An ulcer was found in the intestine, and tuberculosis of a
neighbouring mesenteric gland.   There was tuberculosis of a pharyngeal
gland also, but none elsewhere.   Tubercle bacilli were found and cultivated,
and proved to be of bovine type.

On inquiry the following history was elicited.   The dam could not supply
enough milk for both her young, so one of them was weaned and brought up
by hand on cow's milk, while the other was allowed to suck its mother.   It
was the former that became tuberculous.

*The Comparative Susceptibility of the Goat to Infection
with the Three Types of Tubercle Bacilli.*

Natural Tuberculosis. Up to the present time the type
of tubercle bacillus found in natural tuberculosis in the goat
has not been determined. Griffith's case already mentioned
is still under investigation[1], and in the meantime one can only
infer from experimental investigations that in all probability
in the great majority of cases, if not in all, the tubercle bacillus
is of the bovine type.

Experimental Tuberculosis. Even before 1868 Villemin[2]
had attempted to solve experimentally the question of the
susceptibility of the goat to tuberculosis. With human
tuberculous material he inoculated one of these animals, but
without result to its general health. According to Straus the
first to prove that the goat is not immune to tuberculosis
were Bollinger (1873), Colin (1891), Cadiot, Gilbert and Roger,
Moulé, Siegen and Weber (1893), all of whom produced tuberculosis experimentally in individuals of this species. But this
was before the existence of three types of tubercle bacilli
was suspected.

Recent investigations have shown that the goat reacts to
mammalian tubercle bacilli introduced experimentally very
much like the ox. To infection with the bovine variety
it appears to be even a little more susceptible[3]. To infection
with the human type of bacillus it is as refractory as the calf.

The Bovine Type of Tubercle Bacillus. Injected subcutaneously into the goat large doses of bovine bacilli cause general
miliary tuberculosis which proves rapidly fatal. Even $4\frac{1}{2}$
million tubercle bacilli (contained in a tissue emulsion) have on
more than one occasion produced a fatal result within two or
three months[4]; 1,800,000 bacilli of similar origin have reduced

---

[1] Since the above was written the bacilli have proved to be of bovine type.

[2] *Études sur la tuberculose,* Paris, 1868, p. 554.

[3] In support of this view A. S. Griffith gives a table of results obtained
after injecting equal doses of bovine tubercle bacilli into goats and calves.
While he is no doubt justified in drawing this conclusion, some allowance
must be made for difference in the size of animals injected with identical
doses. *R.C.T. Int Rep.* App. vol. I, p. 47.

[4] *R.C.T. Int. Rep.* vol. I, p. 201 (Goat 2); vol. II, p. 1149 (Goat 5).

an animal to death's door in 47 days[1], and so small a quantity as 5000 has caused general tuberculosis of some severity[2]. Of bacilli from culture, o·o1 mg. on injection has produced "slowly progressing general tuberculosis[3]." On the other hand an amount of culture estimated to contain 1,800,000 bacilli, suspended in salt solution[4], has given rise only to a few tubercles, small and retrogressive in character[5].

From this we see that the goat is highly susceptible to infection with the bovine type of tubercle bacillus, just as the calf is. But like that animal it also has demonstrable powers of resistance, and when the number of infecting bacilli is reduced beyond a certain minimum their injection causes only a local and transitory disease.

To infection through the alimentary canal by the bovine type of bacillus the goat is certainly susceptible, probably a good deal more so than the calf. 10 mg. and even 1·0 mg. doses, which cannot be considered excessive for this animal when given by the mouth, have, under certain circumstances, caused severe ulceration of intestines and fatal general tuberculosis[6].

On another occasion a dose of 1·0 mg. given to an adult goat and also to a young kid produced no apparent disturbance of health during life. But after death caseous nodules were found widely distributed among the glands of the alimentary canal in the adult, and in the kid there were in addition some shallow ulcers in the small intestine, and a large softened nodule in the lung[7].

[1] R.C.T. Int. Rep. vol. II, p. 1149 (Goat 3).
[2] Ibid. vol. I, p. 137 (Goat 6).   [3] Ibid. vol. I, pp. 47 and 208 (Goat 28).
[4] Ibid. vol. II, p. 1149 (Goat 17).
[5] The reader may be reminded that the injection of a given number of tubercle bacilli, if originating in tuberculous tissue and accompanied by an emulsion of the same, is followed by much more severe consequences than the injection of an equal number of bacilli from a young serum culture suspended in some indifferent fluid such as "physiological" salt solution (see p. 287).
[6] R.C.T. Int. Rep. App. vol. II, pp. 699, 701.
These results occurred in goats which were pregnant when they swallowed the bacilli. They remained apparently well for about three months until their kids were born, but after this they went down hill rapidly, one dying of tuberculosis 6½ months after the commencement of the experiment, and the other being killed when moribund exactly four weeks after parturition.
[7] R.C.T. Int. Rep. App. vol I, p. 592.

Smaller doses of 10 to 1 million tubercle bacilli contained in milk or tissue emulsion have sometimes produced progressive disseminated tuberculosis, but as a rule the disease caused by these small doses has been limited to the alimentary canal and the glands connected with it[1].

A. S. Griffith, who fed eight goats with these small doses, remarked on the frequency with which the gastric glands were affected (in five out of eight). In one case there was a typical tuberculous ulcer in the stomach. In another the tonsil was tuberculous[2]. On the other hand the mesenteric glands were tuberculous in two instances only, and in no case was there disease of the intestinal mucous membrane.

Griffith also calls attention to the readiness with which lesions in the goat soften and break down as compared with those in the calf[3], a point which the author can confirm from his own experience.

Tubercle bacilli of the human type seem to be just as incapable of setting up progressive tuberculosis in the goat as in the ox. As in the latter species, so in the goat they cause a local necrotic lesion at the site of the injection of large masses of bacilli, and little tuberculous foci wherever the microbes which become disseminated come to rest. If the injection has been intravenous the number of such lesions in the lungs may be such as to interfere seriously with respiration and to cause death[4]; but after subcutaneous inoculation these disseminated lesions are few and insignificant, and they do not tend to grow or to give rise to others; and the animal, recovering from the slight disturbance of health from which it may at first have suffered, remains to all appearances quite well, and continues to grow at a normal rate.

Subcutaneous injections of such large doses as 10, 25, or 100 mg. of culture[5], or over 100 million bacilli in tissue emulsion[6], have caused only small and retrogressive lesions, with

---

[1] *R.C.T. Int. Rep.* App. vol. ii, pp. 537 and 707.

[2] *Ibid.* App. vol. i, p. 537.   [3] *Ibid.* p. 47.

[4] *Ibid. Fin. Rep.* vol. i, p. 241 (Goat 81). On the other hand tissue emulsion containing 1,000,000 tubercle bacilli of human type has been injected intravenously into a young kid (No. 45) with minimal results. *Ibid. Int. Rep.* vol. ii, p. 1150.

[5] *Ibid. Fin. Rep.* p. 241.   [6] *Ibid. Int. Rep.* p. 1150.

but transient disturbance of health.   When, with these minimal results, we recall the fact that $4\frac{1}{2}$ million or even 1,800,000 bacilli of the bovine type have caused rapidly fatal miliary tuberculosis, we see clearly that the goat belongs to one of those species which differentiate decidedly between tubercle bacilli of bovine and human type.

To the *avian type of tubercle bacillus* the degree of susceptibility of the goat cannot be stated dogmatically, as only a few experiments have been made.   But on the whole one may probably venture to say that this species of animal resists infection with the bacillus in question fairly well, though probably less absolutely than it resists infection with the bacillus of human type; for the goat has withstood large doses of avian bacilli (10–100 mg.) injected subcutaneously without becoming seriously ill, and with little more result than a softening caseous tumour at the seat of inoculation, and caseation of the nearest glands.   But small disseminated tubercles are common, and in one case fatal tuberculosis seems to have been produced.

F. Griffith[1] injected six goats with doses of avian bacilli varying from 10 to 100 mg.   Five of them resisted fairly well, and were in good health when killed from three to five months later.   They all, of course, developed at the seat of inoculation a necrotic tumour which broke down and ulcerated, and several of them were found to have scattered tubercles in the lymphatic glands of the alimentary canal, probably caused by swallowing the discharge from the ulcerating local lesions; but, with one slight exception, there were no lesions in the great organs[2].   Thus these animals may be said to have shown a fairly high degree of resistance.   But the remaining animal (Goat 48), the youngest of the four, after receiving 50 mg. developed a progressive tuberculosis which was approaching a fatal termination when the animal was killed nearly three months after injection.   There were then seen scattered tubercles in the lungs and necrotic foci in the liver.   But the most severe lesions were in the alimentary canal; the mucous membrane of the intestine was pitted and swarming with tubercle bacilli, and the mesenteric glands were caseo-necrotic.   The condition of the gut, Griffith remarks, was no doubt responsible for the animal's weak and emaciated condition.   This result is anomalous and difficult of explanation.   We are told that cultures made from the liver and the prescapular and mesenteric glands were of the avian type, but it is difficult to be sure that the severe intestinal disease, the cause of death in this case, was the result of

---

[1] *R.C.T. Fin. Rep.* App. vol. IV, pp. 190 and 324.

[2] In another animal a few grey tubercles and caseous nodules were found in the lungs and thoracic glands, but a culture, grown from the former situation proved to be of bovine type.

the inoculation and not an independent and spontaneous infection, perhaps caused by the bovine tubercle bacillus, or, it may be, by some other acid-fast bacillus akin to that which causes Johne's disease.

To infection by feeding with avian bacilli the adult goat is resistant. Small foci, or even nodules, may appear in the intestinal mucosa, and some gritty tubercles in the mesenteric or colic glands; but these lesions never attain to any importance, and the animals remain well. But it is otherwise with very young kids. In these, feeding with avian bacilli may cause severe ulceration of the mucous membrane of the intestine and caseation of the neighbouring glands.

F. Griffith fed two kids when five days old each with 50 mg. of avian culture suspended in milk. They were killed in good health 56 days later, and had gained in weight. There was no disseminated tuberculosis in the organs, but the tubercle bacilli had multiplied in the mucous membrane of the intestines and had caused severe ulceration. The mesenteric and ileo-colic glands were enlarged and caseating, and there was slight tuberculosis of the tonsils, and of portal, submaxillary and posterior pharyngeal glands[1].

Tuberculosis in the Sheep.

Although the sheep can quite readily be infected artificially with bovine tubercle bacilli, even when these are given with food, cases of tuberculosis naturally acquired are rarely reported. Koch, 1884, examined one case; McFadyean, 1900, another which he believes to be the first indubitable example recorded in this country. Another was shown by Foulerton, 1892, to the Pathological Society of London.

Slaughter-house statistics concerning tuberculosis in the sheep must be accepted with reserve, for these animals are very liable to become infected with a nematode worm, *Strongylus rubescens*, which, as Villemin pointed out, causes small disseminated pearly-grey nodules in the lungs which may easily pass for tubercles. The condition is exceedingly common, and though, no doubt, inspectors as a rule are well acquainted with it, it seems possible that now and then an exceptional case of this disease may be misunderstood, and may serve to swell the small number of cases of tuberculosis in this species reported from the abattoirs.

[1] *loc. cit.* p. 190.

In a report on tuberculosis in domestic animals in Saxony, published in the year 1895[1], it is stated that, out of 132,578 sheep slaughtered, tuberculosis was detected in 179, or in ·13 per cent. In the abattoirs of one district the proportion of tuberculosis among the sheep was as high as 3 per cent.

In the United States on the other hand tuberculosis among sheep seems to be very rare; and it is stated by Melvin that of nearly 10,000,000 sheep slaughtered under Federal inspection in 1908 only 40, or 0·0004 per cent., were found to be tuberculous[2].

Cases of tuberculosis in the sheep which have been carefully examined are too few to allow of a description of the usual character and situation of the lesions, or of speculation as to the probable portal of entry in the majority of instances.

In Koch's case only the lungs and bronchial glands were available for examination; the former contained tubercular nodules, and the bronchial glands were caseous and calcified. In McFadyean's case there were clusters of caseo-calcareous nodules, very like the so-called "grapes" of the ox, attached to the pleura. In Foulerton's case lungs, liver and kidneys, and mediastinal and cervical glands contained caseous and calcareous nodules.

Tubercle bacilli are probably scarce in the lesions of the sheep. Koch reports that there were few bacilli in the pulmonary tubercles, but that they were more abundant in the bronchial gland. McFadyean could find no tubercle bacilli in preparations made from the lesions in his case, but inoculation of the material into the rabbit caused tuberculosis, and a culture was obtained. Again in Foulerton's case no bacilli could be seen on microscopic examination, but the material of the lesions inoculated into guinea-pigs caused tuberculosis.

The comparative immunity of the sheep to tuberculosis cannot be explained completely. As we shall see, this animal is constitutionally susceptible at least to infection with the bovine bacillus. It can also be infected by feeding. It may be said that the sheep leads an unconfined life in the open air, in

---

[1] Abstract in *Journ. of Comp. Pathol. and Therap.* vol. IX, p. 233.

[2] *25th Rep. Bureau of Animal Industry*, 1908, p. 98.

many cases on mountain pastures, or on moor or downland.
Perhaps for this reason it escapes infection by the air passages.
But how does it escape infection through the alimentary
canal? It is true that it is not often brought into close contact
with cattle, though it feeds at times in the same fields; and
while it changes its feeding grounds often, yet at times, when
on turnips, the ground is very limited and is not changed
until it becomes foul. How then does tuberculosis not spread
from sheep to sheep? The only answer we can suggest is
that such crowding is exceptional. For the most part of the
time the life of the sheep is free and open and spent on clean
ground. It seldom becomes tuberculous from contact with
cattle, and when it does so the disease fails to spread from
sheep to sheep in consequence of the animal's manner of life,
and perhaps too because of the paucity of bacilli in the lesions.

The Comparative Susceptibility of the Sheep to Infection with the Three Types of Tubercle Bacilli.

With regard to the type of the tubercle bacillus which is
the cause of the few instances of natural infection which occur
in the sheep there can be little doubt that it is the bovine
type of bacillus. The culture derived from McFadyean's case,
already mentioned, soon died out, but the results produced by
injecting rabbits with emulsions of the sheep's lesions seem
to indicate clearly that the strain of bacilli was of that type.

Experimental Infection. The small number of experimental
inoculations made on this species have clearly shown it to be
susceptible to infection with the bovine type of tubercle bacillus
and resistant to infection with the human type of bacillus.
Nothing is known as to its capacity to resist infection with
the avian bacillus. Ravenel reported to the British Congress
on Tuberculosis in 1902 the intra-pulmonary injection of four
sheep with emulsions of tuberculous tissues[1]. Two injected
with bovine tubercle bacilli died in a few weeks with tuberculosis
of the lungs, liver, and spleen. The other two, injected with
human material, remained well; and, when killed seven months

[1] *Trans. Brit. Cong. on Tuberculosis*, 1902, vol. III, p. 572.

after the injection, one was found to have a caseous abscess in the lungs, and the other was entirely normal. Dammann and Müssemeier[1], in 1905, showed that sheep may be infected by feeding with bovine bacilli but resist infection by feeding with human tubercle bacilli.

Six young lambs were fed by these authors with tubercle bacilli suspended in milk. Only one received a bovine culture (100 mg.). It died in 44 days of general tuberculosis, with severe ulceration of intestine and great enlargement and caseation of the mesenteric glands. The others received similar doses of human culture, each on a single occasion, except one lamb which was fed three times in this way. All but one remained in good condition, and the other died of an intercurrent traumatic pericarditis. In one of these lambs the disease produced by the tubercle bacilli was limited to a few small retrogressive tubercles in the pharyngeal glands, while in the others there were indeed tubercles disseminated in some of the organs, but these were of low grade and retrogressive in type.

Koch and Schütz, 1902, injected four sheep subcutaneously with 10 and 20 mg. of tubercle bacilli. Two received bacilli of human type and two bacilli of bovine type (perlsucht). The following conclusion was arrived at: Sheep, like swine and calves do not fall ill after injection with bacilli of human tuberculosis, but after injection with bacilli of perlsucht they develop tuberculosis just as calves do; but the extension of the disease seems to take place more quickly in the calf than in the sheep.

REFERENCES. XI

(Chapter XIX)

Tuberculosis in the Pig.

Buchanan, G. S. (1906). Report on the Administration in London with regard to Meat of Pigs affected with Tuberculosis. *Reps. of Medical Inspectors of the Local Government Board*, No. 225, p. 2. Note as to the Prevalence, etc. of Tuberculosis in Pigs.

Cobbett (1907). The Virulence of Tubercle Bacilli of Human Origin for the Pig. *R.C.T. Int. Rep.* App. vol. II, p. 1156.

Deetz (1903). Über die Tuberkulose bei Schweinen im Vergleich mit der bei Menschen und bei Rindern vom sanitätspolizeilichen Standpunkte aus. *Klin. Jahrb.* vol. II.

—— (1903). Zur Frage der Übertragung der Menschentuberkulose auf Schweine, Berlin. Ref. *Centralb. f. Bakt.* vol. XXXIV, p. 119.

Dinwiddie (1902). The Transmissibility of Human and Bovine Tuberculosis. *Journ. of the Amer. Med. Assoc.* No. 5.

—— (1899). *Arkansas Agricult. Expt. Station Bulletin*, No. 57.

---

[1] *Untersuchungen über die Beziehungen zwischen der Tuberkulose des Menschen und der Tiere*, Hanover, 1905, pp. 41, 130, 139.

Eastwood and Griffith, F. (1914).   A Report on Localized Tuberculosis in Swine. *Reps. to the Local Government Board on Public Health and Medical Subjects*, N.S. No. 91.

Griffith, A. S. and F. (1911).   Swine Tuberculosis. *R.C.T. Fin. Rep.* App. vol. III, p. 148.

Griffith, A. S. (1907).   The Pathogenic Effect of Bovine Viruses. *Ibid. Int. Rep.* App. vol. I.   For experiments on pigs see pp. 47, 500, 536, 591, 631, 696 and 706.

—— (1911).   Investigation of Viruses obtained from cases of Human Tuberculosis. *Ibid. Fin. Rep.* App. vol. I.   Inoculation experiments on pigs, p. 44, table, p. 240.   Feeding experiments on pigs p. 49.

Griffith, F. (1911).   Investigation of Avian Tubercle Bacilli. *Ibid. Fin. Rep.* App. vol. IV, p. 168.   For experiments on pigs see pp. 186, 245, 253, 254 and 258.

Kersten and Ungermann (1912).   Untersuchungen über den Typus der bei der Tuberculose des Schweines vorkommenden Tuberkelbazillen. *Tub. Arbeit. a. d. Kaiserl. Gesundheitsamte*, Heft 11, p. 171.

Kossel, Weber and Heuss (1904).   *Ibid.* Heft 1.

—— (1905).   *Ibid.* Heft 3.

Mohler and Washburn (1907).   Tuberculosis of Hogs. *24th Rep. U.S. Bureau of Animal Industry*, p. 215.

—— (1908).   The Causation and Character of Animal Tuberculosis. *Ibid.* 25th Rep. p. 155.

—— (1908).   The Transmission of Avian Tuberculosis to Mammals. *Ibid.* p. 165.

Ravenel, M. P. (1901).   The Comparative Virulence of Tubercle Bacilli from Human and Bovine Sources. *Lancet*, II, pp. 349, 443.

Schroeder and Mohler (1906).   The Tuberculin Test in Hogs, and some methods of their Infection with Tuberculosis. *U.S. Bureau of Animal Industry*, Bulletin No. 88.

Titze (1907).   Fütterungsversuche mit Hühnertuberkelbazillen an Schweinen und an einem Fohlen. *Tub. Arbeit. a. d. Kaiserl. Gesundheitsamte*, Heft 6, p. 215.

Weber and Bofinger (1904).   Die Hühnertuberculose (avian tubercle bacilli found in the mesenteric glands of a young pig), p. 95.

Zwick (1908).   Vergleichende Untersuchungen über die Tuberkelbazillen des Menschen und der Haustiere. *Zeitsch. f. Infectionskrankheiten der Haustiere*, vol. IV, p. 161.

Tuberculosis in the Goat.

Alston, Edgar (1892).   Tuberculosis in a Goat. *Journ. of Comp. Pathol. and Therap.* vol. V, p. 80.

Bulling (1896).   Spontaneous Tuberculosis in a Goat. *Münch. med. Wochenschr.* p. 474.

Cobbett (1907).   *R.C.T. Int. Rep.* App. vol. II, p. 1148.

Editorial Article (1890). Pulmonary Tuberculosis in a Goat. *Journ. of Comp. Pathol. and Therap.* vol. III, p. 275.

—— (1891). Tuberculosis in the Sheep and Goat. *Ibid.* vol. IV, p. 361.

—— (1892). Ditto. *Ibid.* vol. V, p. 61.

Frosch and Hertha (1901). Ein Beitrag zur Kenntnis der Ziegentuberkulose. *Zeitschf. f. Infect. der Haustiere*, vol. VIII, pp. 63–90.

Griffith, A. S. (1907). *R.C.T. Int. Rep.* App. vol. I, pp. 47, 48.

Griffith, F. (1911). *Ibid. Fin. Rep.* App. vol. IV, pp. 173, 189, 324.

Lydtin (1884). Die Perlsucht. *Archiv f. wissensch. u. prakt. Tierheilkunde*, vol. X.

Melvin (1908). *25th Rep. U.S. Bureau of Animal Industry*, p. 98.

Nocard (1890). Pulmonary Tuberculosis in a Goat. *Soc. Cent. de Méd. Vétérin.* Abstract in the *Journ. of Comp. Pathol. and Therap.* vol. III, p. 275.

Thompson, G. F. (1904). Information concerning the Milch Goat. *21st Ann. Rep. U.S. Bureau of Animal Industry*, p. 341.

Thomassen (1892). Tuberculose spontanée chez la chèvre. *Congrès pour l'étude de la Tuberculose.* Paris, p. 650.

Tuberculosis in the Sheep.

Dammann and Müssemeier (1905). *Untersuchungen ü. d. Beziehungen z. d. Tuberculose d. Mensch. u. Tiere*, pp. 41, 130 and 139. M. and H. Schafer, Hanover.

Foulerton (1902). A case of Tuberculosis in a Sheep. *Journ. of Comp. Pathol. and Therap.* vol. XV, p. 102. *Trans. Pathol. Soc. London*, vol. LIII, p. 428.

Koch and Schütz (1902). Menschlichetuberkulose und Rindertuberkulose. *Archiv f. wissenschaftliche u. prakt. Tierheilkunde.* See also *Die Gesammelte Werke von R. Koch*, vol. II, p. 1086.

McFadyean (1900). Tuberculosis in the Sheep. *Journ. of Comp. Pathol. and Therap.* vol. XIII, p. 59.

—— (1902). A case of Tuberculosis in the Sheep. *Ibid.* vol. XV, p. 158.

Melvin, A. D. (1908). The Economic Importance of Tuberculosis of Food-producing Animals. *Internat. Cong. on Tuberculosis, Washington.* See also *25th Report of the U.S. Bureau of Animal Industry*, p. 97.

Ravenel (1902). *Trans. Brit. Cong. on Tuberculosis*, vol. III, p. 572.

CHAPTER XX

THE SUSCEPTIBILITY TO TUBERCULOSIS OF VARIOUS ANIMAL SPECIES (*continued*)

TUBERCULOSIS IN THE RABBIT, GUINEA-PIG, RAT AND MOUSE.

Tuberculosis in the Rabbit.

Natural tuberculosis appears to be very rare, or perhaps one might venture to say unknown, in the wild rabbit. Supposed instances indeed are reported from time to time by sportsmen and others, and a question has actually been asked about it in the House of Commons; but such instances usually turn out on investigation to be cases of coccidiosis; and so far no authenticated case of spontaneous tuberculosis in the wild rabbit is known to the writer. This is the more remarkable for, as we shall see, the laboratory rabbit is exceedingly susceptible to experimental infection with the bovine bacillus, and is by no means immune to that caused by the avian bacillus.

While the wild rabbit is so rarely found to be infected with tuberculosis, the domesticated varieties, especially when kept in institutions where investigation of tuberculosis is going on, are liable sometimes to contract the disease. Koch[1] indeed stated in 1884 that he had found no evidence of spontaneous tuberculosis in many hundred rabbits and guinea-pigs bought for purposes of research, yet when animals of this kind were kept in the same room with others infected with tubercle bacilli solitary cases of spontaneous tuberculosis occurred from time to time. He mentions that he saw seventeen instances of the kind, and this would seem to indicate a considerable frequency of infection under such circumstances. But in all well-conducted establishments with liberal provision for such animals the risk of accidental tuberculosis is really extremely small. Very large numbers of rabbits and guinea-pigs were kept for research by the Royal Commission on Tuberculosis, and yet the writer who examined many of them post-mortem, both after inoculation,

---

[1] *The Etiology of Tuberculosis*, Eng. trans. *loc. cit.* p. 129.

Plate XIII

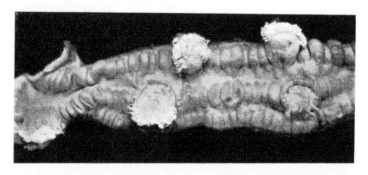

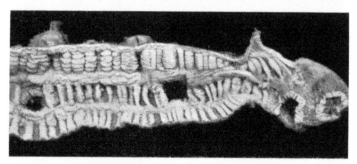

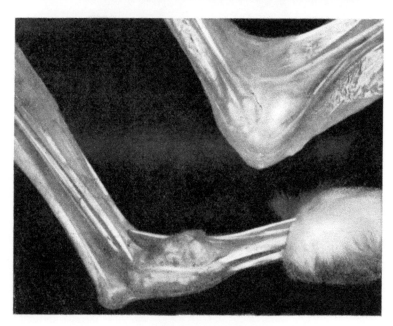

Avian Tuberculosis in Rabbits.

Natural infection.

and when they died of various accidental causes, saw only one case of spontaneous tuberculosis in a rabbit during four and a half years.

Two further instances of the kind came to his notice subsequently in the Cambridge Pathological Laboratory among a small number of rabbits kept near to a tuberculous cow. In them the disease was mainly pulmonary. In addition to these instances the writer has investigated two cases of spontaneous tuberculosis in rabbits kept in a private poultry yard along with fowls several of which were found to be tuberculous. From each of these rabbits tubercle bacilli of the avian type were cultivated. In one of them the disease affected mainly the large intestine, causing ulcers of large size, whose walls, yielding to the intermittent pressure within, came to form aneurismoid dilatations projecting towards the peritoneum. These little pouches, five in number, measured nearly half an inch in diameter, and were covered externally by villous tufts of growth. Several of them contained each a dry incarcerated fæcal pellet. In the second of these animals the tuberculosis was, so far as could be ascertained by macroscopic examination, limited to three joints; namely one humero-radial, one femoro-tibial and one tarso-phalangeal joint.

F. Griffith has informed the writer that he too has seen an instance of spontaneous tuberculosis in the rabbit; and that in this animal also the tubercle bacilli concerned proved to be of the avian type.

Rothe, in 1912, reported an epidemic of tuberculosis in a stock of about 80 or 90 rabbits bred, from a single pair, for purposes of research, in the Sanatorium Heidehaus in Hanover. A great number died and were found to have the usual lesions pointing to inhalation tuberculosis and containing acid-fast bacilli. Inoculation of rabbits and guinea-pigs with portions of the affected organs and, in two cases, with cultures raised from them caused tuberculosis. The bacilli were judged to belong to the bovine type. As to the original cause of the epidemic, it was stated that none of the rabbits had been inoculated with tuberculosis. But it was ascertained that they had been fed with scraps of bread and butter, and the young ones with milk, which however was declared always to have been boiled.

Experimental Infection. The susceptibility of the rabbit to experimental infection with the two types of mammalian tubercle bacilli[1] has already been fully discussed (Chap. XIII). It will therefore suffice to say here that this animal is exceedingly susceptible to the attack of the bovine bacillus—succumbing to the effect of the smallest doses however injected, and being also fairly easily infected by feeding—while it possesses considerable powers of resisting infection with the human type of bacillus. The results of injecting this bacillus, by any method other than the intravenous, are often nil or minimal, but not infrequently lesions of a chronic type appear in the lungs and kidneys; and quite rarely, apparently in unusually susceptible individuals, a progressive tuberculosis may ensue. Intraperitoneal injections of human tubercle bacilli, if the dose be very large, may prove rapidly fatal from tuberculous peritonitis; but the disease hardly ever continues, and if the animal does not die in a few weeks it almost always recovers altogether. Intravenous injections, are, on the other hand, when large frequently followed by death from pulmonary disease. The rabbit then may be said to possess on the whole remarkable power of resisting infection with the human tubercle bacillus, but its resistance is not so high, or so uniform, as that of the ox or goat.

The rabbit is susceptible to experimental injection with the avian type of tubercle bacillus, and may develop tuberculosis even as the result of being fed with this organism. But, according to F. Griffith[2], whose experience was extensive, the virulence of this type is not so great as that of the bovine bacillus, and the disease set up by it, after subcutaneous inoculation at least, is more chronic. Nevertheless large doses injected intraperitoneally may cause rapidly fatal peritonitis, and intravenous injections, as one might suppose, are often followed quickly by death.

[1] See A. S. Griffith, *R.C.T. Int. Rep.* App. vol. I, pp. 436 and 706. *Fin. Rep.* App. vol. I, p. 32, and Cobbett, *Ibid. Int. Rep.* vol. II, p. 1064.
[2] F. Griffith, *Ibid. Fin. Rep.* vol. IV, p. 182.

The lesions caused by different types of tubercle bacilli in the rabbit. Whatever be the method of inoculation the organs most affected are almost invariably the lungs, as is the case in almost all mammals, except the guinea-pig. The liver and spleen have but a small share in the lesions, while the kidneys suffer severely —a distribution which again is in marked contrast to that which occurs in the guinea-pig. An interesting feature of tuberculosis in the rabbit is the comparatively small extent to which the lymphatic glands share in the disease; lesions in them, though not uncommon, are seldom conspicuous, as in the guinea-pig, and are often confined to those nearest the seat of inoculation. On the other hand the joints are particularly susceptible, especially, it seems, to the attack of the avian bacillus[1]. Another peculiarity of tuberculosis in the rabbit, at least of that caused by the mammalian bacillus, is the liability of the pelvis of the tuberculous kidney to become distended with muco-purulent matter containing tubercle bacilli, and of the uterus too, in the female rabbit after intraperitoneal injection, not unfrequently to be filled with caseo-pus. Attention has already been drawn to the frequency with which the functional mammary gland is infected, even after injection of bacilli of human type, and in the male the testes show a like suscepti-bility[2]. After feeding with bovine tubercle bacilli there is very commonly ulceration of the tonsils, and the intestine is similarly affected. The submaxillary and other cervical lymphatic glands are then usually caseous, and the mesenteric glands participate, though usually to a less extent.

The cause of the immunity of the wild rabbit. The high degree of susceptibility to experimental tuberculosis which is exhibited by rabbits when injected with bovine, or even with avian, tubercle bacilli, as well as their liability to contract tuberculosis from either of these micro-organisms when kept in captivity, causes the immunity which the rabbit enjoys in

---

[1] In one of F. Griffith's rabbits injected subcutaneously with 1·0 mg. the only disease beyond the local lesion was tuberculosis of a shoulder joint. Another, similarly injected with 0·001 mg., was in a dying condition 258 days later, and when killed was found to have tuberculosis of nearly all the joints and of the testes, and caseous nodules in the lungs and kidneys (*loc. cit.* p. 183).

[2] A. S. Griffith, *loc. cit. Fin. Rep.* p. 36.

its wild state to appear very remarkable.   This immunity seems the more surprising when one remembers that rabbits frequently come out to feed on pastures where cows have been grazing, or where chickens have been running during the daytime, for we know that from both of these animals when tuberculous the droppings may contain tubercle bacilli.

Several explanations of the immunity of the wild rabbit as contrasted with the laboratory or domesticated rabbit suggest themselves.   Probably the first that will occur to the medical man is that the wild animal is fundamentally healthier; that there is some influence in confinement or domestication which, though it may not obviously impair the general health, nevertheless breaks down the resistance to infection with tuberculosis.   This explanation does not commend itself to the present writer, who has pointed out elsewhere in this book the slight connection which there seems to be between the general health and susceptibility to tuberculosis[1].   It seems to him more likely that the rabbit escapes tuberculosis in infected pastures because it is a very clean feeder provided with an exceedingly sensitive nose which enables it to avoid consuming contaminated grass.   One must remember too that hyper-susceptible as the rabbit is to any kind of injection of bovine tubercle bacilli, it is not so very easily infected by feeding. A considerable number of the rabbits which A. S. Griffith fed with tubercle bacilli of this type escaped infection altogether[2].

[1] (See p. 30.) In the case of the mouse tribe indeed the conditions are reversed. It is the wild field mouse which, as we shall see, is susceptible to tuberculosis while the domesticated white mouse has a much higher resistance (see p. 450).

[2] See *R.C.T. Int. Rep.* App. vol. I, pp. 538 and 592. Of eight rabbits fed once with milk containing tubercle bacilli only one became tuberculous.   The rest escaped infection altogether, and so in another experiment, did one of four which were fed daily with tuberculous milk for thirty-one days.   Griffith, although in summing up (*loc. cit.* p. 706) he classes rabbits with guinea-pigs among the animals very easily infected by feeding, elsewhere (p. 592) admits that "infection through the alimentary tract seems to be effected with less certainty in rabbits than in guinea-pigs."

Another explanation of the immunity of the wild rabbit presents itself, namely, that, being of a different variety from those commonly used in laboratories, it may have higher powers of resisting tuberculosis.   Unfortunately we know very little from actual experiment of the susceptibility of the wild rabbit, but from one of Koch's observations this explanation would

Tuberculosis in the Guinea-pig.

Guinea-pigs, though extremely susceptible to infection both with human and bovine bacilli seldom contract tuberculosis naturally. It is the rarest thing to find a tuberculous guinea-pig among those bought for research. Koch[1] had never seen one, and the writer can say the same. Yet Koch found solitary cases of spontaneous tuberculosis among the guinea-pigs of his laboratory when they were kept in the same room with others infected with tubercle bacilli. Even in laboratories where the best arrangements exist for the separation of the stock animals from those infected, and of the animals of one experiment from those of another, the chance of an individual experimentally infected with one type of bacillus acquiring secondary infection with a bacillus of another type is difficult to exclude altogether ; and the possibility of this accident, though perhaps somewhat remote, must not be ignored, especially in passage experiments where a strain of tubercle bacilli is passed through a series of animals in order to test the stability of its comparative virulence and other type characters.

To experimental infection with either type of mammalian tubercle bacillus the guinea-pig is highly susceptible ; and for this reason, and because it is cheap, hardy, and easy to handle, it is universally preferred to other animals for the purpose of detecting the presence of tubercle bacilli in animal products, when these organisms cannot be found with the aid of the microscope alone. The study of the tuberculous lesions of the guinea-pig therefore is not unimportant ; and especially so since these depart considerably from the characters of tubercle as seen in the majority of animals.

The first point which is worthy of note with regard to the lesions is that their distribution among various organs differs considerably from that which prevails in other mammals. In all those which we have been considering so far the lungs are apt to suffer from tuberculosis more frequently and more

not appear to be sound, for of the instances of spontaneous tuberculosis which he records among the stock animals of his laboratory, one occurred in a rabbit once wild.

[1] *The Etiology of Tuberculosis*, Eng. trans. *loc. cit.* p. 129.

severely than any other large organ, and that too after almost any kind of injection; but in the guinea-pig this is not so; its lungs are seldom affected so severely as other parts[1] unless indeed the infection has been by inhalation. The kidneys too, so liable to tuberculosis in the rabbit, in the guinea-pig (as in birds) generally escape. It is the spleen and the liver (again as in birds), together with the lymphatic glands, which bear the brunt of the disease.

The next point is concerned with the nature of the lesions themselves. Miliary tubercles come but little into evidence, though they may be seen sometimes, as for example on the somatic peritoneum after intra-abdominal injections in severe and acute cases, or in the lungs after infection by inhalation. What gives to guinea-pig tuberculosis its most characteristic and peculiar appearance is its tendency to the formation of extensive areas of necrosis in the liver and spleen, together with great enlargement of these organs, especially the latter.

These necrotic areas in the spleen are whitish like wax. They are often large, and may involve considerable portions, or even nearly the whole, of the organ. In extreme cases there may remain only little irregular areas which retain their original colour, scattered over a spleen otherwise white and waxy and presenting very much the appearance of a piece of Castile soap. In still more extreme cases the whole spleen may be white with the exception of a narrow band of purple tissue along the hilus. In such cases the enlargement is often enormous.

In the liver the necrotic areas are smaller, and are stained yellow or greenish with bile. They are irregular in shape and distributed more or less evenly over the organ, though more frequent along the margins. The surface of the organ, unlike that of the spleen which remains more or less smooth, may become irregular and nodular. In some cases this is the main change, and the organ is then of pale brownish colour.

In cases of shorter duration or lesser severity the increase in size of these organs is more moderate. The spleen may

---

[1] This is true only of lesions tuberculous in the anatomical sense. Death, in acute cases, as we shall see, frequently occurs from excessive pleural effusion and the consequent collapse of the lungs.

Plate XIV

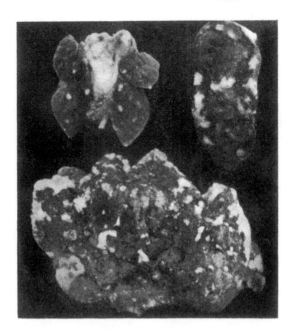

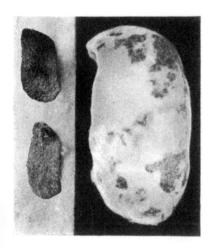
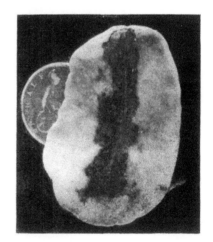

Tuberculosis in the Guinea-pig.

No. 1, showing the common distribution and appearance of the lesions in fatal cases not too acute.

The animal died 67 days after inoculation.

From a specimen by A. S. Griffith.

Nos. 2 and 3, showing enormously enlarged necrotic spleens.

No. 2 shows also normal spleens for comparison of size.

No. 3. The animal died of chronic general tuberculosis 223 days after subcutaneous injection of 0·1 mg. of bovine tubercle bacilli.

From a specimen by A. S. Griffith.

then be rather pale or pinkish in colour, and with a perfectly smooth surface; but more commonly it is dark and somewhat granular, each little granule being formed by an enlarged Malpighian body. In some of these latter may often be seen little central areas of opacity indicating an early stage of caseation, and these may sometimes appear as yellowish points dimly shining through a translucent layer of purple tissue. This is the condition, more or less advanced, which is commonly seen when the animal is killed some six weeks or so after injection of small or moderate doses of bacilli; the large necrotic spleens which sometimes form such a striking feature occurring in cases of greater severity and longer duration, and perhaps especially after injections of bovine bacilli.

When making post-mortem examination of animals infected experimentally it is of some importance to note whether the distribution of the lesions is such as may be expected to occur as the result of an inoculation of the kind which has been employed; otherwise spontaneous tuberculosis, if it existed, would escape recognition as such, and grave error might result.

With any given kind of inoculation the severity and duration of the disease depends mainly on the dose of bacilli, it being always understood that emulsions of tuberculous tissue containing a given number of bacilli are immensely more effective than the same number of bacilli from a pure culture. After intraperitoneal injection death may sometimes occur from tuberculous peritonitis in ten, or even nine, days; but in other cases only a few small lesions may be found after several months.

The extension and development of the lesions will depend partly, of course, on the length of time which has elapsed since inoculation. After five or six weeks, when the injection has been intraperitoneal, and the dose of bacilli, either by chance or design, has been moderate, one may expect to find the pathological picture somewhat as follows: in the abdominal wall at the seat of inoculation, probably, a small caseous focus caused by bacilli which have escaped from the peritoneal cavity along the track of the inoculating needle; secondary to this some enlargement of, and perhaps a caseating focus in, the nearest inguinal glands: the omentum drawn up about the greater curvature of the stomach, and converted into a solid mass, extending from spleen to pylorus, and composed largely of caseating tissue: the portal lymphatic gland enlarged and caseous, and probably also the post-sternal glands—but not the mesenteric which have nothing to do with the drainage of lymph from the peritoneal cavity: the spleen more or less enlarged and granular, containing hypertrophied Malpighian bodies, or perhaps showing small whitish areas of necrosis. Possibly also some yellowish patches of similar nature may be seen along the margin of the liver.

In the case of minimal disease it is important to know where to look for the earliest lesions. After subcutaneous injection these will be found at the seat of inoculation and in the nearest lymphatic glands. When injection has been intraperitoneal the portal lymphatic gland is the most important organ to examine in doubtful cases, since it may sometimes be the only part affected. It lies just behind the pylorus close against the portal vein as this vessel runs along the margin of the foramen of Winslow. Another gland which is affected early is situated in the omentum itself close to the pylorus. The omentum usually suffers severely, but in exceptional cases of minimal severity may be normal, or only show here and there a few translucent tubercles. The spleen should always be examined since it is affected very early, and other lymphatic glands which participate at this stage should not be overlooked, namely the post-sternal and bronchial. Tubercle bacilli are usually fairly numerous, and search for them should never be omitted.

In very acute and rapidly fatal cases death is usually due to pleural effusion and consequent collapse of the lungs. The cause of this is not obvious, for the pleura itself is unaltered, and there may be little or no tuberculosis of the lungs. Possibly it is due to obstruction in the bronchial glands, which are usually affected with comparative severity.

Pseudo-tuberculosis. While the lesions caused in the guinea-pig by tubercle bacilli do not, as a rule, consist very obviously of tubercles, there is another disease, not uncommon

Plate XV

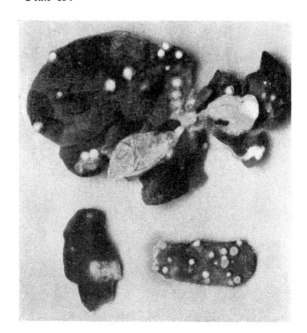

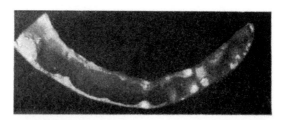

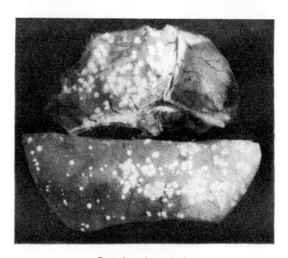

Pseudo-tuberculosis.
No. 1.   Liver, portal gland, lungs and spleen of a guinea-pig.
No. 2.   Appendix of a rabbit.   No. 3.   End of ileum and appendix of a rabbit.

in these animals, which causes changes that, to the student trained in human pathological anatomy only, may appear to correspond more closely with the traditional idea of tuberculosis. This is known as pseudo-tuberculosis, and though its lesions resemble superficially those of tuberculosis in other animals, yet it is caused by a bacillus which is not acid-fast, and, indeed, has no relation at all to the tubercle bacillus, but belongs to the septicæmic group which includes the bacillus of oriental plague.

Infection with this microbe affects, usually, mesenteric glands, spleen and liver. The disease may exist for a long time in the adult guinea-pig as a chronic suppuration of the mesenteric glands, often without any very obvious injury to health; but from this source it is apt to spread to the young as a rapidly fatal general pseudo-tuberculosis.

The pseudo-tubercles in spleen and liver are white and perfectly round, entirely unlike any lesions ever caused in the guinea-pig by true tuberculosis. But the result of experimental inoculation, apart from the rapidity with which it develops, is often so like true tuberculosis—in the production of a necrotic local lesion and caseation of the nearest glands, or of peritonitis with characteristic changes in omentum and mesentery—as sometimes to deceive even those accustomed to examine tuberculous guinea-pigs nearly every day of their lives. Fortunately microscopic examination of smear preparations settles the question at once, and in view of the frequency of pseudo-tuberculosis, we repeat, that this test should never be omitted.

The Comparative Susceptibility of the Guinea-pig to Infection with the Three Types of Tubercle Bacilli.

The Mammalian Tubercle Bacilli. In a previous chapter the guinea-pig was classed with those animals which do not serve to differentiate the two types of mammalian tubercle bacilli; and it has already been said in this section that both types produce severe and fatal tuberculosis in this animal. This statement has now to be qualified somewhat; for though at first sight there would not seem to be much difference in the virulence for this species of animal of these two types of bacilli. yet careful comparison of experiments made with measured doses reveals the fact that the bovine type is slightly, but distinctly, more virulent for the guinea-pig than the human type, and, in any given dose, kills more quickly. The writer once compared the results of 72 intraperitoneal injections of these two types, and the results set out below will be found to justify this statement[1].

Virulence for the Guinea-pig of Tubercle Bacilli of Bovine and Human Type.

	Dose of bacilli	Average duration of life	
		Bovine type	Human type
Intraperitoneal	1·0 mg. 0·1 mg.	13·7 days (18 animals) 18·9 days (20 animals)	19·9 days (18 animals) 23·3 days (16 animals)

The difference in virulence for the guinea-pig of tubercle bacilli of human and bovine type which these figures show was subsequently confirmed by A. S. Griffith, who brought together a more extensive series of observations collected from his own experience. The following table is a simplification of the one published by him[2].

[1] *R.C.T. Int. Rep.* App. vol. II, p. 1134.
[2] *R.C.T. Fin. Rep.* App. vol. I, p. 42. The question whether tubercle bacilli of bovine type were ever to be found in cases of human tuberculosis being *sub judice* at the time of this report, it was felt that the word bovine should not at that period be applied to any tubercle bacilli of human origin, and when two types of tubercle bacilli were found in cases of human tuberculosis they were distinguished provisionally by the terms "virulent" and "slightly virulent" respectively. The choice of these terms was perhaps not very fortunate since they appeared to beg the question whether the former (now known as bacilli of bovine type) are more virulent for *all* animal species than the latter (now known as bacilli of human type). But it is perhaps sufficiently obvious that the virulence referred to was only that exhibited towards such differentiating animals as, for example, the calf and rabbit. Griffith very properly used these provisional terms in his report and he distinguished further between "virulent bacilli of human origin" and "virulent

Method of injection	Dose of bacilli	Average duration of life	
		Bovine type	Human type
Intraperitoneal	1·0 mg. 0·1 mg.	11·9 (15 animals) 16·4 (58 animals)	22·5 (17 animals) 27·9 (40 animals)
Subcutaneous	1·0 mg. 0·1 mg.	49·6 (15 animals) 45·6 (58 animals)	80·9 (30 animals) 65·0 (40 animals)

The Avian Bacillus. As to the susceptibility of the guinea-pig to infection with the avian tubercle bacillus a good deal of uncertainty has prevailed in the past. It is now, however, surely known that, while this animal does not develop a true tuberculosis in the anatomical sense when injected with the micro-organism in question, it may nevertheless die after large doses, especially if these be introduced into the peritoneal cavity. This result is generally ascribed to toxæmia caused by the poisons in the bacilli actually injected, but it is by no means certain that these latter do not multiply in the guinea-pig. Nevertheless it is clear that the avian tubercle bacillus has a low degree of *infectivity* for this species of animal, for not only are moderate doses ineffective, especially when injected

bacilli of animal origin." But now that all are agreed that these two categories are practically identical we need no longer distinguish them, nor continue to use the provisional language of the Appendices to the Reports of the Commission. We are therefore able to simplify Griffith's table considerably by combining his two "virulent" groups into one under the title of "tubercle bacilli of bovine type," and changing the title of his "slightly virulent class" to that of "tubercle bacilli of human type."

But while one freely admits the practical identity of tubercle bacilli of bovine type and human origin with those of bovine type and animal origin, it may be of interest to point out that Griffith's table, as set out in his report, shows that the latter are rather more virulent than the former. This difference of virulence for the guinea-pig is not nearly so marked as that between the bovine and human types, but it comes out distinctly with each dose, and both with subcutaneous and intraperitoneal injections. It is true that the number of experiments made with tubercle bacilli of bovine type and human origin is comparatively small, but the results obtained in them are fully borne out, at least so far as intraperitoneal injections are concerned, by those of the present writer. The latter is therefore inclined to think that the difference though small is a real one.

subcutaneously, but it has not been found possible to infect it by inhalation[1].

Neither Rivolta (1889) nor Maffucci (1892) succeeded in infecting guinea-pigs with avian tuberculous material.

Cadiot, Gilbert and Roger (1890) injected fourteen guinea-pigs intraperitoneally with emulsion of the tuberculous livers and spleens of seven hens, two pheasants and one guinea-fowl. One guinea-pig died of general tuberculosis after 103 days. Of the rest eleven were killed in good condition five months after inoculation. Six of these were found free from lesions, while five had a few tuberculous foci scattered over liver, spleen and lungs. These lesions contained bacilli but appeared to be healing.

Straus and Gamaléia (1891) produced both by subcutaneous and intraperitoneal injection a limited amount of disease, consisting for the most part of an abscess at the seat of injection, marked enlargement of spleen, and tubercle bacilli in the abdominal organs.

Courmont and Dor (1891) noticed that the results of intraperitoneal injection of avian tubercle bacilli into guinea-pigs were very much more severe than those of subcutaneous injection. Twelve guinea-pigs inoculated intraperitoneally with cultures developed general tuberculosis, while eight inoculated subcutaneously remained well.

In more recent times Römer (1903) has observed the occasional production of general tuberculosis in guinea-pigs inoculated with avian tubercle bacilli. Small doses injected subcutaneously produced an abscess at the seat of inoculation, swelling of the lymphatic glands, and nothing more. With larger doses thus injected however a condition like that caused by mammalian tubercle bacilli was not unfrequently seen. When large doses (10 mg.) were injected intraperitoneally the animals died rapidly with symptoms of acute toxæmia. After death effusion into the pleural and peritoneal cavities was found, with great enlargement of spleen; this organ, and sometimes the liver also, being covered by a fibrinous layer in which numerous tubercle bacilli were present. The tendency to tubercle formation was slight.

[1] Weber and Bofinger, *loc. cit.* p. 129.

It is interesting to note that Römer got more severe results with pure cultures than with emulsions of tuberculous tissue. This is contrary to the experience of the Royal Commission when working with bovine and human tubercle bacilli, the *infectivity* of which for the guinea-pig is beyond question. Römer's experience therefore is in favour of the view that the avian bacillus does not kill the guinea-pig by infecting it in the true sense, that is by multiplying in its tissues, but does so by means of the toxins present in the bodies of the bacilli actually introduced. For the superior virulence which emulsions of tuberculous tissues commonly exhibit, as compared with pure cultures, is probably attributable to the protective action of the dead tissue which allows the bacilli favourable conditions for multiplication, and defends them mechanically from their enemies the leucocytes and bactericidal exudates; but such protective action would rather hinder the absorption of toxins, and its absence, as when cultures are used, would favour intoxication, for the fact that the bacilli are then exposed to the direct action of the living tissue facilitates their destruction and the rapid setting free and absorption of the poisons which are contained within them. And lastly we must remember that the numbers of bacilli are commonly far larger when pure cultures are injected than when tissue emulsions are employed.

With Römer's account of the general effect of avian tubercle bacilli on the guinea-pig the majority of modern observers would probably agree. It corresponds closely with the experience of the present writer. It is certainly a mistake to regard the avian tubercle bacillus as harmless for the guinea-pig, though it produces a very different disease from that caused by mammalian tubercle bacilli. It is harmless only in small doses, and when injected subcutaneously.

Weber and Bofinger (1904) after reviewing the subject and investigating the question anew, concluded that the avian bacillus is indeed virulent for the guinea-pig, but they hastened to add that "it never produces tuberculosis in the true sense of the word. It multiplies in the guinea-pig's body; but the increase thus brought about is in the majority of cases limited, and leads only to the formation of a local focus of suppuration.

In exceptional cases the distribution of bacilli is widespread and the animal then dies of toxæmia[1]."

These authors endorse the statement of Courmont and Dor that there is great difference in severity between subcutaneous and intraperitoneal injection. They state that none of the eleven strains of avian tubercle bacilli which they investigated ever produced tuberculosis in guinea-pigs by subcutaneous injection "whether a loop-ful of bacilli or a whole glycerin-serum culture was injected[2]." After intraperitoneal injection, on the other hand, the guinea-pigs were found frequently to have abscesses about as large as peas in the omentum, and sometimes the spleen was enlarged. In a few animals injected with large doses a crop of miliary nodules appeared in the peritoneum and omentum, and in the liver sometimes there were fairly numerous yellowish-grey foci containing bacilli. When the doses were large some animals died emaciated after two to six weeks. This result these authors also attributed to toxæmia, for Grancher and Ledoux-Lebard had already shown that the same result might be obtained by injecting avian tubercle bacilli which had been killed by heat.

It is important to note, as showing the low degree of *infective* power of avian tubercle bacilli for the guinea-pig, that Weber and Bofinger were unable to cause disease in these animals by inhalation; and that feeding them with large quantities only produced little suppurative foci in the Peyer's patches, and in the mesenteric and submaxillary glands.

F. Griffith's verdict (1911), after conducting numerous experiments with avian tubercle bacilli for the Royal Commission, is much the same. He found that after subcutaneous injection of these microbes guinea-pigs never developed progressive tuberculosis, and rarely showed anything more than disease limited to the seat of inoculation and the nearest lymphatic glands. On the other hand, after intraperitoneal injection with moderately large doses guinea-pigs succumbed almost invariably to the toxic effect of the bacilli multiplying in their tissues.

[1] *Tub. Arbeit. a. d. Kaiserl. Gesundheitsamte*, Heft 1, p. 133.
[2] *Ibid.* p. 126.

M. Koch and Rabinowitsch (1907), dissatisfied with the conflicting conclusions of different observers, set themselves to investigate the question anew; and for this purpose injected a large number of guinea-pigs, some with tissue emulsions obtained from a large variety of birds, and others with cultures derived from these sources. Briefly, the severity of the results obtained varied within wide limits. Contrary to the experience of Courmont and Dor and of Römer they found that injections of tissue emulsions caused more severe results than injection of the corresponding cultures. This difference is easily explicable on the very probable assumption that the ratio of average culture dose to average tissue dose varies considerably in the hands of different experimenters.

Subcutaneous injection produced less severe results than intraperitoneal. Nevertheless only seven animals when killed after long periods were found to have *no* trace of tuberculous infection. In about half those injected subcutaneously with culture there was an abscess at the seat of inoculation, and the neighbouring lymphatic glands were enlarged, and in some cases even caseous; in others there were in addition more or less numerous nodules in one or other of the internal organs. The proportion of animals which showed these disseminated lesions was greater when tissue emulsions were used. The authors insist that the larger the dose of bacilli injected subcutaneously the more the post-mortem appearances come to resemble those caused by mammalian tubercle bacilli. In this they agree with Römer.

The bacilli persisted for a long time, and were frequently found after many months, or even, in one case, after a whole year[1]. In some cases at least they were living after these long periods, and cultures were grown from liver and spleen of a guinea-pig which showed no tuberculous lesions whatever when killed 183 days after inoculation of tissue emulsions[2].

After intraperitoneal injection of culture (mostly 1 to 2 mg.) death almost always ensued, in from twenty-two to eighty-one days. The animals as a rule were wasted, and showed for the most part tuberculosis of the omentum and numerous miliary foci in liver and spleen.

The authors observed a certain loss of virulence on long continued cultivation, more marked, they say, than that which occurs under similar circumstances among mammalian cultures. And they add the curious observation that the greater the original virulence the smaller was the loss[3]. The diminution of virulence was more apparent in the case of subcutaneous inoculations than in intraperitoneal ones, possibly because toxins are more effective in the peritoneum than in the subcutaneous tissues.

On the whole, as we have said before, there was great variation of severity in the disease produced by avian tubercle bacilli in the guinea-pig. This the authors, in accordance with their well known views as to absence of precision in the boundaries of the various types, and the existence of intermediate strains, attribute to differences of virulence in the different strains of avian tubercle bacilli. It is not clear from their work that this conclusion is well founded. Some difference in the results must be credited to differences in the susceptibility of different guinea-pigs. Such differences undoubtedly exist. Cadiot, Gilbert and Roger called attention to them. Of two guinea-pigs, they say,

[1] *Virchows Archiv*, 1907, Beiheft zum Bande 190. See table pp. 370 *et seq.*, G.-pig 124, p. 384.

[2] *loc. cit.* G.-pig 66a, p. 380.   [3] *loc. cit.* p. 349.

injected with the same dose of the same material, one may develop local lesions only and the other die of general tuberculosis. Koch and Rabinowitsch endorse this statement, and say they have often seen the same[1]. One would therefore like to be sure that this source of fallacy was eliminated in their work by the use of a sufficient number of guinea-pigs in each case before accepting the conclusion that strains of avian tubercle bacilli differ in virulence from one another[2].

Again, the variation in the severity of the results of injecting guinea-pigs with different strains of avian tubercle bacilli may have been due partly to differences of dose; for Koch and Rabinowitsch, though they carefully measured their doses when using culture, do not seem to have employed any method of estimating the numbers of tubercle bacilli in the tissue emulsions with which many of their experiments were carried out.

Finally Koch and Rabinowitsch came to the conclusion from their own observations, that the usually accepted opinion that the guinea-pig is refractory to avian tuberculosis while the rabbit is susceptible can no longer be maintained[3]. No doubt the power of the guinea-pig to resist infection with avian tubercle bacilli has sometimes been appraised too highly in the past; but we cannot go so far as these authors who recognize but little difference in the effect of inoculating avian tubercle bacilli into guinea-pigs and rabbits respectively[4].

Conclusion.

From the long summary of experiments by various authors which have been reviewed above it may be concluded that the guinea-pig is extraordinarily susceptible to infection with

[1] loc. cit. p. 340.

[2] Of Koch and Rabinowitsch's strains of avian tubercle bacilli the one which had the highest virulence for the guinea-pig (No. 300, loc. cit. p. 338) seems to have been a mixture of avian and mammalian bacilli. It alone, of all their avian strains which were subjected to guinea-pig *passage* increased in guinea-pig virulence: a result more easily explained on the assumption of an elimination of an avian factor of low virulence for the guinea-pig and its replacement by a mammalian factor of high virulence for that animal, rather than on that of a true increase of mammalian virulence in a pure strain originally conforming to the avian type. This view is supported by the work of Koch and Rabinowitsch themselves for, as we shall see, they found that passage of avian bacilli through the guinea-pig does not as a rule produce any increase of guinea-pig virulence.

[3] "Es kann somit auch nach unseren Untersuchungen die häufig in der Literatur wiederkehrende Behauptung, dass das für die Säugetiertuberkulose so hervorragend empfängliche Meerschweinchen sich gegen die Infection mit Hühnertuberkulose refractär zeigt, während hingegen das Kaninchen sich sehr empfänglich erweist, nicht mehr aufrecht erhalten worden" (loc. cit. p. 361).

[4] "Im allgemeinen können wir wohl auch von einer Uebereinstimmung des Impfeffects von Vogeltuberkulosematerial beim Meerschweinchen und Kaninchen sprechen" (ibid. p. 361).

mammalian tubercle bacilli, developing progressive and fatal disease on the introduction of the smallest possible doses, whether injected intraperitoneally or subcutaneously, or administered by inhalation. To infection by feeding it is less susceptible.

Both the human and bovine types of tubercle bacilli are highly virulent for this species, but with equal doses similarly administered bovine bacilli kill more quickly than human.

To true infection with the avian tubercle bacillus this animal is largely, but not absolutely, refractory. It probably never develops a continuously progressive disease, and attempts to infect it by inhalation, the most delicate and easiest mode of infection with small doses, have failed. But when large doses are given, especially when these are injected into the peritoneal cavity, the animal not unfrequently dies. The lesions which may then be seen differ considerably from those of tuberculosis, and are suggestive of toxæmia rather than of active infection. In exceptional cases only is anything like a formation of tubercles to be seen. After subcutaneous injection nothing but local changes as a rule are developed.

Tuberculosis in Rats.

While the rabbit and guinea-pig are instances of animals which possess little or no power of destroying tubercle bacilli (in the former case bacilli of bovine type only) when administered experimentally, and which yet enjoy an almost complete immunity against the disease naturally acquired, the rat, together with the mouse, the dog and the horse are instances of the opposite kind; for, though they are difficult to infect experimentally, all these species are liable sometimes to acquire the disease in the natural manner.

M. Koch and Rabinowitsch have recorded a few cases of spontaneous tuberculosis in the wild brown rat[1]. Fifty of these animals were caught in poultry yards and pheasant preserves known to be infected, and six of them were found to be tuberculous. Cultures obtained from two of these rats

---

[1] *Virchows Archiv*, 1907, Beiheft zum Bande 190, p. 368.

possessed the characters of growth and pathogenic properties of the avian tubercle bacillus. From these experiments one may infer that the disease among rats is commoner than is generally supposed.

But, on the other hand, the rat, or at least the white domesticated variety, seems to have considerable powers of resisting experimental tuberculosis. It survives subcutaneous injection, and, though it slowly succumbs to large doses given intraperitoneally, quite considerable quantities (such as 1 mg. of culture, or several million tubercle bacilli in an emulsion of tuberculous tissue) which would quickly kill more susceptible animals are tolerated, even when injected in this way. Moreover it has not been found possible to infect the rat seriously by feeding, even when avian tubercle bacilli have been employed.

The Lesions produced by Tuberculosis in the Rat. The rat can be infected experimentally, and a fatal disease may be induced by any of the three types of tubercle bacilli; but the dose, as we have said, must be a very large one, and injection must be intraperitoneal. Under these circumstances a progressive general infection is set going, and may slowly prove fatal. But the disease is not like tuberculosis as seen in any other species of animal, except the mouse; the lesions presenting little or no resemblance to tubercles, and being for the most part slight and inconspicuous.

The local lesions produced by the subcutaneous injection of even large doses of tubercle bacilli are insignificant and the neighbouring lymphatic glands remain unaffected; even 50 mg. of bacilli have produced only a little purulent focus of the size of a millet seed. The writer once injected subcutaneously into a rat an emulsion of tuberculous tissue estimated to contain 95,000,000 tubercle bacilli. The animal died from some cause other than tubercle more than a year and a half later, and no changes referable to the injection could be found. After intraperitoneal injection there may be some "soft yellow nodules" or a few "grey translucent tubercles" in the peritoneal cavity (A. S. Griffith), but elsewhere there is an almost complete absence of nodule formation, and, as we have said before, very little cellular new formation of any kind. Sometimes the organs, though full of bacilli, appear to the naked eye perfectly normal, but more usually they are somewhat swollen and congested. The lungs as a rule are voluminous, and marked more or less clearly by irregular grey foci which, by the confluence of their outlying processes, may form a sort of network. The kidneys are often speckled or pitted with minute dark points; the spleen is usually large and congested; and the liver, as a rule, apparently normal. The lymphatic glands seldom show any change.

No matter how large the dose of tubercle bacilli injected adult rats never die quickly, or appear to suffer from any immediate effect. Even a dose of 100 mg. of culture, enormous for so small an animal, has been given without causing any apparent disturbance of health for months. In this respect rats are utterly unlike rabbits, which may sometimes succumb to large intraperitoneal doses of bacilli of a type (human) which does not cause progressive tuberculosis in this species. In rats after large intraperitoneal injections the disease is always progressive; the animal dies in the long run; while the rabbit, under the circumstances we have postulated, either dies quickly or not at all of tuberculosis. In the rat the disease develops very slowly. For a long time the animal may appear as bright and alert as a healthy rat should be. But though there are no immediate symptoms of illness, and lesions of any importance fail, for the most part, to be developed—or rather perhaps because of this failure to react—the bacilli continue to multiply steadily; and at last, it may be after many months, the rat begins to show signs of being ill, becomes thin and ragged, and dies; and its principal organs are found to be swarming with tubercle bacilli.

It would seem that rats are insusceptible to the toxins of the tubercle bacilli; and this view is greatly strengthened by the enormous numbers of these microbes which are found in their bodies after death[1]; for one would suppose that if they

[1] It would be difficult to exaggerate the extent to which tubercle bacilli may swarm in the rat. Smears from some of the organs examined microscopically may appear like preparations from a pure culture. In some cases it is hardly too much to say that the organ seems to consist largely of bacilli. Weber and Bofinger make a very similar statement about the mouse affected with avian bacilli (*Tub. Arbeit. a. d. Kaiserl. Gesundheitsamte*, Heft 1, p. 136).

were as susceptible to the toxins as other animals they would die, like them, before the bacilli could multiply to this extent. Being insusceptible to the toxins the rat seems to tolerate the presence of the bacilli themselves. It makes, as we have seen, the poorest sort of cellular reaction in their neighbourhood, and forms little or no granuloma tissue to act as a barrier between the invaders and the rest of the body. It is extraordinary to what an extent tubercle bacilli may be found in organs apparently healthy, and for what a length of time they may remain there alive without provoking either tubercle formation or caseation. In one case a rat was killed when apparently in good health 574 days after intraperitoneal injection of avian tubercle bacilli, and those organisms were cultivated from both liver and spleen, and yet neither of these organs showed any obvious alterations to the naked eye[1].

The Relative Virulence of the Three Types of Tubercle Bacilli for the Rat.

There is but little difference in the comparative effect of the three types of tubercle bacilli on the rat. The following table of experiments, selected from a considerably larger number scattered through the Appendices to the Reports of the Royal Commission, shows none.

In reading over the post-mortem records however and comparing the lesions produced by one type of bacillus with those caused by another, one becomes aware that affection of the lungs is more frequently mentioned in the case of animals infected with one or other of the mammalian types of bacilli than in that of animals infected with avian bacilli, and that, on the other hand, nodule formation in the peritoneal cavity, after intraperitoneal injections, is more often described in the case of avian than in mammalian infections. The difference, if real, would appear to be but a small one and unimportant, and one must remember that the records in evidence were written by independent observers, of whom one worked with avian bacilli and others with mammalian bacilli. One man is liable to be more impressed by one point, and another by a different point; and the strongest impressions naturally find prominent expression. It would therefore be unreasonable to expect absolute identity of description though the things described do not differ. Weber and Bofinger however have made a very similar statement concerning the mouse, at least so far as feeding infections are concerned. They found, in comparative experiments on this animal with the three types of bacilli,

---

[1] F. Griffith, *R.C.T. Fin. Rep.* App. vol. IV, p. 280, Rat 123.

TABLE XVII. Injections of Rats with Tubercle Bacilli of Human, Bovine and Avian Types.

(Selected from the Reports of the Royal Commission.)

HUMAN

Route	Ref.	No.	Dose in mg.	Result
Subcutaneous	2	82	20	K 204. L.l., few T.B. lungs
	1	48	10	D 74. L.l., few T.B. in organs
	1	55	10	D 454. No lesions anywhere, few T.B. lungs
Intraperitoneal	5	28	100	D 172 ⎫
	5	29	100	D 413 ⎪
	5	37	100	D 113 ⎪
	5	38	100	D 162 ⎬ Inconspicuous lesions. General dissemination of bacilli
	5	34	80	D 97 ⎪
	5	40	74	D 87 ⎪
	5	83	20	D 18 ⎪
	2	49	10	D 53 ⎭
	1	54	10	D 58

BOVINE

Route	Ref.	No.	Dose in mg.	Result
Subcutaneous	3	52	50	D 132. L.l., few T.B. lungs
	2	91	25	K 204. T.B. in organs
	3	50	10	K 217. L.l., T.B. in organs
	3	70	10	D 181. L.l., no T.B. in organs
	3	43	1	K 334. L.l., T.B. in pus
Intraperitoneal	5	39	100	D 33 ⎫
	5	41	100	D 85 ⎪
	5	46	75	D 213 ⎪
	5	33	70	D 52 ⎬ Inconspicuous lesions. General dissemination of bacilli
	5	35	50	D 67 ⎪
	5	30	30	D 258 ⎪
	2	96	10	D 26 ⎪
	2	94	5	D 62 ⎭
	3	39	1	K 251. L.l., T.B.
	3	45	1	K 336. L.l., T.B.
	3	44	1	K 334. Normal, no T.B.
	3	62	1	K 194. Tubercles in omentum. Organs normal, T.B.

AVIAN

Route	Ref.	No.	Dose in mg.	Result
Subcutaneous	4	122	100	K 255. No tub., T.B. gland and spleen
	4	128	20	K 244. No tub., few T.B. spleen
	4	107	10	K 109. L.l., no T.B. in organs
	4	104	10	K 109. No tub., few T.B. in spleen
Intraperitoneal	4	132	200	D 131 ⎫
	4	120	50	D 247 ⎪
	4	121	50	D 164 ⎪
	4	108	50	D 24 ⎬ Inconspicuous lesions. General dissemination of bacilli
	4	127	20	K 82 ⎪
	4	109	10	D 285 ⎪
	4	110	10	D 20 ⎭
	4	105	1	K 109. Some nodules in omentum, T.B. in various organs
	4	102	1	D 376. Few T.B. in spleen and lungs
	4	111	1	K 173. Few T.B. lungs and spleen
	4	124	0·1	
	4	123	0·01	K 574. In good condition. Cultures of T.B. grown from spleen and liver

K = killed. D = died. The number following is the number of days since inoculation. L.l. = local lesion, i.e. at the seat of inoculation. Tub. = tuberculosis.
T.B. = tubercle bacilli.

1 R.C.T. Fin. Rep. App. vol. I, p. 252. 2 R.C.T. Fin. Rep. App. vol. III, pp. 208–209. 3 R.C.T. Int. Rep. App. vol. I, pp. 484 et seq.
4 R.C.T. Fin. Rep. App. vol. IV, pp. 277 et seq. 5 R.C.T. Int. Rep. App. vol. II, p. 1192.

that pulmonary lesions developed earlier and were more severe with either of the mammalian types, while intestinal lesions were more pronounced after infection with the avian type. It is not improbable therefore that a similar difference in the action of mammalian and avian tubercle bacilli may occur in the rat.

Turning now to facts which need no discussion, one finds that the duration of life after intraperitoneal, that is to say the fatal kind of, infection, though varying greatly in the experiments with any one kind of bacillus, on the average is much the same with one type as with another. No one type of tubercle bacillus then, human, avian, or bovine appears to possess for the rat any superiority of virulence over another.

Many attempts were made by the Royal Commission to infect the rat by feeding with cultures of tubercle bacilli, or with the organs of tuberculous animals. All three types of bacilli were employed. But the results were almost entirely negative. A. S. Griffith fed twelve rats with cultures of bovine bacilli, and fourteen with tubercular milk or the organs of acutely infected guinea-pigs. The numbers of tubercle bacilli ingested by many of these animals must have been enormous. None of them developed tuberculosis. The intestines were in every case carefully examined; but in none was there any sign of disease. There was never enlargement of the mesenteric glands, and in two cases only were any lesions observed in them. These took the form of minute grey points, barely visible to the naked eye, which, microscopically examined, were seen to be small areas of necrosis containing tubercle bacilli. Tubercle bacilli, on the other hand, were found in coverslip preparations of the mesenteric glands in seventeen cases. No tubercle bacilli were seen in smears of the large organs[1]. Griffith considered the rat the least susceptible to tuberculous infection of all the many kinds of animal upon which he experimented.

The writer fed nine rats daily for about three months with tuberculous milk together with the most infected organs of guinea-pigs which came to the post-mortem room day by day, some of the latter having been injected with tubercle bacilli of human type and others with tubercle bacilli of bovine type[2].

[1] R.C.T. Int. Rep. App. vol. I, p. 633.
[2] Ibid. vol. II, p. 1190.

These rats must have consumed immense quantities of tubercle bacilli, yet they did not suffer from tuberculosis, or become seriously infected with tubercle bacilli. At most tubercle bacilli were found in apparently normal submaxillary or mesenteric glands, and in two instances a few small white foci containing these microbes were found in the lungs. One animal was fed in this way almost daily for over a year, and yet when killed was found to be quite healthy.

F. Griffith fed four rats on a single occasion with the tuberculous organs of guinea-pigs and rabbits infected with avian tubercle bacilli. The rats remained well, and were killed after many months. Of three it is recorded that all organs and lymphatic glands appeared normal, and that no tubercle bacilli could be seen in them. In the remaining case also the organs and glands were free from obvious changes, but a moderate number of tubercle bacilli were found in the mesenteric gland, and a few in the spleen and kidney[1].

In view of these experiments it is difficult to understand how rats can become infected under natural conditions with avian bacilli, unless one may assume that the susceptibility of the wild brown rat is considerably greater than that of the white rat of the laboratory. Perhaps this may be so, but we do not know. Experiments on the brown rat would probably yield interesting information. In the case of the mouse tribe, as we shall see in the next section, there is some evidence of considerable difference in the power of resisting tuberculous infection in the white mouse and field-mouse respectively, and a similar difference may perhaps exist among different kinds of rats.

Tuberculosis in Mice.

The white mouse reacts to experimental infection with various kinds of tubercle bacilli in much the same way as the white rat. It appears to possess very considerable powers of resistance, and to require large doses before it becomes seriously affected. Given such doses, infection follows with any type of tubercle bacillus, and a slowly developing disease is set up—

[1] R.C.T. Fin. Rep. App. vol. IV, p. 190.

a disease which, as in the rat, is notable for the almost incredible number of bacilli, and the poverty of the lesions, and which ends in death after many weeks or months.

The resistance of the mouse, however, to tuberculous infection is not so great as that offered by the rat. The mouse sometimes succumbs to subcutaneous injection, and generally the lesions in the various organs are more pronounced, especially it seems after injection of avian bacilli; and, quite unlike the rat, the mouse is rather easily infected by feeding. Moreover, according to A. S. Griffith, the mouse, when successfully infected, does not hold out so long as the rat in like circumstances[1].

These statements and most of what follows must be understood to refer to the white or domesticated mouse commonly employed in the laboratory. Concerning other species of mice there is very little information. But there is enough, as we have said before, to warn us that the resistance of the white mouse may not be representative of the whole family. More than thirty years ago, at the very dawn of the study of tubercle bacilli, Koch found that field-mice (species not stated) are considerably more susceptible to tuberculous infection than white mice. This interesting and important observation has never been confirmed, and it is very desirable that the experiments should be repeated. In the meantime, since they stand alone, a brief summary of Koch's experiments on this point may not be devoid of interest.

On one occasion Koch[2] inoculated subcutaneously with a culture raised from the tuberculous lung of a monkey[3] two guinea-pigs, one marmot, six white rats, five white mice, four field-mice, two hedge-hogs, six hens, four pigeons, two sparrows, three eels, five frogs and a tortoise. "Of these animals," he tells us "only the guinea-pigs, the marmot and the field-mice became visibly ill. These were killed fifty-three days after inoculation, and were all found to be highly tubercular....The organs of the field-mouse that have undergone tubercular change have a very characteristic aspect. The inguinal glands are markedly swollen and caseous, the lungs full of grey nodules, of sizes varying from that of a poppy-seed to that of a pin's head; while many

[1] *R.C.T. Fin. Rep.* App. vol. I, p. 47. See also *Int. Rep.* App. vol. I, p. 493.
[2] *The Etiology of Tuberculosis.* In *Microparasites in Disease,* Eng. trans. New Sydenham Soc. p. 166, Exp. 4.
[3] This monkey had developed tuberculosis spontaneously. There is no clue to the type of the tubercle bacilli, but they may be assumed to have belonged either to the human or bovine types, and with some probability to the former.

whitish nodules as large as a millet-seed are distributed uniformly throughout
the liver and spleen, so that they have a very pretty speckled appearance.
The white mice were killed two months later, and on examination it was
discovered that one of the five had a grey nodule in the lung, while the others
were healthy." In another experiment twenty-four field-mice were subcutaneously inoculated in groups of four, each group being injected with a different
strain of tubercle bacilli[1]. Some of the mice died prematurely, others which
died after a survival long enough for the development of tuberculosis were
eaten by their fellows. In the course of four to six weeks they were all dead.
Several animals from each group were available for examination, and "it
was proved that they had all succumbed to extensive tuberculosis of lungs,
liver and spleen."

Subsequently, as a control to this experiment, twelve white mice were
inoculated subcutaneously with one of the cultures used in the experiment
just described. "The mice remained for two months without any symptoms
of illness at all, and in not a single one were tubercular changes found[2]."

As field-mice were found "to respond so certainly and conveniently to
tubercular infection," they were the animals chosen by Koch for some experiments, made with Gaffky, on the therapeutic action of various substances
administered by inhalation. Twenty-four of these animals were for this purpose
inoculated subcutaneously with a culture grown from a phthisical lung. Some
of these animals died a few days later from pneumonia caused by the bactericidal substances administered for therapeutic experiment by inhalation. In
all the rest tuberculosis developed "after a few days," and ran the same course
as in the mice belonging to the first-mentioned experiment[3].

Spontaneous Tuberculosis. Instances of natural infection
with tuberculosis in the mouse have been reported by several
observers but, so far, only with the avian type of tubercle
bacillus.

De Jong[4] (1903) observed tuberculosis caused by bacilli
which appeared to belong to this type in un-inoculated white
mice kept for research in the laboratory.

Weber and Bofinger[5] (1904) found tuberculous lesions in a
grey house-mouse which used to come out and sit in the same
cage with some white mice which had been infected by feeding
with avian bacilli. The same type of bacillus was found in the
organs of the house-mouse.

[1] *loc. cit.* p. 167, Exp. 6. Five of the strains used were of human origin,
one being from a case of lupus. The sixth was from "pearl-nodules" from the
pericardium (presumably) of an ox.
[2] *Ibid.* p. 169, Exp. 11. The strain of bacilli used was cultivated directly
from miliary tubercles in a human lung.
[3] *Ibid.* p. 168, Exp. 7.
[4] Quoted by Weber and Bofinger, *loc. cit.* p. 134.
[5] *Tub. Arbeit. a. d. Kaiserl. Gesundheitsamte*, Heft 1, p. 142.

M. Koch and Rabinowitsch[1] (1907), as we have seen, killed
and examined rats and mice caught in infected poultry yards
and pheasant preserves. Out of 100 mice from such places
eighteen were found to be infected with tuberculosis[2]. From
five of them cultures were grown, and adjudged, by their manner
of growth on artificial media and by their effect when injected
into guinea-pigs and rabbits, to belong to the avian type.

Experimental Infection. We have already referred rather
fully to the experiments of Robert Koch (1884) and need
merely repeat here that he succeeded in infecting field-mice
while he failed almost completely to infect white mice.

Straus[3] (1895) injected, subcutaneously, domesticated mice
(white, grey and black) with cultures of tubercle bacilli of
both human and avian type. In all, ten experiments were
made. They showed in the main that the domesticated mouse
possesses a notable degree of resistance to infection with
avian or human tuberculosis. In several cases however disease
occurred, and in such the mice died at the end of several weeks or
months, without apparent tubercles in the viscera, but with a
voluminous spleen and organs filled with bacilli. No difference
was observed in the action of the human and avian bacilli.

Römer[4] (1903) injected avian and human tubercle bacilli
into mice, and caused general infection. He called attention
to the chronic character of the disease and the enormous
multiplication of bacilli in various organs, and he concluded
that the mouse is tolerant of the toxins of the bacilli.

Weber and Bofinger[5] (1904) made experiments on mice with
avian tubercle bacilli, and succeeded in infecting them, not
only by intraperitoneal injection, but by subcutaneous injection,
and by feeding them with a broth containing tubercle bacilli.
In the latter case death occurred after nine to twelve months,
and lungs and spleen were usually found infected as well as
mesenteric glands. Control feeding experiments were made

[1] *Virchows Archiv*, 1907, Beiheft zum Bande 190, p. 368.
[2] Out of 50 rats so caught only six were tuberculous. Mice therefore
would seem to be more susceptible to spontaneous tuberculosis than rats.
[3] *La tuberculose*, p. 379.
[4] "Tuberkelbazillenstämme," *Beiträge z. expt. Therapie*, Heft 6.
[5] *loc. cit.* p. 133.

with human and bovine bacilli, and with these too it was found possible to infect the mouse.

One grey house-mouse was fed with avian tubercle bacilli. It was killed nine months later, and two small tuberculous foci were found in the lungs.

M. Koch and Rabinowitsch[1] (1907) injected subcutaneously ten mice with emulsions of tuberculous organs from various birds, and succeeded in producing more or less infection. As a rule the only tuberculous changes seen were at the seat of inoculation; sometimes the spleen was swollen; sometimes there were no visible changes at all. Only in one mouse, which died seventy-eight days after injection, were there definitely perceptible tuberculous lesions in spleen, liver and lungs.

Many experiments on mice were made for the Royal Commission from 1902 to 1910, by A. S. Griffith and F. Griffith, and a few by the author. These will be dealt with presently. They show on the whole that the white mouse is possessed of considerable powers of resisting tuberculous infection, as compared for example with the guinea-pig, but that it may be infected with certainty if the dose is sufficient.

The Comparative Susceptibility of the White Mouse to Infection with the Three Types of Tubercle Bacilli.

So far as natural infection is concerned but little is known concerning this subject. The few cases of spontaneous tuberculosis which have been reported in the mouse have been, as we have seen, caused by the avian bacillus (de Jong, M. Koch and Rabinowitsch, Weber and Bofinger).

Experiment has shown that all three types of bacilli may infect the mouse; and probably, as we shall find when we come to examine the evidence in detail, the virulence for the mouse of any one type is much the same as that of another. There are however minor differences, and there is some reason to think that the virulence of the avian tubercle bacillus for this species may be slightly greater than that of the others.

Weber and Bofinger compared the results of feeding mice with avian and mammalian tubercle bacilli respectively.

[1] *loc. cit.* p. 363.

There was not much difference. In either case infection followed the same route; the order in which various organs were involved was the same; only, the lungs were affected earlier when the bacilli belonged to one of the mammalian types and pulmonary lesions were more pronounced than when avian bacilli were employed. On the other hand, in feeding experiments the disease in the intestinal follicles, glands and spleen was more severe with avian than with mammalian bacilli[1].

The investigations of the Royal Commission and of the Gesundheitsamt together cover the ground fairly completely, and where they overlap are in substantial agreement[2]. The following description is based upon their reports.

Subcutaneous Injection. All three types of tubercle bacilli cause only a small lesion at the seat of injection. Of that produced by mammalian bacilli there is little description in the reports. A. S. Griffith writes of "local lesions" and "local tuberculosis" after injections of both human and bovine bacilli, but does not describe them. Of the local lesion produced by avian bacilli the reports have more to say. F. Griffith states that "at the seat of inoculation in the subcutaneous tissues a caseous nodule develops, which softens and is usually discharged through an ulcer in the skin. The nearest lymphatic glands become enlarged and firm but do not caseate." Weber and Bofinger say that in a certain proportion of their animals a small tumour appeared at the seat of inoculation and might attain the size of a pea; sometimes these little tumours softened and discharged pus. Remarkably little is said in the reports about the condition of the internal organs after injections of mammalian tubercle bacilli. This comparative silence is probably significant; there may be but little to say. A. S. Griffith notes in several instances that there was no macroscopic

---

[1] *loc. cit.* p. 147.

[2] It must be understood that the Commission made no systematic efforts to investigate the question now under discussion. Their experiments with the mouse were made for all sorts of purposes, at different times and by various observers. It is to be regretted that no co-ordinated experiments were carried out in order to determine more exactly the relative virulence for the mouse of the three types of tubercle bacilli. The German investigation was concerned mainly with avian tubercle bacilli.

tuberculosis, or that there was local tuberculosis only. In one instance however the present writer recorded a few translucent tubercles in the lungs. Again the descriptions of the lesions caused by avian bacilli are fuller. Weber and Bofinger say that all the lymphatic glands and the intestinal follicles might be swollen, and the spleen and liver greatly enlarged, the latter of a golden colour and frequently beset with little whitish grey points just big enough to be visible. Not unfrequently there was a definite formation of nodules in the liver and spleen. The lungs sometimes had the appearance of marble; ranging over their surfaces there were foci of irregular shape and variable size formed by the confluence of single nodules; and lying more deeply between these were what appeared to be portions of normal lung tissue. Isolated nodules occurred only in small numbers. The larger foci had a lardaceous (*speckig*) appearance, and caseation was never observed[1]. F. Griffith, too, describes nodule formation in the lungs after subcutaneous injection of avian bacilli. He says "the nearest lymphatic glands become large and firm, but do not caseate. The spleen is swollen, and shows grey points beneath the capsule; similar foci may be seen in the liver. The lungs contain nodules, composed of firm grey and greyish-white tissue, which may be so numerous as to completely replace the lung substance." He even goes so far as to compare this condition with what occurs in the rabbit after subcutaneous inoculation of bovine tubercle bacilli[2].

From these accounts, and from the comparative silence of the reports concerning visible lesions after the injection of mammalian tubercle bacilli, it seems reasonable to conclude that the injection of avian tubercle bacilli into the mouse gives rise to more tissue reaction, and especially to more nodule formation, than does the injection of either of the mammalian tubercle bacilli. Nevertheless, a fatal infection may occur with any type of bacillus, and, so far as one can judge from the experiments, as readily with one sort as with another. All accounts speak of the enormous number of tubercle bacilli which may be present in various organs.

[1] Weber and Bofinger, *loc. cit.* p. 135.   [2] F. Griffith, *loc. cit.* p. 185.

Intraperitoneal Injection. Nodule formation has been described occasionally after injections of this kind, even when the bacilli have belonged to one or other of the mammalian types. And the nodules have not been confined entirely to the peritoneal cavity, but have occurred, in some instances, in the thorax also.

A. S. Griffith writes as follows concerning inoculations of bovine bacilli: "A characteristic feature of the disease in these intraperitoneally inoculated mice was the occurrence in the peritoneal cavity of thin-walled nodules, filled with yellow pus composed largely of tubercle bacilli, and similar nodules were sometimes found in the thorax; the lungs were congested, and sometimes partly consolidated and mottled on the surface with grey, or greyish yellow, foci; in one case they were almost completely consolidated, firm and greyish white[1]." F. Griffith described the lesions which followed the intraperitoneal injection of avian bacilli as follows: "The omentum was either slightly thickened or contained a few nodules filled with soft yellow substance. The spleen was enlarged, and occasionally speckled with grey points. The liver was apparently normal. In one mouse, which died in 345 days, the surfaces of the kidneys were pitted. The lungs were usually congested and reddish grey in colour. In rather more than half the mice the lungs contained grey nodules, sometimes numerous, varying up to 4 mm. in diameter[2]."

Feeding. The author failed to infect eight mice which he fed almost daily for many days with tuberculous tissues and tuberculous milk containing mammalian tubercle bacilli[3]. But Weber and Bofinger succeeded, as we have seen, with both human and bovine bacilli[4], and these authors and F. Griffith also were able to infect mice by feeding them with avian bacilli.

Griffith mentions in cases thus infected swelling of Peyer's patches, enlargement and even caseation of the mesenteric glands, swelling of the spleen, and foci in the lungs. In one

[1] *R.C.T. Fin. Rep.* App. vol. I, p. 47. Griffith contrasts this condition with the absence of such lesions in the rat
[2] *loc. cit.* p. 185
[3] *R.C.T. Int. Rep.* App. vol. II, p. 1200.   [4] *loc. cit.* p. 144.

case a mouse (No. 75) died of "general tuberculosis" after 223 days. "The intestinal mucous membrane was speckled with whitish foci; the Peyer's patches were enlarged. The spleen was beset with grey nodules, and there were numerous grey points and tubercles in the liver. The lungs were closely filled with grey nodules[1]."

Inhalation experiments were made by Weber and Bofinger with avian bacilli. The bacilli were observed to multiply in the alveoli of the lungs. In an animal killed after four weeks there were no changes visible to the naked eye, but some nodules were seen under the microscope. In another, killed after three and a half months, the lungs were beset with miliary foci, and the spleen was swollen; and in still another, killed after seven months, there were in the lungs, beside miliary foci, larger yellow nodules, some of which were as big as small peas.

Concerning the minute structure of the lesions caused by avian tubercle bacilli in the mouse Weber and Bofinger state that they begin as typical epithelial-cell tubercles, such as Baumgarten described in rabbits infected with mammalian bacilli, but their further development is very different; there is neither necrosis in the centre, nor, as a rule, infiltration of round cells at the periphery; giant cells are not seen; and the lesion remains at the stage of a pure epithelial-celled tubercle[2]. All observers call attention to the enormous number of tubercle bacilli present in the lesions caused by the avian bacillus. Weber and Bofinger think the bacilli are particularly numerous after intraperitoneal injection. They may then be so plentiful in the lungs as almost to replace the animal tissues, and these authors go so far as to state that it is no exaggeration to say that the organs of the mouse which has died of avian tuberculosis appear to consist for the most part of tubercle bacilli[3]. The bacilli are largely situated in the protoplasm of the epithelial cells, and the latter may become so stuffed with them that in specimens suitably stained nothing but a blue nucleus is seen in a cell otherwise made up of red bacilli. Even the nucleus

---

[1] *loc. cit.* p. 185.   [2] *loc. cit.* p. 142.

[3] *loc. cit.* p 136.

may disappear, and the remains of the cell be indicated only by a clump of bacilli. The situation of the bacilli and their enormous numbers recall the picture presented by the nodules of leprosy.

Weber and Bofinger found this enormous development of the bacilli particularly marked in animals infected with avian bacilli, and in one case in a mouse infected with bovine bacilli. They thought that it did not occur to the same extent in animals infected with human bacilli. This is borne out to some extent by the post-mortem notes of the experiments undertaken for the Royal Commission. But, however, this may be, even the lesions of mice infected with human tubercle bacilli may contain these organisms in very large numbers.

The result of inoculation has been by no means always proportionate to dose of bacilli. It must be understood however that the quantities used have usually been very large for these small animals. A. S. Griffith believed that the mouse is resistant to small doses (of bovine bacilli) injected subcutaneously; and Koch's experiments already described would seem to support this view.

Conclusion.

As to the comparative virulence of the three types of tubercle bacilli for the mouse it will not be possible to come to a definite conclusion until we are in possession of the results of more systematic and exactly co-ordinated experiments. It is because of the absence of such experiments that the various authors have been freely quoted here, and the reader thus given an opportunity of judging the question himself. We shall certainly not be wrong, however, if we conclude that all three types are virulent for the mouse, and produce, when inoculated by any method or given with food in sufficient doses, a peculiar slow tuberculous infection; an infection somewhat similar to that seen in the rat, but probably not quite so deliberate in its progress, and not so strikingly marked by the poverty of the cellular reaction and the absence of lesions resembling the tubercles of other animals; but, on the other hand, equally characterized by the enormous development of tubercle bacilli and their disposition within cells.

Further than this it is difficult to go with safety; but we may perhaps venture to say that there are observations which lead one to suspect that the avian bacillus possesses some slight superiority of virulence for this species of animal over the others; and that this superiority of virulence shows itself in a tendency to provoke lesions of a more obvious kind and more nodular in character, and by an even more wonderful capacity than that possessed by the other types of multiplying in the mouse's cells and tissues.

Even if this distinction is really justified—and we think that it is—the difference in virulence of the three types of bacilli is certainly not great; and if, as seems to be the case, spontaneous tuberculosis in the mouse is commonly caused by the avian bacillus, this is probably because the habits of the mouse render it more liable to contract tuberculosis from the fowl than from other domesticated animals or from man, rather than because of superiority of virulence in the avian type of bacillus.

REFERENCES. XII

(Chapter xx)

Tuberculosis in the Rabbit.

Cobbett (1907). *R.C.T. Int. Rep.* App. vol. II, p. 1067.
—— (1913). Two cases of Spontaneous Tuberculosis in the Rabbit caused by the Avian Tubercle Bacillus. *Journ. of Comp. Pathol. and Therap.* vol. XXVI, p. 33.
Fraenkel and Baumann (1906). Untersuchungen über die Infectiosität verschiedener Kulturen von Tuberkelbazillen. *Zeitschr. f. Hyg.* vol. LIV, p. 247.
Griffith, A. S. (1907). *R.C.T. Int. Rep.* App. vol. I, pp. 437, 538, 592, 706.
—— (1911). *Ibid. Fin. Rep.* App. vol. I, p. 32.
Oehlecker (1907). Untersuchungen über chirurgische Tuberculose. *Tub. Arbeit. a. d. Kaiserl. Gesundheitsamte*, Heft 6, p. 103.
Rothe (1912). Studien über spontane Kaninchentuberkulose. *Veröffent. d. R. Koch-Stiftung*, Heft 4, and *Deutsch. med. Wochenschr.* vol. XXXVIII, p. 642.

Tuberculosis in the Guinea-pig.

Cadiot, Gilbert and Roger (1891). Inoculation de la tuberculose aviaire au cobaye, etc. *Mém. de la Soc. de Biol.* pp. 81, 87.
—— (1890). *Compt. rend. de la Soc. de Biol.* p. 542.
—— (1896). *Ibid.* p. 140.

Cobbett (1907). *R.C.T. Int. Rep.* App. vol. II, p. 1134.
Courmont and Dor (1891). Tuberculose aviaire et tuberculose des mammifères. *Congrès pour l'étude de la tuberculose.* Paris, p. 119.
Grancher and Ledoux-Lebard (1892). Tuberculose aviaire et humaine ; action de la chaleur sur la fertilité et la virulence du bacille tuberculeux. *Archiv. de méd. experiment. et d'anatom. pathol.* vol. IV.
Griffith, A. S. (1911). *R.C.T. Fin. Rep.* App. vol. I, p. 39.
Griffith, F. (1911). *Ibid.* vol. IV, p. 168.
Koch, M. and Rabinowitsch, L. (1907). Die Tuberkulose der Vögel. *Virchows Archiv,* 1907, Beiheft zum Bande 190, p. 246.
Rivolta (1889). *Giorn. di Anat. e Fisiol.* vol. I, p. 22. Abst. in *Baumgarten's Jahresbericht,* 1889, p. 313.
Römer (1903). Ueber Tuberkelbazillenstämme verschiedener Herkunft. *Beiträge zur experimentellen Therapie,* Heft 6.
Straus and Gamaléia (1891). Sur la tuberculose humaine et aviaire. *Congrès pour l'étude de la tuberculose,* p. 66.
—— (1891). Recherches expérimentales sur la tuberculose : la tuberculose humaine, sa distinction de la tuberculose des oiseaux. *Archiv. de méd. experiment. et d'anatom. pathol.* vol. III, p. 457.
Weber and Bofinger (1904). Die Hühnertuberculose. *Tub. Arbeit. a. d. Kaiserl. Gesundheitsamte,* Heft 1, p. 83.

Tuberculosis in Rats and Mice.

Cobbett (1907). *R.C.T. Int. Rep.* App. vol. II, pp. 1190, 1200.
Eastwood. *Ibid. Int. Rep.* vol. IV, p. 152.
Griffith, A. S. (1907). *Ibid. Int. Rep.* vol. I, pp. 483, 493, 633, 706.
—— (1911). *Ibid. Fin. Rep.* vol. I, pp. 46–47, 252–254.
Griffith, A. S. and F. (1911). *Ibid. Fin. Rep.* vol. III, p. 172.
Griffith, F. (1911). *Ibid. Fin. Rep.* vol. IV, pp. 185, 190, 237, 277.
De Jong (1903). XIe Cong. Internat. d'hyg. et démog. Bruxelles.
Koch (1884). *Die Aetiologie der Tuberkulose.* Eng. trans. New Syd. Soc. *Microparasites in Disease,* pp. 164 *et seq.*
Koch, M. and Rabinowitsch. *Virchows Archiv,* 1907, Beiheft zum Bande 190, p. 363.
Römer (1903). Tuberkelbazillenstämme. *Beiträge zur experimentellen Therapie,* Heft 6.
Straus (1895). *La tuberculose et son bacille.* Paris, p. 378.
Weber and Bofinger (1894). *Tub. Arbeit. a. d. Kaiserl. Gesundheitsamte,* Heft 1, p. 133.

CHAPTER XXI

THE SUSCEPTIBILITY TO TUBERCULOSIS OF VARIOUS ANIMAL SPECIES (*continued*)

TUBERCULOSIS IN THE HORSE, ASS, CAMEL, ANTELOPE AND ELEPHANT.

Tuberculosis in the Horse and the Ass.

The horse and the ass were once thought to be immune to tuberculosis; but it is now known that the former suffers from the disease occasionally, while the latter would seem to be not altogether exempt. At one time belief in the immunity of the ass led, not unnaturally, to the proposal to use its blood-serum tentatively for the treatment of the disease in man[1]— just as the similar use of the serum of the dog, also once believed immune, was suggested by Héricourt and Richet. There was indeed considerably more justification for the belief in the immunity of the ass than in that of the dog; for the latter is, as we shall see, attacked by tuberculosis not very unfrequently, while the former is so rarely affected that only a few instances of the disease have ever been reported.

A. *Tuberculosis in the Horse.*

In the horse tuberculosis, though uncommon, cannot be regarded as a rare disease. Many instances are on record. Four were investigated by Koch about 1884; and the number of observations already accumulated ten years later made it possible for Nocard in 1894 to describe the principal forms it assumes in this animal.

---

[1] Viquerat suggested the use of the serum of the mule which had been inoculated with tubercle bacilli. See "Zur Gewinnung von Antituberculin," *Centralb. f. Bakt. u. Parasit.* 1896, Bd. 20, p. 674.

Much interest was taken in the subject about twenty years ago at the Veterinary College in London; and a considerable number of cases were examined by Professor McFadyean and others, and described in the *Journal of Comparative Pathology and Therapeutics*. From these investigations it became evident that many instances of equine tuberculosis must have escaped recognition in the past, for the disease in the horse is apt to cause enormous solid enlargement of spleen and lymphatic glands, sometimes unaccompanied by lesions elsewhere, and probably on this account has often been mistaken for lymph-adenoma, sarcoma, or some such condition. This error was first exposed in 1889, when McFadyean found tubercle bacilli in one of these large spleens; and this observer subsequently studied about forty others, and was able to demonstrate in all but two of them that the disease was really tuberculosis.

The lesions of tuberculosis in the horse are indeed, as Nocard pointed out, very unlike those of other animals such as the ox which naturally form the basis of the veterinary conception of tuberculosis. They may, as was said above, attain enormous proportions and appear like new growths; and this similarity is all the closer because they are usually firm and solid, and show little tendency to caseation. In one case one reads of a liver studded over and throughout with nodules as large as potatoes (Dewer); in another of tumours in the spleen of the size of an infant's head (McFadyean); in others again of lymphatic glands fused into one mass which would have weighed ten to fifteen pounds (Oliver), or which in a certain instance actually did weigh forty pounds (Tailby). In yet another case the sub-lumbar glands formed a tumour so large that it reached from the diaphragm to the pelvis, embracing the aorta, the vena cava and the kidneys.

The enormous enlargement of the spleen already mentioned seems to be rather a common feature of tuberculosis in the horse, and may, as we have said, be the only obvious lesion. The liver however in some instances is also greatly increased in size, and may, like the spleen, be full of large tumour-like masses. Peritoneum, pericardium, and pleura do not escape, and the diease may affect the bones[1].

Tuberculosis in the horse is mainly an abdominal disease; or at least shows signs of having originated in the abdomen (McFadyean, Nocard). The intestinal mucous membrane, especially it would seem that of the ileum, is affected relatively often. The Peyer's patches may be greatly enlarged or even converted into veritable tumours, and some of them may be ulcerated. The enormous enlargement of mesenteric and other lymphatic glands behind the diaphragm, and of the spleen and sometimes also the liver, which has just been described, all go to swell the total of the abdominal form of equine tuberculosis. The lungs, it is true, are found affected relatively often, but in the majority of such cases the disease there is many-centred, and appears to be more recent than that elsewhere. It not unfrequently assumes the form of a secondary miliary tuberculosis, as in one of Koch's cases[2].

There is however, according to Nocard, a pulmonary tuberculosis in the horse which is primary[3]. The description of this form of the disease given by him includes instances in which the pulmonary lesions are multiple, composed of rounded nodules varying in size from a hemp seed to a nut, and disseminated fairly regularly through the pulmonary parenchyma. In such cases it may be thought that the evidence of primary origin in the lungs is not very strong, but there is still another form described by Nocard in which there is a true caseous pneumonia, with dilatation of bronchi and formation of cavities. Cases of this kind however would appear to be uncommon.

It has already been pointed out that tuberculous lesions in

[1] In one of McFadyean's cases all the cervical vertebrae were tuberculous; and in another, recorded by Capt. Lishman in 1914, there was tuberculosis with caseation of the first and second dorsal and last cervical vertebrae.

[2] In this case a tumour, formed by enlargement of the lumbar lymphatic glands, had penetrated the wall of the vena cava inferior, and presented an ulcerated surface within the lumen of that vessel. From thence tubercle bacilli had invaded the blood stream in great numbers, and, as a consequence, multitudes of miliary tubercles had developed in the lungs (*The Etiology of Tuberculosis*, Eng. trans. p. 126).

[3] *Les tuberculoses animales*, p. 175.

the horse show little tendency to become caseous. Caseation however seems sometimes to occur[1]. Calcification too, so common in the lesions of the ox, is rarely seen in those of the horse, but it nevertheless is found occasionally[2].

Tubercle bacilli are often present in the lesions of equine tuberculosis in enormous numbers; and several authors have called attention to this interesting fact (Koch, McFadyean, Pemberthy, Nocard). This abundance presents a marked contrast to the paucity of bacilli seen, even in very acute cases, in the tuberculous lesions of the pig, sheep and calf[3].

[1] McFadyean in one place speaks of caseo-purulent matter from the tuberculous spleen of a horse (*Journ. of Comp. Pathol. and Therap.* vol. xv, p. 156). See also Bowie's case, mentioned in footnote, p. 467.

[2] Straus remarks that calcification, which is the rule in the ox, is quite exceptional in the horse. In one of McFadyean's cases however it is mentioned as occurring in some tuberculous tumours which were present in an enormously enlarged spleen (*Journ. of Comp. Pathol. and Therap.* vol. I, p. 49).

[3] One might, I think, reasonably expect to find some relation between the capacity of an animal to resist tuberculous infection and the number of bacilli commonly present in the lesions when thus infected; though whether one should look to find them numerous in the highly susceptible animals and scarce in the more resistant ones, or vice versa, it would perhaps be difficult to say. Some relationship however was to be expected, but as a matter of fact there would appear to be no rule at all; bacilli being often numerous in both susceptible and resistant animals, and again as often scarce in both categories.

Even in one and the same species of animal the numbers of bacilli present in tuberculous lesions may vary greatly. In man, for instance, as is well known, they are few in the nodules of lupus, in tuberculous synovial membrane, and in the pus of a cold abscess; and again they may be extraordinarily numerous in tuberculous meningitis, or sometimes in the expectoration of pulmonary tuberculosis. In the horse too the bacilli, while usually present in tuberculous lesions in enormous numbers, are sometimes, it would seem, represented only by small numbers; for Nocard states that in some cases of pulmonary tuberculosis the lesions though "très riches en cellules géantes sont très pauvres en bacilles" (*Les tuberculoses animales*, p. 176).

At first sight it might seem that the bacilli are numerous in acute lesions and rare in chronic ones. And though this is often the case, it is by no means always so; in the calf, for example, even in the most acute and severe cases of generalized (experimental) tuberculosis, when death occurs three or four weeks after inoculation, and every organ, almost, is found post-mortem to be densely packed with minute tubercles—even in such cases tubercle bacilli, at least in their usually recognized form, may be difficult to find on microscopic examination.

But in spite of this it would seem, as we have said above, that there are some species of animals in whose tuberculous lesions bacilli are commonly

Portals of entry. It is generally admitted that in equine tuberculosis infection takes place, as a rule, through the alimentary canal. Both Nocard and McFadyean agree about this; but the former, as we have seen already, recognized, in addition to the abdominal form of the disease, another and rarer kind in which the primary lesions are thoracic; and it may be presumed that he believed that in such cases the bacilli enter directly into the lungs.

Markus (1901), who examined thirteen cases of equine tuberculosis, ascribed eight to infection through food, and five to infection through air. In the former it was often found that the bacilli had passed through the mucous membrane without causing a lesion there.

Sources of Infection. It is not easy to understand how the horse acquires tuberculosis. The cases which Nocard observed occurred, for the most part, in large stables, and yet the disease showed no tendency to spread from one animal to another. This is explained by Nocard as follows: tuberculosis soon

numerous while there are others in which they are as regularly scarce. The horse, the rat and the mouse belong to the former class, the pig, sheep and ox to the latter. And here it is that we meet the surprising fact that there seems to be no relationship between the degree of susceptibility of the species and the average number of bacilli in its tuberculous lesions. It is true that the horse, the rat and the mouse, in whose tuberculous lesions bacilli are usually numerous, must be regarded as resistant animals, while the pig, the sheep and the ox, in whom they are usually scanty, are more susceptible. But even these latter are possessed of no mean power of resisting small doses; and when we look to the other end of the scale of susceptibility we find the rabbit, the guinea-pig, and the monkey all very susceptible, with tuberculous lesions in which bacilli are usually present in large numbers. The author has seen, in a case of general tuberculosis in the last-named species, a tubercle in the kidney which when stained in section by the carbol-fuchsin method showed a peripheral ring of crimson visible to the naked eye, composed mainly of tubercle bacilli.

This lack of relationship between the numbers of tubercle bacilli commonly present in the lesions and the general degree of susceptibility of the species of animal would seem to point to a difference in the basic principles on which defence against tuberculous infection is founded in the different species. In one defence appears to depend more on the efficiency with which attack is directed on the bacilli themselves, while in another it seems to depend rather on the power of counteracting the bacterial products. In this respect it is perhaps significant that in the horse and the rat the presence of large numbers of bacilli goes hand in hand with absence of caseation. Both animals one must presume are relatively insusceptible to the necrotizing toxins; but in the one case there is an enormous tissue proliferation, and in the other hardly any.

c.   30

unfits for work, and since a horse which cannot work is too expensive to be kept long, this animal does not long remain diseased before it is sent to the knackers, and consequently the disease seldom becomes so advanced as to be a source of danger to other horses. He might have added, as an additional reason, that, as the lesions of equine tuberculosis are remarkable for their solidity and the absence as a rule of any tendency to caseate and break down, the tubercle bacilli which they contain have little opportunity for leaving the body of their host.

Be the reason what it may, it seems to be generally believed that the horse does not contract tuberculosis, at least in the majority of cases, from other horses. From what animal then does he contract it? Nocard at one time put forward the view that the commonest form of equine tuberculosis, the abdominal, was caused by the avian tubercle bacillus, and it may be inferred that he thought that in such cases infection comes from the common fowl. But, as we shall see, there is very little bacteriological evidence in favour of this view. The opinion commonly held now is that infection in equine tuberculosis comes from the ox. Straus supported this view, and mentioned a case reported by Lehnert in which tuberculosis occurred in a colt which was kept in company with some tuberculous cows. To this view McFadyean also seems to incline, for he calls attention to the undesirability of the practice, which appears to be usual among veterinary surgeons, of administering fresh cow's milk to sick horses, or of giving it to normal ones as a fattening article of diet[1].

If the horse derives its tuberculosis from the cow, under what circumstances is the infection transmitted? Horses and cows do not come much together, except in the pastures when the former are turned out to grass. But at such times there would appear to be a chance of infection, for tubercle bacilli are known to escape with the droppings of tuberculous cattle. It is therefore under these circumstances and from this source that many of the instances of tuberculosis in the horse would appear to arise.

The view which regards equine tuberculosis as derived

[1] *Journ. of Comp. Pathol. and Therap.* vol. IX, p. 190.

from the cow receives strong support from the fact that the tubercle bacilli, isolated from the few cases of equine tuberculosis which have been investigated by modern bacteriological methods, have conformed in the main to the bovine type. But one must hasten to add that no inconsiderable proportion of these strains have, as we shall see later, presented peculiarities of virulence in that they did not attain exactly to the standard of virulence of that type. This would indicate that they had undergone some modification since they left their bovine environment; or in other words that they had changed somewhat in the body of the horse. And since there is reason to think that such modification can take place only very slowly, and since moreover the degree to which equine strains of tubercle bacilli depart from the standard of the bovine type differs considerably in different cases—some being considerably attenuated, while others correspond more or less exactly to the type—it would seem tempting to entertain the belief that those strains which are most attenuated have resided for long periods in the horse, while those which are least, or not at all, attenuated have come comparatively recently from the cow. If this inference is sound then it would seem reasonable to regard those cases of equine tuberculosis which yield the markedly attenuated bacilli as derived in all probability from other cases of equine tuberculosis, and those which yield bacilli of full or approximately full bovine virulence as derived directly from the ox[1].

---

[1] An instance which affords a certain amount of presumptive evidence of transmission of tuberculous infection from one horse to another was recorded in 1889 by Bowie in the *Journ. of Comp. Pathol. and Therap.* vol. II, p. 55. A mare suffered from disease of one kidney and had to be killed. This organ was enormously enlarged. It weighed 32 lbs. On section it presented what appeared to the naked eye to be characters of tuberculosis. There was no disease elsewhere. A year later another mare which occupied the adjoining stall began to lose appetite and condition, and became extremely emaciated. After the death of this animal the abdominal lymphatic glands were found to be greatly enlarged (some of them appear to have been enormous) and caseous. The lungs were densely and uniformly studded with miliary tubercles. Tubercle bacilli were extraordinarily numerous. The diagnosis of the latter case was confirmed by McFadyean. Unfortunately that of the former case is less certain.

Another rather curious instance seems worth mentioning here since it gives a hint at the possibility of a congenital transmission of infection in the

The Comparative Susceptibility of the Horse to Infection with the Three Types of Tubercle Bacilli.

Natural Infection. Investigations of the type of the tubercle bacilli found in the horse have of necessity been few in number, since, as we have seen, the disease is far from common.

Nocard, who gave much attention to the study of equine tuberculosis, seems at one time to have come to the conclusion that the tubercle bacilli which caused it were of the ordinary mammalian kind[1]. But in 1896 he discovered what seems undoubtedly to have been an avian bacillus in the mesenteric glands of a horse affected with the abdominal form of the disease[2]; and about that time he changed his mind concerning the etiology of that form of equine tuberculosis, and concluded that it was caused by the avian type of tubercle bacillus. In 1898 he announced that "whilst primary pulmonary tuberculosis is provoked by a bacillus identical with that of human tuberculosis, it is a bacillus of the avian type, somewhat profoundly modified by its passage through the horse, which causes the abdominal form of tuberculosis in that animal[3]."

· The statement that one form of the disease is caused by the human type of bacillus must not be understood in too literal a

equine species. A mare gave birth to four foals in succession. Two of these developed tuberculosis when yearlings, and another did so when four years old. The first-born also may have been tuberculous, for in its fourth year it "went wrong in the back and had to be shot." No post-mortem examination is recorded, but the knacker remarked that there was a big lump near the kidneys. There is however no direct evidence that the mother of these animals was tuberculous; and she was still living and, presumably, well at the time the report was written (*Journ. of Comp. Pathol. and Therap.* 1888, vol. I, p. 247).

[1] In *Les tuberculoses animales*, published in 1894, he wrote concerning the bacilli of equine tuberculosis (p. 175): "Nous avons vu que l'inoculation au cobaye et les cultures démontrent qu'ils sont identiques aux bacilles qu'on recontre chez les autres mammifères."

[2] In 1896, in the *Bull. de la Soc. Cent. de Méd. Vét.*, he described a strain of tubercle bacilli which he had obtained from a horse with abdominal tuberculosis. This strain is said to have had all the characters of the avian type of tubercle bacillus. It was virulent for the rabbit; produced in the guinea-pig a peculiar form of tuberculosis—characterized by a large smooth red spleen without visible lesions; and caused tubercles in the spleen of a fowl inoculated intravenously.

[3] *Ann. de l'Inst. Past.* 1898, vol. XII, p. 562.

sense; for in 1898, when Nocard wrote, the distinction between human and bovine tubercle bacilli had only been hinted at, while that between avian and mammalian tubercle bacilli was already discerned by the leading bacteriologists. Probably all that Nocard meant to affirm by this statement was that the pulmonary form of equine tuberculosis was due to the *mammalian* tubercle bacillus. He himself at that time certainly regarded all kinds of mammalian tuberculosis as identical, for in the article from which we have quoted he wrote: "On ne conteste plus l'identité de la tuberculose chez toutes les espèces de mammifères" (p. 561).

If then we may read "mammalian" for "human" Nocard was probably not far wrong as regards this part of his statement; for, as we have said, the type of micro-organism found in equine tuberculosis by all recent researches has resembled more or less closely the bovine bacillus. But his affirmation that the abdominal form of the disease in the horse is caused by the avian bacillus cannot be approved, since it receives no shred of support from modern investigations. Such investigations into equine tuberculosis are, it is true, very few in number; but so far no other avian bacillus than that recorded by him has been found in the horse; and, as we shall see later, such attempts as have been made to infect the horse experimentally with this kind of bacillus have not been attended with success.

For the Royal Commission on Tuberculosis five strains of tubercle bacilli from the horse were investigated by F. Griffith[1]. Four of these strains (E I—E IV) were derived from cases of abdominal tuberculosis, the other (E V) came from a case in which the disease may have begun in the lungs[2]. None of these

---

[1] *R.C.T. Fin. Rep.* App. vol. IV, p. 5.

[2] Viruses E I and E V came from cases of general tuberculosis. In the former case the horse had extensive tuberculous lesions in the mesenteric glands and spleen, and miliary tuberculosis of lungs. In the latter case "the lungs were closely infiltrated with irregular tuberculous masses," the spleen contained two firm fibro-caseous tumours about 4 or 5 cm. in diameter, and a mesenteric gland, measuring about 5–6 cm., resembled in structure the tumours in the spleen. E III came from a horse which had enormously enlarged mesenteric glands. E II was derived from the spleen of a horse which had tuberculosis of the mesenteric glands, and E IV from the spleen of a horse in which no lesions were visible elsewhere.

strains of bacilli belonged to the avian type. On the contrary
they all presented a more or less close resemblance to the bovine
type, possessing identical cultural characters, and the same *range*
of virulence for various species of animals, but differing in most
cases, to some extent, from the bovine type in the *degree* of that
virulence.

E I was a typical bovine bacillus—just as virulent for calves
and rabbits as a bacillus derived from the ox itself. E III
had substantially the virulence of the bovine type, but was
probably not quite up to its standard. E II and E IV were
decidedly of low virulence for the ox, rabbit, etc. ; while E v was
virulent for rabbits, but was not tested on calves[1] (see p. 364).

If these strains were to be judged according to the view
put forward above, E II and E IV would be regarded as strains
originally bovine, but modified somewhat in virulence for the
ox, and some other-than-equine animals, by prolonged residence
in the horse; E III would appear to be a similar strain less
modified by shorter residence in this species; while E I would
be a bovine strain, too recently derived from the ox to have
undergone any sensible alteration. To this question we must
return after the facts have been more closely examined[2].

The two least typical of the strains of equine origin, known respectively
as E II and E IV, deserve closer attention. Both were cultivated from
enlarged spleens. E II resembled in cultural characters one of the more dysgonic
of the bovine strains. In pathogenicity however it differed markedly from
the bovine type. Seven calves which were inoculated with it subcutaneously,
in doses of 10 to 100 mg., remained well; and when killed were found to have
developed tuberculosis indeed, but slight in the extent of its distribution,
and which had evidently become chronic or retrogressive in character. The
disease was in fact little if any more severe than that caused in these animals
by tubercle bacilli of human type. In rabbits, when injected into the veins
or peritoneal cavity, it caused fatal miliary tuberculosis : but after subcutaneous
injection the results varied in degree, being on the whole more severe than
those produced by the human, but less severe than those produced by the

[1] Quite recently (1914) Fröhner has investigated the bacilli from a case
of tuberculosis in the horse, and judged them to belong to the bovine type.
The investigation however seems to have been interrupted, owing to the outbreak of war, and the paper contains no bacteriological details.

[2] Very similar to these equine strains of somewhat low virulence were
others derived from the pig (pp. 403, 406) and from certain cases of lupus in
man. Only in this latter case the attenuated strains seemed to belong not
to the bovine type alone, but some of them also to the human type (see
Chapter xxv).

bovine type. In monkeys the disease which it caused was decidedly less serious than that caused by either the bovine or the human type of bacillus. In guinea-pigs and swine fatal tuberculosis followed subcutaneous injection in every case, but less rapidly than after comparable injections of bovine bacilli.

Thus the strain E II differed from the bovine type of tubercle bacillus in being less virulent *for all the animals mentioned.* It therefore did not resemble the human bacillus, nor can it justly be considered to have even approximated to that type; for the human bacillus, while it has but little virulence for the calf, pig or rabbit, is practically as virulent for the guinea-pig and monkey as the bovine bacillus itself. But this strain was at the same time *more* virulent for the pig and the rabbit than the human bacillus, and *less* virulent than that bacillus for the guinea-pig and monkey. In other words its *range of virulence* for various animal species was not at all like that of the human type, but followed that of the bovine type at a generally lower level. Its cultural characters too were, as we have seen, those of the bovine bacillus. The most reasonable view to take of it therefore seems to be that it was a strain descended from the bovine type, but attenuated in virulence by residence in the horse, or for some other reason.

The strain E IV was very similar to E II. In growth however it was rather more luxuriant, and it is said in this respect to have resembled one of the more easily-growing examples of the bovine type. Its virulence, which was very thoroughly tested[1], followed, like that of E II, the range of the bovine type, but at a lower level.

Neither of these attenuated equine strains presented the least resemblance to avian bacilli, and we have endeavoured to show that they cannot be identified with human bacilli. Möllers, it is true, has obtained in Koch's Institute for Infectious Diseases in Berlin an equine strain which he regards as belonging to the human type; but it is perhaps not unreasonable to suggest that this may have belonged to the class we have just been considering.

Zwick (1910) stated that seven cases of equine tuberculosis had, up to that time, been investigated at the Gesundheitsamt. In six the result was already known. The bacilli from all these were virulent (on subcutaneous injection of 10 mg.) for the rabbit, but one was less virulent than the rest. It produced in several rabbits only local tuberculosis. The growth of this strain and of two others recalled that of the human type. The rest possessed all the unmistakable characters of the bovine type.

McFadyean also seems to have previously met with human

---

[1] Namely on six calves, as many monkeys and baboons, and more than fifty rabbits, besides swine and guinea-pigs.

or attenuated equine strains[1].   In 1902 he injected 2 c.c. of an
emulsion made from the tuberculous spleen of a horse, and
showing tubercle bacilli in every field of the microscope, into
the jugular vein of a two-year-old heifer.   The animal became
ill, its respiration increased, and it presented symptoms pointing
to a miliary tuberculosis of the lungs.   It also reacted to
tuberculin.   But the symptoms subsided, and six months after
inoculation the animal was in excellent condition, and to all
outward appearance perfectly healthy.

We may question whether the peculiar strains of tubercle
bacilli of equine origin, which do not conform exactly to any
of the well recognized types, but which resembled the bovine
type more closely than any of the others, were recently of
bovine origin, but modified more or less profoundly by continued
residence in the horse, or whether they represent a true equine
type, with characters firmly impressed and rendered almost
permanent by residence for long ages in the horse itself.

We have seen in a previous chapter that the distinctive
characters of the well known types of tubercle bacilli are, to
say the least, very stable, and that it is difficult, if not impossible,
to alter them artificially by passage through animals.   We may
therefore reasonably assume that if the peculiar strains which
we are now considering, constitute a true equine type they will
prove as stable as the other well known types when exposed to
passage through appropriate animals; while if they have
sprung from bovine bacilli and have had a not too far distant
bovine origin they will prove susceptible to modifying influence, and will return more or less readily to the bovine type
on passage through the calf.   The fact that the strains in question are not identical with one another, but exhibit differences
in the degree to which they depart from the bovine type is in
favour of the latter hypothesis.   On the other hands passage
experiments actually carried out with these strains have had
uncertain results.

[1] In 1902 he wrote as follows: "It appears probable that, whatever be the
usual source of the tubercle bacilli with which horses are occasionally naturally
infected, the bacilli found in the lesions at the time when the horse succumbs
to tuberculosis are less virulent for all animals than those found in the case of
bovine tuberculosis." *Journ. of Comp. Pathol. and Therap.* vol. xv, p. 157.

XXI]

EXPERIMENTAL INFECTION

Several passage experiments were attempted by Griffith with each of these viruses, some in calves, others in rabbits. These resulted in some cases in an increase of virulence; in one experiment with each virus a complete increase up to the standard of the bovine type took place, but in others there was no change. No definite conclusion can be drawn from these experiments and Griffith does not attempt to draw any—for one must recognize that the experiments which had a negative result are just as significant as those which had a positive one.

Experimental Infection. Having described the bacilli found in natural instances of equine tuberculosis, let us now proceed to inquire how the horse reacts to artificial inoculation of tubercle bacilli of various types; and, particularly, let us examine its susceptibility to infection with that type which is peculiar to the horse itself.

Passing over the early work of Chauveau in which it is possible only to guess at the type of bacillus employed, but which established the fact that the horse can be infected experimentally, we come to that of Nocard who seems to have met with considerable difficulty in infecting the horse even by intravenous injection. In 1890 McFadyean caused in this species of animal severe miliary tuberculosis of lungs, which was threatening to cause death on the twenty-first day after inoculation, by injecting intravenously sixty minims of a rather milky emulsion, very rich in tubercle bacilli, and made from the tubercular spleen of another horse.

In 1901 Ravenel reported to the Tuberculosis Congress in London that he had injected two horses, directly into the lung through the thoracic wall, with cultures of tubercle bacilli of human and bovine origin respectively. A marked difference was noted in the effects of the two cultures; while the human one produced only a little local tuberculosis of a non-progressive character, and did not appear to affect the health of the animal, the bovine culture caused some emaciation, quickening of respiration, extensive tuberculosis of the pleura, and changes in the lungs and bronchial glands.

The most extensive experiments which have as yet been made on the horse were those carried out by F. Griffith for the Royal Commission. Their results are set out in the following table (p. 474)

From these experiments we see that the horse, while it may succumb to intravenous injection, resists infection by

TABLE XVIII. *Ponies Injected with Cultures of Various Types of Tubercle Bacilli.*

Mode of Inoculation	Number of Animal	Type of Bacillus	Dose	Result
Intravenous	30	Bovine	10 mg.	Died 20 days. Pulmonary Tuberculosis
	32	Avian	10 mg.	Died 15 ,, Gen. Infect. (Yersin type)
	18	Equine (E II)	10 mg.	Died 40 ,, Gen. Tuberculosis
	24	,, (E IV)	10 mg.	Died 98 ,, Gen. Tuberculosis
Subcutaneous	6	Bovine	50 mg.	Killed 132 days. Small local lesion, caseation of nearest glands
	12	,,	50 mg.	Killed 124 days. Scar at seat of inoculation, caseation of numerous prescapular glands, numerous hard translucent tubercles in lungs, and a moderate number of gritty tubercles in liver and spleen
	1	Human	50 mg.	Killed 116 days. Local tuberculosis only. At the seat of inoculation a series of small softened caseous nodules, and a pea-sized caseous nodule in one of the prescapular glands
	2	Avian	50 mg.	Killed 158 days. A small ulcer at the seat of inoculation, and a caseous nodule in each of two prescapular glands on the same side. No disease elsewhere, except for a "greyish patch" and two greyish nodules in the lungs
	10	,,	100 mg.	Died 38 days. Acute septic peritonitis. The only evidence of tuberculosis being a fibrous-walled cyst at the seat of inoculation and necrosis of several of the prescapular glands
	20	Equine (E II)	50 mg.	Killed 130 days. Small local lesion, caseation in some prescapular and neighbouring glands. A few minute translucent tubercles scattered sparsely in lungs, spleen and liver
	22	,, (E IV)	50 mg.	Killed 125 days. Ill. General tuberculosis
Feeding	26	Bovine	100 mg.	Killed 166 days. Caseo-calcareous tubercles in cervical, mesenteric, and colic glands. Two doubtful nodules in liver, and one in lungs
	8	,,	100 mg.	Killed 132 days. Caseous nodule in one cervical and in each of two mesenteric glands. Lungs liver and spleen contained hard nodules probably parasitic in origin

From experiments by F. Griffith, except No. 1, which was by A. S. Griffith; *R.C.T. Fin. Rep.* App. vol. IV and vol. I, p. 45.

subcutaneous inoculation in a surprising manner, whether the bacilli be of bovine, avian or human type. Even 50 mg. of bovine tubercle bacilli administered in this way produced only a small lesion at the seat of injection, and some caseous patches in the nearest lymphatic glands, and left the internal organs quite unaffected; while in another it caused tuberculosis, widely distributed indeed, but of very moderate severity, and retrogressive in character. Avian and human types of bacilli produced even less effect.

At the Gesundheitsamt in Berlin Titze (1907) fed a foal for two or three months with cultures of avian tubercle bacilli (44 test-tube cultures in all being employed for the experiment). The animal remained perfectly well; its growth was not checked in the least; and when it was killed, after the lapse of nearly a year, there was no trace of tuberculosis found in its body.

The effect of feeding with bovine bacilli (100 mg.) (to return to Griffith's experiments) was minimal.

The resistance shown by the horse to infection with the common types of tubercle bacilli was, as we have said, surprising; especially when we remember that the horse is not entirely immune to naturally acquired tuberculosis. It remains to see what is its degree of susceptibility to infection with the peculiar strains of bacilli derived from members of its own species. Almost the only experiments which bear on this question are those of F. Griffith; unfortunately they are but few in number, and their results are irregular. The intravenous injections give us no help in elucidating this riddle, since not only the equine strains, but bovine and avian strains also caused fatal infection. There remain only two subcutaneous injections of equine bacilli. The strains selected were those with the most marked peculiarities. The dose was 50 mg. One of them (E IV) produced severe illness and general tuberculosis, while the other (E II) caused little more than local lesions limited to the seat of inoculation and the nearest lymphatic glands. The results being thus conflicting the question remains an open one whether or no there is a type of tubercle bacillus specially adapted to live in the horse, but perhaps the evidence is rather in favour of the former alternative.

The high degree of resistance of the horse to experimental tuberculosis, combined with the fact that it suffers
at times from the natural disease remains unexplained. We
shall see that a similar problem arises in the case of the dog.
In that case we shall suggest as a possible explanation the
adjuvant action of some predisposing cause, possibly excessive
infection with intestinal worms, but in the horse any such
predisposing cause would seem to be less likely; the problem
therefore is without solution. It is desirable however to point
out here a fact which may possibly lessen the difficulty by
throwing doubt on its very existence. Griffith's experiments,
for the sake of economy, were carried out exclusively on
Dartmoor ponies, and it is not impossible that these may be
more resistant to infection with tubercle bacilli than more highly
specialized breeds of the genus *equus*. So far one has not heard
of spontaneous tuberculosis in these or other ponies.

Summary and Conclusions.

From the foregoing review of the evidence relating to the
etiology of equine tuberculosis the following facts emerge:
The tubercle bacilli found in lesions of tuberculous horses
resemble the bovine type of tubercle bacillus more closely
than either of the other two types. Some of them, probably
a minority, conform closely to that type, but others depart
from it more or less widely. These latter have the cultural
characters of the type, but are less virulent for all animals
which have been tested, except perhaps the horse itself.

The fact that these strains seem to form a continuous series,
with some identical with the bovine bacillus itself, others
departing widely from it, and others again showing intermediate
properties, make it appear very probable that they have all
arisen from the bovine tubercle bacillus, but at variable
distances of time, and that while some of them have not
resided in the horse long enough to have undergone any sensible
alteration, others have lived longer in their new host and have
become more or less profoundly modified by their change of
environment. It is perhaps natural that in doing so they
should have lost to some extent their power to thrive in their

old host the ox and certain other animals which sometimes afford a home to the bovine tubercle bacillus, and should have thereby become less virulent for these species; but we do not yet know for certain whether these atypical equine strains are more virulent for the horse than the bovine bacillus is—as assuredly they should be if they have adapted themselves specially to live in the body of that animal. The evidence on this point is meagre and uncertain; but perhaps on the whole it inclines towards the side of the hypothesis suggested.

If we may assume provisionally the truth of the view which has been put forward, the further question arises: how far have these peculiarly equine strains advanced towards a new type, or shall we say variety? We have argued in another chapter that the evidence concerning the stability of the three recognized types points to the conclusion that their special characters are so firmly impressed that they cannot be easily altered by changing their environment, and we are inclined on the whole to regard them as varieties. Are the special characters of these equine strains equally stable? Here again the evidence is insufficient, but on the whole it is in favour of a negative answer, and we are inclined provisionally to regard the peculiar equine strains of tubercle bacilli as descended but recently—some more recently than others—from the bovine tubercle bacilli.

The question cannot be decided definitely as yet; but enough experimental work has been done to open up a problem of great interest; and it is to be hoped that some investigator, sufficiently endowed with means for so complex and costly an undertaking, will be found to follow it up to a lasting conclusion.

B. *Tuberculosis in the Ass.*

The ass, as we have said already, has seldom been known to suffer from tuberculosis. Up to 1899, according to Stockman, only one case had been reported in this species, and not more than one or two in the mule. Little more than ten years later Gaultier remarked that spontaneous tuberculosis had been observed in these animals on a number of occasions; but whether on all these the evidence of tuberculosis was conclusive or no it would be difficult to say.

The ass figures among the animals which Chauveau succeeded in infecting experimentally with tuberculosis; and both human and bovine material was found to be effective for infecting it. But it is to be noted that the injections were intravenous, and the material emulsified tissue. Even so the disease produced was not progressive, or even transitory. The tubercles were confined to the lungs; and in order to see them it was said to be necessary that the animals should be killed twenty-five to thirty days after inoculation.

Viquerat (1896) injected more than thirty asses with tuberculosis in the vain attempt to gain an anti-tuberculin for therapeutic use. No details are given, nor are the sources of the infective material mentioned, but the general statement is made that in asses intravenously infected "mechanical[1]" tuberculous foci form in the lungs, but the bacilli do not multiply, and the animal recovers completely and is tubercle-free after thirty-five to forty days.

Johne (1897) injected with culture of tubercle bacilli an ass foal six months old both intravenously and intraperitoneally. The animal was killed forty-seven days later, when tuberculous abscesses were found at both points of inoculation, acute miliary tuberculosis of lungs, and marked swelling of many lymph glands.

Stockman, in 1899, injected with tubercle bacilli two asses and a mule, intravenously, with minimal or negative results.

The doses were small, namely "an ordinary sized platinum loop-ful of culture of tubercle bacilli from an actively growing glycerin-agar culture of five weeks standing." The origin of the culture is not recorded.

Exp. 1, Ass 1 reacted to tuberculin about three weeks after inoculation, but continued in perfect health. After about three months she was sold and remained well.

Exp. 2, Ass 2 also developed a capacity to react to tuberculin shortly after injection, and like its fellow remained well, and put on flesh. It was

[1] "Anämische, mechanische Tuberkelnötchen" is the expression used. Probably the idea of *mechanische* is that the foci were formed by the action of the poisons present in the bacilli introduced, that is to say mechanically and not as the result of any true infection or development of the bacilli in the body of the ass.

killed about five weeks after inoculation, when about two dozen macroscopic
nodules, varying in size from a pin's head to a small pea, were found under
the pleura and in the lung substance. These showed no sign of caseation
and were "very like the pseudo-tuberculous nodules in the lungs of the
sheep." Guinea-pigs, injected, each with 3 c.c. of an emulsion of these nodules,
did not develop "a speck of tubercle, although the inoculated material was
fairly rich in bacilli[1]."

    Exp. 3, Mule. This animal also developed a capacity to react to tuberculin
some time after injection, and like its fellows preserved all the appearances
of health. Five weeks after injection it was killed for the dissecting room.
No complete post-mortem examination was made for fear of spoiling the
organs for dissection, but it is recorded that no distinct nodules were found
in the lungs.

The paucity or absence of evidence of tuberculosis in the
experimental animals which we have just been considering
may be attributed with great probability to insufficiency of
dose, and in the case of Stockman's experiments an additional
reason is supplied in the fact that the bacilli were from cultures,
and were injected suspended in some innocuous fluid. When
what we may reasonably assume to have been larger doses of
emulsified tuberculous tissue were employed for injection into
the veins of the ass, far more serious consequences ensued.
This was the case in some experiments which Stockman
subsequently carried out, and also in a more extensive series
made by Gaultier.

    In Stockman's experiment (No. 4) Ass C received an intravenous injection
of 5 c.c. of an emulsion made from a pea-sized nodule taken from the spleen
of a tuberculous horse. This ass actually died of acute miliary tuberculosis
of lungs, about seven weeks after injection. "The lungs were simply crammed
with tubercles of greyish white colour. The glands were slightly swollen and
congested, but showed no tubercles." At the seat of inoculation, by the side
of the vein, was a caseous swelling the size of a bantam's egg. The other
organs appeared to the naked eye perfectly healthy.

    Gaultier's experiments appeared in 1900. Here again the injections
were intravenous, and the material employed emulsified tissue. This material
was prepared from the lesions of rabbits and guinea-pigs dead of bovine
tuberculosis. Gaultier gives particulars of eleven such experiments. The
animals all became ill, and no less than eight of them *died* of pulmonary
tuberculosis.

    [1] This is a most interesting observation, and is direct evidence that the
lesions were cured. It was one of the surprises which awaited those who
carried out the experimental work of the late Royal Commission that in the
old quiescent tuberculous lesions of man there might be numerous well-formed
tubercle bacilli visible on microscopic examination, and yet the inoculation
of guinea-pigs with the material might prove to be negative.

Stockman, as we have just seen, recorded a fatal case of pulmonary tuberculosis in the ass injected intravenously with an emulsion of tuberculous tissue from a horse. In 1902 he recorded another (Exp. 5). This time the material for injection was obtained from tubercles in the kidney of a cow. The ass fell ill, became much emaciated, and had hurried respiration. Fifty-six days after the injection it was evident that it would not last long; and accordingly it was killed. Post-mortem examination showed that the disease was confined to the lungs and bronchial glands; the former "were simply crammed with grey translucent tubercles."

These results obtained by Stockman and Gaultier may seem at first sight somewhat to conflict with the earlier ones of Chauveau, Johne, and of Stockman himself, and to point to a greater susceptibility of the ass than had hitherto been suspected. But indeed they need not surprise us if we may assume that the doses were larger than those previously employed, or richer in bacilli, even if we hold that the ass is very resistant indeed. For so long as an animal develops a local lesion in response to the immediate irritating action of tubercle bacilli, those bacilli will produce multiple local lesions in the lungs wherever they settle after intravenous injection, and if the dose be large enough these lesions will be sufficient to cause serious impediment to respiration or even to threaten life itself. This is the case even with the ox injected with the human type of bacillus which is quite incapable of producing progressive disease in this species. The ass then in relation to the bovine tubercle bacillus is in the same case as the ox in regard to the human tubercle bacillus. It develops a local lesion at the seat of injection and succumbs to pulmonary tuberculosis after intravenous injection if the dose be a large one; but to other kinds of inoculation it is resistant.

Such results then as were obtained in the experiments which we have been reviewing afford but slight evidence of susceptibility, and indeed rather point to a very unusual degree of capacity for resisting tuberculosis on the part of the animal in question. The ass is indeed a very obstinate animal, and it would appear to resist tuberculous infection as stubbornly as it resists everything else. It is perhaps not too much to say that this species seems to be, of all those belonging to the domesticated mammals, the most resistant to tuberculosis.

To return for a moment to Stockman's experiments: it will be remembered that the contrast between the severe and fatal result produced in experiment 4 (Ass C), and the minimal or negative results caused in experiments 1, 2, and 3, has already been explained on the ground that while the animals in the three experiments last mentioned received small doses of bacilli suspended in some innocuous fluid the other was given an injection of tuberculous tissue. But, as the reader will doubtless have noticed, there is another explanation possible. The minimal results were produced by bacilli of bovine origin, the severe and fatal one by bacilli which came from a species very closely allied to the ass, namely the horse. And it may well be asked: Is not this evidence of a view closely akin to the one we have already been discussing, namely that tubercle bacilli of equine origin are more likely to be virulent for members of the equine family than those derived from other animals such as the ox ?

This we should like to believe; but it must be admitted that in the present instance the evidence carries very little weight. For in Stockman's next experiment (No. 5), as we have already seen, acute pulmonary tuberculosis, which threatened to prove fatal, was caused in an ass by the injection of bovine material. And in Gaultier's experiments also, where the results were almost invariably severe and usually fatal, the bacilli were of bovine origin.

Moreover it would seem from yet another experiment, which has not been mentioned before, that the ass is not particularly susceptible to tuberculous infection from the bacilli from every equine source, though it may be to those from some.

McFadyean (1902) injected intravenously into a donkey an emulsion of caseo-purulent material from the spleen of a horse which had suffered naturally from tuberculosis. The donkey was killed five months after injection, and at the post-mortem examination no trace of tuberculous disease was seen anywhere[1].

[1] McFadyean says of this experience: "One might have supposed that, if the ass species is susceptible to tuberculosis, experimental infection would be obtained with most certainty by using bacilli from the horse as the most nearly related species. It is very doubtful however whether there is any general law of this kind." *Journ. of Comp. Pathol. and Therap.* vol. xv, p. 157.

Tuberculosis in the Camel.

Instances of tuberculosis in the camel have been reported in India by Lingard and Leese, and one has recently been recorded in the Soudan by Archibald. In Egypt the disease has long been thought to exist, and quite recently Mason has investigated an instance in Cairo. In this case rabbits were injected with tissue emulsions, and developed severe general tuberculosis. The bacillus therefore was held to belong to the bovine type, but cultures on glycerin-serum are said to have shown certain peculiarities.

A case of tuberculosis in a camel was recorded in London by Sibley in 1889. The animal died in the Zoölogical Gardens after four years residence there. Its mother is said to have died of a similar disease. Lungs, spleen and liver were affected, and contained nodules varying in size from a pea to a pigeon's egg. They were firm on section, and the smaller ones "were simply one mass of dry caseous material." The pleuræ were beset with fringes and strings of small tubercles "like pearls on a string."

Tuberculosis in a Gnu and an Antelope.

F. Griffith, while working for the Royal Commission, obtained cultures from a gnu and an antelope which had died of tuberculosis in the Zoölogical Gardens in London. It is somewhat surprising to find that these cultures belonged to the human type. But on a general consideration of the tuberculosis of non-domesticated mammals in captivity it would appear that the bacilli are very commonly of this type. This was the case with the elephant reported in the next section, and it seems to be the same, as we shall see, in the monkey.

The strains of bacilli isolated from the gnu and antelope were very thoroughly tested, so that there can be no doubt of their type. They were eugonic in cultural character. The suggestion that they might contain a hidden dysgonic bovine element, the true cause of the disease, was not overlooked, and two passage experiments on rabbits and guinea-pigs were made with the strain from the antelope for the purpose of examining this possibility.   One of these experiments was continued for two years but no alteration of virulence occurred, thus proving that the strain contained no bovine bacilli[1].

Tuberculosis in the Elephant.

Dammann and Stedefeder (1909) reported a case of tuberculosis in an elephant which had been sent for treatment of a wound of the foot to the Veterinary School in Hamburg. This animal died of septicæmia, and at the post-mortem examination tuberculosis was found in the lungs and in the bodies of several vertebræ.   A strain of tubercle bacilli was cultivated, and grew luxuriantly.   It was infective for guinea-pigs, but rabbits inoculated with the spleens of these animals did not develop tuberculosis.   This strain therefore seems to have belonged to the human type.

REFERENCES. XIII

(Chapter XXI)

Tuberculosis in the Horse and Ass.

Burnett (1890).   Tuberculosis in the Horse.   *Journ. of Comp. Pathol. and Therap.* vol. III, p. 66.
Bowie (1889).   A Case of Equine Tuberculosis.   *Ibid.* vol. II, p. 55.
Campbell (1888).   Tuberculosis (Lymphadenoma) in the Horse.   *Ibid.* vol. I, p. 162.
Cooke (1890).   A Case of Tuberculosis in the Horse.   *Ibid.* vol. III, p. 69.
Dewer (1890).   A Case of Tuberculosis in the Horse.   *Ibid.* vol. III, p. 365.
Editorial Article (1900).   The Susceptibility of the Ass to Tuberculosis. *Ibid.* vol. XIII, p. 76.
—— (1890).   Equine Tuberculosis.   *Ibid.* vol. III, p. 256.
—— (1892).   Equine Tuberculosis.   *Ibid.* vol. V, p. 164.
—— (1896).   Equine Tuberculosis.   *Ibid.* vol. IX, p. 173.
Fally and Liéneau (1902).   Tuberculose généralisée chez un cheval. *Recueil de Méd. Vét.* sér. 8, vol. IX, p. 58.
Faulkner (1891).   Two Cases of Equine Tuberculosis.   *Journ. of Comp. Pathol. and Therap.* vol. IV, p. 65.

[1] *R.C.T. Fin. Rep.* App. vol. IV, p. 149.

Freer (1888).   Equine Tuberculosis.   *Ibid.* vol. I, p. 246.

Fröhner (1914).   Bovine Tuberkulose beim Pferd.   *Monatshefte f. prakt. Tierheilkunde*, vol. XXVI, Heft 1 and 2, p. 5.

Gaultier (1900).   *Journ. de Méd. Vét.* Feb.   Abst. in *Journ. of Comp. Pathol. and Therap.* vol. XIII, p. 76.

Griffith, F. (1911).   Investigation of Tubercle Bacilli derived from the Horse.   *R.C.T. Fin. Rep.* App. vol. IV, p. 4.

—— (1911).   Experimental Infection of the Horse with Bovine Tubercle Bacilli.   *Ibid.* p. 137.

—— (1911).   Experimental Infection of the Horse with Avian Tubercle Bacilli.   *Ibid.* p. 187.

Hill, G. C. (1896).   A Case of Equine Tuberculosis.   *Journ. of Comp. Pathol. and Therap.* vol. IX, p. 228.

Johne (1897).   Ein Infectionsversuch mit Tuberkulose bei einem Esel.   *Zeitsch. f. Tiermed.* Bd. I, p. 360.

Lishman, Capt. T. (1914).   Tuberculous Osteitis of the Vertebrae in a Horse.   *Journ. of Comp. Pathol. and Therap.* vol. XXVII, p. 256.

McFadyean (1888).   Tuberculosis in the Horse.   *Ibid.* vol. I, pp. 51 and 335.

—— (1889).   Tuberculosis in the Horse.   *Ibid.* vol. II, p. 349.

—— (1890).   Two Cases of Experimental Tuberculosis in Equidae.   *Ibid.* vol. III, p. 70.

—— (1892).   Tuberculosis in the Horse.   *Ibid.* vol. V, pp. 246, 342.

—— (1896).   Equine Tuberculosis.   *Ibid.* vol. IX, p. 190.

—— (1898).   Injection of Equine Tuberculous Material into a Cow.   *Ibid.* vol. XI, p. 244.

—— (1902).   The Susceptibility of the Ass to Tuberculosis.   *Ibid.* vol. XV, p. 156.

Markus (1901).   Tuberkulose beim Pferd.   *Holl. Zeitsch. f. Tierheilk.* vol. XXVIII, pp. 97, 484–5.   *Baumgarten's Jahresbericht*, vol. XVII, p. 422.

Mettam (1890).   A case of Tuberculosis in the Horse.   *Journ. of Comp. Pathol. and Therap.* vol. III, p. 69.

Möllers (1912).   *Report of the Xth International Tuberculosis Conference.* Rome, p. 95.

Nocard (1888).   *Compt. Rend. Cong. pour l'étude de la Tuberculose.*

—— (1894).   *Les tuberculoses animales.* Paris, p. 171.

—— (1896).   Le type abdominal de la Tuberculose du Cheval est d'origine aviaire.   *Bull. de la Soc. Cent. de Méd. Vétérinaire*, p. 248.   See also *Recueil de Méd. Vétérinaire*, 1896, also *Abstract in Journ. of Comp. Pathol. and Therap.* vol. IX, p. 173.

—— (1898).   Tuberculose humaine et tuberculose aviaire.   *Ann. de l'Institut Pasteur*, vol. XII, p. 562.

Oliver (1889).   A Case of Equine Tuberculosis.   *Journ. of Comp. Pathol. and Therap.* vol. II, p. 258.

Ravenel (1891).   The Comparative Virulence of the Tubercle Bacillus from Human and Bovine Sources.   *Trans. Brit. Cong. on Tub.* vol. III, p. 562.

Röder and Robert (1892). Uebertragung der Tuberkulose vom Rind auf das Pferd. *Bericht ü. d. Veterinärwesen i. Kgr. Sachsen*, p. 92.

Rutherford (1890). A Case of Lymphadenoma (Tuberculosis) in the Horse. *Journ. of Comp. Pathol. and Therap.* vol. III, p. 269.

Smith (1890). Tuberculosis in the Horse. *Ibid.* vol. III, p. 183.

Stockman (1899). Experimental Tuberculosis in the Ass. *Ibid.* vol. XII, p. 125.

—— (1902). Experimental Tuberculosis in the Ass. *Ibid.* vol. XV, p. 146.

Straus (1895). *La Tuberculose et son bacille.* Paris, p. 335.

Tailby (1891). A Case of Equine Tuberculosis. *Journ. of Comp. Pathol. and Therap.* vol. IV, p. 66.

Titze (1907). Fütterungsversuche mit Hühnertuberkelbazillen an Schweinen und an einem Fohlen. *Tub. Arbeit. a. d. Kaiserl. Gesundheitsamte*, Heft 6, p. 215.

Viquerat (1896). Zur Gewinnung von Antituberculin. *Centralb. f. Bakteriol. u. Parasit.* vol. XX, p. 674.

Wostenholm and Kelynack (1892). A Case of Equine Tuberculosis. *Journ. of Comp. Pathol. and Therap.* vol. V, p. 166.

Zwick (1910). Ueber die Beziehungen zwischen Säugetier- und Hühnertuberkulose, insbesondere über das Vorkommen von Hühnerbazillen beim Pferd. *Beiheft z. Centralb. f. Bakt. etc.* Ref. vol. XLVII, p. 190.

Tuberculosis in the Camel.

Archibald (1910). Acid-fast Bacilli in a Camel's Lung, the Gross Lesions of which closely resembled Miliary Tuberculosis. *Journ. of Comp. Pathol. and Therap.* vol. XXIII, p. 96.

Mason (1912). Some observations on Camels in Egypt. *Ibid.* vol. XXV, p. 109.

Sibley (1889). Camel with Tuberculosis. *Trans. Pathol. Soc. Lond.* vol. XL, p. 460.

Tuberculosis in the Elephant, Giraffe and Antelope.

Dammann and Stedefeder (1909). Tuberculous Disease in an Elephant. *Deutsch. tierarztl. Wochenschr.* p. 345. Abst. in the *Journ. of Comp. Pathol. and Therap.* vol. XXII, p. 258.

Griffith, F. (1911). Tuberculosis in a Gnu and an Antelope. *R.C.T. Fin. Rep.* App. vol. IV, p. 151.

Myers (1891). Tuberculosis in a Giraffe. *Journ. of Comp. Med. and Vet. Archives*, vol. XIII, p. 181.

CHAPTER XXII

THE SUSCEPTIBILITY TO TUBERCULOSIS OF VARIOUS ANIMAL SPECIES (*continued*)

TUBERCULOSIS IN THE DOG, CAT AND MONKEY

Tuberculosis in the Dog.

Before the discovery of the tubercle bacillus it was commonly believed that tuberculosis did not occur in the dog. And moreover this supposed immunity was at one time thought by some to be due to an anti-tuberculous principle residing in the blood of the animal, and it was even proposed to use its serum as a cure for consumption[1]. But the dog is not immune; and, as we shall see, instances of tuberculosis in this species are by no means very uncommon.

Even before the time of Koch's discovery cases of canine tuberculosis were reported from time to time; but the diagnosis was necessarily very uncertain. About an instance, however, recorded by one Malin as early as 1839, there is great probability. A woman afflicted with phthisis had a pet dog which for a whole year was in the habit of devouring its mistress' expectoration. The animal developed a cough with purulent sputum and died. The woman procured another dog which exhibited the same gastronomic habits as the other. It also fell ill and died; and "on opening the thorax the two lungs were found to be entirely destroyed by suppuration[2]." This case is so like others which have been reported since, and

---

[1] Richet and Héricourt, "Immunité contre la tuberculose, conférée par la transfusion péritonéale du sang de chien," *Études sur la tuberculose*, publiées sous la direction du professeur Verneuil, vol. II, 1890. "Expériences sur la vaccination antituberculeuse: Traitement de la tuberculose par le sérum de chien," *Compt. rend. de la Soc. de Biolog.* 1890–1892, 1893. Héricourt, "Traitement de la tuberculose par les injections sous-cutanées de sérum de chien," *Compt. rend. du Congrès pour l'étude de la tuberculose*, 2e session, 1891.

[2] *Gaz. méd. de Paris*, 1839, p. 634. Quoted by Straus, *La tuberculose*, p. 603 (footnote).

in which the diagnosis has been satisfactorily confirmed, that we can hardly doubt that it was a case of tuberculosis[1].

That the dog is susceptible to *artificial* infection was demonstrated for the first time by Villemin[2], 1868, and confirmed by Koch in 1882. Nevertheless belief in the immunity of this species to tuberculosis continued for a long time to be held.

The first authentic case of spontaneous tuberculosis in the dog, according to Straus, was that described in 1882, in Italy by Brusasco[3]. This observer placed the diagnosis beyond doubt by successfully transmitting the disease to rabbits. In 1885 Nocard demonstrated the presence of tubercle bacilli in a dog whose disease was described by Andrieu. Three years later two cases were recorded by Petit[4]. Stockman contributed an instance in this country in 1892, and about the same time various authors published a good many others. But the latter were not numerous; and in 1895 Straus was only able to collect about 100 cases.

Some rough sort of idea may be formed of the extent to which tuberculosis occurs among dogs from the statistics of certain veterinary schools in Germany and France. But it must not be forgotten that these figures do not apply to the general canine population at large, but only to such as, on account of sickness or some other reason, are brought to the veterinary hospitals.

In the Veterinary Clinic in Berlin, between 1886 and 1894, forty cases of tuberculosis were recorded by Fröhner[5] among 70,000 dogs examined there. In Dresden, in 1893, Eber[6] saw eleven cases among 400 dogs. In Leipzig thirteen were found to be tuberculous among 1100 brought to the Clinic to be

---

[1] Straub also, in 1845, wrote on tuberculosis in the dog. "Tuberculose beim Hund," *Repertor.* 1845 (mentioned in the Bibliography of Cadiot's *La Tuberculose du Chien*). The author has not been able to obtain his paper.

[2] *Études sur la tuberculose*, Paris, 1868, p. 548.

[3] See Straus, *loc. cit.* p. 352.

[4] *Journ. de Méd. Vét.* Paris, 1888. Trans. in *Journ. of Pathol. and Therap.* vol. I, p. 60.

[5] Friedberger and Fröhner, 1896, *Pathologie und Therapie der Haustiere*, Die Tuberkulose des Hundes, vol. II, p. 495.

[6] Eber, "Die Tuberkulose des Hundes und der Katze," *Ergebn. d. allgem. Patholog. u. pathol. Anatom.* von Lubarsch and Oestertag, 1894–5.

destroyed[1]. And in Saxony, about the end of the century, among the dogs slaughtered there at the rate of 300 to 500 a year, 0·16 (1900) to 0·2 per cent. (1899) were found to be infected with the disease[2].

It is in France however that the largest amount of canine tuberculosis has been reported. Cadiot, between 1891 and 1893, found forty instances among 9000 dogs brought to the veterinary school of Alfort (Paris); while Petit[3], who succeeded him there, discovered no less than 152 among 2717 dogs which perished from one cause or another in the same clinic in the years 1900–1904.

In Copenhagen canine tuberculosis would seem to be comparatively common. Jensen came across fifteen cases there in eleven months; and Bang was able to place at his disposal the notes of thirteen others[4].

In Holland it is said by Schornagel[5] that up to quite recently only a few cases had been reported; but this observer was able to collect eleven among 568 dogs brought to his clinic to be disposed of.

It may be interesting to compare the percentages of infection in various places which are to be obtained from the figures quoted above; they are therefore set out in the following table. But their value is only for comparison, and they must not be taken to represent the frequency of tuberculosis among the canine populations of the various localities mentioned, but, as we have said before, only that among such dogs as, on account of illness or other causes, are brought to the veterinary institutions. Probably the true frequency of canine tuberculosis is less than that shown by these figures; on the other hand one observes that the most recent figures are the largest, and this suggests that many a case during the earlier period escaped recognition.

[1] Berichte über das Veterinärwesen im Königreich Sachsen." Quoted by Titze and Weidanz, *loc. cit.*

[2] *Ibid.*

[3] " Sur les rapports qui existent entre la tuberculose de l'homme et celle des carnivores domestiques (Chien et Chat)," *Recueil de Méd. Vét.* vol. LXXXII, p. 713.

[4] Abst in *Journ. of Comp. Pathol. and Therap.* vol. IV, p. 103, 1891.

[5] Schornagel, 1914, *Untersuchungen über elf Fälle von Hundtuberkulose,* Inaug. Diss. Beijers, Utrecht.

Tuberculosis in Dogs brought to Veterinary Schools.

Locality	Author	Date	Percentage tuberculous
Berlin	Fröhner	1886–1894	0·06
Paris	Cadiot	1891–1893	0·44
Saxony	Titze and Weidanz	1899–1900	0 16–0·2
Leipzig	Eber	1904–1905	1·2
Utrecht	Schornagel	1914	1·9
Dresden	Eber	1891–1892	2·75
Paris (Alfort)	Petit	1900–1904	5·6*

* The average at Alfort varied in different years from 2·98 in 1901 to
9·11 per cent. in 1904.

Distribution of the Lesions. Tuberculosis in the dog may
be widespread and severe, so as to cause death, or induce the
owner to have the animal destroyed; or it may be a secondary
disorder of small importance, found only after decease from
other causes.

The lesions are sometimes very large and they are usually
confined to one or a few organs. Acute miliary tuberculosis,
according to Straus, is rare—and this is what one would expect
in a species, the general power of resistance of which (as
shown by the results of experimental infection) is very considerable. Schornagel, however, records one instance of acute,
and three of chronic, miliary tuberculosis out of the eleven cases
which he examined[1].

The lungs are attacked very commonly. According to
Straus and also to Friedberger and Fröhner, canine tuberculosis
is mainly a pulmonary disease. These organs are sometimes
affected with caseous pneumonia, at others they are studded
with tuberculous nodules. They may contain large cavities,
or be riddled with smaller ones[2].

Jensen recorded pulmonary tuberculosis in nineteen out of
the twenty-eight cases examined by himself and Bang. Eber
found this condition in nine out of eleven, and Petit and
Basset in twenty-five out of thirty-two cases. Adding these

[1] He gives a beautiful photograph of acute miliary tuberculosis of liver.
[2] Petit, *Recueil de Méd. Vét.* 1905, vol. LXXXII, p. 716.

together we get fifty-three cases of pulmonary disease among seventy-one tuberculous dogs; that is to say pulmonary disease was present in seventy-five per cent. Cadiot who summarized the literature up to date in 1892 found pulmonary tuberculosis in twenty-five out of thirty-two cases, that is in nearly eighty per cent.[1]

The lymphatic glands are apt to be attacked with especial severity, and sometimes form large tumours which may have even a sarcomatous aspect[2]. Sometimes the thoracic glands are tuberculous when no corresponding disease is detected in the lungs (Cadiot); and, on the other hand, the lungs may be affected without visible disease in the bronchial glands. When the mesenteric glands are tuberculous the intestinal mucous membrane often shows no trace of disease.

Among the abdominal organs the liver is most often affected. Next come the kidneys. Curiously enough the spleen seems seldom to be involved[3].

The serous membranes are attacked with relative frequency, especially the pleura and pericardium. Of tuberculous pericarditis Cadiot saw six cases[4].

Tuberculosis of the heart itself is said by this authority to be more frequent in the dog than in any other species of animal[5]. Both he and Jensen had each seen two cases, and one has recently been reported by Bull in Australia. On the

---

[1] Schornagel (1914) only met with five cases among the eleven recorded by him.

[2] As for example the bronchial glands in a case figured by Cadiot (*La tuberculose du Chien*, p. 28); or those of one photographed by Schornagel (*loc. cit.* figs. I and II); or the perigastric glands in a case described by Petit and Basset; or the mediastinal glands in one recorded by Guérin (*Recueil de Méd. Vét.* 1910, vol. LXXXVII, p. 277).

[3] Among thirty-two cases of tuberculosis in dogs recorded by Petit and Basset, the various organs were affected as follows: lungs in twenty-five, liver in fourteen, kidneys in nine, spleen in one, pleuræ in nineteen, pericardium in fifteen, peritoneum in ten, tracheo-bronchial glands in seventeen, mesenteric in five.

Straus gives a coloured plate showing a liver studded with yellow nodules many of which seem to be about half-an-inch in diameter (*loc. cit.* p. 359).

[4] Cadiot, *La tuberculose du Chien*, p. 34.

[5] *Ibid.* p. 38.

other hand Petit and Basset point out that they only observed
the myocardium affected once in thirty-two cases[1].

Tuberculous ulcers on head and neck, probably caused by
wounds received in fighting have been described by Petit (1905).

Sources of Infection. Numerous instances of tuberculosis
have been recorded in dogs whose owners were consumptive;
and it is definitely stated in the case of several of the animals,
as in that of one already referred to, that they were in the
habit of consuming the sputum of their owners[2]. Nine of the
tuberculous dogs examined by Cadiot belonged to keepers of
restaurants or public houses, where the animals had access to
expectoration scattered on the floor, or were exposed to infected
dust caused by sweeping out the premises. Cadiot himself
thought that in half his cases there was evidence that infection
had come from a human source. On the other hand in one of
the cases recorded by Thomassen the dog belonged to a butcher,

---

[1] For this case see Petit, "Sur la tuberculose du chien: Tubercle de la
paroi inter-auriculaire," *Recueil de Méd. Vét.* vol. LXXXI, p. 762. An instance
of cardiac tuberculosis in a bulldog was recorded by Hobday and Belcher
(1908), and another in a bull-terrier by Schlesinger (1912). Tuberculous
pericarditis in a dog was recently seen by the author in Cambridge.

If tuberculosis of the heart is really commoner in the dog than in other
animals—and this would seem to be the case, at least if we include the
pericardium with the heart itself—one would be inclined to think that this is
because the dog habitually puts a greater strain on that organ than almost
any other animal, for it appears to delight in violent and rapid movement
above all the rest.

The horse also "rejoiceth in his strength." In him tuberculosis is uncommon: but one would like to know whether, when it does occur in this
species and especially in the racehorse, the equine heart, like the canine,
suffers relatively more severely than that in other animals.

We have already seen that certain organs upon the functional activity of
which large demands are made, such as the mammary glands of the cow and
rabbit, and perhaps also the climbing muscles of the monkey, are more liable
to tubercle than the corresponding organs of other animals which are more
sparingly used; and it seems as though the dog's heart might be added
to the list of overworked organs which are relatively susceptible to tuberculosis.

[2] This is said to have occurred in cases recorded by Malin, Brusasco,
Czokor, Andrieu, Bourgougnon, Johne, Beugnot, Peters, Guérin, Jewtichiew,
Filleau and Petit, Benjamin and Nocard. In one of Czokor's cases it is stated
that the phthisical owner was in the habit of allowing the dog to sleep with him
in his bed, and a similar statement is made in the case described by Beugnot.
(Quoted by Cadiot, *loc. cit.* p. 9.)

and it seems probable that it contracted tuberculosis by eating tuberculous offal; and a similar instance is given by Jensen.

Dogs therefore would appear to derive their tuberculosis from both human and bovine sources; and this view is, as we shall see, supported by the bacteriological evidence.

Portals of Invasion. Experimental Tuberculosis. In consequence of the comparative frequency with which in tuberculous dogs the lungs and bronchial glands are the principal, or indeed the sole, seat of the disease Straus believed that canine tuberculosis is caused mainly by inhalation[1]. But he admitted that infection might occasionally occur through the digestive tract[2]. The mesenteric glands are sometimes the seat of disease which has the appearance of being primary; and one of Jensen's cases is said to have been an excellent example of food-borne tuberculosis[3]. Petit seems to have held that tuberculous infection in the dog *usually* occurs through the digestive tract[4].

Arloing had some success with feeding experiments in 1903. In two of his cases tuberculosis spread from the intestinal tract to the spleen and lungs.

On the other hand several observers have failed to infect dogs by feeding them with tuberculous material or pure cultures, and others have produced only minimal lesions. Tappeiner in 1877, and again in 1881, fed dogs for several weeks with

[1] "Le chien, comme l'homme, paraît surtout s'infecter par la voie respiratoire" (*La tuberculose,* p. 355).

[2] "L'ingestion fréquemment répétée de crachats de phthisiques, de viscères d'animaux tuberculeux paraît néanmoins pouvoir entraîner chez le chien une tuberculose abdominale primitive" (*Ibid.* p. 360).

[3] This was the dog, already mentioned, which belonged to a butcher, and which no doubt had many opportunities of consuming tuberculous offal.

[4] For his opinion see *Recueil de Méd. Vét.* 1895, vol. LXXXII, p. 716, and also his contribution to the discussion of Guérin's paper where he speaks more guardedly (*Ibid.* 1910, vol. LXXXVII, p. 278). In experimental researches, in conjunction with Leudet in 1904, Petit had found reason to believe that the dog may be easily infected by the alimentary route, while he failed to produce tuberculosis experimentally by inhalation (*Recueil de Méd. Vét.* vol. LXXXI, p. 298). From the experiments Petit and Leudet conclude as follows:

"Il resulte en particulier de nos expériences que nous avons facilement réalisé la transmission naturelle au chien, par la voie digestive, de la tuberculose humaine."

tuberculous sputum without results. Again Zugari in 1889 failed in similar experiments, although he fed his dogs with tuberculous sputum, or with the tuberculous organs of animals for several months.

A. S. Griffith, sometimes in conjunction with F. Griffith, fed twenty-nine dogs, for the Royal Commission, with varying doses of tubercle bacilli from cultures; and though some of his animals were puppies, and some were fed with large doses such as 50 to 100 mg. of bacilli, or with one to ten million tubercle bacilli suspended in milk, the disease produced was only minimal. No definite lesions developed in the intestinal mucosa, and only a few small retrogressive foci in the mesenteric or pharyngeal glands. In addition minute grey tubercles or other small lesions were not uncommon in the lungs[1].

About the same time Chaussé (1910) entirely failed to produce macroscopic lesions in twenty-two dogs which he fed, some with pure cultures of tubercle bacilli both human and bovine in type, others with tuberculous sputum, or organs of tuberculous cattle. Microscopic lesions however were present in the mesenteric glands in the great majority of cases, and emulsions of these glands caused tuberculosis when injected into guinea-pigs

The dog then is difficult to infect seriously by means of experimental feeding with tuberculous material. But one must remember that the dog is difficult to infect by other portals also—Leudet and Petit failed to infect dogs which they caused to receive tubercle bacilli by inhalation, and, as we shall see in a moment, subcutaneous injection did not succeed in the hands of the Royal Commission in producing severe or progressive disease.

The question then, so far as the problem of the portal of

[1] R.C.T. Int. Rep. App. vol. I, pp. 537, 592, 632, 707, and vol. III, p. 91 (see ante, p. 164).

The present writer made only a few feeding experiments on dogs for the Royal Commission, one of which however led to death from a tuberculous lesion in the lungs bursting into the pleural cavity and causing pyo-pneumo-thorax. This result was so exceptional that it was thought possibly due to an accidental insufflation of tubercle bacilli into the lung during the experimental feeding (see p. 499). Two somewhat similar results were obtained at the Gesundheitsamt (see p. 500).

infection is concerned, is not: Is it easy or difficult to infect
the dog by feeding, but rather Is it easier or more difficult to
infect it by feeding than by inhalation ? Findel, who has
investigated this question directly answers it very definitely in
favour of the latter of these alternatives. He succeeded in
producing fairly widespread miliary tuberculosis of lungs by
causing dogs to inhale tubercle bacilli in very minute doses,
while he failed to produce any lesions by feeding them with
far larger quantities of bacilli. Titze and Weidanz at the
Gesundheitsamt however failed, as we shall see, to produce
very severe results even by inhalation.

In conclusion then it may be said that experiment has
revealed considerable and somewhat unexpected difficulty in
transmitting tuberculosis to the dog either by feeding or,
sometimes, even by inhalation. Some predisposing cause would
appear to be necessary before an infection with tubercle bacilli
assumes a progressive character. The difficulty of causing
serious infection artificially is especially well established in the
case of feeding experiments, and Petit's opinion that tuberculosis
in the dog is *usually* caused by bacilli which enter the body
through the alimentary canal is probably too dogmatic. That
it sometimes occurs in this way, however, seems probable as
for example in the butchers' dogs mentioned by Thomassen
and Jensen. Even the healthy intestinal mucosa of the dog
is not entirely impervious to tubercle bacilli, as Ravenel and
A. S. Griffith have shown when they fed dogs with these
bacteria and found the microbes in many cases some hours
later in the mesenteric glands. It is possible that when the
mucous membrane is no longer healthy its permeability is much
increased. We must remember that the dog is often badly
infested with intestinal worms; and it may be that it is under
these circumstances, and owing to the consequently increased
absorption of tubercle bacilli, that tuberculosis of intestinal
entry can arise.

Whether pulmonary tuberculosis can arise in the dog in
consequence of absorption of tubercle bacilli through the intestinal wall, and without the mucous membrane itself or the
mesenteric or other abdominal lymphatic glands participating

obviously in the disease cannot as yet be finally decided. Griffith's experiments lend some slight support to this view. But we must remember that it is complicated by the further question whether in feeding experiments it is not possible for some of the bacilli to enter the lungs directly through the trachea owing to slight accidents in the performance of deglutition. This question has been discussed already (p. 165). Moreover against the view that mesenteric glands can transmit tubercle bacilli in numbers sufficient to produce pulmonary tuberculosis without themselves participating in the disease is the fact that in certain cases, of which the intestinal origin is not disputed, these glands have borne their fair share of the lesions.

Finally the most probable conclusion which we can draw at present concerning this question of the portals of entry of tubercle bacilli in canine tuberculosis seems to be that while some cases are caused by bacilli which penetrate the intestinal mucous membrane, the majority are caused by bacilli which enter the lungs through the air passages.

Experimental infection by means of subcutaneous and intraperitoneal injection will be dealt with fully when we come to discuss the relative susceptibility of the dog to infection with the three types of tubercle bacilli. It will then be seen that it has been found impossible, so far, to cause severe tuberculosis by subcutaneous injection, but that by intraperitoneal injection a severe and fatal tuberculous peritonitis, and even a general tuberculosis may be set up fairly readily, especially in young animals.

In 1884 Koch published the results of the successful infection of three dogs in this way[1]. In 1902 de Jong also succeeded

---

[1] One animal becoming ill was killed after five weeks, and was found to be suffering from severe tuberculous peritonitis and general tuberculosis of lungs, liver and spleen. Another became ill, but apparently recovered. In order to find out whether it had become immune, it was injected again—this time with a larger dose, and a third dog was injected at the same time as a control. Both these animals fell ill. One actually died, the other was killed when ill and weak. The same pathological conditions were found in these animals as in the one first mentioned (*The Etiology of Tuberculosis*, Eng. trans. p. 176).

in the use of this method, and, as we shall see in a moment, severe and fatal results were produced with it by the Royal Commission.

The Comparative Susceptibility of the Dog to Infection with the Three Types of Tubercle Bacilli.

Natural Infection. Very little work has been done towards determining the types of the tubercle bacilli which occur in cases of naturally acquired tuberculosis in the dog. In 1908 Zwick[1] investigated cultures from two cases. The one yielded a strain which had the cultural characters of the human type and failed to cause tuberculosis in rabbits; from the other was grown a strain which had the characters of the bovine type.

In 1909 Römer[2] from one of two cases isolated a bacillus of the bovine type, which was virulent for rabbits, and in the same year Joest obtained a strain of the same kind.

In 1912 Malm[3] stated that in five cases of canine tuberculosis which he investigated he found only bacilli of bovine type.

Schornagel in 1914 investigated eleven cases of natural tuberculosis in the dog. From three of them no cultures were obtained, and there is nothing to indicate the type of bacillus concerned. From four of the remaining cases eight strains of tubercle bacilli were cultivated which had low virulence for calf, goat and rabbit, and clearly belonged to the human type. From two cases the cultures obtained belonged to the bovine type. In the case of the remaining two the evidence of type was somewhat conflicting. The strains were considered by Schornagel to be transitional (*Übergangsformen*), but it appears to the present writer more probable that they were ordinary members of the human type[4].

[1], [2] and [3] cited by Schornagel.

[4] In the case of strain No. v cultural characters, and goat and rabbit injections were all consistent with the view that the strain belonged to the human type. Only the calf experiment was anomalous. 55 mg. were subcutaneously injected into one of these animals; when killed six months later it was found to have, besides tuberculous changes at the seat of inoculation

Thus we must conclude that the dog may become infected with both the human and the bovine tubercle bacillus. This is supported by the results of experimental investigation which we shall examine in a moment. But whether, under natural conditions, infection with one type of bacillus is commoner than that with the other there is as yet not sufficient evidence to determine. In no case of spontaneous disease has the avian bacillus been found to be present.

Experimental Injection with Human and Bovine Bacilli. In de Jong's experiments, already mentioned, both human and bovine tubercle bacilli were injected intraperitoneally with positive results. Leudet and Petit successfully injected the dog with human tubercle bacilli. Koch, in his experiments referred to above, used "a pure culture of miliary tubercle from a human lung." It is clear then that the dog may be successfully infected experimentally with the human as well as with the bovine type of tubercle bacilli. In this respect it differs from almost all the lower animals, monkeys, guinea-pigs, rats and mice, and possibly many foreign wild animals kept in our menageries, excepted. This important point has been, as we shall see, amply confirmed both by the work of the Royal Commission, and of the Gesundheitsamt.

In the course of the lengthy investigation carried out by the former body many experiments with human and bovine tubercle bacilli were made on the dog for various objects and at different times. They have been collected together from the various Appendices of the Reports of the Commission and

and prescapular gland, "slight tuberculosis of pleura and peritoneum," along with non-tubercular disease of kidneys and liver. Now pleura and peritoneum are not the parts attacked by preference in an infection spreading from a subcutaneous inoculation. In the author's opinion therefore one should not overlook the possibility that this was a case of spontaneous infection.

In the other case, No. VII, cultural characters, and calf and rabbit injections combined to show that the strain was one of human type. Only a goat, which received 20 mg. of culture *intravenously* died after twenty-nine days of acute miliary tuberculosis of lungs. There is really nothing very surprising in this. Human tubercle bacilli are quite capable of killing calves, goats and rabbits when injected into the blood stream; nor need the dose be very large. Doubtless a good deal will depend on the size of the animal (not mentioned in this case) and the fineness of the emulsion. (For the details of the experiment criticized here see table opposite p. 75 of Schornagel's dissertation.)

tabulated for the first time.   But the table, including as it does sixty animals, is too long to be reproduced here.   Nearly all these experiments were made by A. S. Griffith.   The animals were of various ages, some quite young puppies.   Thirteen were inoculated by subcutaneous injection, fourteen by intraperitoneal injection, and thirty-three were infected by feeding. In about two-thirds of the experiments the bacilli employed belonged to the bovine type, and in the other third to the human type.   (Some experiments with avian bacilli will be dealt with separately.)

Subcutaneous Injection of pure cultures in doses varying from 1 to 25 mg. of bacilli produced only a mild type of disease in the dog.   A small abscess would develop at the seat of inoculation, and after a time discharge its contents, leaving a sinus.   The lesion however tended to heal completely; so that after some months when the animals came to be killed nothing more than a scar as a rule remained at the seat of inoculation.   Meanwhile the lymphatic glands became enlarged and there might be a good deal of periglandular infiltration.   These glandular lesions would soften and ulcerate through the skin, leaving behind sinuses or, ultimately, only a scar.   After death a few minute grey tubercles were commonly found in the lungs, liver or kidneys.   These little disseminated lesions were quite inconsiderable, and never assumed a progressive form.   The animals which possessed them remained in good general condition; and the disease was in no case severe, and never fatal, either in grown dogs or in puppies.   There was no difference in the severity of the disease set up in this way by the bovine and human types of bacilli respectively.

Intraperitoneal Injection produced a much more severe type of disease, and death usually occurred when the dose was as much as, or more than, 10 mg.   Thus of three puppies which received, two of them 10 mg. and one 50 mg., and one adult which received the larger of these doses, intraperitoneally, all died of general tuberculosis within one or two months.   One adult which received 10 mg. in this way survived and was found, when killed 413 days after injection, to have general tuberculosis.   These results were produced with tubercle bacilli of the human type.   Only four experiments were carried out with bacilli of bovine type, but the results were very similar to those we have already considered.   One young dog which received 10 mg. of bovine bacilli died thirty-seven days later of tuberculous peritonitis and general tuberculosis.   One puppy died of tuberculous peritonitis after a dose of 1 mg.   One grown dog which received the same small dose survived, and when killed five months later was found to have developed only a few tubercles scattered in lungs and liver, and some doubtful foci in the kidneys.   The peritoneum was normal.

Infection by Feeding caused, as a rule, disseminated lesions, but these were, for the most part, trivial, and the disease did not assume a severe type.   There was however one exception: a dog, after being fed with 10 mg. of tubercle bacilli of human type, slowly fell ill, and died after ninety-four days, with pulmonary tuberculosis and pyo-pneumothorax[1]. This result was so exceptional that a suggestion was entertained that it might have been caused by an accidental entry of tubercle bacilli directly into the lungs at the time of the experimental feeding. Titze and Weidanz, as we shall see in a moment, had a very similar experience.

These experiments showed clearly that the dog's powers of resisting experimental infection with tubercle bacilli are very considerable, and that neither type of mammalian bacillus is specially virulent for him. The dog may however under certain circumstances be infected with a progressive and fatal tuberculosis, and in such cases one type of bacillus has been found as virulent as the other.

At the Gesundheitsamt, while the researches of the Royal Commission were going on, a German investigation of the degree of susceptibility of the dog to experimental infection with the two types of mammalian tubercle bacilli was carried out by Titze and Weidanz. The results support and supplement the work of the Commission. They demonstrate clearly that the dog possesses great powers of resisting artificial infection with tubercle bacilli by whatever channel they are administered, while at the same time they show that it may sometimes be made to develop severe tuberculous disease. They found no difference in virulence for the dog between the human and bovine types of tubercle bacilli.

The German investigators found, like the Royal Commission, that subcutaneous injection produced at the seat of injection a lesion which ulcerated and then tended to heal. Progressive disseminated disease did not occur, and the dogs remained well; but sometimes a few little grey tuberculous foci were seen in the lungs or one of the other organs.

Even *intravenous injection* did not always produce progressive disease. Four animals were injected in this way with 1 mg. of bacilli. One killed in good condition six-and-a-half months later was found to have developed a chronic tuberculous pleurisy; another fell ill and lost appetite and weight for a time, but, recovering both, continued to improve until it was killed five-and-a-half months after injection. In the lungs were found some nodules which appeared to represent tubercles which had healed, but in which tubercle bacilli could not be

---

[1] Dog 1. *R.C.T. Int. Rep.* App. vol. II, p. 1178. The pharyngeal glands were normal; the mesenteric glands showed minute white foci scattered in their cortices, but no tubercle bacilli could be found in them on microscopic examination. There were several tuberculous nodules in the lungs, one as large as a pigeon's egg, and this one had softened and opened into the pleura.

demonstrated either by microscopic examination or by injection of guinea-pigs. On the other hand two animals developed severe disease which proved fatal. One of these, a bitch, injected at the beginning of pregnancy, died of general tuberculosis fifty-nine days later, and the other succumbed to pulmonary tuberculosis 144 days after the injection of tubercle bacilli.

Intraperitoneal injections, which yielded such striking results to the Royal Commission, were not employed at the Gesundheitsamt.

Titze and Weidanz made some interesting experiments by inhalation. Six animals were used, and the doses varied from 1 to 5 mg. of bacilli; but it must be understood that the quantities which actually entered the lungs were considerably less than these amounts, since a considerable part necessarily remained behind in the apparatus. It is rather surprising to find that severe disease was not in any instance caused in this way. Sometimes a few small tuberculous foci were found when the animals came to be killed, and in other cases all the organs appeared to be sound.

Attempts to infect by administering the bacilli with food as a rule either failed completely, or at most produced a few little grey foci of disease in the mesenteric glands. But one experiment was followed by serious results, and merits more detailed consideration. To eight puppies when only four days old was administered by means of a feeding bottle a quarter of a broth culture of tubercle bacilli emulsified in cow's milk. Three of these animals were found when killed to be quite sound; five developed more or less pulmonary disease. In three this was of no great severity, but in the remaining two it proved fatal. One of these latter died five weeks after the experimental feeding, shortly after receiving 5 c.c. of tuberculin by the mouth. A small cavity, as large as a hazel nut, together with numerous grey tubercles, with yellow centres and as large as pin heads, and which in some places were confluent, was found in the lungs. In the other fatal case the animal died, twenty-five days after infection, with its lungs beset with numerous small cavities, and presenting on section an appearance like that of a sponge. The exceptional nature of these severe pulmonary lesions led the authors to believe that they might have been caused by bacilli which had entered directly into the air passages at the moment of the experimental feeding. They recalled the fact that the puppies had resisted this unnatural method of alimentation, and had taken the infected milk not without protest, accompanied even by some slight choking. In order to test this hypothesis they fed some puppies in a similar manner with milk blackened with Chinese ink. The animals were killed immediately after and traces of the milk were found in the pouches of Morgagni in the larynx, and on the vocal cords, thus showing that the escape of particles of fluid administered by the mouth into the air passage is not an improbable occurrence under the circumstances of experimental feeding. It will be remembered that when we were discussing the question of the portals of tuberculous infection in man it was pointed out that A. S. Griffith had suggested a similar explanation for the pulmonary tubercles which commonly occurred in the dogs which he subjected to experimental feeding with tubercle bacilli, p. 165.

In 1910 Sticker succeeded in infecting dogs by intraperitoneal injection, both with human and bovine bacilli, and he came to the conclusion that these animals are more susceptible to the human than to the bovine type of bacillus.

In the same year Schrum was able to infect dogs by subcutaneous, intraperitoneal and intravenous injection. But the disease showed little tendency to be progressive, no matter which type of bacillus was used, and Schrum came to the conclusion, as others had done before him, that the dog possesses considerable powers of resisting infection with tubercle bacilli of all kinds[1].

It has been suggested by Link, that the dog may owe its high powers of resisting tuberculous infection to repeated exposure to infection with small doses in early life. In answer to this it was pointed out by Titze and Weidanz that the power of resistance possessed by the dog is inherent and not acquired, for it is present already in the young puppy.

Avian Tubercle Bacilli. To infection with avian tubercle bacilli the dog is still more highly resistant than it is to infection with mammalian tubercle bacilli. Even intravenous injection, and in large doses too, provokes remarkably little change. Long ago Straus and Gamaléia[2] pointed out that intravenous injection of the dog differentiates very clearly between avian and mammalian tubercle bacilli; and F. Griffith's experiments, made for the Royal Commission, fully confirm this. In some of his experiments he injected doses of 10 and even 50 mg. of avian bacilli intravenously into grown dogs and puppies with little or no result. The table on p. 502 shows this very clearly.

It is interesting to note that while avian tubercle bacilli do not produce disease in the dog, they survive for a long time in its body. Thus in the case of Dog No. 164, while "all organs

[1] Schrum calls particular attention to the fact that in all his eight dogs, the lungs, broadly speaking, were the only seat of tuberculous lesions (*Inaug. Diss.* Bern p. 60).

[2] "Sur la tuberculose humaine et aviaire," *Compt. rend. du Congrès pour l'Étude de la tuberculose chez l'homme et chez les animaux,* 1891. As a matter of fact it is much better to inject fowls (intravenously) and guinea-pigs (subcutaneously) for this purpose.

Intravenous Injection of Human and Avian Tubercle Bacilli into Dogs[1].

Human Tubercle Bacilli				Avian Tubercle Bacilli			
No.	Age	Dose	Result	No.	Age	Dose	Result
				162	Puppy	50 mg.	Killed 146 days. Two small grey nodules in one kidney
				164	Adult	50 mg.	Killed 142 days. No Tub.
				154	Puppy	10 mg.	Killed 174 days. No Tub.
3	Puppy	1 mg.	Died 33 days. Gen. Tub.	152	Puppy	1 mg.	Killed 194 days. No Tub.

and glands were free from tuberculous lesions" (142 days after injection), cultures sown from the liver, kidneys and spleen in each case developed colonies of avian tubercle bacilli.

The Danger of Tuberculosis being communicated by the Dog to Man. The close association between man and the dog need hardly be insisted on, nor the frequency with which this animal is the intimate playmate of children. Moreover, as we have seen, the tubercle bacilli with which the dog is infected is often of the human type. The danger is all the greater because tuberculosis in the dog is usually of the "open" kind, the disease being often pulmonary, and cavities not uncommon; moreover, according to Petit, cutaneous ulcers, "incredibly rich in tubercle bacilli," may sometimes occur.

Tuberculosis in the Cat.

The cat is the associate of man almost as much as the dog, and is especially the playmate of young children; yet feline tuberculosis has received but little attention from pathologists. Its importance however as a danger to man is minimized by the fact that the cat, as we shall see, appears to be susceptible only to the bovine form of tuberculosis.

[1] For Dogs Nos. 162, 164, 152, 154, see F. Griffith, *R.C.T. Fin. Rep.* App. vol. IV, p. 282. For Dog 3 see A. S. Griffith, *R.C.T. Fin. Rep.* vol. I, p. 245.

A case of tuberculosis in the cat was recorded by Filleau and Petit early in 1888; two more cases were reported later in the same year—one by Nocard in France, and the other by McFadyean in this country; and a considerable number have been recognized since at various veterinary schools. Without making any particular search the writer has seen three cases during the last year or two at Cambridge. Feline tuberculosis is certainly not very uncommon.

Exactly how common it is would be difficult at present to say; some rough idea may however be gathered from the following figures. Jensen, 1891, saw twenty-five cases at the Veterinary School in Copenhagen in less than two years. Abel of Leipzig is said by Hess to have found nine tuberculous cats among 400 which he examined there. Petit examined 366 cats which died or were killed in the Veterinary School of Alfort (Paris) during the five years 1900–1904, and found, in round numbers, about two per cent. tuberculous. Friedberger and Fröhner concluded, from a review of veterinary statistics, that about one per cent. of the sick cats of Berlin were tuberculous.

Several cases are recorded in which the tuberculous cats belonged to persons who were themselves consumptive; and in some it is definitely stated that the animals consumed human tuberculous sputum. It was so in a case recorded by Filleau and Petit[1]. But such stories are not nearly so common

---

[1] This fact should warn us not to accept too readily similar testimony concerning the dog. The evidence of this kind in the case of the dog is however much more considerable than it is in the case of the cat. Filleau and Petit's case however is of considerable interest since the cat is alleged to have contracted tuberculosis from eating sputum, and to have recovered. The facts are as follows: the cat lived in a pathological laboratory attached to a hospital where there were consumptive patients. It developed a liking for sputum, and was in the habit of consuming the refuse of what was sent to the laboratory for examination. This habit was not discouraged, and the cat was kept under observation to see what would happen. After a time the animal became ill, and presented all the symptoms of a chronic grave disease. It had a muco-purulent discharge from the nose in which tubercle bacilli were found; it suffered from cough and sneezing, and was expected to die. But it became pregnant and about the same time began to recover; and presently giving birth to a kitten it suckled it, and still continued to improve for five months. It was then bitten by a mad dog and had to be killed. Post-mortem examination showed a collection of small calcareous nodules in one lung, and no disease elsewhere. *Journ. de Méd. de Paris*, Jan. 1888.

as in the case of the tuberculous dog. Friedberger and Fröhner
believed that human tuberculosis provided the source of infection for tuberculosis in cats[1]. But in the light of more
recent investigations this cannot be accepted, for it has, as
we have said, been definitely shown (by experiments which
will be reviewed presently) that the cat is not susceptible to
infection with tubercle bacilli of the human type.

According to the German authorities the lungs are the
organs which chiefly suffer; and with this Straus, and Petit and
Basset concur. But all these authors agree that the mesenteric
glands also are frequently attacked, and that the kidneys are
liable to suffer. Liver and spleen, curiously enough, seem to
be seldom affected, and the serous membranes to suffer less
often than in the dog. But, as in the latter, cutaneous lesions
sometimes occur, and when they do so may be swarming with
tubercle bacilli[2].

As to the portal of entry in feline tuberculosis it seems
probable that this is usually in some part of the alimentary
canal. It is true that the lungs are often the seat of disease.
But one cannot always be sure that the lesions there are
primary; and, after all, the proof of entrance through the air
passages is not so much the mere presence of comparatively
advanced disease in the lungs, as the presence of this condition
in *the absence of equally old disease in the mesenteric glands*. In
Jensen's series of cases while the lungs were affected in sixteen,
the mesenteric glands were tuberculous in fourteen; and in
five cases the disease was confined entirely to these glands.
The intestinal mucous membrane, as in the dog, is said to be
seldom the seat of visible tuberculous lesions; only once was
Jensen able to detect a lesion here. Nocard however records
intestinal ulceration in two cases[3].

---

[1] "Wie beim Hunde dürften in der Regel tuberculöse Menschen (Eigen-
thümer) die Infectionsquelle bilden," *loc. cit.* p. 500.

[2] Petit and Cognot, 1902. Charmoy, 1912. *Recueil de Méd. Vét.* vol.
LXXXIX, p. 17.

[3] In McFadyean's case tuberculosis was confined to the lungs and bronchial
glands, and in Hess's case there was marked tuberculosis in both lungs. (*Proc.
N. Y. Path. Soc.* N.S. vol. VII, p. 104.) In one of Nocard's cases there was
acute peritonitis caused by the bursting of an intestinal ulcer, and the lungs

The Comparative Susceptibility of the Cat to Infection with the Three Types of Tubercle Bacilli.

Natural Infection. As to the type of bacillus to be found in cats affected with tuberculosis naturally acquired but little is known for certain. F. Griffith, in the single case investigated by him, found that the bacillus was of the bovine type; and this was also the type found in two cases examined by the author.

Experimental Infection. The cat is included among the various animal species to which Villemin succeeded in transmitting tuberculosis by inoculation. Viseur (1874) infected cats by feeding them with tuberculous material. Koch (1884) produced similar results in these animals by inoculation. Nocard fed four kittens and their mother with cultures of these micro-organisms, and thereby transmitted an acute disease to the kittens and a more chronic one to the cat[1]. In these early experiments it is not always possible to distinguish the type of bacillus employed, but we know that the material used by Viseur was the tuberculous lung of a cow[2].

were almost normal; so that it is practically certain in this case that the intestinal disease was primary. In the other case there was diarrhœa during life; and after death all the mesenteric glands were found to be hypertrophied and the majority caseous and softened, the cæcum was ulcerated, and the spleen, curiously enough if it is true that it is affected but seldom, was crammed with miliary tubercles. (*Recueil de Méd. Vét.* 1888; vol. LXV, and 1889, vol. LXVI.)

[1] Nocard, art. "Tuberculose," *Dict. pratique de méd. Vét.* vol. XXI, p. 508. Quoted by Straus, *loc. cit.* p. 363.

[2] In Koch's experiments the source of the tubercle bacilli was sometimes human and sometimes bovine, and yet no difference in the result in the two cases is recorded. This is very extraordinary, because as the experiments of the Royal Commission have shown, the difference is as well marked in the cat as in the ox or any other of the differentiating animals. Koch's experiments on cats were briefly as follows: Two, inoculated with tuberculous material derived, either directly or indirectly, from a case of bovine tuberculosis, developed rapidly fatal tuberculosis. Two, inoculated with the lung tubercles of a monkey which died of spontaneous tuberculosis, are said to have died tubercular. Four cats were injected with various pure cultures: One from a case of human miliary tuberculosis, another from a case of phthisis, a third from a "perl" nodule in an ox, and a fourth from a tuberculous monkey. Thus it is almost certain that tubercle bacilli both of human and bovine type were employed in these experiments, and yet Koch merely remarks that all the animals showed tuberculous changes. (*The Etiology of Tuberculosis,* Eng. trans. pp. 161–163 and 177.)

TABLE XIX. *Experiments showing Comparative Susceptibility of Cats to Human and Bovine Tubercle Bacilli.*

(Royal Commission on Tuberculosis.)

Mode of Injection	Human Type				Bovine Type			
	Ref. No.	Description	Dose of culture in mg.	Result	Ref. No.	Description	Dose of culture in mg.	Result
Subcutaneous	1	25	Cat	50	D 29 days. Local caseous tumour, nearest glands caseous, T.B. in apparently normal organs	2	26	Cat	1	K 35 days. Miliary tuberculosis in lungs, few tubercles elsewhere
	1	33	Cat	10	K 98 ,, Local caseous tumour and inguinal gland	2	28	Cat	1	D 49 ,, Ditto
	1	47	Cat.	10	D 74 ,, Local lesion only	2	32	Kit.	1	D 17 ,, Gen. Tuberculosis
	1	55	Kit.	1	K 88 ,, ,, ,, ,,	2	66	Cat	1	D 70 ,, ,,
	1	65	Kit.	1	K 162 ,, ,, ,, ,,	2	68	Kit.	1	D 25 ,, ,,
	1	67	Kit.	1	K 162 ,, ,, ,, ,,	2	84	Kit.	1	D 21 ,, ,,
	1	23	Kit.	0·01	D 72 ,, Local lesion, glands normal, small grey foci in liver	2	78	Cat	1	K 74 ,, Severe pulmonary tuberculosis, tubercles in liver
						2	80	Kit.	0·1	D 34 ,, Gen. Tuberculosis
						2	76	Cat	0·1	D 22 ,, ,,
						2	82	Kit.	0·01	D 39 ,, ,,

Method	No.	Exp. No.	Animal	Dose	Result
Intraperitoneal	I	29	Cat	50	D 77 days. Local tuberculosis, few tubercles in lungs
	I	37	Cat	50	D 56 „ Slight gen. tub.
	I	27	Cat	10	K 86 „ very ill. Local tub. only
	I	31	Cat	10	D 94 „ Numerous yellowish-grey nodules in lungs
	I	69	Kit.	10	K 146 „ No tuberculosis
	I	71	Kit.	10	K 146 „ „
	4	9	Cat	10	K 116 „ Minute „ grey foci mesentery, several grey nodules in left lung
	I	61	Kit.	1	K 162 „ Minute transparent tubercles in omentum
	I	63	Kit.	1	K 162 „ Ditto
	I	59	Kit.	1	D 23 „ No visible lesions, few T.B. lungs, liver, spleen
	2	34	Cat	1	D 39 days. Gen. Tuberculosis
	2	36	Kit.	1	D 17 „ „
	I	11	Cat	1	D 17 „ „ very ill. Gen. Tub.
	I	13	Cat	1	K 36 „ „
Feeding	I	41	Cat	50	K 108 „ No tuberculosis
	I	39	Cat	50	K 110 „ „
	I	35	Cat	10	K 95 „ „
	I	73	Kit.	50, 50, and 14 mg. on 3 successive occasions	K 99 „ „
	I	75	Kit.		K 99 „ „
	I	77	Kit.		K 99 „ „
	3	86	Cat	10	K 71 „ Few tubs. in lungs
	3	88	Cat	10	K 73 „ Tub. mes. glds., widely disseminated tuberculosis
	3	38	Cat	1	K 111 „ One tub. mes. glds.
	3	46	Cat	1	K 48 „ One tub. mes. glds., one ileo-colic gld.
	3	48	Kit.	1	K 47 „ Tub. mes. glds., small ulcers in intestine. Tuberculosis of lungs
	3	50	Kit.	1	K 74 „ Grey tubs. in lungs
	3	52	Kit.	1	K 121 „ Tub. mes. glds., Tubercles and nodules in lungs

1 R.C.T. Fin. Rep. App. vol. I, pp. 246–249 and 268.   2 R.C.T. Int. Rep. App. vol. I, p. 422.
3 R.C.T. Int. Rep. App. vol. I, pp. 618–620 and 687–688.   4 R.C.T. Int. Rep. App. vol. II, p. 1187.

The susceptibility of the cat to the three types of tubercle bacilli was worked out for the first time incidentally by the Royal Commission. The great majority of the experiments were done by A. S. Griffith, and the most important are collected together here from the various Appendices to the Reports of the Commission.

These results may be briefly summarized. Tubercle bacilli of bovine type injected, either subcutaneously or intraperitoneally, in small doses (·01 to 1·0 mg.) caused invariably rapidly fatal general tuberculosis. Similar doses of bacilli of human type had little or no effect. Only a small local lesion was seen under the skin, or, after intraperitoneal injection, a few minute grey tubercles in the omentum. Moreover doses which for these small animals can only be regarded as enormous, namely, 10 or 50 mg. of bacilli, injected intraperitoneally were, as a rule well borne. Slight general tuberculosis, it is true, was recorded in one case (Cat 37) and some nodules or tubercles in the lungs of two others, but nothing like acute general tuberculosis or progressive disease of more chronic type was set up by this type of bacillus.

It is true that five out of the ten cats which received these large doses, including the three which were injected with 50 mg., died within one to three months of the injections; and it is conceivable that these may have succumbed to the poisons in the bacilli. But cats are difficult to keep confined in laboratory cages, and are liable to die from more or less obscure causes, and it is not unlikely that the death of these animals was unconnected with the injections; nevertheless when one compares this mortality among the animals which received large doses with the much smaller mortality among those which received small doses by injection or were fed with bacilli, it seems possible that the five cats in question may have succumbed to tuberculous toxæmia.

To infection by feeding with bovine tubercle bacilli the cat is susceptible. Tubercles appear in the mesenteric glands and sometimes in the lungs. In a single case ulcers were noted in the intestine. These effects were produced with moderate doses (1 mg.). With 10 c.c. widely disseminated tuberculosis is recorded in one case, and a few tubercles in the lungs in another. Clearly the cat may be infected by feeding with bovine tubercle bacilli, but is not very highly susceptible. Of the human type of bacillus on the other hand large doses (10 and 50 mg.) have been given in this way without effect.

From all these experiments one may safely conclude that the cat differentiates very sharply between the two types of mammalian tubercle bacilli.

It is less easy to be dogmatic with regard to the susceptibility of the cat to infection with the avian type of bacillus. F. Griffith attempted to infect ten cats with bacilli of this type by intravenous, subcutaneous, or intraperitoneal injection and one by feeding, doses from 0·1 to 10 mg., in the last case the organs of a rabbit, which had died of an injection of avian bacilli, being used. Few and inconspicuous were the lesions recorded, yet seven out of the ten cats injected died in from sixteen days to two-and-a-half months. Some of them may possibly have died of an intercurrent disease, for, as we have said already, cats are difficult to keep confined in laboratory cages. But the mortality was so much higher than that of the cats infected with human bacilli and kept under identical conditions that in this case there seems to be very little doubt that some of them, at least of those which received intraperitoneal injection, died from multiplication and dissemination of the bacilli without the formation of anatomical tubercles or other obvious lesions. For four animals injected in this way died, and though no tubercles were seen in their organs, in three of the cases these contained numerous tubercle bacilli[1].

Tuberculosis in Monkeys.

Anthropoid apes, baboons, various other monkeys and lemurs are, as is well known, very liable to become infected with tuberculosis when kept in captivity. The disease spreads readily from one to another when a number of individuals are living in the same cage; their susceptibility must therefore be

---

[1] *R.C.T. Fin. Rep.* App. vol. IV, p. 188. Kittens 56 and 60 died sixteen days after injection of 1 and 5 mg. of bacilli respectively, and Cat 62 died seventy-three days after injection of 1 mg.

great; and yet they are not known to suffer from the disease in their natural state (Straus, von Dungern, and Baermann and Halberstaedter). De Haan (1903) examined the bodies of over thirty monkeys which died of various causes in Java without finding any that were tuberculous.

The lesions found in tuberculous monkeys are not unlike those seen in man. They become caseous and soften; cavities may appear in the lungs, and ulcers in the Peyer's patches of the intestine; miliary tuberculosis is common. R. Koch, who examined eight cases of spontaneous tuberculosis in these animals, drew attention to certain differences between simian and human tuberculosis. He pointed out that in monkeys the disease is seldom confined to one organ as is so often the case in man, but usually is generalized; moreover caseation is followed rapidly by softening, so that the lesions often come to contain a thin pus, and are apt to take the form of multiple abscesses rather than of tubercles. This is however by no means always the case.

Another point of distinction which seems worthy of mention is the liability of the skeletal muscles of the monkey to be involved in a general tuberculosis. This occurs, at least in experimental infections, and the writer has twice seen numerous little irregular caseous foci widely scattered in the leg muscles of *Macacus rhesus*.

The Comparative Susceptibility of Monkeys to Infection with the Three Types of Tubercle Bacilli.

Spontaneous Infection. It seems probable that two, or perhaps three, of the eight tuberculous monkeys examined by Koch were infected with the bovine type of tubercle bacillus; for he states that the disease proved transmissible to cats and rabbits[1]. But too much must not be made of this since Koch at that time (1884) seems to have failed to distinguish between localized non-progressive lesions, such as the human type of tubercle bacillus produces in the rabbit, and the severe generalized disease which is caused in that animal by the bovine bacillus, and he may merely have referred to local lesions in the case of the cat.

---

[1] *The Etiology of Tuberculosis,* Eng. trans. *loc. cit.* pp. 162 and 171.

Plate XVI

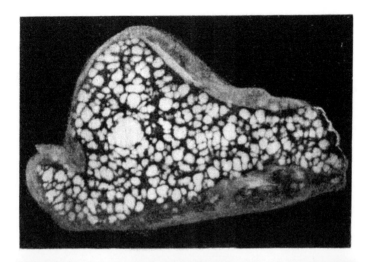

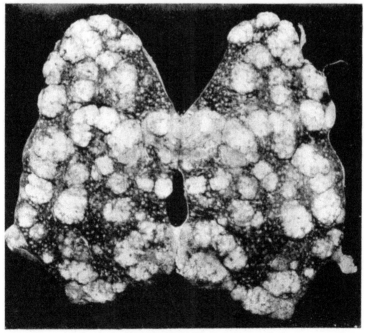

No. 1. Tuberculosis in the Spleen of a Monkey.
No. 2. Tuberculosis in the Spleen of a Baboon.

From preparations by A. S. Griffith.

Indeed it would seem probable from more recent work that the great majority of instances of tuberculosis in monkeys are caused by bacilli of the human type. Rabinowitsch (1907) examined forty-five tuberculous monkeys which died in the Zoölogical Gardens in Berlin. These included an orang-outang and a chimpanzee. Twenty-seven strains of tubercle bacilli were cultivated from these monkeys, and tested for comparative virulence by inoculation of rabbits, and, in special cases, other animals. Nineteen of the strains were judged to belong to the human, and only three to the bovine type[1].

F. Griffith investigated a case of spontaneous tuberculosis in a chimpanzee, and another in a rhesus monkey. In each case the tubercle bacilli cultivated proved to be of the human type.

The present writer obtained strains of tubercle bacilli from two ring-tailed lemurs which died in captivity of spontaneous tuberculosis. These strains also proved to be of the human type.

Though the type of tubercle bacillus found in monkeys is nearly always the human, it by no means follows that this type is more virulent for these animals than the others. As a matter of fact experiment has shown that there is no difference in virulence for monkeys between the human and the bovine types. The cases of spontaneous simian tuberculosis examined have come for the most part from zoölogical gardens where the chance of infection from other animals (except in the case of carnivores) is small, while the possibility of infection from human visitors cannot be excluded. Probably however the disease commonly spreads from monkeys infected before arrival. However this may be, it seems that opportunity for infection with a particular type of bacillus, rather than superior virulence of that type, plays the dominant rôle in simian tuberculosis.

[1] The five other strains were as follows: From one case human tubercle bacilli were cultivated from the lung and bovine from the spleen; from three other cases were cultivated strains which were held to be transitional (*Übergangsformen*). Two of these appeared to be intermediate between the human and bovine types, and one intermediate between the human and avian types. Another strain, cultivated from a case of general tuberculosis, was judged to be purely avian. It must be understood that Rabinowitsch, while recognizing in general the existence of three types of tubercle bacilli, does not hold them to be so sharply defined or so distinct from one another as do most of those who have given as much attention as she has to the subject.

Experimental Infection. Since Koch's announcement of the distinction between human and bovine tubercle bacilli in 1901 a number of researches on monkeys have been made. Grünbaum (1901) showed that the chimpanzee is capable of being infected with bovine tuberculosis. Nocard (1902), de Jong (1902), Ravenel (1902), and de Schweinitz, Dorset and Schroeder (1902) were able to infect monkeys both with human and bovine tuberculous material, and by feeding as well as by one or other kind of inoculation. All these observers came to the conclusion that the disease set up by the bovine bacillus is more severe and more rapidly fatal than that caused by the human bacillus.

On the other hand Alan Macfadyen (1903), who infected sixteen monkeys, some with human and others with bovine tuberculous material and most of them by feeding, could find nó difference in the severity of the disease caused by these two kinds of infective agents. Those animals which were fed with sputum, it is true, developed ulceration of the intestine, while those fed with bovine material did not, but this difference was probably attributable to other bacteria present along with the tubercle bacilli in the sputum.

Beck (1903), in a limited number of experiments, found the disease set up by human tuberculous material *more* severe than that caused by bovine.

Kraus and Grosz (1907) attempted to produce cutaneous tuberculosis in monkeys by applying cultures to scarified areas of skin. They succeeded in producing such lesions, both with human and bovine tubercle bacilli, but with the former bacillus the lesions remained limited to the seat of inoculation and healed, while with the latter a progressive and fatal tuberculosis ensued.

On the whole then it would seem that the majority of those observers whose work we have been considering are inclined to the view that the bovine bacillus is rather more virulent for the monkey than the human. The difference, if there is one, is however not great, and it would require a number of very carefully correlated experiments, carried out with animals of the same species and age, and infected with comparable doses measured with exactness, before it could be completely established.

Some experiments more or less satisfying these conditions were carried out for the Royal Commission by A. S. Griffith, who gives the following table of his experiments on twenty-seven rhesus monkeys subcutaneously inoculated with cultures of human and bovine tubercle bacilli. In all cases the disease was allowed to terminate naturally; and since in none of them was it complicated by other disorders, the duration of life after injection (as shown in the penultimate columns of the table) may be taken as a convenient measure of the severity of the tuberculous disease in each case.

Rhesus Monkeys subcutaneously injected with Cultures of Bovine and Human Tubercle Bacilli[1].

Dose in mg.	Bovine Type			Human Type		
	Number injected with each dose	Survival in days	Result	Number injected with each dose	Survival in days	Result
10	one	35	G.T.	one	30	G.T.
1·0	five	27–45	,,	six	25–45	,,
0·1	two	26 and 56	,,	one	54	,,
0·01	two	36 and 53	,,	one	32	,,
0·001	one	45	,,	two	48 and 54	,,
0·00001	—	—	—	one	49	,,

G.T. = General tuberculosis

This table gives no indication whatever of any difference in severity of the disease caused in monkeys by comparable doses of bovine and human tubercle bacilli respectively. In the one case eleven monkeys died of general tuberculosis in a space of time which varied from twenty-six to fifty-six days; while in the other twelve monkeys died from the same cause in a space of time which varied from twenty-five to fifty-four days. If we take all the cases of infection with each type of bacillus

[1] *R.C.T. Fin. Rep.* App. vol. I, p. 43.

together irrespective of dose[1], we find that the average length of survival was, in the case of the bovine infections, 39·9 days, and in the case of the human something just short of forty days. Well might Griffith conclude from these experiments that "the human tubercle bacillus is as virulent for the monkey as the bovine tubercle bacillus."

On baboons of various kinds many experiments were carried out by Griffith on behalf of the Commission. Some were fed and others subcutaneously inoculated, bacilli both of human and bovine type being employed. The doses used were however not strictly comparable, and in some cases the animals died prematurely or were killed, so that no exact comparison of the virulence of the two types of bacilli for these animals is possible. The experiments however showed that baboons can easily be infected with either type of mammalian tubercle bacilli, whether administered with food or subcutaneously injected, and this much can be added: no difference in the virulence for these animals of the two types of bacilli came to light.

Lemurs were found to be very susceptible to experimental infection with bovine tubercle bacilli. With human tubercle bacilli no experiments were undertaken, but since two of these animals which died of spontaneous tuberculosis were found, as we have seen, to be infected with human tubercle bacilli, one can confidently affirm that these animals also are susceptible to infection with both types of mammalian tubercle bacilli.

With the chimpanzee no less than nine comparable experiments were made by the Royal Commission[2]. In all cases the disease was allowed to terminate naturally.

These experiments show clearly that the chimpanzee is very susceptible to infection both with human and bovine

---

[1] This is permissible because the number of animals infected with each dose of human and bovine bacilli respectively is about the same; and because in the monkey differences of dose do not make very much difference.

[2] Six of these were carried out by A. S. Griffith and three by the author. The first table is taken mainly from Griffith's Report (*R.C.T. Fin. Rep.* App. vol. I, p. 44), but one additional experiment which was omitted in the original is added (see *Ibid. Int. Rep.* vol. II, p. 1169). The experiments included in the second table are: Chimpanzees No. 2 and No. 14 from the *Int. Rep.* vol. I, pp. 444 and 649, and Chimpanzee No. 3, *Ibid.* vol. II, p. 1170.

tubercle bacilli. There does not appear the least indication that one type is more virulent for this species than the other.

The rapidity with which feeding infection proved fatal, in comparison with that caused by subcutaneous injection, is worthy of note, and is in distinct contrast to what occurs in the ox and guinea-pig, and indeed in nearly all other species.

Chimpanzees Injected subcutaneously with Cultures of Tubercle Bacilli.

Dose in mg.	Bovine type			Human type		
	Chim-panzee	Length of survival	Result	Chim-panzee	Length of survival	Result
1·0	No. 5	55 days	G.T.	No. 1	50 days	G.T.
1·0	No. 4	79 ,,	G.T.	—	—	—
0·001	No. 16	87 ,,	G.T.	—	—	—
0·00001	No. 24	107 ,,	G.T.	No. 7	90 days	G.T.

Chimpanzees Fed with Cultures of Tubercle Bacilli.

Dose in mg.	Bovine type			Human type		
	Chim-panzee	Length of survival	Result	Chim-panzee	Length of survival	Result
1·0	No. 2	56 days	G.T.	No. 3	77 days	G.T.
1·0	No. 14	63 days	G.T.		—	—

Von Dungern and Smidt (1906) in Sumatra carried out on the gibbon some comparative experiments with tubercle bacilli of human and bovine type, with the express purpose of finding out whether these animals, so nearly related to man, are more susceptible to infection with the one type than with the other. Two kinds of gibbon were used, a larger, *Hylobates syndactylus*, or siamang, and a smaller, *Hylobates agilis*, or unco.

The bacilli actually injected were cultivated in the Gesund-heitsamt in Berlin, and consisted of four separate strains—two of ordinary human type and human origin, and two of bovine type, one of which was of bovine and the other of porcine origin. The bacilli were grown on glycerin-broth, in flasks containing 100 c.c., and the fluid was removed and the bacilli still in the original flasks were carried out to Sumatra in the refrigerating chamber of the ship, and used as soon after arrival as possible.

The first series of experiments comprised subcutaneous injections, and the animals were allowed to die of the infection, which resulted. The results may be seen in the following table, the details of which are abstracted from the original paper.

Subcutaneous Injection of Tubercle Bacilli into Gibbons.

Human type					Bovine type				
Species No.	Weight in grms.	Dose in mg.	Result		Species No.	Weight in grms.	Dose in mg.	Result	
Unco 1	1·200	5	G.T.*	days 37	Unco 3	1·750	10	G.T.*	days 65
Unco 2	3·000	10	G.T.*	63	Unco 4	3·500	10	G.T.*	51
Siamang 1	3·250	10	G.T.*	46	Siamang 2	1·500	10	G.T.*	35
					Siamang 3	2·300	10	G.T.*	38
					Siamang 4	2·700	10	G.T.*	42

G. T. = general tuberculosis.   * = died.

The authors concluded that there was no difference in the action of the two kinds of tubercle bacilli on the higher apes. The histological character of the lesions caused by one was identical with that of those caused by the other.

Six feeding experiments were carried out on the siamang; three with tubercle bacilli of human type and human origin, and three with tubercle bacilli of bovine type. One animal in each group died, after fifty-one and eighty-four days respectively, but showed no tubercular changes.. The remaining four developed tuberculosis[1]. Of these one small animal infected with bovine bacilli died after fifty-seven days, while the remaining three were alive after three months, and had to be killed in order to complete the experiments, as the authors were about to leave Sumatra.

There does not seem to have been any notable difference in the severity of the disease produced by the bovine and human tubercle bacilli respectively; but in the case of those animals which were infected with the former type the ileum was ulcerated and the mesenteric glands caseous; while in that of those infected with the latter there were no tuberculous lesions in the intestines or in the lymphatic glands connected with them. This difference was probably fortuitous[2].

Let us now turn to the question whether the monkey is susceptible to infection with the avian tubercle bacillus. Rabinowitsch, in her investigation of spontaneous tuberculosis among the monkeys in the Zoölogical Gardens in Berlin, which has been alluded to already more than once, found one case from which the strain of bacilli isolated appeared to be of the avian type, and there was another case which yielded a strain of bacilli with characters which seemed to be intermediate between the avian and human types. From this one would suppose that the monkey is susceptible to infection with the avian bacillus.

On the other hand there is very strong experimental evidence which shows that the susceptibility of the monkey to infection of this kind is very slight. Thus Héricourt and Richet failed in two attempts to infect monkeys with avian tubercle bacilli.

---

[1] In each of the two gibbons infected by feeding with bacilli of human type there was a caseous nodule in one lung and a caseous bronchial gland on the same side; other lesions, in the liver and spleen, appeared to be more recent, and as already stated the intestines and mesenteric glands were free from tuberculous lesions. The authors considered that the pulmonary lesions were primary, and came to the conclusion that they must have been caused by bacilli aspirated into the lung along the air passages.

[2] In Macfadyen's experiments on the rhesus already referred to the effect on the intestine was just the opposite. See p. 512. In man the human type of bacillus seems to be more liable to cause intestinal ulceration than the bovine. (See Table of Origins, R.C.T. Int. Rep. App. vol. II, pp. 9 et seq.)

515

More recently Kraus and Grosz (1907) were unable to produce cutaneous tuberculosis in these animals by the application of avian bacilli to scarified areas of skin, though they succeeded in doing so by the similar use of bovine or human bacilli[1].

Very conclusive evidence on this point is afforded by the work of F. Griffith for the Royal Commission, which shows that monkeys, while they succumb to intravenous injection of avian tubercle bacilli, do not develop severe or progressive disease when subcutaneously inoculated or fed with them.

In these experiments nineteen young rhesus monkeys were injected or fed with avain tubercle bacilli in culture or tuberculous tissue[2].

Seven monkeys were injected intravenously with cultures in doses varying from 1 to 100 mg. One seems to have died prematurely, of cold. In one the inoculation was partly (or more probably wholely) subcutaneous. Five died of pulmonary disease in 18–34 days. The disease was acute, without lesions of a definitely tuberculous character. The lungs were congested and œdematous, the spleen swollen, and the liver and kidneys pale. Such results as these we have seen already more than once can be caused by intravenous injection of tubercle bacilli which are not really infective for the species of animal used (*e.g.* human type in calf, rabbit, etc.).

Two monkeys were injected subcutaneously with emulsions of tuberculous tissue containing fairly numerous bacilli. Both died after fifty-five and fifty-six days respectively. The cause of death is not explained. But it is stated that they showed only local tuberculosis, and in one case a single translucent tubercle in the lung.

Five were injected subcutaneously with culture (four in doses of 10 mg. and one with 1·0 mg.). Of these four were killed more than 100 days later when quite well. At the postmortem examinations two showed nothing but a small scar at the seat of inoculation; in one there were two tubercles in the

---

[1] See also Rabinowitsch, p. 651.

[2] *R.C.T. Fin. Rep.* App. vol. IV, pp. 188 and 250–251. In the above account the present writer has followed Griffith's table rather than his summary concerning one or two points of small importance where there seems to be some disagreement.

lungs, and in each of the other two there was a caseo-purulent nodule in the wall of the cæcum containing numerous bacilli. The fifth developed spontaneous mammalian tuberculosis and was killed when very ill[1].

Five monkeys were fed with culture in doses varying from 1 to 500 mg. They were all quite well when killed 112 to 151 days afterwards. At the post-mortem examinations no definite tuberculous lesions were seen. The bodies of three of these monkeys were perfectly normal. Two showed mesenteric glands containing one or two yellow purulent nodules. It is interesting to note that no tubercle bacilli could be seen on microscopic examination of these lesions, though cultures of avian tubercle bacilli were grown from them in both cases.

F. Griffith[2] also inoculated a chimpanzee with avian tubercle bacilli. The dose was 50 mg. of bacilli, injected under the skin of the back. The animal remained alive and well for nearly two years, but succumbed at last to an attack of diarrhœa. The post-mortem examination showed no trace of tuberculosis, and the only sign of the inoculation was a few scars in the skin of the back. Four rabbits inoculated with the culture at the same time as the chimpanzee developed tuberculosis, thus showing that the bacilli were living.

Summary.

Tuberculosis in monkeys which die in captivity is almost always due to the human type of tubercle bacillus. This is to be ascribed to the conditions of life under which the animals exist, and not to any greater susceptibility to infection with human than with bovine bacilli. Comparative experiments with comparable doses have shown no difference in this respect. Eleven animals injected subcutaneously with human bacilli

---

[1] Tuberculosis was general, but most severe in the lungs, while at the seat of inoculation was only a smooth walled cystic tumour, and in the neighbouring lymphatic glands only a single tubercle. From the lungs, bronchial glands, and spleen typical mammalian cultures were isolated, virulent for rabbits and guinea-pigs; while from the local lesion cultures of both avian and mammalian tubercle bacilli were obtained.

[2] *loc. cit.* p. 191.

succumbed after periods which averaged 39·9 days, while twelve similarly inoculated with bovine bacilli survived on the average almost 40 days. Other experiments, far more numerous, but less precisely adapted to resolving this question, have afforded confirmatory evidence.

As to the anthropoid ape, a considerable body of experimental evidence is available, considering the rarity and costliness of these animals, and the reluctance which one naturally feels for destroying creatures which attach themselves with such evident affection to their owners. These experiments show a remarkable equality of susceptibility to the two types of mammalian tubercle bacilli; an equality which, as we shall see, is not paralleled in the case of man.

While the two types of mammalian tubercle bacilli show equal virulence for monkeys in general the avian bacillus is in this respect distinctly inferior. While one or more cases of spontaneous disease have been attributed to this type, experiments have clearly shown that its virulence for the monkey is of a low order, and that it is unable to produce severe or progressive disease on subcutaneous injection or when taken into the stomach.

REFERENCES. XIV

(Chapter XXII)

Tuberculosis in the Dog and Cat.

Arloing (1903). *Compt. rendus de la Soc. de Biol.* p. 480.

Andrieu and Nocard (1885). Transmission de la Tuberculose de l'homme aux volailles et au chien. *Bullet. de la Soc. centrale de Méd. Vétérin.* p. 98.

Basset (1910). De la tuberculose des carnassiers domestiques. Chien et Chat. *Bullet. de la Soc. centrale de Méd. Vétérin.* vol. LXIV, p. 257.

Bernheim (1891). Tuberculose du chien. *Congrès pour l'étude de la tuberculose.* Paris, p. 650.

Bourgougnon (1888). A Case of Transmission of Tuberculosis from Man to the Dog. *Journ. de Méd. de Paris.* Abst. in *Journ. of Comp. Pathol. and Therap.* vol. I, p. 169.

Brusasco (1882). Tuberculosi miliare per contagione diretta dall' uomo ad una cagna. *Il medico veterinario*, p. 1. Quoted by Straus (*loc. cit.* p. 352).

Bull, L. B. (1914). Tuberculosis in Dogs. *Veterinary Journal*. London, vol. LXX, p. 34.

Cadiot, Gilbert and Roger (1891). Notes sur la tuberculose du chien. *Bullet. de la Soc. centrale de Méd. Vétérin.* vol. IX, pp. 108, 250, 587. *Compt. Rendus de la Soc. de Biol.* Jan. 1891, p. 20.

Cadiot (1892). Sur la tuberculose du chien. *Bullet. de la Soc. centrale de Méd. Vétérin.* vol. X.

—— (1894). Sur la tuberculose du cœur chez le chien. Tuberculose de l'encéphale. *Ibid.* vol. XII.

—— (1893). *La tuberculose du chien.* Paris.

Chantmesse et Le Dantec (1891). Tuberculose spontanée du chien. *Congrès pour l'étude de la Tuberculose.* Paris, p. 650.

Charmoy (1912). Tuberculose primitive de la face chez une Chatte. *Recueil de Méd. Vétérin.* vol. LXXXIX, p. 17.

Chaussé (1909). Expériences d'ingestion de matière tuberculeuse chez le chat. *Compt. Rendus de la Soc. de Biol.* 1909, p. 450.

—— (1910). La tuberculose mésentérique occulte réalisée expérimentalement chez le chien. *Recueil de Méd. Vétérin.* vol. LXXXVII.

Cobbett (1907). The Virulence of Tubercle Bacilli of Human Origin for the Dog. *R.C.T. Int. Rep.* App. vol. II, p. 1174.

—— (1907). The Virulence of Tubercle Bacilli of Human Origin for the Cat. *Ibid.* p. 1186.

Craig (1910). Tuberculosis in a Scotch Terrier. *Veterinary Journal.* November.

Czokor (1888). Tuberculose. *Oest. Zeitsch. f. Wissensch. Vet. Kunde.* vol. II, p. 48. Ref. in *Baumgarten's Jahresbericht,* 1888, p. 213.

Douville (1914). De la tuberculose des carnivores domestiques (chien et chat). *Rev. gén. de Méd. Vétérin.* vol. XXIII, pp. 473 and 537.

Eber (1893). Beitrag zur Kentniss der Tuberkulose bei Hund und Katze. *Deutsch. Zeitschf. f. Tiermedizin,* vol. XVII, p. 295.

—— (1904–5). Die Tuberkulose des Hundes und der Katze. *Ergebn. d. allgem. Pathologie u. pathol. Anatom. von Lubarsch u. Ostertag.*

Filleau and Petit (1888). A Case of Transmission of Pulmonary Tuberculosis from Man to the Cat. *Journ. de Méd. de Paris.* Jan. 1888. Transl. in *Journ. of Comp. Pathol. and Therap.* vol. I, p. 60.

Findel (1907). Vergleichende Untersuchungen über Inhalations- und Fütterungs-tuberkulose. *Zeitsch. f. Hyg. und Infect.* vol. LVII, p. 104.

Fröhner (1895). Statistische Mitteilungen über die Häufigkeit der wichtigsten innern Krankheiten beim Hund. *Monatshefte f. prakt. Tierheilkunde,* vol. VI.

Griffith, A. S. (1907). Inoculation Experiments on Dogs. *R.C.T. Int. Rep.* App. vol. I, p. 397. 1911. *Ibid. Fin. Rep.* vol. I, pp. 45 and 244–246.

—— (1907). Feeding Experiments on Dogs. *Ibid. Int. Rep.* vol. I, pp. 537, 542, 573–576, 592, 595, 616–618, 639, 696–702, 707.

Griffith, A. S. (1911). Feeding Experiments on Dogs. *Ibid. Fin. Rep.* App. vol. I, pp. 49 and 288.

—— (1907). Inoculation Experiments on Cats. *Ibid. Int. Rep.* App. vol. I, p. 422. 1911. *Ibid. Fin. Rep.* App. pp. 46 and 246–249.

—— (1907). Feeding Experiments on Cats. *Ibid. Int. Rep.* App. vol. I, pp. 537, 452, 577–581, 592, 595, 618–620, 639, 687–688 and 707. 1911. *Ibid. Fin. Rep.* App. pp. 268.

Griffith, F. (1911). Inoculation Experiments on Dogs with Cultures of Avian Tubercle Bacilli. *Ibid.* vol. IV, p. 191.

—— Infection Experiments on Cats with Avian Tubercle Bacilli. *Ibid.* p. 188.

—— Bovine tubercle bacilli cultivated from the mesenteric glands of a Cat infected with casual tuberculosis. *Ibid.* p. 151.

Guérin (1910). Un nouvel exemple de transmission de la tuberculose humaine chez le chien. *Bullet. de la Soc. centrale de Méd. Vétérin.* vol. LXIV, p. 277.

Héricourt and Richet (1890). De l'immunité conférée à des lapins par la transfusion péritonéale du sang de chien. *Études exp. et clin. sur la tuberculose.* Publiées sous la direction du professeur Verneuil. Vol. II, pp. 381 and 678. And 1892. *Ibid.* vol. III, p. 139.

Hess, A. F. (1908). A Case of Tuberculosis in a Cat. *Proc. New York Path. Soc.* N.S. vol. VIII, p. 104.

Hobday and Belcher (1908). Two Interesting Cases of Tuberculosis. *The Veterinary Journal.* Oct.

Jatta and Cosco (1905). *Ricerche speriment. sulla Tuberculosi dell' uomo e dei bovini.* Roma.

Jensen (1891). Tuberculose hos Hunden og Katten. *Maanedscrift for Dyrlaeger,* vol. III, p. 295. Ref. *Baumgarten's Jahresbericht.*

—— (1891). Tuberkulose beim Hund und bei der Katze. *Deutsch. Zeitschf. f. Tiermedizin,* vol. XVII, p. 295. Abst. in *Journ. of Comp. Pathol. and Therap.* vol. IV, p. 103.

Johne (1889). Ein Fall von Uebertragung der Tuberkulose vom Menschen auf den Hund etc. *Deutsch. Zeitschf. f. Tiermedizin,* vol. XV, p. iii.

De Jong (1902). *De eenheid der zoogdiertuberkulose.* Leyden.

Koch (1884). The Etiology of Tuberculosis. Transl. in *Microparasites in Disease.* New Sydenham Soc. For experimental transmission of tuberculosis to dogs and cats see pp. 176, 177 (dogs), 161–163, 176–178 (cats).

Leudet and Petit (1904). Résultats d'expériences d'inoculation de la tuberculose humaine au chien. Infection naturelle de ce dernier par les voies digestives. *Recueil de Méd. Vétérin.* vol. LXXXI, p. 298.

Link (1904). *Archiv f. klin. Med.* Heft 3.

McFadyean (1888). A Case of Spontaneous Tuberculosis in a Cat. *Journ. of Comp Pathol. and Therap.* vol. I, p. 156.

Malin (1839). Transmission de la phtisie aux animaux. *Gaz. Méd. de Paris*, p. 634. Quoted by Straus, *loc. cit.* p. 604, footnote.

Malm (1912). Ueber die sogennanten bovinen und humanen Typen des Tuberkelbazillus. *Centralb. f. Bakt. etc. Orig.* vol. XLV, p. 42.

Marcus (1888). Zur Prophylaxie der Tuberculose. *Deutsch. Med. Wochenschr.* p. 301.

Nocard (1888). A Case of Tuberculosis in a Cat. *Recueil de Méd. Vétérin.* Oct. 1889.

—— (1889). A Case of Tuberculosis in a Cat. *Ibid.* Feb. 1889. Abst. of these two papers in *Journ. of Comp. Pathol. and Therap.* vol. II, p. 1889.

—— (1891). Notes sur la tuberculose du chien et du chat. *Bullet. de la Soc. centrale de Méd. Vétérin.* vol. XLV, pp. 108, 250 and 589.

Peters, A. (1889). A Case of Tuberculosis in the Dog. *Journ. of Comp. Med. and Surg.* Ref. *Baumgarten's Jahresbericht*, vol. V, p. 313.

Petit (1901). Péricardite Tuberculeuse du chien. *Bullet. de la Soc. centrale de Méd. Vétérin.* vol. XIX, p. 264.

—— (1901). Tuberculose du Chien. *Ibid.* p. 457.

—— (1904). Tuberculose du Chien. *Recueil de Méd. Vétérin.* vol. LXXXI, p. 762.

—— (1905). Sur les rapports qui existent entre la tuberculose de l'homme et celle des carnivores domestiques (Chien et Chat). *Ibid.* vol. LXXXII, p. 713.

Petit and Basset (1900). Notes sur la tuberculose du Chien. *Recueil de Méd. Vétérin.* June and July.

—— (1901). The same continued. *Ibid.* Ser 8, vol. VIII, pp. 5, 85 and 163.

Römer (1909). Ueber Tuberkulose beim Hund. *Arbeit. a. d. pathol. Inst. z. Tübingen*, vol. VII, p. 50.

Schlesinger (1912). Miliary Tuberculosis in a dog with Ulcerative Endocarditis. *American Veterinary Review*, vol. XVI.

Schornagel (1914). *Untersuchungen über elf Fälle von Hundtuberculose.* Inaug. Diss. Beijers, Utrecht.

Schrum, E. (1910). *Ueber Hundtuberkulose.* Inaug. Diss. Bern. H. Gent & Co.

Siedamgrotsky (1871). Tuberculose beim Hund. *Sächs. Jahresbericht.*

Sticker (1910). Lymphosarcomatose und Tuberkulose beim Hunde. *Archiv f. wissensch. u. prakt. Tierheilkunde*, vol. XXXVII (suppl. vol.).

Stockman (1892). A Case of Tuberculosis n the Dog. *Journ. of Comp. Pathol. and Therap.* vol. V, p. 164.

Straus and Gamaléia (1891). *Compt. rend. du Congrès pour l'étude de la tuberculose chez l'homme et chez les animaux.*

Tappeiner (1897). Quoted by Titze and Weidanz, *loc. cit.* p. 81.

—— (1881). *Deutsch. Archiv f. klin. Med.* vol. XXIX.

Thomassen (1888). Sur la tuberculose animale en Hollande. *Compt. rend. du Congrès pour l'étude de la tuberculose chez l'homme et chez les animaux.*

Titze and Weidanz (1908). Infectionsversuche an Hunden mit Tuberkelbazillen des Typus bovinus und Tuberkelbazillen des Typus humanus. *Tub. Arbeit. a. d. Kaiserl. Gesundheitsamte,* Heft 9, p. 79.

Villemin (1868). *Études sur la Tuberculose.* Paris, p. 548.

Viseur (1874). Faits nouveaux de transmission de tuberculose par la voie digestive chez les animaux domestiques. *Bullet. de l'Acad. de Méd.* p. 890.

Weyl, Th. (1888). Spontane Tuberkulose beim Hunde. *Centralb. f. Bakteriol.* etc. vol. VI, p. 689.

Zugari (1889). On the Passage of Tubercle Virus through the Alimentary Canal of the Dog. Ref. *Baumgarten's Jahresbericht,* vol. V, p. 257.

Tuberculosis in Monkeys.

Baermann and Halberstaedter (1906). Experimentelle Hauttuberkulose bei Affen. *Berl. klin. Wochenschr.* No. 7.

Beck (1903). Beiträge über die Unterscheidung der Bazillen von menschlicher und tierlicher Tuberkulose, namentlich nach Infection verschiedener Tiere. *Festschrift f. Robert Koch,* p. 611. Fischer, Jena.

Cobbett (1907). *R.C.T. Int. Rep.* App. vol. II, p. 1164.

Dieulafoy and Krishalber (1883). De l'inoculation du tubercle sur le Singe. *Archiv. de physiologie norm. et pathol.* p. 24.

von Dungern and Smidt (1906). Ueber die Wirkung der Tuberkulosestämme des Menschens und des Rindes auf anthropoide Affen. *Arbeit. a. d. Kaiserl. Gesundheitsamte,* vol. XXIII, p. 570.

Gratia (1903). *XIth Internat. Cong. on Hyg. and Demog.* Brussels.

Griffith, A. S. (1907). *R.C.T. Int. Rep.* App. vol. I, pp. 49 and 52.

—— (1911). *Ibid. Fin. Rep.* App. vol. I, p. 43.

Griffith, F. (1911). *Ibid. Fin. Rep.* App. vol. IV, p. 167.

Grünbaum (1901). Die Uebertragbarkeit der Perlsucht auf Affen. *Verhandl. d. Tuberkulose-Kommission d. Gesellsch. Deutsch. Natürforscher u. Aertze.* Hamburg.

De Haan (1903). Experimentelle Tuberkulose bei Affen. *Virchows Archiv,* vol. CLXXIV, p. 1.

Héricourt and Richet (1891). De l'état réfractaire du singe à la tuberculose aviaire. *Compt. rendus de la Soc. de Biol.* p. 802.

Imlach (1884). Report on the Transmissibility of Bovine Tuberculosis through milk to young animals. *British Medical Journal.*

De Jong (1902). *La Semaine Médicale.*

Koch, R. (1882). Die Ätiologie der Tuberkulose. *Berlin. klin. Wochenschr.*

—— (1884). Über die Ätiologie der Tuberculose. *Mitteilungen aus dem Kaiserlichen Gesundheitsamte,* vol. II.

Koch, R. (1886). Translation of the above in *Microparasites in Disease*. New Sydenham Society. For tuberculosis of monkeys see p. 128.

Kraus and Grosz (1907). Ueber experimentelle Hauttuberkulose bei Affen. *Wiener klin. Wochenschr.* No. 26.

Macfadyen, A. (1903). Virulence of Bovine and Human Tuberculosis for Monkeys. *Lancet*, p. 745.

Nocard (1902). *Presse Vétérinaire.* Ap. May, Nov.

Rabinowitsch, L. (1906). Untersuchungen über die Beziehungen zwischen der Tuberkulose des Menschen und der Tiere. *Arbeit. a. d. Patholog. Inst. zu Berlin.* Hirschwald, Berlin.

—— (1907). Ueber spontane Affentuberkulose. *Deutsch. med. Wochenschr.* p. 866 and *Virchows Archiv*, vol. cxc, Beiheft, p. 196.

Ravenel (1902). The Intercommunicability of Human and Bovine Tuberculosis. *Univ. of Pennsylvania Medical Bulletin.*

De Schweinitz, Dorset and Schroeder (1902). Virulence of Bovine Tuberculosis for Monkeys. *International Tuberculosis Conference, II.* Berlin, p. 366. Experiments concerning Tuberculosis, Pt. II, p. 66.

—— (1905). Experiments on Monkeys. *U.S. Dept. of Agriculture, Bureau of Animal Industry.* Bulletin No. 52.

Straus (1895). *La Tuberculose et son bacille.* Paris.

CHAPTER XXIII

THE SUSCEPTIBILITY TO TUBERCULOSIS OF VARIOUS ANIMAL SPECIES (*continued*)

Tuberculosis in Birds.

Before the discovery of the tubercle bacillus the very existence of tuberculosis in birds was in doubt. "Rien n'est plus problématique que l'existence de la tuberculose chez les oiseaux[1]" wrote Villemin in 1868, and nine years later Zundel still regarded it as questionable. The caseo-necrotic lesions which are now known to be caused by tubercle bacilli were in those days variously ascribed to animal parasites (Villemin), or to moulds which had entered the air sacs, and were called lympho-sarcoma (Roloff), tuberculo-diphtérie (Léniez), or by the noncommittal term scleroma. Paulicki, indeed, (1872) and Arloing and Tripier (1873), called attention to the similarity of the caseo-necrotic lesions in birds to those

[1] *Études sur la tuberculose*, p. 524.

of tuberculosis in mammals; but it was not until the discovery of tubercle bacilli in such lesions by Koch that the doubt was finally cleared up.

Tuberculosis is now known to be very widely distributed among many species of birds kept in captivity in zoölogical gardens, or under conditions of domestication. The common fowl is the principal sufferer, but other birds living with it do not escape. Turkeys, guinea-fowls, peacocks and pheasants (hand reared) are often found to be infected; and geese and ducks, though less susceptible, do not altogether escape. The caged parrot not unfrequently is attacked by tuberculosis, and a few instances of the disease have been recorded in the canary.

Bland-Sutton and Gibbes (1884) examined the birds which died in the Zoölogical Gardens in Regent's Park and found many tuberculous. According to these authors the birds most liable to tuberculosis when living in captivity are the common fowl, peacock, guinea-fowl, tragopan, grouse, pigeon and partridge. The rhea, too, they say, is particularly susceptible to tuberculosis. Sibley (1888), who afterwards examined the birds dying in these gardens, added to the list the canary, corn-crake, finch, goose, guan, swan, owl and vulture. Shattock, Seligmann, Dudgeon and Panton (1907), who obtained their material from the same source, mention among others the cormorant, gannet, several Indian ducks and many other foreign birds.

M. Koch and L. Rabinowitsch (1907), who investigated the mortality among birds in the zoölogical gardens in Berlin, saw no less than 118 tuberculous out of a total of 459 birds of various kinds which died there. They found one or more instances of tuberculosis in 10 out of 15 different orders of birds, and since of the remaining 5 orders only a very few examples or none at all were available for examination, they suggested that in all probability every kind of bird is liable to tuberculosis.

Bland-Sutton and Gibbes thought that tuberculosis affects almost exclusively the birds which feed on grain, and spares the flesh-eaters, and the waders and other water-fowl which live

principally on fish. But Sibley disputed this, and indeed
Bland-Sutton and Gibbes themselves found two instances
of tuberculosis in birds of prey, namely in a falcon and an
eagle. M. Koch and Rabinowitsch also have found tuberculosis
in birds of this class. In fact they place these birds high in the
order of susceptibility which they give as follows: fowls, birds
of prey, marsh-fowl, domestic water-fowl, pigeons, sparrows.

Of considerable interest is the statement that ducks and geese,
though often living in close contact with fowls, very commonly
escape tuberculous infection. The truth of this, apparently,
cannot be doubted. Poulterers whom the writer has questioned
on the subject, though freely admitting that they frequently
see tuberculosis in fowls, turkeys and pheasants, do not seem
to have met with the disease in geese and ducks.

In this connection the following experience related by Straus[1] is so interesting that one cannot resist the temptation to quote it:

A certain Dr Pomay, senior physician to the Orphanage Hériot at Boissière,
had the opportunity of observing a severe epidemic of tuberculosis which
for several years affected certain of the birds at a farm where they kept about
six hundred fowls and chickens. Straus himself on several occasions examined
fowls which Pomay brought to his laboratory, and was able to satisfy himself
that they really were suffering from tuberculosis. Now together with the
fowls lived turkeys, ducks and geese, eating the same food, drinking the
same water, and sleeping in the same sheds. Of the turkeys, 92 in all, 80
died of tuberculosis; but of the ducks and geese not one fell ill, and though
many were killed for food no tuberculous lesions were noticed in any of them.

Though these birds commonly escape tuberculosis when
living under the ordinary conditions of domestication they
nevertheless, as we have seen, contract tuberculosis in zoölogical
gardens. They therefore do not enjoy a complete constitutional
immunity, and it would be interesting to know why they escape
under ordinary conditions.

Although tuberculosis is common among domesticated
birds, ducks and geese excepted, and probably attacks every
avian species living in zoölogical gardens, yet among wild
birds it seems to be extremely rare. Very few instances are
on record. Shattock, Seligmann, Dudgeon and Panton
described a case in a lapwing which was captured in a moribund
state in Scotland, and of which the specimen is now in the

[1] *loc. cit.* p. 397.

College of Surgeons[1]; Hammond Smith recorded a case in a kestrel[2], and quite recently a partridge sent to the Cambridge laboratory by a poulterer was found to be suffering from tuberculosis. The lesions in this case were very like those seen in the domestic fowl[3].

Tuberculous lesions were found in a sparrow by A. S. and F. Griffith. The bird was shot for examination when observed feeding on a heap of refuse thrown out from a yard where some fowls which had been experimentally infected with the disease were kept. From this sparrow a strain of tubercle bacilli was isolated which proved, on investigation of its cultural characters and comparative virulence, to be of the avian type[4].

On the other hand some wild pigeons shot by Sibley when feeding in infected poultry yards, or in the Zoölogical Gardens, as well as others obtained by Shattock and his collaborators under similar circumstances, were free from tuberculosis. But the number of these observations is too few to lend much weight to a negative conclusion. More convincing is the almost universal testimony of game keepers and sportsmen. E. A. Wilson, while he was working for the Grouse Commission, examined about 2000 of these birds picked up dead on the moors of Scotland, Cumberland and Wales without coming across any instance of tuberculosis.

Tuberculosis then is rare in the wild bird. It is common under the conditions of domestication and captivity. One might be tempted to apply to avian tuberculosis Dr Philip's aphorism concerning tuberculosis in man; namely that it is "a vicious by-product of an incomplete and ill-formed civilization[5]."

But the real significance of the fact that tuberculosis is common in civilized man and in domesticated and captive

---

[1] These authors give a plate illustrating this case on p. 8 of their paper.

[2] *The Field*, April 18, 1908.

[3] Unfortunately the bird arrived when the writer, to whom it was sent, was absent and on his return it was too late to raise a culture of tubercle bacilli.

[4] Privately communicated.

[5] Dr R. W. Philip. Addresses to the International Congress at Rome, 1902, *Brit. Med. Journ.* p. 873.

Plate XVII

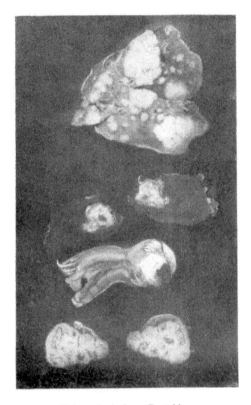

Tuberculosis in a Partridge.

Natural infection.

Liver, lungs, Peyer's patches in caeca close to their openings and spleen.

animals, while it spares the primitive savage and the birds
and beasts which live a wild free life, is often misunderstood.
Civilization is spoken of as though, by some mysterious softening
influence, it increases the susceptibility to tuberculous infection
by undermining the stamina of the race. Probably selective
breeding for special qualities among certain animals has done
this to some extent, as for example the production of varieties
of poultry which lay an unnaturally large number of eggs,
or of cattle whose cows yield an excessive quantity of milk.
But the simple truth, as far as poultry at least is concerned,
is that the disease is caused by overcrowding. The birds
are forced to feed off ground which is grossly contaminated
with their own droppings. If, then, a bird infected with tuberculosis is introduced among them, it is small wonder that the
disease spreads to the others; for tuberculosis in the fowl is,
as we shall see, mainly an abdominal and intestinal disease,
and tubercle bacilli have been proved to pass out with their
dejecta.

The case of the sparrow mentioned above shows that the
wild bird has no superior powers of resistance. It commonly
escapes tuberculosis because its food is cleaner, and if tuberculosis should happen to occur among its tribe it has little
tendency to spread because there is little chance of the tubercle
bacilli contaminating the food of the birds as long as they
are free.

The Character and Distribution of the Lesions. In the
common fowl, and in most of the birds when affected with
spontaneous tuberculosis, the lesions are large, and conspicuous
by advanced caseation[1]. Liver and spleen are, as a rule, the
organs most severely attacked; lungs are affected less often
and to a much smaller extent; kidneys, though not entirely

[1] On this point Sibley made the following interesting observations: "It would
seem that the tissues of the avian tribe offer a soil in which tubercle develops
to a much more extensive degree than in the human subject, and that the
life-energy of the bird is greater, withstanding a more prolonged strain upon its
molecular constitution before the dissolution of the individual....Not only is
caseation very extensive, but there is frequently considerable tissue formation
previous to complete degeneration, so the nodules were large compared to the
size of the animals: in fact the disease closely approached a neoplasm in its
nature." *Trans. Path. Soc. Lond.* vol. XXXIX, p. 471.

exempt, are seldom diseased. Bones on the other hand frequently take their share of the lesions.

In the liver the lesions vary in size from small miliary foci to nodules as large as a pea, a small cherry, or even a walnut—Koch declared one, in the liver of a fowl, to be as big as a small apple. They project as rounded masses from the surface of the organ. The larger ones are irregular in outline, and nodular, as though they grew by addition of small tubercles to the periphery. M. Koch and Rabinowitsch say that some of the masses may show concentric lamination. The lesions in the spleen are like those in the liver.

The tuberculous nodules are whitish in colour, or stained yellowish or greenish by bile. Caseation is a marked character, but softening is rare. Calcification seldom occurs, and probably never to anything like the extent often seen in old tuberculous lesions in man or the ox.

All writers have remarked on the hardness of the caseo-necrotic material found in birds. French authors speak of this substance as "masse vitreuse." And, while others compare it to boiled potato, Koch and Rabinowitsch say that this suggests something far too soft to be compared with what is sometimes more like cartilage. To the present writer (if a comparison is necessary) it seems more like old and rather dry putty—a simile which at least has the advantage of avoiding the unpleasantness of comparing pathological products with articles of diet.

Many authors have remarked that the tuberculous nodules shell out very cleanly from the surrounding tissue—"like a kernel from a nut," as Weber puts it. This is undoubtedly the case; but it probably has more to do with the normal structure of birds' organs than with any peculiarity of their pathological products. For it seems that these organs are extremely soft, needing far less supporting, or connective, tissue than do those of mammals, and especially those of carnivora whose bodies have to be constructed so as to be able to stand considerable violence[1]. The reason of this

---

[1] The cat undoubtedly owes its proverbial nine lives to the toughness of its viscera, as any experimental pathologist can testify who has endeavoured to pound up its organs.

Plate XVIII

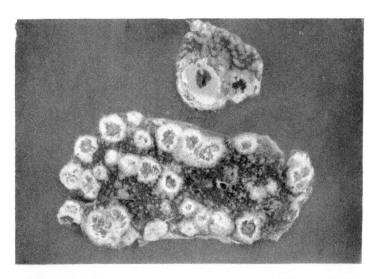

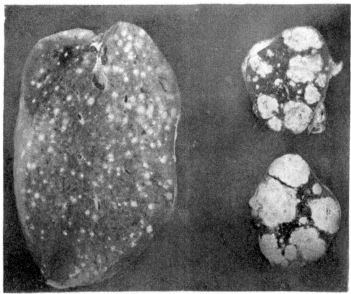

Tuberculosis of Liver and Spleen of two Fowls.

Natural disease.

XXIII]
SUSCEPTIBILITY OF VARIOUS ORGANS
531

no doubt is that the organs of birds, owing to the great development of the bony thorax, enjoy an altogether exceptional degree of external protection.

The lungs are much less liable to tuberculous disease than the liver or spleen. Weber and Bofinger, speaking of the common fowl, say that, as a rule, these organs are free from disease. For his part the writer is inclined to think that they are affected to some extent oftener than is generally supposed. He has seen pulmonary tubercles several times in a limited number of cases which have come before him, and in one of them the lungs were the seat of the *principal* disease. F. Griffith found the lungs affected in six out of seven birds, including both of two fowls, and two out of three pheasants examined by him. Turning now to birds of various species kept in zoölogical gardens Koch and Rabinowitsch found the lungs affected in 78 out of 120 tuberculous birds—that is in 65 per cent. In twelve of these the lungs were the only parts affected; namely in four birds of prey, two geese, a pigeon, a canary and various foreign birds. Cavities have not been observed in the lungs of birds.

Liver and spleen are, as we have said, the organs most severely affected when tuberculosis attacks birds. Sibley found that the spleen was more often affected than the liver. Weber and Bofinger, on the other hand saw the liver more often involved than the spleen. The truth is both organs are usually attacked together. Koch and Rabinowitsch found both organs affected in 85 out of 118 tuberculous birds of all sorts. The liver was affected in 101, and the spleen in 88. In 16 the liver was tuberculous without the spleen being affected, and in three the spleen was tuberculous without the liver being involved.

The kidneys are seldom tuberculous in the birds of the farmyard. Koch and Rabinowitsch found them tuberculous in ten of their cases from zoölogical gardens. F. Griffith mentions a minute grey tubercle in one kidney of a tuberculous fowl examined by him; and the present writer has seen a good many small tubercles in the kidneys of a fowl with severe and widely generalized tuberculosis elsewhere. The tubercles were in the substance as well as on the surface of the organ, and being of an ivory white colour they showed up very clearly on the dark red tissue.

Tubercles in the heart wall were twice observed by Koch and Rabinowitsch, and have been seen by the present writer, namely in the fowl just mentioned.

In one case Koch and Rabinowitsch found the testes affected, and in five they saw the ovaries tuberculous.

Tuberculosis of brain and spinal cord they never came across.

The skin is rarely affected in birds, if we except the parrot tribe, but lesions may sometimes occur about the head and on the feet.

The alimentary canal is very commonly the seat of disease in the tuberculous common fowl. Koch and Rabinowitsch found tuberculous lesions there in 71 per cent. of the tuberculous birds of this family which they examined; and it is probably even commoner in the fowls of the farm-yard. Among other orders of birds it is less common, as the table already quoted from these authors shows.

Sibley states that any part of the alimentary canal from mouth to cloaca, not excepting the crop, œsophagus and gizzard, may be the seat of tuberculous changes; but the seat of election is the neighbourhood of the cæcal openings, and especially the lymphoid follicles which are situated in the cæca close to these openings[1].

The lesions commonly take the form of nodules which project towards the peritoneal surface, and appear to arise in the outer part of the wall of the gut. These nodules vary in size. Commonly they are of the dimensions of a shot or a small pea, but larger nodules may often be seen, and some as large as a walnut or a pigeon's egg have been described. Arloing found one which weighed 600 grammes attached to the intestine of a fowl.

The mode of origin of these nodules has been disputed. Shattock, Seligmann, Dudgeon and Panton, F. Griffith, and

[1] See wood-cut in Sibley's first paper, *Trans. Path. Soc. Lond.* 1888, vol. XXXIX, p. 467.

Weber and Bofinger have all found the earliest lesions seen in feeding experiments in the mucous membrane of the villi. The authors last named think that the lesions begin in small ulcers in the mucous membrane, and spread outwardly while the ulcers themselves may heal and leave only little scars to mark their site. But Koch and Rabinowitsch dispute this and hold that the nodules commence in aggregations of lymphoid tissue which lie in the outer part of the intestinal wall. The bacilli, according to their view, pass through the intact mucous membrane, and set up primary lesions in these foci, just as in mammals tuberculosis may be primary in mesenteric glands. At a later period the nodules may ulcerate through the mucous membrane, and indeed in advanced cases usually do so[1].

Lymphatic glands, as we know them in other animals, are little if at all developed in birds. Owen, 1886, said the lymphatic glands in birds are few. Bland-Sutton wrote to the author: "There are no lymphatic glands in birds." In Bronn's *Thierreich* H. Gadow states that in birds there are no lymphatic glands in the mesentery, and none in the inguinal region or axilla, indeed subcutaneous lymph glands do not exist except a few in the upper part of the breast and, sometimes, on the wing. On the other hand lymph follicles are numerous in the intestine[2]. Ellenberger and Baum make a very similar statement[3]. Koch and Rabinowitsch could find no bronchial glands with certainty, and the writer has never been able to detect any mesenteric glands, even in birds with intestinal tuberculosis, in which, if in any, they should be apparent. In the mesentery, however, along the vessels little tuberculous nodules are not at all uncommon. Sibley mentions them and says they are always to be seen when the intestine itself is involved. A good photograph of them may be seen in V. Moore's paper[4]. Possibly these arise in little collections of lymphoid tissue.

---

[1] This seems to have been the opinion of Sibley also. *loc. cit.* p. 464.
[2] *Die Klassen des Thierreichs*, 1891, vol. VI, Vögel, p. 814.
[3] *Comp. Anat. and Physiol. of Vertebrates*, 1886, vol. II, p. 180.
[4] *Journ. of Med. Research*, vol. IX, p. 536.

In the neck of the fowl two little chains of glandular bodies may be seen running from the head to the thoracic opening. They are loosely attached to the deeper surface of the skin and have no definite relation to the great vessels. These bodies are said by Shattock, Seligmann, Dudgeon and Panton to be thymus glands. They not unfrequently are the seat of tubercular disease. Tuberculosis has several times been observed in them by the writer, and A. S. Griffith tells him that he has often seen them involved. Tuberculous nodules in the necks of birds, doubtless situated in these glands, are mentioned by Bland-Sutton and Gibbes, by Sibley, and also by Koch and Rabinowitsch. An excellent photograph of tuberculous lesions in these structures in the case of a Roller is given by Shattock and his collaborators[1].

Tuberculosis of bone-marrow appears to be rather common among domestic fowls, though Koch and Rabinowitsch do not seem to have seen it often among the various species of birds in the Berlin gardens. Sibley drew particular attention to it, and he described a case of tuberculosis in a peacock in which " several tumours of a caseous nature, many as large as walnuts, were found in various parts of the body. These were nearly all attached to the fibrous tissue surrounding bones such as the inferior angle of the scapula, one perforating the vertical plate of the sternum, another on the inner surface of the ribs. The right knee-joint was beset with large masses, one the size of a walnut being attached to the surface of the patella[2]." He also mentions caries of the vertebræ in two other cases, in one of which there was a large abscess containing two ounces of fluid. In another there was disease of the hip joint chiefly confined to the acetabulum, the floor of which was replaced by fungating masses of granulation tissue projecting into the interior of the pelvis.

In a fowl seen by the present writer the bone-marrow throughout the skeleton was largely transformed into caseous masses, very similar to those found in the livers and spleens of tuberculous birds. The disease had become so advanced

[1] *Proc. Roy. Soc. of Medicine,* 1907–8, vol. I, Path. Section, p. 19.
[2] *Trans. Path. Soc. Lond.* 1890, vol. XLI, p. 335.

in one femur that it had led to spontaneous fracture. But so much tuberculous callus had formed around the broken ends of the bone that the condition had passed without being detected during life. The bird was killed because it was obviously ill, and the fracture was then found to be of some standing, for the broken ends were quite rounded. Tuberculous disease was extensive in liver and spleen, and it was in this case that the heart and kidneys were affected.

F. Griffith has recorded bone tuberculosis in fowls artificially infected.

All observers from Robert Koch onwards have remarked on the great number of tubercle bacilli found in the lesions of birds, and on the fact that they are very largely contained within cells.

The Parrot Tribe. The first to recognize tuberculosis in parrots were Fröhner and Eberlein. Fröhner (1895) found that out of 700 parrots treated for various complaints at the Veterinary School in Berlin 170 (or 25 per cent.) were tuberculous.

In zoölogical gardens on the other hand, according to Shattock, Seligmann, Dudgeon and Panton, tuberculosis is relatively uncommon in the parrot tribe, and M. Koch and Rabinowitsch found only two instances of tuberculosis among the 39 birds of this kind which died in the Berlin gardens and were examined by them. We see then that tuberculosis is common in the parrot chiefly when kept as a pet and brought into intimate contact with human beings.

The disease as seen in parrots is unlike that which occurs in the common fowl, and indeed in most other birds. According to Cadiot, Gilbert and Roger, it occurs most commonly in the skin of the head, attacking such parts as the eye-lids, the nasal orifices, the root of the beak, the tongue or the floor of the mouth. Warty or horny outgrowths appear on the affected parts. The internal organs may be free from tuberculosis, but when these are affected it is the lungs, rather than the abdominal organs, which suffer most. This at least is the type of disease commonly seen in the pet parrot. In the few parrots which have died of tuberculosis in zoölogical gardens and have been examined the disease has been of the abdominal type, as in most other birds[1].

The lesions of the skin which have just been described are in all probability primary; and are attributed to infection of small scratches or abrasions caused by rubbing the beak violently on the perch or bars of the cage in order to cleanse it from particles of food, or, as Koch and Rabinowitsch suggest, to get rid of lice from a portion of the body which cannot be reached in the usual way.

The Tubercle Bacilli found in Avian Tuberculosis

The earlier investigations of the bacilli found in tuberculous birds were made chiefly on the fowl and the pheasant, and from them it soon became evident that the tubercle bacillus concerned was of a special kind, and differed in important particulars from those found in man and other mammals. As this bacillus was found in other birds also it was natural to regard it as the one cause of tuberculosis in the avian kingdom, and to call it the avian tubercle bacillus. But the name is not strictly logical for, since Cadiot, Gilbert and Roger, in 1894, found in some tuberculous parrots tubercle bacilli which were virulent for guinea-pigs but which failed to infect rabbits and fowls, it has been clear that this bird at least may be infected with a tubercle bacillus which is different from that found in the common fowl, and is like that seen in certain mammals—a bacillus which is now recognized as the human tubercle bacillus. This bacillus has been found recently by M. Koch and Rabinowitsch in some other birds also; so it can no longer be said that all birds when tuberculous are infected by the same kind of bacillus. Nor is the bacillus which infects the great majority of them confined entirely to birds, for it has been found occasionally in rabbits and mice. The title avian tubercle bacillus then obviously is not strictly appropriate; and it has been proposed to call the bacillus which is found in nearly but not quite all tuberculous birds, and is the only

---

[1] Koch and Rabinowitsch's two instances will be found on p. 436 of their paper already quoted.

one which attacks the common fowl (*Gallus domesticus*),
B. tuberculosis typus gallinaceus; and the Germans commonly
speak of it as the Hühnertuberkelbazillus.

But after all it is quite exceptional for any bird to be
infected with any other type of tubercle bacillus than this;
and it is equally rare for this bacillus to infect any creature
which is not a bird. Therefore the title avian tubercle bacillus
is quite as appropriate as those which are generally accepted
for the other types; for tuberculosis in man is not invariably
caused by the human type of tubercle bacillus, and the human
type of bacillus may infect other animals besides man, namely
monkeys and guinea-pigs. The bovine type of bacillus too
is by no means confined to the ox, but is the bacillus which
is responsible for nearly all the tuberculosis in mammals,
man and monkey excepted, and, as we shall see, may infect
the parrot, at least, among birds. The title avian tubercle
bacillus then is no worse than its neighbours, human tubercle
bacillus and bovine tubercle bacillus, which are too firmly
established to be displaced. It is too convenient to be given
up lightly, and it is probably by this time as firmly rooted
as the others. It seems likely then that, in spite of their
defects, all three titles will stand together, and continue to
be used.

Of the many instances of tuberculosis in birds which have
been investigated bacteriologically an overwhelming majority
have yielded tubercle bacilli of the avian type. M. Koch
and Rabinowitsch isolated 95 strains of tubercle bacilli from
70 birds of various kinds. The majority of these strains clearly
belonged to the avian type; but many were held to be more
or less atypical. These authors, as we have pointed out before,
do not see so sharp a distinction between the three types of
tubercle bacilli as do most other authorities, and are inclined
to recognize transitional strains. From their strains of avian
origin they selected 35 for closer investigation because they
showed some peculiarity. Five of them were found to belong to
the human type. These came from three birds, already referred
to, namely from two African eagles and a species of jay. Two
more strains had the cultural characters of human tubercle

bacilli, and many others were, as we have said, thought to show more or less deviation from the avian type[1].

F. Griffith examined a few birds which died of tuberculosis in the Zoölogical Gardens, London. Strains of tubercle bacilli were obtained from nine of them, namely from three fowls, three pheasants, a pigeon, a demoiselle crane and a Senegal touracou. All these strains proved to be typically avian in type.

In the tuberculous parrot, as we have said, the human type of bacillus has been found repeatedly since Cadiot, Gilbert and Roger first discovered in these birds a tubercle bacillus incapable of infecting fowls and rabbits. Straus, Mursajeff, Delbanco and Hutyra and Marck have all shown that parrot tuberculosis can be transmitted to the guinea-pig—that is to say that the bacillus concerned is not of the usual avian kind.

Experiment has shown that the parrot is susceptible of artificial infection with all three types of tubercle bacilli[2]. The question of the relative virulence of the types for this family of birds was investigated by F. Griffith, who concluded from his experiments that the bovine is the most virulent of the three. Weber, Titze and Weidanz also examined the point and came to the same conclusion, adding that the avian type proved to be the least virulent.

But the difference in virulence for these birds of the various types of tubercle bacilli is probably small; and the reason why it is the human type of bacillus rather than one of the others which is commonly the cause of tuberculosis in the parrot is to be sought, not in the comparative virulence of the three types of bacilli, but in the conditions of life of the birds, which make it exceedingly unlikely that they should come in contact with avian or bovine tubercle bacilli, and at the same time not unfrequently expose them to infection from human sources. In this connection it is interesting to observe that the only two tuberculous parrots which Koch and Rabinowitsch received from the Berlin Zoölogical Gardens (where, it is needless to say, the conditions of life are different

[1] *loc. cit.* p. 465.
[2] A. S. Griffith was able to infect the parrot with human bacilli.

from those of the ordinary pet parrot) were infected by the avian type of bacillus[1].

Canaries have occasionally been found to suffer from spontaneous tuberculosis. And as these birds are often kept as pets within our houses the question has naturally arisen whether they too, like the parrot, are liable to be infected with the human type of tubercle bacillus. So far as the writer is aware there is no clear case on record, though, as we shall see from experimental evidence, canaries are probably susceptible to infection with this type of bacillus.

Max Wolff in 1904 reported a case of tuberculosis in a canary whose cage was regularly cleaned out by a servant who suffered from phthisis, and from whom, it was naturally suspected, the bird might have caught the disease. Inoculation of guinea-pigs, however, with the infected organs failed to produce tuberculosis. In order to test the susceptibility of canaries to human tuberculosis, Wolff kept a number of them in his surgery which was frequented by many tuberculous patients, but none of the birds contracted the disease.

Attempts to inoculate these birds experimentally with human tubercle bacilli have succeeded, but not invariably. Gärtner successfully infected canaries with these bacilli. Koch and Rabinowitsch fed four canaries, two with human and two with avian tubercle bacilli. The experiments showed that the birds were susceptible to infection with either type, but the lesions produced by the avian bacilli were more severe than those caused by the human.

Weber, Titze and Weidanz (1908) fed eleven canaries, some once, others twice, with human tubercle bacilli, but without result. On the other hand, of two canaries which they fed with avian bacilli one developed severe tuberculosis; the other died of some intercurrent disorder twenty-five days after the experimental feeding, with no tuberculous lesions but with tubercle bacilli in the liver. In another experiment eleven canaries were fed with bovine tubercle bacilli and contracted tuberculosis, but others fed at the same time with avian bacilli suffered from a more severe type of disease, and the authors

[1] *loc. cit.* p. 436.

concluded that these birds are more susceptible to infection with avian than with mammalian tubercle bacilli.

The only spontaneously tuberculous canary examined by Koch and Rabinowitsch was found to be infected with the avian type of bacillus[1].

Experiments with other birds have given uncertain results. Koch and Rabinowitsch, who, as we have seen, found tubercle bacilli of human type in three birds of prey, attempted to infect young hawks by feeding them with bacilli of this kind; but the results were negative. Weber, Titze and Weidanz were equally unsuccessful with six starlings which they attempted to infect, some with human, others with bovine, and others again with avian tubercle bacilli. On the other hand a finch which they fed with avian bacilli died of tuberculosis. Sixteen sparrows, fed on a single occasion with bovine tubercle bacilli, were killed five months later and found to be free from tuberculosis. A case of spontaneous tuberculosis (avian) in a sparrow has already been referred to.

Now while some birds, notably those belonging to the parrot family, and probably also the canary and certain birds of prey are susceptible to the attack of mammalian tubercle bacilli it is quite certain that the common fowl and the pigeon are not. Innumerable attempts have been made to infect these birds by feeding them on sputum, or by inoculating them with human or bovine tuberculous material. A few apparently positive results have been obtained now and again, as for example by Nocard, and by Cadiot, Gilbert and Roger. These results are in sharp contrast to those of the majority of such experiments, and especially of the more recent ones. They are probably explicable on the assumption that the results of spontaneous infection with avian bacilli were mistaken for those of artificial infection with mammalian bacilli—a mistake very easy to make in the earlier days of such investigation.

Among those who were unable to infect the fowl or pigeon with mammalian tubercle bacilli Weber and Bofinger mention Villemin, Martin, Palamidessi, Rivolta, Maffucci, Straus and

[1] loc. cit. p. 444.

Gamaléia, Gärtner, and Auclair, Lannelongue, and Achard; and to these may be added Weber and Bofinger themselves, Shattock, Seligmann, Dudgeon and Panton, V. Moore, Koch and Rabinowitsch and the Royal Commission. Nocard himself also in certain extensive feeding experiments with sputum obtained only negative results.

Inoculation experiments performed for the Royal Commission with pure cultures of tubercle bacilli of human and bovine type have shown that even large doses produce in the fowl no lesion whatever, or at the best the most minimal of local changes around the bacilli· injected. An exception to this rule must be made in the case of intravenous injection, for A. S. Griffith[1] found that 50 milligrammes of mammalian tubercle bacilli thus injected will often cause fowls to succumb; not indeed from an anatomical tuberculosis, but with signs of anæmia and emaciation, and with tubercle bacilli scattered widely throughout the body. This effect, however, is attributable, not to a true infection, but to the effect of toxins in the bacilli injected; for Griffith has found that similar effects may be produced if the bacilli injected have previously been killed by exposure to steam at 100° C. It is presumed the toxins act locally, and that the reason why intravenous injection of mammalian bacilli is followed by serious consequences, while the subcutaneous or intraperitoneal injection of these organisms is not, is because by its means the bacilli and their toxins are distributed to situations, namely the lungs, where the local action of the latter is dangerous to life.

While the fowl is so highly resistant to experimental infection with tubercle bacilli of either of the mammalian types it is easily infected with those of avian type. Feeding experiments, it is true occasionally fail, but intravenous, intraperitoneal or subcutaneous injection produces, according to A. S. Griffith, invariably, general tuberculosis which would ultimately prove fatal, even when so small a dose as a ten-millionth part of a milligramme of culture is used.

With the pigeon it is much the same as with the fowl, though the evidence is less extensive. Shattock, Seligmann,

---

[1] *R.C.T. Final Report*, App. vol. I, p. 47.

Dudgeon and· Panton succeeded in infecting pigeons with avian tubercle bacilli, but they failed to infect them by feeding with sputum. This was not because the sputum bacilli failed to penetrate, for they were demonstrated in apparently unaltered spleens by the injection of the emulsified organs into guinea-pigs. This was the case even so long as eight weeks after injection. Thus they showed that human tubercle bacilli are able to remain alive for considerable periods in the tissues of birds which they are unable seriously to harm, a fact which had been pointed out previously by Gärtner who showed that these bacilli might remain alive in the body of the hen for as much as three months.

How do Birds become infected with Tuberculosis; and through what Portals of Entry?

The possibility that avian tuberculosis may be hereditary has attracted a good deal of attention. And with it is connected the important practical question whether tuberculosis can be introduced into a healthy stock of poultry by the importation of brood eggs from infected stocks. The question of hereditary transmission of tuberculosis in general has been discussed in an earlier chapter and its relation to birds in particular was there considered[1]. It will be sufficient therefore to deal with the question very briefly here. Hereditary transmission was accepted by Sibley. Tubercle bacilli have actually been seen in the egg by Gärtner, F. Griffith and Koch and Rabinowitsch. But this does not mean that hereditary transmission is the rule, or even a common mode of propagation of the disease. The authors last mentioned believe that the possibility of hereditary transmission of tuberculosis has been demonstrated, but what part it plays in nature, they say, they do not venture to estimate. Among the birds of the Zoölogical Gardens, which provided the material for their investigation, they were of opinion that "it played as good as none." Weber and Bofinger take a similar view.

Infection by inhalation is thought by Koch and Rabinowitsch to occur in a limited number of cases; but the rarity of important lesions in the lungs of domestic fowls

[1] p. 120.

would suggest that this manner of infection plays a very secondary part in this family. In parrots on the other hand pulmonary tuberculosis is often primary, and infection through the air passages is probably in this species the rule.

Infection through the skin of the head occurs, especially in the parrot, and to some extent in farm-yard fowls also. In the former it is undoubtedly caused by their habit of rubbing their beaks on their perches.

Nearly all writers on the subject believe that infection through food is the common means by which tuberculous disease is spread among poultry. In support of this view it may be urged that (a) intestinal lesions are commonly present in tuberculous fowls, while liver and spleen, and not lungs, are the organs which principally suffer, (b) that fowls may be easily infected experimentally by feeding, and (c) that a ready means of contamination of food with tubercle bacilli is provided by the bacilli which tuberculous fowls pass out with their droppings. About this last point there can be no doubt. It was proved by Mohler and Washburn, and has been confirmed by Weber and Bofinger and by others. It cannot be doubted, as we have said before, that in the great majority of cases tuberculosis is spread among fowls by their being fed on ground grossly contaminated in this way.

But the introduction of tuberculous infection into a healthy stock is not likely to occur in this way, for when it is desired to introduce new blood, as is frequently the case, eggs and not birds are usually purchased. It is here that the possibility of hereditary transmission assumes some practical significance. We do not know as yet precisely how much importance to attribute to this mode of transmission, but while we do not think it is great, we cannot deny the possibility of its existence.

But it has recently been suggested that there is another way in which tuberculous infection may be carried from one poultry yard to another, namely by infected mice. If mice are really very susceptible to infection with avian tubercle bacilli, this means of transmission is probably of considerable import- ance. For these little creatures are not unfrequent travellers in search of food, and may be imported in bundles of hay or sacks of corn, and it is well known that hens will kill and eat mice when they get the chance. The transmission of infection by mice was put forward by Weber and Bofinger, who showed that these animals may be infected by feeding them with avian tubercle bacilli, and it was strongly supported by M. Koch and Rabinowitsch. Mice are, as we have seen, among the very limited number of mammals which are susceptible to experimental infection with avian tubercle bacilli; and a few instances of their spontaneous infection with this type of microbe are on record (see p. 452). The possibility of transmission of infection by mice seems then to have been demonstrated. And it is conceivable that rats (p. 443) also and perhaps sparrows may play a similar part.

Perhaps the most practical inference which we can draw from the study of the etiology of avian tuberculosis is that poultry should be fed as far as possible on clean ground, and not on soil grossly contaminated with their droppings, as is frequently the case. It is no doubt in many cases difficult or impossible to carry out this precaution. But in some cases at all events it should be possible to fence off a small space to which the birds could be admitted for feeding, and from which they would be rigidly excluded as soon as their food had been picked up.

In conclusion it may be pointed out once more that while the tuberculosis of the parrot, being caused as it is almost always by the human type of tubercle bacillus, is to be regarded as a possible source of infection for man, the tuberculosis of the poultry yard, so far as we know, does not present any serious danger to him, and is to be combated chiefly on the ground of its economic importance.

REFERENCES. XV

(Chapter XXIII)

Tuberculosis in Birds.

Bland-Sutton and Gibbes (1884). Tuberculosis in Birds. Trans. Pathol. Soc. Lond. p. 477.

Cadiot, Gilbert and Roger (1891). Contribution à l'étude de tuberculose aviaire. Tuberculosis Congress, Paris. Also several papers in 1891–1898 in the Compt. rendus de la Soc. de Biol.

Cadiot (1894). Sur la tuberculose du perroquet. *Recueil de Méd. Vétér.* vol. XII, pp. 196 and 710.

Courmont and Dor (1891). Tuberculose aviaire et tuberculose des mammifères. See *ante*, p. 460.

—— (1891). De la tuberculose osseuse chez les poules. *Compt. rendus de la Soc. de Biol.* p. 554.

Delbanco (1903). Zur Anatomie der Papageien-tuberkulose. *Biologische Abteilung d. Ärztl. Vereins, Hamburg.*

Ellenberger and Baum. *Handbuch der Vergleichende Anatomie der Haustiere.* Berlin. (Quoted by Koch and Rabinowitsch, p. 285.)

Fröhner (1893). Zur Statistik der Verbreitung der Tuberkulose unter den kleinen Haustieren in Berlin. *Monatshefte f. prakt. Tierheilkunde,* p. 51.

Gärtner (1891). Über die Erblichkeit der Tuberkulose. *Zeitschr. f. Hygiene,* vol. XIII, p. 101.

Gadow, Hans (1891). Article "Birds" in *Bronn's Klassen u. Ordnungen des Thierreichs,* vol. VI, p. 814.

Griffith, A. S. (1911). Experiments on Parrots and Fowls with Tubercle Bacilli of Human Origin. *R.C.T. Fin. Rep.* App. vol. I, pp. 47 and 259.

Griffith, F. (1911). Investigation of Avian Tubercle Bacilli obtained from Birds and Swine. *Ibid. Fin. Rep.* App. vol. IV, p. 167.

Hammond-Smith (1908). Tuberculosis in a Kestrel. *Field,* April 8th.

Hutyra and Marek (1905). Spezielle Pathologie und Therapie der Haustiere, vol. I. G. Fischer, Jena.

Koch, R. (1884). The Etiology of Tuberculosis. New Syd. Soc. p. 128.

Koch, M. and Rabinowitsch (1907). See *ante*, p. 460.

Kruse (1893). Über das Vorkommen der sogenannten Hühnertuberkulose beim Menschen und bei Säugetieren. *Ziegler's Beiträge zur Patholog. Anat.* vol. XII, p. 544.

De Lamellerée (1886). De la contagion de la tuberculose par les poules. *Gaz. méd. de Paris,* p. 376, and *Semaine méd.* 1887, p. 239. (See Straus, *La Tuberculose,* p. 398.)

Maffucci (1889). Tuberkulöse Infection der Hühner-embryonen. See *ante*, p. 135.

Moore, Veranus A. (1904). The morbid anatomy and etiology of avian tuberculosis. *Journ. of Med. Res.* vol. XI, p. 521.

—— (1906). A study of avian Tuberculosis. *Zeitschr. f. Infectionskrankheiten, u.s.w. der Haustiere,* vol. I, p. 333.

Mursajeff (1900). Versuche über die Infection der Tauben mit Säugetiertuberkulose. *Wratsch,* No. 19.

—— (1901). Über die Empfänglichkeit der Tauben für die Tuberkulose der Vögel und der Säugetiere. *Ibid.* No. 28.

Nocard (1898). See *ante*, p. 372.

Owen (1866). *Comp. Anat. and Physiol. of Vertebrates,* vol. II, p. 180.

Paterson (1897). A method of producing Immunity against Tuberculous Infection. *Lancet,* II, p. 1106

Paulicki (1872). *Beiträge zur vergleichende Anatomie.* Berlin. (Quoted by Koch and Rabinowitsch.)

Rabinowitsch, L. (1904). Die Geflügeltuberkulose und ihre Beziehungen zur Säugetiertuberkulose. *Deutsch. med. Wochenschr.* No. 46.

Shattock, Seligmann, Dudgeon and Panton (1909). The Relation between Avian and Human Tuberculosis. *Proc. Roy. Soc. of Med.* Dec.

Sibley (1888). Tuberculosis in Fowls. *Trans. Pathol. Soc. Lond.* p. 464. Also *Lancet,* April 1890.

Straus (1895). See *ante,* p. 460.

Straus and Gamaléia (1891). See *ante,* p. 460.

—— (1891). See *ante,* p. 460.

Straus and Wurtz (1888). Sur la résistance des poules à la tuberculose par ingestion. *Congrès pour l'étude de la tuberculose.* Paris, p. 328.

Villemin, (1868). *Études sur la tuberculose.* Paris, p. 518.

Weber (1906). Die Tuberkulose der Vögel. *Kolle und Wassermann, Handbuch der pathog. Micro-organismen.* Supp. vol.

Weber and Bofinger (1904). Die Hühnertuberkulose. See *ante,* p. 373.

Weber, Titze and Weidanz (1908). Über Papageien- und Kanarienvogeltuberkulose. *Tub. Arbeit.a. d.Kaiserl. Gesundheitsamte,* Heft 9, p. 59.

Wolff, Max. (1904). *Report of the Second Congress of Tuberculosis Specialists.* Berlin.

Zürn (1882). *Die Krankheiten des Hausgeflügels,* p. 198. (Quoted by Straus.)

CHAPTER XXIV

TUBERCULOSIS IN MAN: THE TYPES OF TUBERCLE BACILLI WHICH CAUSE IT

To describe the many ways in which tuberculosis attacks man and the various lesions which it causes in him does not come within the scope of this book. All that will be attempted here is to give some account of the anatomical differences which characterize in general the lesions in man and the ox, and to discuss the etiological relationship of the bovine tubercle bacillus to each of the various forms of human tuberculosis.

The Contrast which exists in general between the Lesions of Human and Bovine Tuberculosis not due to Differences in the Bacilli which cause them.

It is well known that considerable differences exist in the lesions caused by tuberculosis in man and the ox

Plate XIX

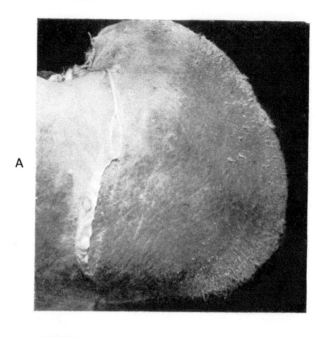

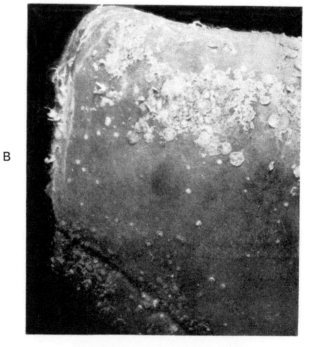

Livers of two Tuberculous Calves.

A. Showing hypertrophied villous processes.
B. Showing "duck-weed" tubercles developed in these process

respectively.   The disease in the latter is known in Germany
as *perlsucht*, and in this country sometimes goes by the name
of "grapes."   These terms imply pedunculated, or at least
prominent, rounded outgrowths, and are not in the least
applicable to the disease as it occurs in man.   It may be
said in general that the lesions in the ox are hypertrophic while
those in man are degenerative.   In the former growth predominates, and we see enormous solid lymphatic glands, and nodules
of various size projecting from the serous linings of cavities or
from the surfaces of the organs.   In the latter we find, for the
most part, abscess in glands, ulceration of mucous membranes
and of joint surfaces, or cavitation of the lungs.   There is of
course endless variety, but in the ox, on the whole, as we
have said, growth predominates, and in man disintegration.

It was natural enough to suppose, in the absence of direct
evidence, that these differences in the tuberculous lesions of
man and the ox were due to differences in the agents which
caused them; and, in 1881, Creighton believed himself able to
detect a bovine origin in certain cases of human tuberculosis,
which he saw in Addenbrooke's Hospital, Cambridge, on the
grounds that the lesions showed anatomical peculiarities.   One
form taken by the serous outgrowths in bovine tubercle has
been likened to duckweed.   It occurs on the surface of the
liver, where the little outgrowths, which might form "pearls"
or "grapes" if they were situated elsewhere, become flattened
by the pressure of the diaphragm and expand into thin discs
in which some resemblance has been seen to the plant's round
flat leaves which float on the surface of the water.   Such
"duckweed" growth Creighton detected in one or more of his
human cases, and he thought that this was evidence that the
disease was the bovine variety of tuberculosis.

We now know that in this he was mistaken, and that
anatomical differences in the tuberculous lesions in man and
the ox are not due to differences in the bacilli which initiate them,
but to differences in the animals which develop them.   This is
shown by the fact that in monkeys and guinea-pigs—animals
which are susceptible to infection both with the human and
the bovine tubercle bacillus—no difference can be seen in the

lesions produced by these microbes. Neither in man himself have the lesions which have been shown to be due to the bovine bacillus been found to differ in any way from those caused by the human bacillus. It may even be confidently asserted that the differences which characterize the tuberculous lesions in the human and bovine species respectively are due to differences of anatomical structure in man and the ox, and in the nature of the responses made to the irritation set up by the bacilli and their products in their respective hosts. In almost every animal species indeed the lesions of tuberculosis, as we have seen, have their characteristic differences, independent of the type of bacilli; witness the necrotic areas in the enlarged livers and spleens of the guinea-pig and the tendency of that animal to die, when the disease is acute, of pleural effusion, the enormous lymphadenomatous spleens of the horse and the comparative insignificance of the tuberculous lesions in the rat.

Thus we see the tuberculous lesions of each species of animal have their peculiarities. The characteristic features of those which occur in the ox seem to be due, to a large extent at least, to the presence of numerous little villous processes situated on the serous membranes, which are not developed to a like extent in other animals and the function of which is, presumably, the regulative absorption of fluid from the serous cavities. They can easily be seen on the serous membranes of the normal ox if these be examined under water. They may become greatly hypertrophied in tuberculosis; and in these hypertrophied villi tubercles are apt to develop. Such is the origin of the outgrowths which characterize bovine tuberculosis —of the "grapes" and "pearls" which are seen attached to the margins of the lung, or protruding in bunches from the costal pleura. Such too is the origin of the "duck-weed" growth on the surface of the liver.

These villous processes so prominent in the ox are but slightly developed in man; and it is, in the writer's opinion, to this anatomical difference in the two animal species that the differences in their tuberculous lesions are largely to be attributed. Other and physiological differences, of course, play their part. The extent to which the cellular tissues respond, or

Plate XX

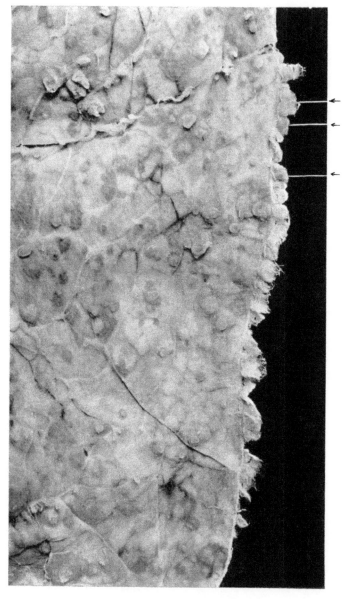

Tubercles forming in the hypertrophied villous processes and fringes
of a Heifer's Lung.

Experimental infection.

Plate XXI

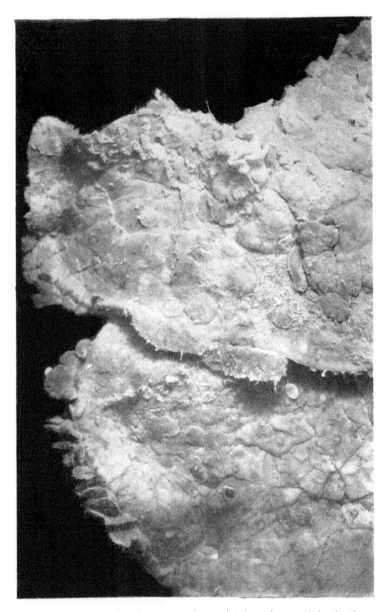

Another instance showing more advanced tuberculous nodules in the hypertrophied fringes of a Heifer's Lung.

Inoculation of bacilli of bovine type obtained from a case of general tuberculosis in a child.

are indifferent, to the action of the toxins will no doubt determine how far growth is carried before degeneration and disintegration take place; and the extent to which calcification
advances also will depend upon like causes.

The Comparative Susceptibility of Man to Infection with the Three Types of Tubercle Bacilli.

The controversy which arose on the question of the relation
of human to animal tuberculosis about the year 1901, in
consequence of Koch's too confident announcement to the
Tuberculosis Congress held in London, has already been described
in an earlier chapter (p. 190). Since that time many very
thorough and conclusive investigations of the subject have been
carried out, particularly those conducted by a Committee of
the Gesundheitsamt in Berlin under the successive leadership
of Kossel and Weber, by Park and Krumwiede in the United
States, and by a Royal Commission in this country.

These investigations have dispelled all doubt as to the
liability of man to infection with bovine tubercle bacilli.
Without question he becomes so infected at times. But, as we
shall see, such infections are the exception, are confined for the
most part to certain kinds of tuberculosis, and are limited,
as a rule, to the early periods of life; and it remains true that
the great majority of all cases of tuberculosis (recognized as
such during life) at all ages taken together are due to the
human type of tubercle bacillus, and are derived directly from
other cases of tuberculosis in man.

This is admitted practically by everyone who has studied
the subject; there remain now only some differences of opinion
as to the exact proportion of cases caused by tubercle bacilli
of bovine and human type respectively in various kinds of
tuberculous disease, as for example in lupus, or in the tuberculosis of bones and joints or in that of lymphatic glands. Under
these circumstances the best course for us to pursue seems to
be to consider the evidence as to the type of bacillus concerned
in the production of each of the main groups into which human
tuberculosis may be divided. We shall therefore consider the
subject under the following heads: (1) pulmonary tuberculosis,

(2) tuberculous meningitis, (3) general tuberculosis, (4) abdominal and mesenteric-gland tuberculosis, (5) bronchial-gland tuberculosis, (6) tuberculosis primary in two or more sets of lymphatic glands, (7) cervical-gland tuberculosis, (8) tuberculosis of bones and joints, (9) tuberculosis of skin.

I.   *Pulmonary Tuberculosis.*

Tuberculosis affecting principally the lungs, or limited, broadly speaking, to those organs, or to them and the bronchial glands and pleura, or, if involving any other organs, then doing so in a secondary manner—this kind of tuberculosis, commonly called phthisis, will be dealt with in this section.   It is far more often the cause of death than all other kinds of tubercle put together, claiming as it does in Europe more than three-quarters of the deaths attributed to tuberculosis of all kinds[1].

From the etiological point of view phthisis is even more important than this statement implies, for it is admittedly the main source of infection for all other kinds of tubercle.   It is therefore in this kind of tuberculosis of greater interest than in any other to know what proportion of cases, if any, have a bovine origin.

In considering the evidence as to the types of tubercle bacilli which cause phthisis we shall have to distinguish between that derived from cases investigated post-mortem and in which the bacilli were derived from the lungs themselves, and that derived from the investigation of sputum; for however careful may be the precautions taken to prevent the accidental contamination of sputum with tubercle bacilli which by chance may be present in food, evidence derived from this source can never be so completely satisfactory as that derived from investigation of the lung itself.

[1] In England and Wales pulmonary tuberculosis accounted for 71 per cent. of all deaths attributed to tuberculosis.   In Ireland to 75 per cent. of these deaths.   In Prussia to 89·6 and in U.S.A. to 86·1 per cent.   These figures are taken from a table contained in the report of an address delivered by Dr Schmid of Bern at the International Congress held at Rome in 1912 (see *Rep. of Congress,* p. 463).   Another paper dealing with the same subject was communicated to the Congress by Dr Hamel of Berlin and may be found in the same volume p. 113.   According to the Report of the Registrar General for E. and W. for 1911 "phthisis" accounted for 74 per cent. of the total deaths from tuberculosis.

Plate XXII

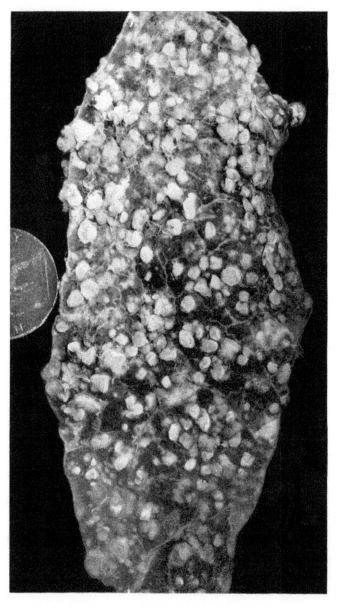

Early tubercles (68 days) projecting from the surface of a Calf's Lung.

Experimental infection.

Plate XXIII

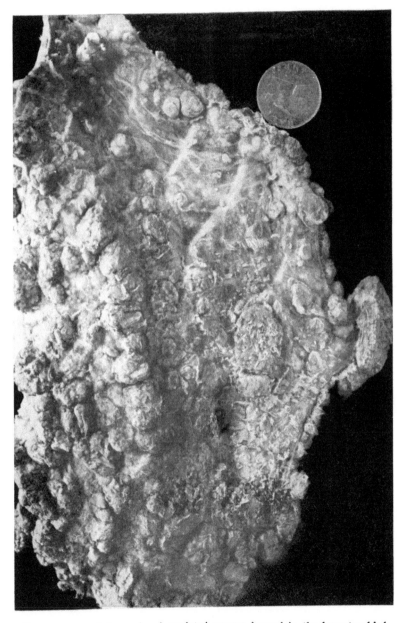

Tuberculous nodules and pedunculated masses formed in the hypertrophied villous processes and fringes of a Heifer's Lung.

Experimental infection.

There is another class of evidence also which demands separate treatment, namely that derived post-mortem from the investigation of tuberculous glands, or organs other than the lungs themselves. This kind of evidence is of great weight, but it can never be conclusive, because bacteriological investigation both here and abroad has abundantly shown that occasionally in the same individual a lesion in one part may be caused by a bacillus of bovine type while one in another part is caused by one of human type. We shall therefore take the evidence in the following order: A. Investigation of tubercle bacilli taken from tuberculous organs (1) from the lungs themselves, (2) from some other part; and B. Investigation of tubercle bacilli derived from sputum.

A. Investigation of Tubercle Bacilli taken from Tuberculous Organs.

The Royal Commission on Tuberculosis finally classified fourteen of their cases under the heading "Primary Pulmonary Tuberculosis[1]." In thirteen of these the bacilli investigated came from the lungs themselves, and in one from a bronchial gland. In all these cases the bacilli proved to be of human type.

In four of the thirteen cases tubercle bacilli from some affected part or parts in addition to those from the lungs were also investigated and these too proved to be of the same type.

One of the cases, H 45[2] deserves mention on account of the early age of the patient. This was a child just one year old who developed acute phthisis after an attack of measles. The disease proved fatal two and a half months after the onset of the illness; and at the post-mortem examination a large multilocular cavity and several smaller ones were found in the lower lobe of the right lung, and the bronchial and mesenteric glands were caseous. From a bronchial gland tubercle bacilli of human type were cultivated.

In another of the cases the disease may have begun in a bronchial gland. This case was known as H 22[3]. It occurred in a girl of sixteen years. After

[1] R.C.T. Fin. Rep. p. 10 and Int. Rep. App. vol. II, p. 4 et seq. and Fin. Rep. App. vol. I, p. 99. H 4, here included, was rejected by the Royal Commission as an early and incomplete experiment. No cultures were obtained, but inoculation of calves with portions of the tuberculous lung showed that the bacilli could not have belonged to the bovine type.

[2] Ibid. Int. Rep. App. vol. II, pp. 5 and 813.   [3] Ibid. pp. 4 and 535.

death both lungs were found to be riddled with cavities and the pleura greatly thickened on one side, but the lesions in the bronchial glands were obviously of long standing, and perhaps older than those in the lungs. These glands were very numerous, and most of them considerably enlarged. Some were caseous, others contained calcareous nodules so hard as to resemble little stones, and in others there were collections of stony grains which could not be cut through with the knife. One held a soft nodule composed of whitish putty-like matter containing numerous grains and enclosed in a thin papery membrane.

It may be of interest to note, in connection with the question, raised at the beginning of this chapter, of the correlation, if any, of the character of the lesions and the type of tubercle bacillus found in them, that in this case, in which only tubercle bacilli of human type were present, "several growths much resembling the so-called grape-like bodies common in bovine tuberculosis were seen on the pleura[1]."

In addition to the fourteen cases accepted by the Royal Commission as instances of "primary pulmonary tuberculosis" there are two which, though probably of abdominal origin, ought not to be excluded from the category we are now considering, inasmuch as they, or at least one of them, may perhaps be regarded as instances of pulmonary tuberculosis or phthisis in the commonly accepted meaning of the term. These yielded, the one a bovine bacillus and the other, not indeed from the lung itself but from a mesenteric gland, a mixture of human and bovine bacilli. These two cases therefore demand further consideration.

H 59[2], a male child, aged two and three-quarter years, died after eight months' illness commencing apparently in an attack of measles. The symptoms were mainly abdominal, such as vomiting, diarrhœa and enlargement of abdomen, but there were enlarged glands to be felt in the neck, and physical signs in the lungs; and ultimately the child died of pneumothorax. At the post-mortem examination numerous small ulcers were found in the intestine, and the mesenteric glands were greatly enlarged, caseous and softened; the cervical glands contained a number of yellow foci; the lungs were said to show extensive tuberculous infiltration, with emphysema and small cavities; a small piece sent to the laboratory was found to be packed with yellowish tubercles, occasionally separate but mostly confluent, forming irregular caseating areas. There was a pea-sized caseous nodule in the cerebellum. Cultures derived from lungs, mesenteric glands, cervical glands and cerebellum were all of bovine type.

The other case was known as H 49[3]. It has already been fully discussed in Chapter XVI which dealt with the question of stability of type among tubercle

[1] *loc. cit.* p. 4.
[2] *R.C.T. Int. Rep* App. vol. II, pp. 12 and 940.
[3] *Ibid.* p. 839.

bacilli (p. 330). It will be sufficient therefore to remind the reader that it was obviously a case of phthisis in which severe mesenteric disease of old standing was discovered after death, in a young man eighteen years of age. Both lungs were extensively diseased and contained numerous hard tuberculous nodules of a somewhat fibrous type. Several mesenteric glands were enlarged to the size of haricot beans, and calcareous. They were so hard that it was difficult to break them up in a mortar, even with a heavy pestle.

It is very unfortunate that, owing to premature death of the animals inoculated, no cultures of tubercle bacilli were obtained from the lungs in this case. But an atypical strain was obtained from the mesenteric glands, and this was ultimately proved to be a mixture of bacilli belonging both to the human and bovine types.

There is, of course, no evidence in this case that the bovine bacilli took any part in the pulmonary disease. They may have been present in the mesenteric glands only, as "harmless lodgers," residing in lesions made by human bacilli; or the pulmonary lesions may have been the consequence of an independent infection.

Both these cases are included in the table which follows.

From the Gesundheitsamt in Berlin Weber[1], summarizing all the cases investigated there up to April 1907, gives the following figures:

Adults.   Pulmonary Tuberculosis (Phthisis) **22**.

Children.   Pulmonary Tuberculosis (Phthisis, Caseous Pneumonia, Caseous Bronchitis), General Miliary Tuberculosis, Tuberculous Meningitis, **18**.

But this classification, as regards the children at least, does not suit our present purpose; and if we wish to confine our attention to instances of pulmonary tuberculosis, we must make our own selection of cases. This we are able to do from the short summaries of the cases published[2]. Having selected the cases we must subdivide them according to the source of the bacilli investigated. This done we find eight cases in which sputum was the source of the bacilli examined. These we leave for the next section. There remain then fourteen adult cases, in seven of which the bacilli investigated were provided by the lungs themselves, and seven in which they came from a bronchial or mesenteric gland, and eight in children, including three which belong to the first of these subdivisions,

---

[1] *Tub. Arbeiten, etc.* Heft 6, pp. 7 and 8.
[2] *Ibid.* Heft 3, p. 50, Table V, and Heft 6, p. 51, Table VIII.

and five which belong to the second[1].   All these cases without exception yielded tubercle bacilli of human type.

Beitzke (1907) in the Pathological Institute in Berlin, investigated the tubercle bacilli from twenty-five consecutive fatal cases of tuberculosis in children under nine years of age.   An interesting point in his series is the large proportion of cases in which there was "cavernous tuberculosis of lungs" or "caseous pneumonia," especially in children under two years of age, no less than eight out of sixteen under this age, and nine out of the whole twenty-five being so described.

These nine cases may fairly be considered as instances of phthisis, and to them have been added two further cases in which the disease, though generalized (as indeed it was to some extent in certain of the others) was more severe in the lungs than elsewhere.

In only two of these cases did the lungs themselves provide the bacilli investigated.   In both of these the micro-organisms proved to be of human type.

In the remaining nine cases the bacilli investigated came from a bronchial or mesenteric gland, and in one case from the peritoneum also.   Eight of them yielded strains of tubercle bacilli of human type, and one a strain of bovine type.

This latter case occurred in a ricketty child, eighteen months old, which died of acute caseous pneumonic tuberculosis of the lungs, and empyema. There were also a few tubercles in liver and spleen and slight ulceration of the intestines.   Bronchial and mesenteric glands were enlarged, but the former alone were caseous.   Beitzke draws attention to the fact that this was a case of pulmonary phthisis, and is evidently of opinion that it was the result of a respiratory invasion.   The strain of bovine bacilli was obtained from the bronchial glands.

Rothe (1911) following up the work of Gaffky at the Institute for Infectious Diseases in Berlin, examined the bronchial and mesenteric glands taken, without selection, from 100 children

[1] In order to make our figures conform as nearly as possible to those of Weber we have included one or two cases in which the pulmonary disease appears to have been secondary to mischief elsewhere, and several where there were severe complications such as meningitis, but have excluded all cases where the pulmonary disease seems to have been only a secondary part of a general miliary tuberculosis.   In none of the excluded cases were bovine tubercle bacilli found.

not exceeding five years of age, who died of various causes. Twenty-one of these children were found to be infected with tubercle; and of the twenty-one, eight were described as cases of pulmonary tuberculosis. The remainder do not concern us for the moment. Seven of the eight pulmonary cases yielded strains of tubercle bacilli of human type and one a strain of bovine type.

This latter case was that of a ricketty child who suffered from whooping cough and died of pneumonia at the age of thirteen months. At the post-mortem examination some caseous disease of the left lung, and tuberculosis of a bronchial gland were discovered. The mesenteric glands were swollen, and, though not obviously tuberculous, infected one guinea-pig out of four injected with an emulsion of them. Two strains of tubercle bacilli were raised in culture, one from a guinea-pig injected with bronchial glands and another from a guinea-pig injected with mesenteric glands. Both strains proved to be of bovine type. The former, subcutaneously injected into a calf, caused progressive tuberculosis.

Ungermann (1912) in the Gesundheitsamt in Berlin made a comprehensive study of the tubercle bacilli found in lymphatic glands of children who died from all sorts of causes. The material was obtained post-mortem from the Kaiser-und-Kaiserin-Friedrich-Kinderkrankenhaus, and was entirely unselected. Nevertheless tuberculosis was the principal or an accessory cause of death in twenty-nine out of 171 children, and in another ten the glands were tuberculous, or at least proved capable of transmitting tuberculosis to guinea-pigs. Among the tuberculous cases were eight which were described as pulmonary tuberculosis. In six of these cases the age was below five years and in two between five and sixteen. All yielded tubercle bacilli of human type.

In Eastwood and F. Griffith's similar investigations, made in 1914 in the Local Government Board's laboratories, the bodies of 150 children, ranging in age from two to ten years, and irrespective of cause of death, were examined, with the result that ninety-four showed evidence of infection with tubercle bacilli. Of these, twenty-one may perhaps be reckoned as cases of pulmonary tuberculosis. From four of these cases of pulmonary tuberculosis in children strains of tubercle bacilli were obtained from the lungs. All proved to be of human type. From the remaining seventeen cases the cultures investigated were raised from bronchial, mesenteric or cervical glands, and often from two or more of these groups. All but one of these also yielded tubercle bacilli of human type.

The remaining case (H 37) yielded a bovine bacillus. It is a little difficult to classify. It has been accepted on the ground that the lungs "contained moderately numerous discrete tubercles and nodules up to ·5 c.c. in diameter" although it is scarcely probable that it would have been regarded during life as a case of pulmonary tuberculosis. Rather it would have appeared to be one of abdominal tuberculosis with some generalization. A bronchial gland showed a caseous focus; the mesenteric glands were enlarged and caseous generally, and there were numerous tubercles on the peritoneum. Both sets of glands yielded bovine bacilli.

There were in addition four cases in which some nodules, presumably tuberculous, were present in the lungs, but from which no cultures could be obtained by inoculation of guinea-pigs with emulsions either of lungs or lymph glands.

Among the forty-five children dead of any cause examined for the Local Government Board by A. S. Griffith in Cambridge (1914) there were twenty-four which showed evidence of infection with tubercle bacilli. Six of these Griffith classified as instances of primary pulmonary tuberculosis. The ages varied from 15 months to 11 years. Cultures of tubercle bacilli were obtained from the lungs as well as from glands in three cases, and in the other three cultures were obtained from sources other than lungs. In all cases the bacilli proved to be of human type.

Taking all these investigations together we get the following results. Out of twenty-six cases of pulmonary tuberculosis in adults (if we may exclude one in which both types of tubercle bacilli were found in a mesenteric gland) not one yielded a bovine tubercle bacillus. While among sixty-five children there were four in which the bacilli were of this kind and sixty-one in which they were of human type. In one of the bovine cases the bovine bacilli were found in the lungs themselves, but in two others they were demonstrated only in the bronchial and, in one case, only in the mesenteric glands.

Eber has recorded two cases of phthisis, the material from which ultimately produced tuberculosis in calves. The method he adopted was a simultaneous intraperitoneal and subcutaneous injection into the calf of an emulsion of the organs of a guinea-pig infected with the original material. This method

PULMONARY TUBERCULOSIS.

(i) *Tubercle Bacilli from Lungs.*

Authors	Adults			Children up to 12 years	
	Type of bacillus			Type of bacillus	
	Human	Bovine	Mixture	Human	Bovine
Royal Commission ...	12	o	—	1	1
Gesundheitsamt, Berlin	7	o	—	3	o
Beitzke	—	—	—	2	o
Eastwood and F. Griffith	—	—	—	4	o
A. S. Griffith	—	—	—	3	o
Total	19	o	—	13	1

(ii) *Tubercle Bacilli from some other Organ or Gland.*

Authors	Human	Bovine	Mixture	Human	Bovine
Royal Commission ...	—	—	1	1	o
Gesundheitsamt, Berlin	7	o	—	5	o
Beitzke	—	—	—	8	1
Rothe	—	—	—	7	1
Ungermann	—	—	—	8	o
Eastwood and F. Griffith	—	—	—	16	1
A. S. Griffith	—	—	—	3	o
Total	7	o	1	48	3

he believed to be specially suited to bring about an adaptation of the bacilli to their new environment. The first case was one of phthisis in a young man. The calf injected with the guinea-pig organs developed a chronic tuberculosis of the peritoneum, and pleura. A goat simultaneously injected with the same material failed to develop tuberculosis. The second case was also one of phthisis, but complicated with meningitis, and in an older patient. Injection of an emulsion of the organs of the guinea-pig infected with the meningeal tubercles into a calf caused general tuberculosis.

Weber criticized these experiments adversely, pointing out that determination of type of tubercle bacilli can only be effected satisfactorily by careful and toilsome researches with pure cultures carried out by exact methods. In the second case, the injection of meningeal tissue does not show the kind of bacillus which was the cause of the lung disease. This criticism seems on the whole sound; and Eber's cases have not been included in our table. They are discussed more fully in the chapter on "Stability of Type" (p. 322).

B. *Investigation of Tubercle Bacilli from Sputum.*

With regard to the evidence as to the types of tubercle
bacillus concerned in the causation of pulmonary tuberculosis,
which is based on the investigation of the bacilli found in
sputum, we have already pointed out that it is weakened by
the possibility that now and again the latter may perchance
be contaminated with bovine bacilli derived from food.   Such
bacilli, contained in milk or butter, may, if adequate care be
not taken, either pass directly into the sputum, or, perchance,
take up a lodging in some corner such, for example, as a crypt
in the tonsil (just as diphtheria bacilli are believed to do) and
contaminate the sputum as it passes through the pharynx.
Such a source of contamination as this latter, if it really exists,
will be a particularly pernicious source of possible error; for it
will be likely to exercise its misleading influence even though
the investigation be repeated; on the other hand, in such cases
the bovine bacilli will not appear alone.

It may perhaps be said that errors arising from these sources
are not likely to be frequent.   But while this is readily granted it
does not eliminate the danger altogether.   For the question
after all is not so much what proportion of cases of pulmonary
tuberculosis are caused by bovine bacilli? but whether any
at all are so caused.   Under these circumstances errors, even
though they are unfrequent, will be liable falsely to reverse
the judgment.

On the other hand investigation of sputum is comparatively
easy.   It is somewhat surprising that this method of research
received Koch's sanction; though, as we shall see, he was
fully alive to its dangers and to the necessity of using strict
precautions when it was employed.

At the International Congress on Tuberculosis, held in 1908
at Washington, Koch[1], calling attention, not for the first time,
to the overwhelming importance of pulmonary tuberculosis as
compared with all other kinds of tuberculosis, and saying that
it constituted eleven-twelfths of the whole, maintained that

---

[1] *Report of the Tuberculosis Congress held at Washington in* 1908, vol. II, pt.
II, p. 743.

"up to date in no case of pulmonary tuberculosis had the tubercle bacillus of bovine type been definitely demonstrated."

Arloing then challenged this statement, and claimed that he himself had discovered an instance of the kind. The original source of the strain of bacilli in this case was the contents of a cavity; and the strain itself "possessed all the cultural characters of the bovine bacillus and, when injected into animals of the bovine species produced generalized tuberculosis."

Koch would not admit this evidence as conclusive on account of the possibility of accidental contamination with milk or butter or other food substances, which must always be kept in view. "Even if bovine tubercle bacilli," he said, "are found in a cavity after death the possibility must always be thought of that the patient, in the course of his last hours, may have inhaled particles vomited from the stomach, or retained in the mouth. One isolated instance of this kind (referring to Arloing's case) has not the necessary power of proof." He also rejected the de Jong-Stuurmann case which will be referred to later, and at the same time he attacked, not without just cause, the elaborate experiments which the Royal Commission had carried out with the mixed sputa of a large number of patients. Koch was, then, keenly alive to the possibility of sputum becoming contaminated with bovine bacilli contained in milk or other food, and rightly insisted that one sputum only should be examined at a time[1]. He also objected, and again not without justice, to the investigation being carried out by means of "passage" experiments. For this method is, as we have seen, surrounded by serious pitfalls and difficulties, and though, unfortunately, necessary for trying the question of stability of type, should not be used to ascertain the original virulence of a strain. Especially is this so when there is, as in the case of sputum investigations, any risk of even minimal contamination with bovine bacilli; for should a few

[1] Koch himself had set the bad example when in experiments made in collaboration with Schütz and communicated to the British Congress on Tuberculosis in 1901 he fed four young cattle with mixed sputa almost daily for four months. But the truth is the results of this method when negative, that is when the cattle do not become infected, as in Koch's case, are very impressive, it is only when they are positive that they are unconvincing.

bacilli of this kind have accidentally found their way into the sputum, though they might not be numerous enough to make their mark in original experiments, they were bound to gain preponderance in the end if the contaminated strain was passed through a series of animals more susceptible to infection with the contaminating bacillus than with the other. To experiment with mixed sputa, or by the method of passage, we may therefore say, is gratuitously to open the door to experimental error. This argument is undoubtedly of great weight and we may pass over the experiments of the Royal Commission made with mixed sputa without further comment, except to say that the fact, which emerged from the experiment known as Sputum B, namely that four calves might be fed almost daily for three or four months, with the mixed sputa of many patients, and consume during this time 20 or 30 litres of this material without developing anything more than minute calcareous foci in some of the lymphatic glands connected with the alimentary canal is very strong testimony to the rarity of the bovine bacillus in such material. The sputum was collected with all reasonable precautions, and the results serve to show that these are as a rule effective.

But while reasonable precautions may get over the difficulties in the great majority of cases, the weakness of sputum investigations is that you can never feel sure that these precautions may not have failed in a particular case. If bovine bacilli were *frequently* found in sputum in spite of all precautions one might feel confident that they were really present in the lungs, for precautions which have proved so effective in very searching tests, such as the one we have just mentioned, could hardly fail so often. But if the finding of such bacilli is a *rarity*, and only occurs, let us say, once in a hundred times we cannot feel so sure that they have not come by contamination of the sputum, for precautions, however ample, cannot be held to be absolute or exempt from the possibility of occasional failure.

Moreover if tubercle bacilli may under certain conditions take up their residence in tonsilar crypts it is clear that no precautions such as are described below can be expected to protect completely against risk of contamination from this source.

The question of the precautions necessary to make sputum investigation of value was discussed in 1908 at a meeting of the Gesundheitsamt at which Koch was present, and there was then drawn up a plan of procedure, which was simplified and improved at a subsequent meeting held in 1910[1]. The principal precautions recommended in this plan referred to the danger of the sputum becoming contaminated with milk and butter, and it was laid down that such articles of diet were to be withheld from the patients for two days before taking the sample of sputum. The sputum itself, after being repeatedly washed in water, was to be injected into guinea-pigs, and cultures raised from these animals.

But perhaps the most important point insisted on was that in the event of bovine bacilli being found in any case a second investigation should be made with a fresh sample of sputum, and the investigation repeated as often as possible. Moreover it was urged that every endeavour should be made to follow the case up to the end; and if an opportunity for post-mortem examination occurred, an investigation of the bacilli contained in the organs of the patient should be made.

It may be pointed out that such repetition of the investigation of the tubercle bacilli in sputum affords substantial security against errors which otherwise might be caused by direct contamination with food containing tubercle bacilli; for the extreme rarity with which bovine bacilli have been found in sputum in the course of numerous experiments carried out by various observers shows that the precautions usually employed are almost invariably successful; and it may justly be held that an accident which, it is thus shown to be very exceptional, if it occurs at all, cannot in all reasonable probability occur on two or more consecutive occasions. But while repetition thus provides satisfactorily against the danger of *direct* contamination from food it does little to guard against the danger, if in fact such exists, of contamination with bacilli originally introduced in food and which have taken up a more or less temporary lodging in the tonsilar crypts.

---

[1] *Tub. Arbeit. a. d. Kaiserl. Gesundheitsamte*, Heft 12, pp. 1 and 2.

But there is a point of even greater importance than those we have just been considering, attention to which alone can guard against the danger last referred to, and which cannot be dispensed with as a precaution against errors due to direct contamination with food-borne bacilli. This is the adequate investigation of the cultural characters of the strains in question. It is obvious that, if bovine bacilli get by accident into sputum from a case of phthisis caused by human bacilli, the resulting culture is likely to be a mixed one, and it is of the greatest importance that the fact of the strain being a mixture should not escape the attention of the observer; for a mixed strain has nothing like the significance that a pure bovine strain has. It is essential therefore that whenever a strain of tubercle bacilli derived from sputum proves virulent for rabbits and calves the most careful attention should be given to ascertaining whether or no human tubercle bacilli are present along with the bovine. Now a mixture such as we are considering will have the virulence (more or less) of the bovine type for differentiating animals such as calves and rabbits. What distinguishes it from a bovine strain is that it has the cultural characters of the human type. The only way therefore to detect the presence of human bacilli in a mixture which is virulent for these animals is to determine correctly the cultural characters of the strain. This is by no means so simple a matter as it is sometimes thought; for, as we have shown in a previous chapter, the true characters may remain hidden owing to imperfections in the culture media, and in any case the investigations of cultural characters if adequate cannot be otherwise than long and tedious; and in the end the verdict remains a matter of judgment.

Having now considered the dangers inherent in the method, and the precautions devised to avoid them, let us pass on to review the results obtained by the investigation of the tubercle bacilli in sputum.

In Germany investigations were carried out according to the plan recommended by the Gesundheitsamt by Dieterlen (50 cases), Möllers (51 cases), Kossel (46 cases), Weber and Dieterlen (9 cases) and Lindemann (41 cases). In all 197 cases were investigated; of these 195 yielded only tubercle bacilli of human type, and two yielded mixed strains containing bacilli both of the human and of the bovine type.

In America Park and Krumwiede (1911) investigated the type of tubercle bacilli obtained from the sputum of 296 cases of phthisis, and found only tubercle bacilli of the human type.

In Japan Kitasato (1909) made a similar investigation in 152 cases, in 60 of which the examination was repeated, and again no tubercle bacilli other than those of the human type were found.

In this country Bulloch (1911) examined 23 cases with a like result. Cruickshank· (1912) obtained cultures by the antiformin method from the sputum of nearly 60 cases of phthisis. All the strains were eugonic, but they were not tested on animals; and for this reason they cannot be included in the table which follows. A. S. Griffith (1911) examined for the Royal Commission the sputum from 29 cases and succeeded in finding two infected with bovine bacilli. To these we must refer again in a moment.

After the work of the Commission had come to an end at Stansted Griffith (1914) returned to the question at Cambridge, and investigated by the same methods as before the sputum from 148 additional cases of phthisis. In the meantime some recent work on bone and joint tuberculosis, to which we must refer again in its proper place, had suggested the probability that there was an unusual proportion of bovine infections in Edinburgh. Griffith therefore obtained a portion of his material from that city The results were as follows: from the Brompton Hospital, London, sputum was obtained from 105 cases, and yielded only tubercle bacilli of human type; but from the Victoria Hospital, Edinburgh, one patient out of forty-three examined yielded an unmixed strain of tubercle bacilli of bovine type.

The literature of the subject had been reviewed for the Gesundheitsamt by Dieterlen in 1910, and a tabular list of the investigations in which the type of tubercle bacilli present in sputum had been definitely determined was drawn up by Möllers in the following year. This list was extended by

Lindemann in 1912 and again by A. S. Griffith in 1914[1]. The following table is taken from Griffith's paper with some minor alterations[2].

Tubercle Bacilli found in Sputum.

Authors	No. of cases	Classification of bacilli		
		Human	Bovine	Mixed
Various authors	88	87	1	—
Dieterlen	50	50	0	—
Kitasato	152	152	0	—
Park and Krumwiede	296	296	0	—
Möllers	51	51	0	—
Jancsó and Elfer	5	5	0	—
A. S. Griffith (Royal Commission)	29	27	2	—
Kossel	46	45	0	1
Bulloch	23	23	0	—
Weber and Dieterlen	9	9	—	—
Lindemann	41	40	—	1
A. S. Griffith (London cases) ...	105	105	0	—
,, (Edinburgh cases)	43	42	1	—
Total	938	932	4	2

Lindemann's list contained records of 790 cases, of which one yielded a doubtful strain (Mohler and Washburn[3]), and two mixed strains. These latter are of little importance since the bovine bacilli may have been present only as "harmless lodgers," or may have gained access to the sputum after it had left the lungs. Only three cases are admitted to have yielded bovine bacilli alone. Two of these were those of A. S. Griffith

[1] *Brit. Med. Journ.* 1914, I, p. 1171. Griffith condensed Lindemann's list by adding together the cases contributed by the first fifteen authors mentioned by the latter. For details of this group, labelled "Various Authors" Lindemann's table may be consulted (see *Tub. Arbeit. etc.* Heft 12, p. 73).

[2] The alterations are the following: the de Jong-Stuurmann case is admitted to be a bovine infection; and the cases ascribed to the Royal Commission are credited to Griffith himself.

[3] Mohler and Washburn, 1907, A Comparative Study of Tubercle Bacilli from Varied Sources, *U.S. Dep. of Agriculture, Bureau of Animal Industry,* Bull. 96. For criticism of this case see Kossel, *Centralb. f. Bakt.* Abt. I, Ref. XLIII, 3, and Dieterlen, *Tub. Arbeit. a. d. Kaiserl. Gesundheitsamte,* Heft 10, p. 111. This case is not included in the table above.

already mentioned. The third was the famous case of de Jong-Stuurmann about which there has been a good deal of controversy.

This case is summarized as follows by Bulloch: the patient was a peasant girl, aged twenty-seven, whose sputum contained many tubercle bacilli. This sputum was injected into a guinea-pig, and cultures were obtained from the animal. The cultures, injected intravenously into a healthy calf, caused death in three weeks from generalized tuberculosis. Two other calves also succumbed to inoculation with this virus. Bulloch points out that only one sample of sputum was examined, and notes that it is to be regretted that no attempts were made to determine whether the infection was a pure one with the bovine bacillus only.

We need not delay over this case since the recent and more thoroughly investigated cases of A. S. Griffith hold the field. If these are accepted the de Jong-Stuurmann case can be admitted without demur.

Griffith's list brings the total up to 938 cases and adds, as we have seen, one more instance of bovine infection. Thus, putting his two investigations together, there are in all three cases which yielded from the sputum bacilli of bovine type only. These, standing as they do in such contrast to all the rest must be critically examined. Let us begin with those investigated for the Royal Commission[1].

H 127. The patient was a young man, twenty-one years old, who had been a butcher's assistant. The sputum examined was obtained on four separate occasions, at intervals of 76, 117 and 118 days respectively. Cultures were obtained from all four samples—on two occasions directly by means of the antiformin method, and at other times from guinea-pigs inoculated with the sputum.

Seven strains of tubercle bacilli in all were thus obtained. They all grew on artificial media like bovine bacilli, and produced severe general tuberculosis in rabbits (twenty in number) when injected subcutaneously. Four calves were injected subcutaneously. Of two of these, injected with cultures raised from the first sample, one was killed when very ill forty-eight days after injection, but the other developed only "slight general tuberculosis, apparently retrogressive." This result is plausibly attributed to high resisting power on the part of this particular calf; for two rabbits inoculated at the same time with the same strain, and receiving 10 mg. subcutaneously, died, in fifty-two and fifty-eight days respectively, of general tuberculosis. The other two calves were injected subcutaneously with culture raised from the third sample of sputum and developed acute general tuberculosis.

[1] *R.C.T. Fin. Rep.* App. vol. i, pp. 8, 167, 168, 182, 183.

Thus all four samples of sputum from this case were proved to contain tubercle bacilli which were virulent for rabbits, and in the case of two of them the bacilli were shown to be virulent for calves also.

H 128.   A young man aged twenty-one suffered from consolidation without cavities affecting the whole of the right lung and the apex of the left.   He eventually died of pulmonary disease.

Two samples of sputum were examined, the second being taken after an interval of four months.   From these samples three strains of tubercle bacilli were isolated in culture—one from the first sample obtained from a guinea-pig inoculated with the sputum, and two from the second sample, the one taken directly from the sputum, by means of the antiformin method, and the other from a guinea-pig which had been inoculated with it.   All three strains "grew like bovine bacilli," and produced severe general tuberculosis in rabbits.   One strain from each sample of sputum was injected subcutaneously into calves and caused severe general tuberculosis.

Thus we see that the animal experiments made with the sputum of these two patients were very thorough.   Not only was the virulence tested on rabbits, but in the case of two strains from each of the patients it was tested also on calves. These experiments, of course, prove beyond doubt that bovine bacilli were present in the sputum of each patient; and the fact that their presence was demonstrated on four occasions in the case of the one patient, and on two occasions in the case of the other, shows that they were not there in consequence of a direct accidental food contamination.

When we come to the question whether the bovine bacilli were alone, or accompanied by bacilli of human type, we are on more difficult ground, and its discussion we shall defer for a moment until we have described the third case in which bovine bacilli were found; but we may note in passing that in these two cases the cultural characters of the bacilli in question were studied in no less than ten different strains, and that in each they appeared to be of the bovine type.

It would have been still more satisfactory if post-mortem examinations could have been obtained in these cases, and investigation made of the bacilli in the lungs themselves.   The importance of this was kept clearly in mind, but though both patients died during the period of investigation in neither case could an examination be obtained.

Lastly we must examine the evidence concerned with the more recent case.

The patient was a girl of sixteen and a half, with dullness at both apices and, to a lesser extent, over the right lower lobe. There were some indications of a cavity at the right apex. The girl seems to have improved a good deal under treatment and expectoration is said to have ceased, at least for a time. She however died suddenly at her own home a little more than a year and a half after the onset of her illness; but from what cause it is not stated. No post-mortem examination was made.

No less than five samples of sputum were investigated from this case. From the first cultures were obtained directly by the antiformin method and indirectly from a guinea-pig inoculated with the sputum. A calf inoculated with 50 mg. of the direct culture developed slight general tuberculosis of a retrogressive type, but rabbits injected intravenously at the same time with small doses died of general miliary tuberculosis. In consequence of the apparent discrepancy in the results of the injections of the calf and rabbit, a second calf was injected, also subcutaneously, with 50 mg. This animal became very ill and, having been killed about nine weeks after inoculation, was found to have "severe general miliary tuberculosis of all organs and glands, identical in every respect with the general tuberculosis produced by tubercle bacilli of bovine origin." The culture obtained from a guinea-pig was injected into rabbits and produced fatal general tuberculosis.

Both these strains, grown on the various culture media commonly used, were "dysgonic and identical in cultural characteristics with tubercle bacilli of bovine type."

From the second sample of sputum, taken about two months after the first, two strains of culture were raised through guinea-pigs. "They were identical in cultural characteristics with those isolated from the first specimen of sputum." These strains were tested by inoculation of a goat and two rabbits, and in all of these animals they caused fatal general tuberculosis.

Rabbits also injected with a dilute suspension of the sputum itself developed fatal general tuberculosis.

The third specimen of sputum was received about a month after the second. The sputum was diluted and injected into a calf (·5 c.c. sputum intravenously), a goat (·25 c.c. sputum subcutaneously), four rabbits and two guinea-pigs. All these animals except the guinea-pigs died of acute general tuberculosis. The guinea-pigs were killed before the end was reached and cultures were obtained from them. These also were dysgonic like the others. One of them was injected subcutaneously into a rabbit (10 mg.) and produced general tuberculosis.

The fourth sample of sputum was received after the lapse of another month. The conditions under which the specimen was collected were however not considered quite satisfactory and no animals were inoculated with it. But a culture obtained directly by the antiformin method grew like the others. "There was no sign of the presence of human tubercle bacilli."

The fifth and last sample: Strains of tubercle bacilli were obtained in culture both directly from the sputum, and from a guinea-pig injected with it. Both strains "were dysgonic and identical in cultural characters with those obtained from the first four specimens." One of them injected into rabbits (10 mg. subcutaneously) caused death from general tuberculosis.

Thus Griffith demonstrated the presence of bovine tubercle bacilli in the sputum of three patients suffering from pulmonary

tuberculosis of the common type. The facts do not admit of
any doubt. In each case the bovine bacilli were demonstrated
repeatedly, in samples of sputum taken at considerable intervals.
Moreover, everything was done which is humanly possible to
test for the presence of human tubercle bacilli without any
evidence of them coming to light[1]. Such tests however, as we
have already pointed out, must depend on the study of cultural
characters, for there is no objective test, such as inoculation
of certain animals provides in the case of the bovine bacillus,
which will serve to detect the presence of human bacilli in a
mixture of the two types. We do not desire in the least to
impugn the correctness of Griffith's conclusions. They depend,
as we have insisted, in the last resort on the observer's judgment. But judgment in such matters rests on experience, and
no man has a better, or, probably, as good, claim to experience
of this kind as A. S. Griffith. We have therefore reason to trust
his judgment, and we accept his conclusions, and hold that his
work has demonstrated that an occasional case of phthisis—
perhaps one in a hundred or so—is caused by the bovine bacillus.
But at the same time we think that this position will be greatly
strengthened when we have *post-mortem* evidence of the presence
of bovine tubercle bacilli in the lesions of the lungs themselves.

Summary and Conclusions.

Bacteriological investigation of the lung tissues themselves
in cases of pulmonary tuberculosis in adults have not been very
numerous, but, so far as they have gone, they have revealed
only the presence of tubercle bacilli of human type.

---

[1] The question is further complicated by the existence of dysgonic bacilli
possessing low virulence for rabbits and calves. Of such we are likely to hear
more in future. They have already been found, as we shall see, by A. S.
Griffith in a considerable number of cases of lupus, and one is described by
Eastwood and F. Griffith, obtained from a mesenteric gland in a case of tuber-
culosis of spine and rib in a boy of nearly ten years of age (*Loc. Gov. Bd.
Reports on Public Health and Medical Subjects*, N.S. No. 88, p. 74). (See also
Appendix III, p. 680 of this volume.)

If there really are in existence tubercle bacilli of human type which grow
dysgonically, as some think there would seem to be small means of recognizing
their presence when they are mixed with bacilli of bovine type. (P.S. Griffith
has recently found them in sputum, and identified them by their production
of pigment on serum. See App. p. 681.)

Investigations of the tubercle bacilli in sputum from consumptive patients number close on a thousand. Nearly all observers have found only tubercle bacilli conforming to the human type. Two observers, Kossel and Lindemann, have each obtained an atypical strain which they judged to be a mixture of human and bovine bacilli. De Jong, some years ago, found a bacillus in sputum which he believed to be bovine, so also did Arloing in the contents of a cavity examined after death. A. S. Griffith has definitely proved the presence of bovine bacilli in the sputum of three representative cases of phthisis, and has done all that is humanly possible to prove that the bovine bacilli were not accompanied by human bacilli in these cases. It must therefore be admitted as practically certain that the bovine bacillus is occasionally responsible for a case of phthisis. But such cases are rare. Taking the figures from all sources together they appear to amount to less than one in 200, or, if we prefer to take Griffith's figures alone as more applicable to Great Britain, to about 1·7 per cent. of all cases of phthisis.

In young children it is probably not very uncommon for the lungs to become infected with bovine bacilli. In such cases the pulmonary disease is commonly part of a tuberculosis more widely spread, and usually there is evidence, in ulceration of intestine, caseation of mesenteric glands or peritoneal tubercles, of intestinal origin.

The extent of the pulmonary lesions in such cases varies. Miliary tubercles, caseous nodules, and even small cavities have all been described. But it is probable that few of these cases would be classed during life as "pulmonary tuberculosis"; rather, it seems, they would appear to be instances of abdominal tuberculosis with more or less generalization.

2. *Tuberculous Meningitis.*

Tuberculous meningitis, looked at from the pathological standpoint, appears usually as part only of a more or less general tuberculosis, starting very commonly in the bronchial or some other lymphatic glands, and spreading ·by means of the blood stream to various organs and tissues including the membranes of the brain[1]. The latter are seldom, if ever, involved alone, but the disturbance produced by implication of the central nervous system is so great that whenever the meninges are involved the case appears from the clinical point of view to be essentially one of meningitis, and is labelled as such. It is therefore under this heading that we shall consider such cases; relegating to another category other instances of general tuberculosis in which the meninges are not known to have been involved.

In a considerable number of cases of tuberculous meningitis the tubercle bacilli have been subjected to investigation by modern methods. The Royal Commission in their Final Report classify three only under this heading; but the abstracts of the post-mortem examinations which are published make it clear that either the meninges or the brain itself were involved in no less than nineteen of their cases.

From eleven of these nineteen cases the tubercle bacilli investigated were taken from the meningeal tubercles themselves, or from the brain, or cerebro-spinal fluid. In the remaining eight cases a bronchial, or mesenteric gland or one of the great organs was the source of the cultures. Of the strains of bacilli of direct meningeal or cerebro-spinal origin eight proved to be of human type and three of bovine type, while of those of indirect origin six proved to be of human type and two of bovine type. In one of these cases, H 60, the meninges themselves, the lung and the mesenteric glands all yielded bacilli of human type, while the bronchial glands yielded a mixture of human and bovine types.

Among Rothe's series of cases, which we have already referred to in connection with pulmonary tuberculosis, tuberculous meningitis is mentioned only once. This infrequency is probably to be explained by the fact that a large proportion of the twenty-one children, in whose bodies tuberculous lesions

---

[1] Steinmeyer (1914) who has recently made a statistical examination of the post-mortem material of the General Hospital at Hamburg-Eppendorff, stated that tuberculous meningitis was always secondary to tuberculosis elsewhere, and that in 44·69 of the cases it was part of a general tuberculosis.

were discovered after death, died of some other cause, such as one of the specific fevers, and therefore the tuberculosis was in an early stage and not widely disseminated. The single case of meningitis yielded, both from bronchial and mesenteric glands, tubercle bacilli of human type.

Park and Krumwiede (1911) among the cases of tuberculosis which they investigated classified twenty-seven under "Generalized Tuberculosis including Meninges" and another thirty-one, in which there was no autopsy, under "Tubercular Meningitis." Thus altogether there were fifty-eight cases in which meningitis was present[1]. The results of the investigation of the tubercle bacilli are given as follows:

Type of disease	Over 16 yrs		5–16 yrs		Under 5 yrs	
	Type of bacillus		Type of bacillus		Type of bacillus	
	H	B	H	B	H	B
Gen. tuberculosis including meninges	1	—	—	—	25	1
Tubercular meningitis (no autopsy)	1	—	2	—	26	2

There was also a case of a child who died of tuberculous meningitis when thirteen months old, and from whom a bacillus of bovine type was cultivated from the cerebro-spinal fluid and one of human type from a mesenteric gland[2].

Thus there were fifty-nine cases in all. But for our present purpose it is necessary to divide them into two groups according to the source of the bacilli which were investigated; and when we turn to the detailed accounts[3] of these cases in order to see whether the bacilli came from the meninges or cerebro-spinal fluid, or from some lesion remote from the brain we meet

[1] *Collected Studies, Res. Lab. Dep. of Health, N.Y.* 1911, p. 75.
[2] Case M. H. strains 634 and 651, mentioned at foot of table on p. 76 and again on p. 98.
[3] *Ibid.* pp. 88 *et seq.*

with difficulty. We cannot find details of more than fifty cases[1].

From these fifty cases we must rule out nineteen in which only the cultural characters of the bacilli were determined, no animal inoculations being made. From all these nineteen cases the bacilli isolated were judged to possess the cultural characters of the human type. The remaining thirty-one cases are incorporated in the table which will presently follow. They include all the instances of infection with bacilli of bovine type.

Of the thirty-one cases there were twenty-seven in which the bacilli were obtained directly from meningeal tubercles or from cerebro-spinal fluid. Twenty-three of these yielded bacilli of human type and four yielded bacilli of bovine type. From one of these latter however a culture of human type was obtained from a mesenteric gland[2]. There were also four cases from which the bacilli came from some part other than meninges or cerebro-spinal fluid; all of these yielded bacilli of human type.

It is remarkable how very young were the majority of the children examined by Park and Krumwiede. No less than fifteen were twelve months or under, and fourteen between the age of one and two years.

Among the cases investigated in the Gesundheitsamt by Kossel, Weber and Heuss[3] and by Weber and Taute[4], we find ten in which tuberculous meningitis or tuberculosis of the brain, was present along with more or less tuberculosis elsewhere. In nine of these cases the bacilli were obtained from the meningeal or cerebral tubercles, as well as from other parts. Of these, seven yielded bacilli of human type and two bacilli of bovine type. In one case the only strain of bacilli investigated came from bronchial and mesenteric glands. It proved to be of bovine type. The oldest of these patients was seven years of age.

---

[1] The omission of these nine cases is not of much importance since all of them were instances of infection with human tubercle bacilli; that is to say they were similar in this respect to an overwhelming majority of the cases, and therefore the omission of them makes very little difference to the ratio of human to bovine infections.

[2] Case M. H. mentioned on previous page.

[3] *Tub. Arbeiten, etc.* Heft 3, p. 51.   [4] *Ibid.* Heft 6, p. 50.

Thus altogether we have ten cases of general tuberculosis with meningitis or cerebral tubercle, in three of which the infection was with bovine bacilli and in seven with human bacilli. These latter include one (No. 74) in which the meningeal tubercles yielded a strain of human type while the mesenteric glands yielded one of bovine type.

In the series of children whose lymphatic glands were examined for tubercle bacilli, after death from various causes, by Ungermann in the Gesundheitsamt (1912) there were, as we have already seen, thirty-nine cases in which tuberculous infection was found. Of these thirty-nine children, twelve suffered from tuberculous meningitis. The bacilli in the meningeal tubercles themselves were not investigated, but only those in the various groups of lymphatic glands. From these in every instance the bacilli isolated proved to be of human type. In one case only is the age definitely stated to be over five years. In another, the age is given in one place as *two* years and five months and in another as *ten* years and five months. This case therefore we have been unable to include in the tabulated results.

It will be remembered that Eastwood and F. Griffith, on behalf of the Local Government Board, examined for tubercle bacilli the various groups of lymphatic glands taken post-mortem from a large number of children who had died of all sorts of causes. Among these were found ninety-four instances of infection with tubercle, and among these meningitis is mentioned, either as having been diagnosed during life or found after death, thirty-four times. In one case (No. 100) the diagnosis "meningitis" was not confirmed at the post-mortem examination, and in seven others diagnosed as meningitis there is no mention in the post-mortem notes of confirmatory evidence. For this reason, and because it is not clear that the word meningitis was intended necessarily to imply *tuberculous* meningitis, these eight cases have not been included in our table. There remain then twenty-six cases in which definite meningeal tuberculosis was found after death. Three of these cases yielded tubercle bacilli of bovine type, one from bronchial and mesenteric glands, one from mesenteric glands and liver, and the third from liver and spleen. From the remaining twenty-three the tubercle bacilli were of human type. The tubercle bacilli were isolated mostly from various lymphatic glands, and in no case did the cultures investigated come from the meningeal tubercles themselves. All the children were under ten years of age.

Case 96 is of interest as an instance of infection with bovine tubercle bacilli causing an almost pure meningitis. A male child died just under three years of age. At the post-mortem examination there was "well-marked tuberculous meningitis with classical distribution and tubercles easily visible." But elsewhere there was remarkably little evidence of tuberculosis to be seen. There were indeed traces of old pleurisy and in the lungs some emphysema and bronchitis, but no evidence that these lesions had a tuberculous origin. The bronchial glands were small and failed to infect guinea-pigs. The tubercle bacilli had probably entered through the intestine, for, though there was no ulceration and the mesenteric glands appeared normal, the latter when injected produced tuberculosis in guinea-pigs. The liver was the only organ which showed any change of a tuberculous character. Beneath its capsule were a few grey foci, and injection of an emulsion of part of the organ produced tuberculosis in guinea-pigs. The bacilli from both liver and mesenteric glands were of the bovine type.

Of the eight cases omitted for reasons mentioned above, one (No. 47) yielded a bovine bacillus from bronchial and mesenteric glands.

Of the forty-five cases of tuberculosis which, as we have seen, were investigated for the Local Government Board by A. S. Griffith there were eighteen in which there was tuberculous meningitis. In none of these cases were the tubercle bacilli isolated from the meninges themselves or from the brain, but they were derived in the main from lymphatic glands and, in a few cases, from organs other than the brain. Three cases yielded bovine tubercle bacilli, and one a mixed culture.

In this latter case[1] three strains of tubercle bacilli were isolated from two guinea-pigs injected with the emulsified bronchial glands. Two of these strains were pure cultures of bovine tubercle bacilli, while the third was pronounced to be a mixture of human and bovine tubercle bacilli. This is a very curious result. The other fourteen cases yielded strains of human tubercle bacilli only.

Mitchell (1914) investigated the tubercle bacilli obtained from the lymphatic glands of twelve children who died in the

[1] No. 31, *loc. cit.* pp. 131 and 163.

Tuberculous Meningitis.

Source of bacilli tested	Authors	Over 16 years Type of bacillus		5–16 years Type of bacillus		Under 5 years Type of bacillus	
		H	B	H	B	H	B
Meningeal tubercles, brain or cerebro-spinal fluid	Royal Commission ...	—	—	2	0	6[2]	3
	Park and Krumwiede ...	—	—	—	—	23	4[3]
	Kossel, Weber, etc.[1] ...	—	—	1	0	6[4]	2
	Mitchell	—	—	—	—	0	1
	Total	—	—	3	0	35	10
Some lymph gland, or organ other than brain	Royal Commission ...	—	—	1	0	5	2
	Park and Krumwiede ...	—	—	—	—	4	0
	Kossel, Weber, etc.[1] ...	—	—	—	—	0	1
	Ungermann	—	—	1	0	10	0
	Eastwood and F. Griffith	—	—	11	1	12	2
	A. S. Griffith	—	—	2	1[5]	12	3
	Mitchell	—	—	1	—	2	2
	Total	—	—	16	2	45	10
	Grand total ...	—	—	19	2	80	20

[1] Kossel, Weber and Heuss, *loc. cit.* Heft 3, p. 50, and Weber and Taute, *ibid.* Heft 6, p. 51.

[2] Including H 60, in which cultures from the meninges, lungs, and mesenteric glands were of human type and those from bronchial glands a mixture of both human and bovine types. Including also H 13 classed by the Commission as having yielded a mixed virus, but on grounds which seem to the writer insufficient (see chapter on "Stability of Type," p. 331).

[3] Including case M. H. in which a culture from the meninges was of bovine type and one from the mesenteric glands of human type. A somewhat surprising combination (*loc. cit.* p. 98).

[4] Including case 74 in which the meninges yielded a culture of human type and the mesenteric glands one of bovine type.

[5] Including case 31 which yielded, through guinea-pigs injected from a bronchial gland, three strains of tubercle bacilli of which "two were pure cultures of bovine tubercle bacilli, and one a mixed culture of human and bovine tubercle bacilli" (*loc. cit.* p. 132).

Hospital for Sick Children in Edinburgh. In six of these children there was tuberculous meningitis. Five of them were under five years of age. Two yielded bovine bacilli—from mesenteric, and mesenteric and cervical glands respectively; another yielded bovine tubercle bacilli from the meninges themselves; while three yielded tubercle bacilli of human type from two or more sets of lymphatic glands.

It is remarkable how strong is the evidence afforded by the researches of Ungermann, of Eastwood and F. Griffith, and of A. S. Griffith in favour of the conclusion that the common portal of entry of the infection in tuberculous meningitis is afforded by the air passages and not the alimentary canal. Again and again one finds in the notes of all these observers that the bronchial glands were affected severely, and the mesenteric glands to a much lesser extent or not at all. It is remarkable too how constantly in these cases of infection through the air passages the tubercle bacilli turned out to be of the human type. On the other hand there is a respectable minority of cases of meningitis in which there can be no reasonable doubt that the bacilli passed in through the intestinal mucosa. Such cases have sometimes been found to be due to the bovine type and sometimes to the human type of bacillus[1].

Conclusion.

From the table on p. 575 it is clear that the great majority of cases of tuberculous meningitis are caused by the human type of tubercle bacillus. It is quite certain however that a minority, perhaps about 18 per cent., are caused by bovine bacilli. Bacilli of this type have been isolated from tubercles in the meninges themselves and from cerebro-spinal fluid by several observers, English, German and American.

The great majority of cases are caused by tubercle bacilli which have been inhaled into the air passages of the lung, and have left evidence of the route they have followed in the bronchial glands. In such cases the bacilli seem to be always of the human type. A minority of cases are due to tubercle bacilli

---

[1] No. 45, reported by A. S. Griffith, is a good example of the latter.

which have found their way in through the intestines, and
have left evidence of their passage in the mesenteric glands.
Some of these cases are caused by bovine and others by human
tubercle bacilli.

3. *General Tuberculosis (not including Meningitis).*

It is not easy to frame a definition of general tuberculosis
which will serve for the due selection of cases for this section.
On the one hand one wishes to include all cases in which there
is evidence of widespread distribution of bacilli by the blood
stream, and on the other to exclude such cases as show a
predominant infection of any one organ, such as would cause
them to appear during life as, let us say, pulmonary tuberculosis,
or meningitis rather than general tuberculosis. It would be
obviously undesirable to include under this heading a severe
case of lung disease because there were a few tubercles
in the spleen; for the clinical aspect of the case cannot be
ignored in making our selection. But, naturally, there are all
degrees of dissemination and if we are to pass over the minor
ones the question arises where are we to draw the line. Some
investigators, such as Park and Krumwiede make their own
classification, but the majority give little help towards framing
a class of general tuberculosis such as we are aiming at; and it
must be understood that in this review of the work of various
authors the writer is, as a rule, responsible for the selection of
cases put into this class, and, it must be added, to some extent
for that of the other classes also.

It is difficult to avoid some overlapping. A given case
may be interesting from more than one of its points of view.
It may be a very pronounced case of general tuberculosis, and
yet, perhaps on account of disease in a joint, one which it would
not be right to exclude from the category of bone and joint tuberculosis. Instances however of a case being included in more
than one class are few, and whenever a repetition occurs attention is directed to the fact that the case has appeared before.

Among the cases investigated by the Royal Commission are
six which may fairly be considered instances of general tuberculosis, and in the records of which there is no mention of

meningitis or of disease preponderant in any one organ.   All these cases occurred in children under five years of age.   The bacilli from three of them were found to be of bovine type, while those from the other three were of human type.

This is a remarkably high proportion of bovine infections, and is, as we shall see, in marked contrast to the results of other authors.   It is however easily explained by the fact that during a large part of the Commission's labours cases of primary abdominal tuberculosis were deliberately sought out and selected for investigation.   All these six cases showed evidence of infection through the alimentary tract[1].

Park and Krumwiede classify twenty-eight of their cases as general tuberculosis without meningitis, twenty-five being children under five years of age.   The tubercle bacilli obtained from six of the latter were of bovine type.   Those isolated from the remaining twenty-two cases were of human type.

Rothe, in his series already referred to, described five cases as miliary tuberculosis.   The ages varied from eight months to three years.   All yielded tubercle bacilli of human type.

Among Ungermann's cases are five labelled either general tuberculosis or miliary tuberculosis.   The ages varied from four months to nearly four years.   The tubercle bacilli from all these cases proved to be of human type.

From the cases investigated by Eastwood and F. Griffith eleven may be selected as instances of general tuberculosis without meningitis.   Ten of these yielded tubercle bacilli of human type, and one tubercle bacilli of bovine type.   This latter was evidently a case of intestinal invasion.   Both bronchial and mesenteric glands were affected, but the latter were the more severely diseased, and there was also tuberculous peritonitis.   The child was two years and three months old.

Of the cases investigated by A. S. Griffith for the Local Government Board there are four which may be included in the class we are now considering.   All yielded tubercle bacilli of human type.

---

[1] The three cases which yielded bovine bacilli are H 14, H 32, and H 89. The first two will be found in vol. II, App. *Int. Rep. R.C.T.* and the last in vol. I, *Fin. Rep.*

Among Mitchell's cases are four described as general tuberculosis, and in which there is no mention of meningitis. All occurred in young children, and all yielded from various lymphatic glands tubercle bacilli of human type.

General Tuberculosis (without Meningitis).

Authors	Over 16 yrs Type of bacillus		5–16 yrs Type of bacillus		Under 5 yrs Type of bacillus	
	H	B	H	B	H	B
Royal Commission ...	—	—	—	—	3	3
Park and Krumwiede ...	2	0	1	0	19	6
Rothe	—	—	—	—	5	0
Ungermann	—	—	—	—	5	0
Eastwood and F. Griffith	—	—	6	0	4	1
A S. Griffith	—	—	3	0	1	0
Mitchell	—	—	—	—	4	0
Total	2	0	10	0	41	10

Conclusion.

From this table we see that sixty-three cases of general tuberculosis without meningitis have been investigated, and that 10, or nearly 16 per cent. of them, have yielded bacilli of bovine type. If we were to add the 122 cases of meningitis, which included 22 (or 18 per cent.) bovine infections, we should have in all 185 cases of which thirty-two yielded bovine bacilli, thus giving a proportion of bovine infections in general tuberculosis of all kinds of 17·3 per cent. These numbers probably over-represent the proportion of bovine infections in such cases, owing to the method by which the Royal Commission cases were selected. Almost all the instances of infection with bovine bacilli have occurred in children under five years of age.

4. *Primary Abdominal Tuberculous Infection.*

We have next to consider cases of primary abdominal tuberculosis, characterized particularly by disease of mesenteric glands, and in some cases also by that of intestines and peritoneum. Several cases of primary abdominal tuberculosis which led to general tuberculosis and in some instances to meningitis have already been considered under another heading, and it is difficult to know whether to include them in this category also. To do so would doubtless create a more comprehensive group of that kind of tuberculosis which begins with invasion through the intestinal mucosa; but, on the other hand, it would tend to give a false impression of the relative importance of the part played by bovine tubercle bacilli, for, as we shall see, infection with that type of organism is relatively much commoner in this class of tuberculosis than in those we have already considered, so that to repeat some of these cases would be to duplicate an undue proportion of bovine infections. On the whole it has appeared best to avoid repetition as far as possible and we have consequently excluded them.

We shall therefore consider in this section only those cases in which the mesenteric glands contained lesions obviously older and more advanced than those, if any, present in bronchial and cervical glands, and in which there was no very serious generalization beyond the abdominal cavity; and to these we must add a few cases in which there was no obvious tuberculous disease anywhere, but in which it was proved, after death from causes other than tuberculosis, that the mesenteric glands alone were infected with tubercle bacilli.

The Appendices to the Reports of the Royal Commission contain ten cases which conform to this definition. Of six cases under five years of age two yielded tubercle bacilli of human type and four tubercle bacilli of bovine type. In three cases between the ages of five and sixteen this proportion was reversed, two yielding tubercle bacilli of human type and one tubercle bacilli of bovine type. There was in addition a case of tuberculosis in a man, seventy years of age, who was found after death to have tuberculosis of the mesenteric and retro-peritoneal glands, and intestinal adhesions, but no tuberculosis elsewhere.   In this case A. S. Griffith obtained from a mesenteric gland a culture of human type and from a retro-peritoneal gland one containing bacilli of both human and bovine types.   Taking all the ten cases together we find a proportion of about 50 per cent. of bovine infections.

If we were to include all cases showing evidence of infection through the intestinal portals whether complicated with tuberculous meningitis or serious pulmonary disease or no, we should have in all twenty-eight cases of which thirteen yielded bovine bacilli, thirteen human bacilli and two (adults) mixtures of both these types.   Thus the exclusion of cases with preponderant disease in pia mater or lungs does not alter the proportion of human and bovine infections.

In 1907 Weber drew up a summary of all the cases investigated up to that time at the Gesundheitsamt.   These included twenty cases of "primary intestinal and mesenteric tuberculosis" among children, and six cases of the same kind, and three of peritonitis, and one of tuberculosis of the retro-peritoneal glands among adults.   Of the twenty cases in children thirteen yielded bovine bacilli and seven human bacilli; while of the ten adults nine yielded human bacilli and one a mixed culture.

If we exclude the cases of meningitis and general tuberculosis which have already been dealt with, there remain twenty-three cases of which eight were adults, eight children between five and sixteen years, and seven infants under five years of age. Among the adults one (H 33) yielded a mixture of bacilli, and the rest bacilli of human type: of the children five yielded bovine and three human bacilli: while of the infants four yielded bovine and three human bacilli.   Thus of the cases under sixteen years, 60 per cent. yielded bovine bacilli.

Park and Krumwiede include under the heading Abdominal Tuberculosis only seven of their cases.   There were however many other instances of tuberculosis which appeared to have begun in the abdomen, but these had led to serious disease elsewhere and had been relegated to other categories.   Of the seven cases three were found to be infected with human tubercle bacilli and four with bovine tubercle bacilli.

Of Rothe's cases it is only possible to include two in this

class. There was no visible tuberculosis in either; but in each the mesenteric glands proved infective to guinea-pigs, while the bronchial glands did not. In both cases the tubercle bacilli proved to be of human type.

In Ungermann's paper precise information is given as to the relative degree of severity of the disease in the various groups of lymphatic glands; so that it is easy to assign the cases to one of three classes, according as bronchial, mesenteric, or cervical glands are alone or principally affected, or to a fourth class in which two or more of these groups of glands are more or less equally involved. Cases which showed tuberculosis of lungs, meningitis, or general miliary tuberculosis have already been picked out. There remain three cases which can be regarded as instances of primary abdominal tuberculous infection. In all these cases death was independent of tuberculosis. In two of them definitely tuberculous lesions were limited to the mesenteric glands; while in the third all three groups of glands appeared normal, but on injection the mesenteric alone caused tuberculosis. The tubercle bacilli from two of these cases (both infants) were of human type. Those from the remaining case, a child of six years who died of sepsis, and in whose body three caseous mesenteric glands were found, were of bovine type.

In Eastwood and F. Griffith's series there are eight cases which may be regarded as instances of primary tuberculous infection of mesenteric glands. In three of these there was no obvious tuberculosis anywhere, the children having died of diarrhœa and wasting, heart disease or accident, but in each case injection of mesenteric glands into guinea-pigs caused tuberculosis, while injection of bronchial glands failed to do so. Cultures were obtained in each of these cases from guinea-pigs inoculated with the mesenteric glands. In two cases the strain of bacilli proved to be of bovine, and in one of human type. In one case, where the cause of death was heart disease, tuberculous lesions were found in the mesenteric glands but not elsewhere. These glands yielded a strain of bacilli of bovine type. Four were cases of tuberculous peritonitis. Of these, three yielded bacilli of bovine, and one bacilli of human type.

In one of these cases infected with bovine tubercle bacilli there was some tuberculous broncho-pneumonia.

In the series of cases investigated by A. S. Griffith for the Local Government Board are three which may be regarded as instances of primary mesenteric tuberculosis without serious dissemination. One of these died of "tabes mesenterica," one of broncho-pneumonia apparently non-tuberculous, and the third of an accident. The bacilli from the first and last of these cases proved to be of bovine type, while that from the second case were found to be of human type.

One of Mitchell's cases was an instance of tuberculous peritonitis in a child a year and five months old. The caseous mesenteric glands yielded a culture of bovine tubercle bacilli.

Abdominal Tuberculosis.

Authors	Adults over 16 yrs			Children 5–16 yrs		Infants under 5 yrs	
	Type of bacillus			Type of bacillus		Type of bacillus	
	Human	Bovine	Mixture	Human	Bovine	Human	Bovine
Royal Commission ...	—	—	1[1]	2	1	2	4
Park and Krumwiede ...	1	0	0	1	1	1	3
Gesundheitsamt (Weber)	7	0	1	3	5	3	4
Rothe	—	—	—	—	—	2	0
Ungermann	—	—	—	—	1	2	0
Eastwood and F. Griffith	—	—	—	—	3	2	3
A. S. Griffith	—	—	—	—	—	1	2
Mitchell	—	—	—	—	—	0	1
Total	8	0	2	6	11	13	17

Conclusion.

Taking all cases of abdominal tuberculosis and excluding such as had developed preponderant disease elsewhere than

[1] A culture of human type was obtained from the mesenteric glands of this case, and one containing both bovine and human bacilli from a retro-peritoneal gland.

in the abdominal cavity, and which have already been dealt with in other classes, and excluding also the (two) cases in which both types of bacilli were present, we find that rather more than half, or to be more precise nearly 51 per cent., were caused by bovine tubercle bacilli. But the proportion is greatly affected by the relative number of adults and children examined; for among the adults there was no case of pure infection with bovine bacilli, and among the children and infants considerably more than half, or nearly 60 per cent., were of this kind.

5. *Tuberculosis of Bronchial Glands.*

We must next consider certain cases of tuberculous infection where the bronchial glands are affected, either alone, or to an obviously greater extent than the mesenteric or cervical glands. And again, in order to avoid inclusion of cases which have already been considered under another heading, instances showing general tuberculosis, meningitis or marked pulmonary disease will have to be omitted. This omission limits us very largely to cases where tuberculosis of bronchial glands is discovered unexpectedly, after death from other causes than tuberculosis.

Among the cases which the Royal Commission investigated there is only one which falls under this head. This was (H 21) a girl who died at the age of sixteen of heart disease, and in whose body caseous bronchial glands were found without sign of tuberculosis elsewhere. The tubercle bacilli cultivated from these glands proved to be of human type.

One of the cases investigated at the Gesundheitsamt was of this kind (H 55)[1]. In a child of four and a half years, who died of colitis and convulsions, cervical mesenteric and bronchial glands were all enlarged, but the bronchials alone were caseous and partly calcareous. A strain of tubercle bacilli raised from a guinea-pig injected with an emulsion of these glands proved to be of human type.

Four of Rothe's cases fit into this group—all children under two years of age who died of some cause other than tuberculosis.

[1] *loc. cit.* Heft 3, p. 79.

In one case (No. 4) some of the bronchial glands were calcareous. In another (No. 8) these glands looked suspicious and provoked tuberculosis in guinea-pigs, while in the two remaining (Nos. 56 and 68) nothing is said of their appearance but they caused tuberculosis when injected. There does not appear to have been any tuberculous infection in these four cases, except in the bronchial glands. The bacilli from all of them were of human type.

Among the cases investigated by Ungermann four come under this heading. One alone died of tuberculosis. The extent of the disease in this case[1] is not recorded. The bronchial glands were enlarged and caseous, the mesenterics slightly enlarged and the cervicals apparently normal. All three sets of glands caused tuberculosis in guinea-pigs. In two cases the bronchial glands were the only parts visibly affected with tubercle; while in the remaining case an apparently normal bronchial gland caused tuberculosis on injection. The tubercle bacilli from all these cases proved to belong to the human type.

Four cases may be claimed for this class from Eastwood and F. Griffith's series. All occurred in children between the ages of four and seven years who died of various causes unconnected with tuberculosis. In one the majority of the bronchial glands were enlarged up to the size of thrushs' eggs. There was a small caseous nodule and a few minute tubercles in the lungs, and some sparsely scattered tubercles in the spleen. In another, besides a caseo-calcareous nodule as large as a pea in a bronchial gland, there was in addition a nodule of much the same size in the lungs. In the third case a calcareous bronchial gland was the only part visibly affected, while in the fourth, in which death had occurred at the age of four from " anæmia," an apparently normal bronchial gland proved infective on injection. The bacilli derived from this latter case proved to be of bovine type, while those from the other three were of human type. In the case where a bovine bacillus was derived from an apparently normal bronchial gland the mesenteric glands, which also were unaltered in appearance, were injected into guinea-pigs with negative results.

[1] H XI, *loc. cit.* Heft 12, p. 179.

From A. S. Griffith's cases four may be selected for inclusion in this group. The ages ranged from eleven months to six years. None of them died of tuberculosis. In one there was a doubtful looking focus in a bronchial gland which proved infective, and there were also some caseo-purulent foci in the spleen, but these did not produce tuberculosis on injection. The child aged eleven months had died of broncho-pneumonia. In one case the bronchial glands were caseous, and no other parts were affected, and in the two remaining cases apparently normal bronchial glands provoked tuberculosis on injection into guinea-pigs, while the mesenteric glands failed to infect. The bacilli in every case belonged to the human type.

Thus out of the eighteen cases investigated by various authors there is only one in which the bronchial glands contained a bovine tubercle bacillus; and that was in a case where there was no visible sign of tuberculosis either in these glands or elsewhere.

Bronchial Gland Tuberculosis.

	Type of bacillus	
Authors	Human	Bovine
Royal Commission ...	1	0
Gesundheitsamt (Weber)	1	0
Rothe	4	0
Ungermann	4	0
Eastwood and F. Griffith	3	1
A. S. Griffith	4	0
Total	17	1

Conclusion.

Primary tuberculosis of the bronchial glands is caused in the great majority of cases by the human tubercle bacillus. The evidence of the preponderance of infection with human tubercle bacilli in cases of bronchial gland tuberculosis would be greatly increased if we were to include cases of general tuberculosis, meningitis, etc. in which there is evidence of primary disease in these glands.

6. Tuberculosis apparently Primary in Two or more Groups of Lymphatic Glands.

In the various series of cases that we have been considering a good many instances of early tuberculosis may be found which cannot be placed in any of the foregoing classes, because the tuberculous disease, while limited more or less completely to lymphatic glands, is not confined to, or even predominant in, any one group of glands, but affects two or more groups to very much the same extent, so that one cannot guess at the portal of entry, or must assume an invasion through more portals than one. These cases must therefore be considered under a separate heading.

One of the cases investigated by the Royal Commission, and already referred to in the section on abdominal tuberculosis, may be referred to again here; but it is not included in the table which follows. A girl child aged nearly four years died of tuberculosis. The case was described as one of "primary mesenteric tuberculosis and generalized tuberculous adenitis." Bronchial, mesenteric, cervical and inguinal glands, all were affected. It was difficult to say whether the disease in the bronchial or mesenteric glands was the more advanced. Abdominal disease, however, predominated over thoracic, for while there was extensive ulceration of the intestine and some peritoneal adhesions, there were but some seven or eight shot-sized tubercles in the lungs. The tubercle bacilli from both bronchial and mesenteric glands were of the human type. This seems to have been a case of a double, perhaps simultaneous, infection through the bronchial and intestinal portals.

Among the cases investigated in the Gesundheitsamt up to 1907 and summarized by Weber were two which may be held to have belonged to the class we are now considering. In one of them caseo-calcareous bronchial and mesenteric glands were the only tuberculous lesions found in a woman who died from carcinoma at the age of sixty-nine. A strain of tubercle bacilli raised from a guinea-pig infected from a mesenteric gland proved to be of human type. The other was the case of a child who died at the age of six and a half years from intestinal tuberculosis, and from whose bronchial and mesenteric glands bovine tubercle bacilli were cultivated[1].

[1] This was H 84 (loc. cit. Heft 6, p. 73). It seems not unlikely that in this case the tuberculous disease began in the bronchial glands; for while some of these were as large as small walnuts and caseous, the mesenteric

Of Rothe's cases there were two in which both bronchial and mesenteric glands were infected with tubercle bacilli to much the same extent, and in which there does not appear to have been any tuberculosis elsewhere.   In one case the infective glands were normal in appearance while in the other both groups were caseous.   The bacilli cultivated from each of these cases were of human type.

Of Ungermann's cases six may perhaps be put into this class, though in four there was no visible tuberculous disease; the reason for their inclusion being that two or more sets of apparently normal or suspicious looking lymphatic glands when emulsified and injected into guinea-pigs caused tuberculosis. The other two cases might perhaps have been placed in another class had particulars been given, for they died of tuberculous disease; but in what organ is not stated[1]. One of these six cases yielded a bovine type of tubercle bacillus from cervical, bronchial, and mesenteric glands, all of which appeared to be normal.   The child had succumbed to diphtheria when nearly four years old.   The remaining five cases yielded strains of tubercle bacilli of human type.

Among the cases investigated by Eastwood and F. Griffith are two which may be included in this section.   In one death was due to accident, in the other to typhoid fever.   The age in each case was five years.   In neither were the glands obviously tuberculous, though the mesenteric were enlarged. In one cervical, bronchial and mesenteric, and in the other bronchial and mesenteric glands yielded cultures of human tubercle bacilli.

Two of A. S. Griffith's cases fall into this group.   One, a boy of eight and a half years who died of shock following operation for tuberculous spine, showed calcareous nodules in

glands were only swollen and reddened, while in a few of them there were a few small fresh tubercles.   On the other hand there was no pulmonary or pharyngeal tuberculosis from which the intestines might have received their infection and the latter were very severely ulcerated indeed.   The writer considered whether this case should not have been placed in the previous class of bronchial gland tuberculosis, but on the whole it seemed to him best to treat it as one of probable double infection.

[1] Cases XVIII and XXVIII, *loc. cit.* Heft 12, pp. 183 and 194.

bronchial and mesenteric glands. Culture and inoculation experiments with these nodules gave negative results—the tubercle bacilli in them were, presumably, dead; but an apparently normal cervical gland injected into a guinea-pig caused tuberculosis, and a culture raised from this animal proved to be of human type. The other case occurred in a child aged two who died of measles. Caseous bronchial and mesenteric glands were found after death, and these yielded cultures of tubercle bacilli of bovine type.

Tuberculosis of Two or more Groups of Lymphatic Glands.

Authors	Type of bacillus	
	Human	Bovine
Gesundheitsamt (Weber)	1	1
Rothe	2	0
Ungermann	5	1
Eastwood and F. Griffith	2	0
A. S. Griffith	1	1
Total	11	3

7. *Tuberculosis of Cervical Glands.*

When tuberculosis occurs in one or more of the cervical glands, the disease, as it is seen during life, usually seems to be limited to those structures, and deep-seated mischief is, as a rule, hardly suspected. But post-mortem examination has shown that it is the exception for tuberculosis to be limited to these glands, even in those who die of causes which have nothing to do with tuberculosis and in whom the tuberculous infection is in an early stage. Quite commonly bronchial or mesenteric glands, or both, are tuberculous as well as the cervicals. This comes out very clearly from the investigations of Ungermann for the Gesundheitsamt in Berlin, and from those of Eastwood and F. Griffith, and of A. S. Griffith for the Local Government Board in this country.

The cervical glands (using the term in its more comprehensive sense) transmit lymph from the nose, mouth and pharynx, and thus belong both to the respiratory and the alimentary systems.   They are therefore liable to receive bacilli both from the air and the food.   But, to judge from the relative frequency with which bovine tubercle bacilli are found in these glands when diseased—a frequency which corresponds to that found in abdominal tuberculosis, rather than to what occurs in tuberculosis of the lungs and bronchial glands—it is probable that food-borne infections greatly predominate.   Exactly why this should be is a little hard to say. Perhaps it is because bacilli wrapped up in food material are more apt to cling about carious teeth or to lodge in depressions in the surface of the tonsils than are those which are carried in the air stream.

It is probable that the tonsils afford the main portal of entry for the tubercle bacilli which reach the cervical glands. Tuberculosis in these structures is not unfrequent, though it does not attract much attention during life owing to the absence of definite symptoms.   Professor Pybus has recently compiled a list of ten separate investigations in which a total of 762 hypertrophied tonsils removed during life were tested by inoculation.   No less than 6·7 per cent. of these inoculations caused tuberculosis.

The question of the type of bacilli found in glandular tuberculosis has received more attention in this group than in any other.   This is doubtless because the cervical glands are pre-eminently accessible to surgical interference, and thus material for their investigation is provided more abundantly than is the case with any other group   Moreover to many minds the pathological study of a case of disease loses much of its interest when the patient ceases to live, though it is obvious that during life investigation can only be incomplete.

Weber, summarizing in 1907 the work done up to that time in the laboratories of the Gesundheitsamt, Berlin (including the investigations of Kossel, Weber and Heuss, Weber and Taute, and Oehlecker) reported altogether the results of investigating the types of tubercle bacilli found in tuberculous cervical glands removed from eighteen persons. In a considerable majority of the cases the bacilli were of human type. From two adults the bacilli were of this kind, and from sixteen children they were of human type in ten cases and of bovine type in six cases.

Burckhardt (1910) investigated the bacilli from nine cases of cervical gland tuberculosis. Five persons over fifteen years of age all yielded bacilli of human type, and of four children between five and sixteen three gave bacilli of human type and one bacilli of bovine type.

The Royal Commission about the same time included in their Second Interim Report nine cases in which the type of tubercle bacilli isolated from cervical glands, removed by operation during life, was determined. One of these cannot be included in the table which follows because the age is not recorded. The bacilli obtained from it were of human type. To the rest may be added another case in which the bacilli investigated came from axillary glands, the cervicals having been removed previously. These nine cases all occurred in children between one and twelve years of age. Six of them (including the axillary case) yielded bacilli of human type and three bacilli of bovine type.

Other investigations have yielded a higher proportion of bovine infections. In America Theobald Smith and Brown (1907) found tubercle bacilli of bovine type in tonsils removed during life from three children suffering from tuberculosis in their cervical glands. As these cases were admittedly selected for publication as instances of bovine infection they obviously do not help to determine the relative frequency of such infection, and they are not included in the table which follows.

Lewis (1910), working at Smith's suggestion and under his immediate supervision, made a study of the tubercle bacilli cultivated from cervical glands removed during life from seventeen persons of various ages. In two cases injection of the glandular material failed to infect guinea-pigs. In the remaining fifteen cases cultures were obtained from inoculated animals. Of these cultures six proved to be of human and nine of bovine type. This gives a ratio of 60 per cent. of bovine infections, which is much higher than that found by the Royal Commission or by the Gesundheitsamt (namely 33·3 per cent.). Lewis seems to have added three cases later, for Park and Krumwiede in summarizing the literature make eighteen in all, seven of which yielded human and eleven bovine bacilli[1]   These authors also obtained from Lewis the ages of his cases (which had not been previously communicated) and thus enabled the figures to be grouped according to age, and to be compared with those of other authors.

The proportion of infections with bovine bacilli in Lewis's cases was very high in early life, and diminished rapidly with age; thus while three cases under five years of age all yielded bacilli of bovine type (100 per cent.), nine between five and sixteen yielded seven bovine and two human strains (75 per cent.), and six over sixteen years of age yielded one bovine strain and five human (17 per cent. of bovine infections).

Litterer (1910), also working in America, examined the bacilli obtained from eleven cases and found those from five to be of human type, and those from six to be of bovine type. As he does not give the ages of the patients from whom the glands were obtained it is not possible to place them in our table.

Park and Krumwiede (1911), working for the Department of Health of the City of New York, undertook a more extensive investigation.   The cervical glands removed by operation from fifty-three persons were examined by these authors, and the type of tubercle bacilli which they contained determined.   To these cases may be added two more in which the primary focus of the disease was cervical, though the glands which actually furnished the bacilli investigated were axillary.

Of these fifty-five cases thirty-four (including the two last mentioned) yielded tubercle bacilli of human type and twenty-one bacilli of bovine type.   Again we find the proportion of bovine infections diminishing rapidly with age; for while nineteen children under five years of age gave 70 per cent. of bovine infections, twenty-seven aged from five to sixteen gave only 30 per cent., and among nine adults there were no instances of bovine infection.

[1] *Collected Studies*, Dep. of Health, N.Y. vol. v, p. 138.

So far we have been considering operation cases, examined during life—cases, that is to say, which would appear to the clinical observer as instances of primary tuberculosis of cervical glands. Let us turn now for a moment to cases where these glands have been examined after death, whether this occurred from tuberculosis or from some other cause. At the Gesundheitsamt Ungermann (1912) made, as we have seen already, an investigation of the types of tubercle bacilli found in the lymphatic glands of children who died from various causes in a general hospital. Among 171 cases he found thirty-nine in which one or more, and usually several, of the various groups of lymphatic glands were either visibly tuberculous, or at least capable of causing tuberculosis when injected into animals. In twenty-nine of these fatal cases tuberculosis was the principal, or at least an accessory, cause of death. In ten death was due to measles, scarlet fever, or some cause unconnected with tuberculosis. Among the twenty-nine cases in which death was due to tuberculosis the cervical glands were visibly tuberculous in thirteen, suspicious in appearance and infective on inoculation in twelve, and apparently normal but infective in three. Among the ten cases in which death was due to other causes than tubercle the cervical glands were visibly tuberculous in one (No. 6), suspicious and infective in two, and normal but infective in one. Only in seven of the thirty-nine cases in which there was evidence of tuberculous infection elsewhere were the cervical glands neither visibly tuberculous nor infective. It is therefore extremely common for these glands to be involved when there is tuberculous disease in some other situation. It is also a remarkable fact that in this series of cases, which included 132 children who died of all sorts of causes other than tuberculosis, there was not one in which the cervical glands were the sole, or even the principal seat of tuberculous disease; nor were these glands ever affected without the bronchials and mesenterics, and often both these groups of glands, being involved also. It would appear then that the cervical glands are seldom affected alone, although this frequently appears to be the case to the clinical observer.

In one of these cases only did the cervical glands yield bovine bacilli. This was a case, already mentioned in the last section, in which, after death from diphtheria at the age of nearly four years, cervical, bronchial and mesenteric glands, though apparently normal in appearance, proved on injection into guinea-pigs to be capable of setting up tuberculosis.

In Weber and Taute's cases are two of general miliary tuberculosis in which tubercle bacilli from cervical glands, along with those from other organs, were investigated[1]. One of these, aged four years, yielded a strain of tubercle bacilli of human type, and the other, aged three years and nine months, yielded one of bovine type.

Among the fatal cases investigated by the Royal Commission were five in which the tubercle bacilli from cervical glands, together with those from other parts, were studied. Three yielded human bacilli and two bovine bacilli.

These cases having all proved fatal from tuberculosis, either general, or dominant in some organ other than cervical glands, have already appeared in other sections and will not be included in the table which follows. We have excluded also the cases of Ungermann and of Weber and Taute which have just been reviewed. They would never during life have been classed as examples of cervical gland tuberculosis. Out of a total of thirty-nine cases thus excluded only four yielded bacilli of bovine type. Among the thirty-five which died of tuberculosis bovine bacilli were only found in three (8·6 per cent.), we may therefore conclude that when the cervical glands are involved as part of a severe tuberculous infection centred elsewhere, the disease is commonly caused by the human type of tubercle bacillus.

Let us now return to the study of tubercle bacilli found in lymphatic glands removed during life. Thus far we have seen that the proportion of bovine infections found in cervical gland tuberculosis has varied from 44 per cent. in the United States to 26 per cent. in Germany. The proportion, as we have seen, is very different at different ages, and

---

[1] *Tub. Arbeit. etc.* Heft 6, p. 52 (cases 68 and 70).

these numbers are consequently dependent partly on the age constitution of the different groups of cases. Too much therefore must not be made of their exact size, but we may conclude broadly that in these countries and in England the proportion of bovine infections in cervical gland tuberculosis found up to this time had been well under 50 per cent.

Very different is the conclusion drawn from some recent researches carried out in Scotland. In that country A. P. Mitchell (1914) made a study of the tubercle bacilli to be found in tuberculous cervical glands of children under thirteen years of age. The material, removed by operation during life, came from Edinburgh and its neighbourhood. Seventy-two cases were examined, and of these no less than sixty-five were held to have been caused by the bovine bacillus, and only seven by the human bacillus. Thus 90 per cent. were found to be bovine infections[1].

Since these results are so different from those we have just reviewed it will be desirable to give some description of the methods employed. The glandular material removed by operation was injected into guinea-pigs, and from these animals the strains of tubercle bacilli were obtained in artificial culture. These strains having been obtained, their cultural characters and virulence for animals were studied.

Mitchell tells us that for determining cultural character he used egg medium, both with and without glycerin, together with glycerin-agar and glycerin-serum. He seems to have relied largely on the egg medium, and glycerin-broth and glycerin-potato do not seem to have been used at all. Virulence was tested on rabbits, intravenous injection, in doses of 0·01 and 0·1 mg., being mainly employed[2]. Sometimes subcutaneous injection of 5 or 10 mg. was substituted for intravenous injection with the larger dose. With regard to these experiments it is to be regretted that Mitchell did not give particulars of the post-mortem examinations in such detail as the novelty of his conclusions would appear to demand. He seems to have considered it sufficient to give a general description of the changes produced in these animals by the bacilli which he classed as bovine and human respectively, and to have inferred that in every case the lesions corresponded with one or other of these pictures. He tells us that he met with no difficulty in classifying his strains according either to their cultural characters or their virulence, and in every case the verdict based on the one criterion corresponded with that based upon the other.

[1] *Brit. Med. Journ.* 1914, I. p. 125. Mitchell subsequently added eight more surgical cases, six of which yielded bovine and two human bacilli, thus bringing his total number of cases up to eighty, with an incidence of bovine infection of 88 per cent. These additional cases all occurred in children under thirteen years of age, but as no details of age are given it is not possible to include them in the table which follows. (" A Bacteriological Study of Tuberculosis in the Lymph Glands of Children," *Edin. Med. Journ.* 1914, N.S. vol. XIII, p. 213.)

[2] Compare pp. 276 and 277.

38—2

Mitchell himself was well aware of the discrepancy between his results and those of other observers elsewhere; and he alleged in explanation (a) the fact that his material came largely from very young children, and (b) the great prevalence of tuberculosis among the cows of Edinburgh and its neighbourhood, and "the almost universal practice" which prevails there of feeding children with unsterilized milk[1].

As to the first of these explanations, Mitchell is undoubtedly right in drawing attention, as we have seen American authors had already done, to the importance of the age constitution of any group of patients yielding material for investigations. Bovine infections are without doubt much commoner in younger children than in older ones or adults, and many of Mitchell's strains of bacilli came from young children. This explanation then might apply to Mitchell's results as a whole, but it cannot be made to explain the discrepancy which remains after his results are analysed according to the ages of the patients; for no other observer whose work we have reviewed has found, *at corresponding age periods*, anything like so high a percentage of bovine infections as the 87 per cent. found by Mitchell in children between five and sixteen, or the 93 per cent. found by him in children under five. The most remarkable part of Mitchell's results is the very high rate of bovine infections at the higher of these ages.

With regard to the second explanation it may be pointed out that the practice of feeding children on unsterilized milk is not confined to Edinburgh, but is common everywhere; and that, while the milk supply of Edinburgh may be as bad as Mitchell represents it to be, that of other places also leaves much to be desired. It is hard to believe that in these respects Edinburgh is so much worse than other cities in other countries as Mitchell's figures would imply if this is the true explanation of the discrepancy. Nevertheless if there really is anything

---

[1] In many of his cases, Mitchell tells us he was able to trace the infection directly to a cow with a tuberculous udder, and he devotes part of the paper we are now considering and the whole of another which followed it ("The Milk Question in Edinburgh," *Edin. Med. Journ.* 1914) to showing that tuberculosis is extraordinarily common among the cows of Edinburgh and its neighbourhood.

like 90 per cent. of bovine infections in the cervical gland tuberculosis of children in Edinburgh and its neighbourhood (and, as we shall see, it is not in this kind of tuberculosis alone that Edinburgh is exceptional, for an even greater contrast to other cities is presented by her in the domain of bone and joint tuberculosis) we shall be obliged to believe that this is due to differences in the quality of the milk and the methods of infant feeding in this as compared with other places. And indeed such a conclusion would be highly satisfactory; for such causes are removable. In the meantime what is wanted is independent confirmation of the facts alleged, and a comparative investigation, by one and the same observer, of the incidence of bovine tuberculosis in certain selected cities. This want, as we shall proceed to show, has already been partly supplied by the work of A. S. Griffith.

This author has recently (1915) published an important study of the tubercle bacilli concerned in tuberculosis of the cervical glands, and has kept in mind the possibility that the proportion of bovine infections may differ in different localities. For this reason, while the greater part of the material which served him for his investigation came from various places in England, some of it was obtained from Edinburgh and Glasgow.

The material investigated consisted of lymphatic glands removed by operation from 110 persons of various ages. In two cases the glands were axillary, in one femoral, and in 107 cervical.

In the case of ten patients the glands were not macroscopically tuberculous, and these did not cause tuberculosis when injected into guinea-pigs. There remain then 100 patients with glands definitely tuberculous to the naked eye. Of these patients twenty-nine yielded glands which when emulsified and injected into guinea-pigs failed to provoke tuberculosis[1].

From the remaining seventy-one cases the glands removed yielded tubercle bacilli in cultures. Of these cases Griffith,

[1] This, as Griffith points out, while it does not, of course, prove that the patients were cured of the disease—for the latter might be active elsewhere—nevertheless shows that the infective process had come to an end in those particular glands; and it indicates in a rather striking way the natural tendency to cure which exists in glandular tuberculosis. These ten cases do not stand alone, but merely add to the evidence of this fact which has been accumulating for some years.

in drawing up his statistical statement, excludes three: namely, one because the glandular disease was secondary to tuberculosis of the lungs, and two because the disease was in the axillary glands, the cervicals being unaffected. The case in which the glands investigated were femoral is included because the cervical glands also were tuberculous.

After these exclusions have been made there remain sixty-eight cases of tuberculosis apparently primary in cervical glands. Of these thirty-five yielded bacilli of human type and thirty-three bacilli of bovine type. This gives a proportion of bovine infections at all ages of about 48·5 per cent., which is only a little higher than the figure deduced from American investigations, but in Griffith's series there is a larger proportion of adults. If we confine ourselves for the moment to cases under sixteen years, we find that Griffith's figures give a proportion of bovine infections equal to 61 per cent. while Lewis's figures together with those of Park and Krumwiede give one equal to a little over 53 per cent.

Turning now to the question whether the proportion of bovine infections differs in England and Scotland, and if so to what extent, we find that the proportion in question works out in Griffith's series at 41 per cent. in England and 70 per cent. in Scotland. But let us eliminate the adult cases (over sixteen years) of which there are a good many in Griffith's series and none at all in Mitchell's. This done there remain of Griffith's cases twenty-seven English cases with fifteen instances of bovine infection and fourteen Scottish cases with ten instances of bovine infection. This gives the proportion of bovine infections in cervical gland tuberculosis under sixteen years of age as 55·5 per cent. for England and 71·4 per cent. for Scotland. This certainly supports Mitchell's position, though we could wish that the number of Scottish cases was larger. The figure 71·4 per cent. for Scotland is certainly high, but it is not equal to that found by Mitchell which the reader will remember was 90 per cent.

Tubercle Bacilli in Cervical Glands (removed by Operation).

Locality	Authors	Adolescents and adults, 16 years and over			Children 5–16 years			Infants under 5 years		
		Type of bacillus			Type of bacillus			Type of bacillus		
		Human	Bovine	Per cent.	Human	Bovine	Per cent.	Human	Bovine	Per cent.
Germany	Gesundheitsamt in 1907 ... Burckhardt ...	2 5	0 0		4 3	3 1		6 —	3 —	
	Total	**7**	**0**	*0*	**7**	**4**	*36*	**6**	**3**	*33*
U.S.A.	Lewis ... ... Park and Krumwiede	5 9	1 0		2 19	7 8		0 6	3 13	
	Total	**14**	**1**	*6·6*	**21**	**15**	*42*	**6**	**16**	*73*
England	Royal Commission A. S. Griffith (English cases)	— 18	— 6		5 12	2 9		1 0	1 6	
	Total	**18**	**6**	*25*	**17**	**11**	*40*	**1**	**7**	*87·5*
Scotland	A. S. Griffith (Scottish cases) Mitchell*	1 —	2 —		3 4	7 26		1 3	3 39	
	Total	**1**	**2**	*66*	**7**	**33**	*84*	**4**	**42**	*90*

* Mitchell gives his results as follows:

Children 5 to 12 years of age: Children under 5 years of age:
    Human bacilli 4   Human bacilli 3
    Bovine bacilli 30   Bovine bacilli 35

But from the particulars which he gives in a table just above this statement (p. 18 of his reprinted paper), it appears that four cases of bovine infection in children aged from 4 to 5 years were inadvertently included in the former, instead of the latter, group.

In order to show at a glance how the figures stand for different countries, there has been drawn up the following condensed table in which are combined the figures for all ages under sixteen years.

Tuberculosis in Cervical Glands removed by Operation.
In persons under 16 years of age.

Country	Type of bacillus		Percentage of bovine infections
	Human	Bovine	
England	18	18	**50**
(Griffith only) ...	*12*	*15*	*55*
Scotland*	**11**	**75**	**87**
(Griffith only) ...	*4*	*10*	*71*
(Mitchell only) ...	*7*	*65*	*90*
United States ...	27	31	**53**
Germany	13	7	**35**

* Not including Mitchell's eight additional cases.

Conclusion.

Numerous investigations have shown beyond all doubt that much of the tuberculosis of cervical glands is caused by bovine tubercle bacilli.   In the face, however, of great discrepancies in the results obtained by different investigators it is difficult to make a precise statement as to the proportion of cases so caused.

The discrepancies alluded to are most marked when the results obtained in different countries are compared with one another.   It would appear that infection with bovine tubercle bacilli, as compared with infection with human tubercle bacilli, is much commoner in Scotland than in England and the United States; and that in all these countries it is commoner than in Germany.   Probably this is the case.   There is already a considerable amount of evidence in support of such a conclusion. But it can hardly as yet be said to be proved conclusively—

the amount of work is as yet too small; sample cases may not always be representative; human judgment is not infallible; (and it is a matter which, as we have argued elsewhere, is partly dependent on judgment). Our conclusion on this point therefore must at present be regarded as provisional.

On the other hand we are on surer ground in speaking of the proportion of bovine infection in this kind of tuberculosis in all countries taken together. This we believe to be in the region of 50 per cent. if we include all cases irrespective of age. But it is doubtless very much higher than this in early life, and under five years of age it is probably more like 75 per cent. In adolescence on the other hand it is comparatively small.

8. *Tuberculosis of Bones and Joints.*

Tuberculosis of the spinal column and of various bones and joints forms a not unimportant member of the groups of diseases which are caused by tubercle bacilli; for though the loss of life for which it is directly responsible is but a small fraction of that caused by all kinds of tuberculosis, the amount of suffering and deformity produced by it is large[1].

Little is known of the portal of entry in this kind of tuberculosis, though it is sometimes assumed to be the intestine; but post-mortem examinations in cases of this sort are relatively uncommon, and the distribution of tuberculous lesions in the various lymphatic glands has not been sufficiently studied. Some information on this point however may be gathered from recent contributions made to the *Reports of the Local Government Board* by Eastwood and F. Griffith and by A. S. Griffith. Together these contain details of eight fatal cases in children in whom some bone or joint was the seat of tuberculous disease. In four of these cases both bronchial and mesenteric glands were involved more or less equally; in two the mesenteric, and in two the bronchial glands were solely or

---

[1] The number of deaths referred to this cause in the Report of the Registrar General for 1911 was 1061, which is about one-fiftieth of the total number of deaths attributable to tuberculosis of all kinds. These deaths occurred at all ages, the majority being between five and twenty-five years, and the maximum mortality occurring between fifteen and twenty.

mainly affected. Thus the evidence for thoracic and abdominal origin respectively was equally divided.

To these cases may be added one (H 7 M.C.) investigated by the Royal Commission and already referred to in another section. The patient had tuberculous disease of the ankle joint and died of general tuberculosis and meningitis at the age of three. Post-mortem examination revealed an ulcer in the small intestine, enlargement and caseation of the mesenteric glands, and some tuberculous peritonitis. Tubercle bacilli cultivated from the mesenteric glands in this case proved to be of bovine type.

Another case, examined by the writer, may perhaps be added though it may be questioned whether the disease in gland and bone respectively resulted from one and the same infection. The patient was an elderly man who died of tuberculosis of the vertebral column. In one of his mesenteric glands was a calcareous nodule, of the size of a large pea, and of stony hardness. If we take these ten cases together we find that the balance of evidence inclines rather towards the side of invasion through the intestine than to that through the respiratory passages; as a matter of fact we have four examples of the one kind and two of the other, with four cases neutral. These cases are altogether too few to found a conclusion upon, but we shall probably not be wrong if we hold that bone and joint tuberculosis may be caused by bacilli which have entered through *either of* these portals. This conclusion is in harmony with that which we have already formed concerning general tuberculosis, which, like tuberculosis of the bones and joints, must be due to an invasion of the blood stream.

The type of bacillus concerned in the kind of tuberculosis which is now under consideration has already been determined in a number of cases. Most of the investigations have been made during the life of the patient, with material removed by operation; and the great majority of them have yielded results of singular uniformity, instances of bovine infection being remarkably rare.

But once again we find a report from Edinburgh which differs widely from the rest; and this time the difference is even greater than that which we have already examined in the case of cervical gland tuberculosis. For this reason the details of the evidence demand our close attention.

The Royal Commission examined material taken at operations from fourteen cases of tuberculosis of bones and joints. The majority of the patients were adults over thirty years of age; only six were under fifteen. In all cases the bacilli were of human type[1]. To these may be added the case of ankle joint tuberculosis in the child mentioned above in which the bacilli investigated came from mesenteric glands removed after death. This case alone yielded a bovine bacillus.

In the Gesundheitsamt Oehlecker and others investigated material removed by operation from thirty-eight cases of bone and joint tuberculosis[2]. Eleven of these occurred in adults and twenty-seven in children. Thirty-seven yielded bacilli of human type and one tubercle bacilli of bovine type. The virus in this latter case presented certain peculiarities, and, obtained afresh from the patient from time to time, fluctuated in virulence. For reasons, which will become evident as we proceed, the details of this case are discussed in the next chapter (p. 629). The tuberculosis in this case had attacked a metacarpal bone of a child whose age when the investigation began was eight years.

In America Park and Krumwiede examined material removed from eighteen cases of bone and joint tuberculosis. The patients were of various ages. One was over sixteen, ten were between five and sixteen, and seven under five years of age. In all the disease was found to be caused by tubercle bacilli of human type.

Returning again to Germany we observe that Burckhardt found a slightly higher proportion of bovine infections. Twenty-nine cases were examined by him with the following results. Of ten cases over sixteen years of age, nine were found to be

---

[1] This includes H 16 J. H., which the Commission classified as a mixed virus, on grounds which seem insufficient to the writer, who carried out the investigation. This virus is one of those which underwent change on *passage*. It has already been discussed at length in Chap. XVI, p. 335. That it was a mixed virus at a certain stage of its history there can be no doubt whatever, but the writer submits that there is no evidence of a bovine constituent in it as it existed in J. H.

[2] *Tub. Arbeit. etc.* Heft 6, pp. 7 and 8, and p. 159.

infected with bacilli of human type, and one with bacilli of bovine type. Of fourteen cases in which the ages ranged from five to sixteen years, twelve were found to be infected with bacilli of human type and two with bacilli of bovine type. Four cases under five years of age, and one in which the age is not recorded (and which consequently cannot be included in the table which follows) were found to be infected with tubercle bacilli of human type.

Möllers investigated twelve cases in the Robert Koch Institute in Berlin, partly under the eyes of Koch himself. Four of the patients were between five and sixteen years, and the rest over sixteen. In all these cases the disease was found to be caused by the human type of tubercle bacillus.

Turning now to cases which were investigated after death we find that among those examined for the Local Government Board by Eastwood and F. Griffith there were seven in which there was tuberculosis of one or more bones or joints, and that among those investigated for the same authority by A. S. Griffith was one other of this kind. It must be understood that in these cases the bacteriological examination did not include the infected bones or joints themselves, but was confined mainly to lymphatic glands, or to one of the great organs.

Of the seven cases investigated by Eastwood and F. Griffith two failed to yield any tubercle bacilli, emulsions of visibly tuberculous as well as of apparently normal lymphatic glands failing to provoke tuberculosis in guinea-pigs into which they were injected. One case, in which tuberculous pneumonia had proved fatal in a boy of nine years who suffered with hip disease, yielded from bronchial and mesenteric glands tubercle bacilli of human type. One case, aged nearly ten years, in which death was due to lardaceous disease of liver and kidneys following spinal caries and tuberculosis of a rib with a discharging sinus, yielded an atypical strain of bacilli which combined the limited virulence of the human type with the feeble growth of the bovine type[1]. Three cases in which the

[1] H. 99, the case which yielded an atypical culture is of special interest, not for this reason only, but because the tuberculous disease seems to a very large extent to have become arrested. The spinal disease appeared at the

ages ranged from two and a quarter to four and a half years, and in two of which death was due to meningitis and in the other to tuberculous pneumonia, the tubercle bacilli obtained from bronchial or mesenteric glands proved to be of human type.   In these cases knee, hip, and spine respectively were affected with tuberculosis.

A. S. Griffith found only one case of bone or joint disease included in his series.   This was in a boy of eight and a half years who died of shock following operation for tuberculosis of the vertebral column, and who was found to have calcareous nodules in the bronchial and mesenteric glands.   These glands, emulsified and injected into guinea-pigs, failed to infect, and cultures could not be obtained from them directly; but a guinea-pig inoculated with the substance of an apparently normal cervical gland developed tuberculosis, and from it was grown a culture of tubercle bacilli of human type.

Most of these cases investigated post-mortem have appeared in one or other of the tables in the preceding sections; they will however reappear in the table which follows; for cases of bone and joint tuberculosis in which the type of tubercle bacillus concerned has been investigated are so few that these cannot be spared.

Thus far we have collected of bone or joint tuberculosis 113 cases, in one of which the bacilli were atypical, and in five only of bovine type.   This gives a proportion of bovine infections of 4·4 per cent. (or if we were to leave out Burckhardt's cases of only 2·35 per cent.).   Bovine infections were relatively commoner in children under sixteen (5·2 per cent.) than in persons of greater age (2·9 per cent.) but they showed no preponderance in children under five years of age.

post-mortem examination to have become healed. There were a good number of small caseo-calcareous foci in the spleen, but an emulsion of this organ failed to infect guinea-pigs. Bronchial glands appeared normal, and failed to infect when injected, but the mesenteric glands, some of which were moderately enlarged and contained some miliary, caseo-calcareous yellow tubercles, infected one guinea-pig out of four into which an emulsion of them was injected. It seems as if the tuberculous disease, though of old standing and extensive, had all but come to an end, and but for a discharging sinus from a tuberculous rib which seems to have brought on lardaceous disease the boy might have recovered.

In strong contrast to these results are those of J. Fraser (1912), who investigated seventy cases of bone and joint tuberculosis in the Research Laboratory of the Royal College of Physicians in Edinburgh. This observer found nearly 60 per cent. of bovine infections (or more precisely 58·6 per cent. of pure bovine infections, or 63 per cent. if we include mixed cases), for of these seventy cases forty-one yielded bovine bacilli alone, twenty-six human bacilli alone, and three both bovine and human bacilli.

Fraser, like Mitchell in a similar case before him, was of course fully aware that his results were very different from those of previous investigators; and he advanced similar reasons in explanation. Firstly he pointed out that many of his cases occurred in young children, in whom, when affected with other kinds of tuberculosis, bovine bacilli have been found much more frequently than in older persons. Let us examine the details a little more closely and see how far this explanation holds good. Forty-seven of Fraser's cases were under five years of age, and of these thirty-two—or 68 per cent.—yielded bovine bacilli only, and three gave mixed cultures. Twenty were between five and sixteen years of age, and in nine of these— or in 45 per cent.—the bacilli were of the bovine type. Three were over sixteen, and all of these yielded bacilli of human type. This explanation then is valid up to a certain point— Fraser's series contained a large proportion of cases in young children; and in the young children the proportion of bovine infections was higher than in older ones. But it is utterly inadequate to get over the discrepancy between his results in general and those of other observers, for it does not touch the difficulty that while he found, between the ages of five and sixteen, 45 per cent. of pure bovine infections, the others had found only 6¼ per cent.

Fraser himself recognized this, and went on to base his explanation in the main on the greater prevalence of tuberculosis among the dairy cattle of Edinburgh than among those of other lands, and on the relative frequency with which infants there are fed on unsterilized milk.

But, as we have said when critically reviewing the Edinburgh

results obtained in the kindred case of cervical gland tuberculosis, it is difficult to believe that the conditions of the milk
supply of Edinburgh, and the manner of feeding infants there,
however bad they may be, can account for so great a difference
in the relative amounts of human infection with tubercle
bacilli of human and bovine type there and elsewhere as
Fraser's results would imply. The difficulty in this case is
greater than in that of cervical gland tuberculosis. For while
in the latter Mitchell claimed for Edinburgh a proportion of
bovine infections among children which was less than twice as
great as that which had been found elsewhere, Fraser's results
would lead us to infer that, so far as bone and joint tuberculosis
is concerned, the proportion is about eleven times as great.

If these explanations then seem inadequate there remains for
consideration one which cannot be left entirely out of sight. It
is possible that different observers unconsciously adopt different
criteria in judging the type of bacillus. It must be remembered
that a statement as to the type of micro-organism is not a
statement of observed fact, but an inference from observations,
and that the judgment of the observer has played a part in
arriving at it. That in such a case as this different observers
should judge differently from similar facts will not appear
surprising to the reader if he is able to agree with the view
which has been put forward in an earlier chapter as to the
difficulties which lie in the way of correct determination of
type, due, among other things, to unavoidable variations of
culture media and to differences of susceptibility of individual
rabbits. We ought to remember too, as illustrating these
difficulties, that even now there is not entire unanimity as
to the existence of two distinct types, and that some highly
experienced observers (e.g. M. Koch and Rabinowitsch) see very
indeterminate limits to them.

It will probably be conceded that the amount of evidence
required to support any new conclusion is in proportion to
the novelty of that conclusion; and that the more unexpected
that conclusion is so much the more fully should the evidence
be set out. In view therefore of the great discrepancy between
Fraser's results and those of other observers it is to be regretted

that he did not publish his experiments in full. He tells us indeed that he relied for identification of type on morphological and cultural characters and on the injection of rabbits. These animals were injected intravenously with 0·01 mg. of culture. No details are given of the results of these injections, but it was stated, in answer to Möllers, who criticized this investigation adversely[1], that in every instance where bovine bacilli were identified the injections produced general tuberculosis[2]. But what we should like to learn is the extent to which the disease was generalized in each rabbit, and what was the type of the lesions; for we know that from time to time a considerable amount of disease of a chronic type may be produced in the lungs and kidneys of rabbits by tubercle bacilli of human type (see p. 272).

The plain truth is Fraser's conclusions are so novel that they appear to us to need confirmation before they can be finally accepted. Nevertheless, taken in conjunction with the investigations of Mitchell on cervical gland tuberculosis, they make out a case for the view that the relative frequency of infection from bovine sources varies in different places. And though it seems to us improbable that it should vary to such an extent as Fraser's results would imply, yet it is possible that there are what one might perhaps call "pockets" of bovine infection, and that it was into one of these that by chance he had dipped[3].

One more word may be said concerning the question whether there is an excess of bovine infections among the inhabitants of Scotland as compared with those of England and Germany. A comparatively high ratio of infections with bovine bacilli to those with human bacilli may be due either to (a) a real excess of infections with bovine bacilli or to (b) a deficiency of infections with human bacilli. Now in Scotland it cannot be due to the latter cause, because the death-rate from phthisis, which as we have seen is caused almost entirely with bacilli of human type, is higher in Scotland than in England. On

---

[1] *Deutsch. med. Wochenschr.* 1913, p. 1826, and *Lancet*, 1913, II, p. 1075.
[2] *Lancet*, 1913, II, p. 1430.   [3] See also Appendix II, p. 679.

the other hand it may well be due to a real excess of bovine infections in Scotland; for we find that the death-rate from all kinds of tuberculosis other than phthisis (which as we have said includes practically all the instances of bovine infection) claims a greater share in the death-rate from all kinds of tuberculosis in Scotland (32 per cent.) than in England and Wales (29·2 per cent.) and in Prussia (10·4 per cent.).

Tuberculosis of Bones and Joints (Surgical and Post-mortem).

Authors	Adults over 16 years		Children 5–16		Infants under 5 years		
	Type of bacillus		Type of bacillus		Type of bacillus		
	Human	Bovine	Human	Bovine	Human	Bovine	Atypical
Royal Commission ...	8	0	5	0	1	1	—
Park and Krumwiede ...	1	0	10	0	7	0	—
Oehlecker	9	0	12	1	12	0	—
Burckhardt *	9	1	12	2	4	0	—
Möllers	8	0	4	0	0	0	—
Eastwood and F. Griffith and A. S. Griffith	0	0	2	0	3	0	1 †
Total ...	35	1	45	3	27	1	1
Fraser	3	0	11	9	12	32	3 ‡
Grand Total ...	38	1	56	12	39	33	4

Several of the cases have appeared in previous tables under other headings such as Meningitis, General Tuberculosis, etc.

* One case, in a child, could not be included because the age was not given. The bacilli proved to be of human type.
† The strain of tubercle bacilli derived from this case possessed the virulence of the human type and the cultural characters of the bovine type.
‡ Mixed cultures of human and bovine bacilli.

Conclusions.

Bone and joint tuberculosis appears in most countries to be due largely to tubercle bacilli of human type. The contribution made by infection from a bovine source would appear from the evidence available, which is admittedly somewhat meagre, to be on an average in various countries, excluding Scotland, small.

In Edinburgh and neighbourhood a very much larger share has been claimed for bovine infection, amounting roughly to 60 per cent. of the cases in children. This claim needs confirmation. It seems to us unlikely that there should be so great a difference between Edinburgh and other great cities. Possibly some "pocket" of bovine infection had been tapped. Nevertheless a substantial case has been made out both in the case of tuberculosis of bones and joints, and in that of cervical glands for the view that the relative proportion of infections with tubercle bacilli of bovine and human type differs considerably in different places.

P.S.   For some quite recent work see Appendix, p. 679.

REFERENCES.   XVI

(Chapter XXIV)

Pulmonary Tuberculosis.

Beitzke (1907).   Ueber die Infection des Menschen mit Rindertuberkel-bazillen. *Virchows Archiv*, Beiheft zum Bande 190, p. 58.

Bulloch (1911).   Horace Dobell Lecture. Roy. Coll. of Physicians.

Cobbett (1907).   *R.C.T. Int. Rep.* App. vol. II, pp. 4, etc.

Cruickshank (1912).   On the Direct Cultivation of Tubercle Bacilli from Tuberculous Tissues. *Brit. Med. Journ.* Nov. 1912.

Dieterlen (1910).   Untersuchungen über die im Auswurf Lungen-kranker vorkommenden Tuberkelbazillen. *Tub. Arbeit. a. d. Kaiserl. Gesundheitsamte*, Heft 10, p. 101.

Eber (1905).   Experimentelle Uebertragung der Tuberkulose vom Menschen auf das Rind. *Brauer's Beiträge zur Klinik der Tuber-kulose*, vol. III, p. 257.

—— (1907).   Zwei Fälle von erfolgreicher Uebertragung tuberkulösen Materials von an Lungenphthise gestorbenen erwachsen Menschen auf das Rind. *Deutsch. med. Wochenschr.* p. 378.

Griffith, A. S. (1911).   *R.C.T. Fin. Rep.* App. vol. I, pp. 8, 100, etc.

—— (1914).   Further Investigations of the Type of Tubercle Bacilli occurring in the Sputum of Phthisical Persons. *Brit. Med. Journ.* I, p. 1171.

Kitasato (1909).   Die Tuberkulose in Japan. *Zeitsch. f. Hygiene*, vol. LXIII, p. 517.

Koch, R. (1908).   The Relation of Human and Bovine Tuberculosis. *International Congress on Tuberculosis*, Washington.

Kossel (1913). Die tierische Tuberkulose in ihren Beziehungen zur menschlichen Tuberkulose, besonders zur Lungenschwindsucht. *Veröff. d. R. Koch-Stiftung z. Bekämpfung der Tuberkulose,* Heft 8–9, p. 1.

Kossel, Weber and Heuss (1904 and 1905). Vergleichende Untersuchungen über Tuberkelbazillen verschiedener Herkunft. *Tub. Arbeit. a. d. Kaiserl. Gesundheitsamte,* Hefte 1 and 3.

Lindemann (1912). Untersuchungen über den Typus der im Auswurf Lungenkranker vorkommenden Tuberkelbazillen. *Tub. Arbeit. a. d. Kaiserl. Gesundheitsamte,* Heft 12, p. 11.

Mietzsch (1910). *Arbeit. a. d. Gebiete d. pathol. Anatom. u. Bakt. a. d. Pathol.-anatom. Inst. z. Tübingen,* vol. VII, pp. 306–309.

Möllers (1911). Ueber den Typus der Tuberkelbazillen im Auswurf der Phthisiker. *Veröff. der R. Koch-Stiftung,* Heft 1, Leipzig.

Park and Krumwiede (1909, 1910, 1911). The Relative Importance of the Bovine and Human Types of Tubercle Bacilli in Human Tuberculosis. *Collected Studies from the Research Laboratory, Department of Health, City of New York,* vols. IV, V and VI.

Rabinowitsch, L. (1906). Untersuchungen über die Beziehungen zwischen der Tuberkulose des Menschen und der Tiere. *Arbeiten aus dem Pathologischen Institut zu Berlin.*

—— Marcus. Zur Identitäts Frage der Tuberkelbakterien verschiedener Herkunft. *Zeitsch. für Tuberkulose,* vol. IX, p. 457.

Schmid (1912). Die Tuberkulosesterblichkeit der Schweiz und die zur Bekämpfung der Tuberkulose daselbst im letzten Jahrzehnt gemachten Anstrengungen. *Internat. Tuberc. Conference,* Rome, p. 457.

Schroeder (1908). Ueber das Vorkommen von Perlsuchtbazillen im Sputum der Phthisiker und ihre Bedeutung für die Therapie der chron. Lungentuberkulose. *Brauer's Beiträge z. Klinik der Tuberkulose,* vol. XI, p. 219.

Smith, Th. (1898). A Comparative Study of Bovine Tubercle Bacilli and of Human Bacilli from Sputum. *Journ. of Experim. Med.* vol. III.

Sprengler (1905). *Deutsch. med. Wochenschr.* No. 31.

—— (1907). *Ibid.* No. 9.

Stuurmann (1903). Inaug. Dissertation, Leiden.

Weber (1907). Vergleichende Untersuchungen über Tuberkelbazillen verschiedener Herkunft, III. Vorwort. *Tub. Arbeit. a. d. Kaiserl. Gesundheitsamte,* Heft 6, p. 1.

—— (1907). Bemerkung zu der Arbeit von Eber, "Zwei Fälle," etc. *Deutsch. med. Wochenschr.* p. 381.

Weber and Dieterlen (1912). Untersuchungen über den Typus der im Auswurf Lungenkranker vorkommenden Tuberkelbazillen. Virulenzprüfung von mittelst der Antiforminmethode gezüchteten Tuberkelbazillen. *Tub. Arbeit. a. d. Kaiserl. Gesundheitsamte,* Heft 12, p. 1.

Tuberculosis of the Mammary Glands.

(Chapter XVIII)

Beuder (1891). *Baumgarten's Jahresbericht*, vol. VII, p. 809.

Cooper, Sir Astley (1829). *Illustrations of Diseases of the Breast*, Pt. I, p. 73.

Deaver (1914). *Am. Journ. of Medical Sciences*, vol. CXLVII, p. 157.

von Eberts (1909). *Ibid.* vol. CXXXVIII, p. 70.

Hebb (1888). *Trans. Path. Soc. Lond.* vol. XXXIX.

Lane (1890). *Brit. Med. Journ.* II, p. 690.

Mandry (1891). Die Tuberkulose der Brüstdrüsen. *Brunn's Beiträge zur klinischen Chirurgie*, vol. VIII, Heft I, p. 179. (Abst. in Baumgarten, vol. VII, p. 809.)

Scott (1904). Tuberculosis of the Human Breast. *St Bartholomew's Hospital Reports*, vol. XL, p. 97.

Shattock (1889). *Trans. Path. Soc. Lond.* vol. XL, p. 391. (Contains many references to papers and articles not mentioned here.)

Shield (1895). *Diseases of the Breast.*

Surgical Tuberculosis (other than Lupus).

Arloing (1908). Internat. Congress at Washington.

Beitzke (1907). Ueber die Infection des Menschen mit Rindertuberkulose. *Virchows Archiv*, vol. CXC. Beiheft.

Burckhardt (1910). Bacteriologische Untersuchungen über Chirurgische Tuberkulose. *Deutsche Zeitschr. f. Chir.* vol. CLX.

Cobbett (1907). *R.C.T. Int. Rep.* App. vol. II.

Creighton (1881). *Bovine Tuberculosis in Man.* Macmillan and Co.

Eastwood and F. Griffith (1914). The Incidence and Bacteriological Characteristics of Tuberculous Infection in Children. *Reports to the Local Government on Public Health and Medical Subjects*, N.S. No. 88, p. I.

Fibiger and Jensen (1907). Ueber die Bedeutung der Milchinfection für die Entstehung der primären Intestinaltuberkulose. *Berl. klin. Wochenschr.* Nos. 4 and 5.

Fibiger (1908). Untersuchungen über die Beziehungen zwischen der Tuberkulose und den Tuberkelbazillen des Menschen und der Tuberkulose und den Tuberkelbazillen des Rindes. *Berl. klin. Wochenschr.* p. 42.

Fraser, J. (1912). The Relative Prevalence of Human and Bovine Types of Tubercle Bacilli in Bone and Joint Tuberculosis occurring in Children. *Journ. of Experimental Medicine*, vol. XVI, p. 432.

—— (1913). The Etiology of Bone and Joint Tuberculosis. A reply to the criticism of Möllers. *Lancet*, II, p. 1430.

Gaffky (1907). Zur Frage der Infectionswege der Tuberkulose. *Tuberculosis*, vol. VI, p. 437.

Goodale (1906). The Examination of the Throat in Chronic Systemic Infections. *Boston Med. and Surg. Journ.* Nov. 1906.

Griffith, A. S. (1911). *R.C.T. Fin. Rep.* App. vol. 1.

—— (1914). Tuberculous Infection in Children, and its Relation to the Bovine and Human Types of Tubercle Bacilli. *Reports to the Local Government Board on Public Health and Medical Subjects,* N.S. LXXXVIII, p. 105.

—— (1915). Cervical Gland Tuberculosis. *Lancet,* I, p. 1275.

Jancsó and Elfer (1910). Vergleichende Untersuchungen mit den praktisch wichtigeren säurefesten Bazillen. *Brauer's Beiträge,* vol. XVIII.

Koch, R. (1908). *International Congress on Tuberculosis,* Washington.

Kossel, Weber and Heuss (1904 and 1905). Vergleichende Untersuchungen über Tuberkelbazillen verschiedener Herkunft. *Tub. Arbeit. a. d. Kaiserl. Gesundheitsamte,* Heft 1 and 3.

Lewis (1910). Tuberculous Cervical Adenitis. *Journ. of Exp. Medicine,* vol. XII, p. 82.

Litterer (1910). Medical Record.

Mitchell, A. P. (1914). The Infection of Children with the Bovine Tubercle Bacillus. *Brit. Med. Journ.* I, p. 125 (deals with cervical lymph glands).

—— (1914). A Bacteriological Study of Tuberculosis of the Lymph Glands in Children. *Edinburgh Medical Journal,* Sept.

—— (1914). The Milk Question in Edinburgh. *Edinburgh Medical Journal,* April.

Mohler and Washburn (1907). A Comparative Study of Tubercle Bacilli from Varied Sources. *U.S. Dept. of Agriculture, Bureau of Animal Industry,* Bull. No. 96.

Möllers. Zur Aetiologie der Knochen- und Gelenktuberkulose. *Veröffentlichen der Robert Koch-Stiftung,* Heft X.

—— (1913). *Deutsch. med. Wochenschr.* p. 1826. Abst. in the *Lancet,* II, p. 1075.

Oehlecker (1907). Untersuchungen über chirurgische Tuberculosen. *Tub. Arbeit. a. d. Kaiserl. Gesundheitsamte,* Heft 6, p. 88.

Park and Krumwiede (1909, 1910, 1911). The Relative Importance of the Bovine and Human Types of Tubercle Bacilli in Human Tuberculosis. *Collected Studies from the Research Laboratory, Department of Health, City of New York,* vols. IV, V, and VI.

Pybus (1911). Some Infections of the Tonsils. Hunterian Lecture. *Lancet,* May 15, p. 1011.

Smith and Brown (1907). Studies in Mammalian Tubercle Bacilli, No. IV. Bacilli Resembling the Bovine Type from Four Cases in Man. *Journ. of Med. Research,* vol. XVI, p. 435.

Ungermann (1912). Untersuchungen über die tuberkulöse Infection der Lymphdrüsen im Kindersalter. *Tub. Arbeit. a. d. Kaiserl. Gesundheitsamte,* Heft 12, p. 109.

Weber and Taute (1907). Weitere Untersuchungen etc. mit besonderer Berücksichtigung der primären Darm- und Mesenterialdrüsentuberkulose. *Tub. Arbeit. a. d. Kaiserl. Gesundheitsamte,* Heft 6, p. 15.

614

CHAPTER XXV

TUBERCULOSIS IN MAN: THE TYPES OF TUBERCLE BACILLI WHICH CAUSE IT (*continued*)

9. *Lupus.*

From our present point of view lupus is of special interest because the tubercle bacilli which have been isolated from the majority of cases of the disease which have been bacteriologically investigated, in this country at least, have proved to be more or less atypical. Thus lupus, as in other ways, stands somewhat apart from other kinds of tuberculosis. In them, as we have seen, the tubercle bacilli conform, closely enough, to one or other distinct type, the human or the bovine; now and then an atypical strain is met with, but it turns out as a rule, when adequately investigated, to be a mixture of these types. Pure atypical strains of tubercle bacilli are rarely seen in all the various deep-seated forms of tuberculosis. But in lupus, as we have said, it is otherwise; according to A. S. Griffith, who has very specially devoted himself to the bacteriological study of this disease, atypical strains are the rule.

These grow like ordinary tubercle bacilli—some like the bovine, others like the human type; but, whether bovine or human in cultural characters, they possess a virulence which in varying degree is lower than that of the type to which their mode of growth would seem to assign them; and, so far, such strains have been limited, almost exclusively, to cases of lupus[1].

That tubercle bacilli derived from lupus should be peculiar was no more than was to be expected, for lupus itself is a peculiar disease, and differs in several respects so much from other kinds of tuberculosis that some have found it difficult to believe it can be due to exactly the same bacilli. The ways in which lupus differs from other kinds of tuberculosis

[1] For a closer examination of this point see Section III of the Appendix (p. 682).

are as follows: it is an extraordinarily refractory and persistent disease, and though accessible to remedies often defies treatment. It has very little tendency to spontaneous cure, such as we have seen in other kinds of tuberculosis, and often continues to spread for many years, or even for life. In other respects it shows a remarkably low degree of virulence. It spreads very slowly, and seldom extends to the internal organs; and, what is more remarkable, seems commonly to spare even the neighbouring lymphatic glands, though it may be secondary to disease in these structures[1]. Its peculiarities, in short, are that it is at once a very intractable and persistent, and a constitutionally mild disease[2].

Straus, writing about lupus in his book published in 1895, made a remarkable forecast. After describing the main peculiarities of the disease, and laying stress on its slow course, the small effect it produces as a rule on the general health, the richness of the lesions in giant cells and their poverty in bacilli, he goes on to suggest that it may be due to an attenuated variety of tubercle bacillus[3].

The forecast has, in a sense, come true, but perhaps not in that sense which Straus intended. The tubercle bacilli obtained from the majority of cases investigated are, as we have said, atypical. Their virulence is distinctly low—lower than that of the type to which otherwise they would seem to belong. The bacilli found in lupus, then, *are* attenuated. But this does not prove that lupus is *caused* by bacilli of low virulence; for it may equally well be that lupus attenuates the virulence of the bacilli which cause it. To this point we shall presently return.

---

[1] Treves mentions among the complications of lupus the occurrence of tubercular (caseous) disease of the nearest lymphatic glands. "But this," he adds, "considering the true nature of lupus, is surprisingly rare." *System of Surgery*, vol. I, p. 717. Pulmonary tuberculosis may sometimes precede lupus; but it probably supervenes in persons suffering from lupus no more commonly than it occurs in ordinary persons.

[2] The number of deaths attributed to lupus in England and Wales in 1911 was fifty-six.

[3] "Faut-il y voir une forme spéciale, atténuée, de la tuberculose, due à une variété de bacilles moins virulents que ceux qui produisent la tuberculose franche?" *La tuberculose*, p. 741.

With this question of type of bacillus is closely bound up
another: Is the lupus lesion caused by direct inoculation of skin,
or is it but a local manifestation of a blood-borne infection[1]?   If
the latter it is clear that, in view of the constitutional mildness
of the disease, we must postulate either (a) a bacillus of low
virulence from the start, largely incapable of causing mischief
in organs other than the skin, or (b) a patient with peculiar, and
one might perhaps say patchy, powers of resistance—susceptibile
to tuberculosis in the skin, but able to resist infection in the
internal organs.   If, on the other hand, the lesion is due to
external inoculation two alternatives present themselves, either
(c) a bacillus of low virulence incapable of causing further
disease by metastasis and capable, as a rule, only of extension by
continuity, or (d) a normal virulent bacillus, which for some
reason connected with its new environment becomes attenuated,
and which seldom causes deep-seated disease owing to anatomical
peculiarities in the skin itself.   To this latter view, it will be
seen, we tend to incline, though we would not be thought to
deny that there may be something peculiar in the constitution
of the patient liable to lupus.   It is just conceivable that, for
some unknown reason, a skin inoculation of any kind may be
less liable to cause constitutional infection than one elsewhere.   The skin being the frontier most open to attack has
perhaps a stouter barrier interposed between it and the blood
stream than any other; the reader will no doubt call to
mind the fact that in the days before vaccination cutaneous
inoculation provided a more or less safe means of administering so virulent a virus as that of variola, even to young
children.

But these questions cannot be conveniently discussed at
this stage.   We have mentioned them now only to excite
interest in the somewhat lengthy and detailed account, which
will follow, of the results which have been achieved by
experimental investigation.

---

[1] Straus believed it to be due to direct inoculation, for he says: "On
voit donc que le lupus est un type complet de tuberculose locale, résultant
probablement, dans la majorité des cas, d'une inoculation externe," *loc. cit.*
p. 741. For other opinions see footnote, p. 654.

Experimental investigation. Koch was the first to isolate cultures of tubercle bacilli from cases of lupus; and with them he produced tuberculosis in animals. Thus he proved, what until then was only a matter of inference, namely that lupus was but one of the many manifestations of tuberculosis. This was in the early eighties, when as yet there was no hint of the existence of various types of tubercle bacilli, and Koch does not seem to have noticed any peculiarities in his lupus cultures. But from what one can gather from the account of his experiments, regarded in the light of knowledge acquired since that time, it seems probable that some of the strains of tubercle bacilli which he then obtained were of the bovine type; for he records the fact that out of eighteen rabbits, inoculated in the anterior chamber of the eye with material from five different cases of lupus, some died "with extensive tuberculosis of lungs, liver, spleen and kidneys[1]."

Nothing further of importance seems to have come to light regarding the tubercle bacilli in lupus until the Royal Commission investigated their first case of that disease in 1905, and discovered in it an atypical strain of tubercle bacilli which was placed, by the investigator who carried out the experiments for the Commission, in a class by itself as being incapable of complete identification either with the human type or the bovine type[2]. The Commissioners themselves clearly recognized the anomalous nature of this virus[3].

This case[4], known as H 53, was as follows: A young girl, fourteen years old, had suffered, at the time the investigation began, for about four years from lupus of the skin over the right hip. An operation was performed in January, 1905, and scrapings of lupoid tissue sent to one of the laboratories of the Royal Commission. With these scrapings guinea-pigs were inoculated, and from one of these animals a strain of tubercle bacilli was obtained in artificial culture.

This strain grew fairly well on various media, but on the whole it possessed the cultural characters of one of the less

---

[1] *The Etiology of Tuberculosis, loc. cit.* p. 161.

[2] *R.C.T. Int. Rep.* App. vol. II, p. 1059.

[3] *Ibid. Int. Rep.* p. 30.   [4] *Ibid.* p. 884; also 882 A and 1128.

dysgonic examples of the bovine type. Eastwood, who also examined it, placed it in his bovine Class III, and A. S. Griffith, who subsequently reinvestigated the strain, agreed in this[1].

The strain corresponded with the bovine type also in that it produced general tuberculosis in rabbits and calves. But, though this was the case, it was clear that its virulence was not up to the standard of the type. For rabbits indeed, injected intraperitoneally, it seemed at first to be as virulent as ordinary bovine bacilli, but closer scrutiny of the results showed that on the average it killed rather less quickly; and further investigation by A. S. Griffith, using other methods of inoculation, especially subcutaneous injection, clearly showed that its virulence for these animals was not normal. For the calf there could, from the first, be no question that its virulence was not that of the bovine type, though it was clearly higher than that of the human type. It produced indeed a chronic general tuberculosis of mild type.

Three calves were injected subcutaneously with 50 mg. of the bacilli. These animals after some slight indisposition regained their general health and remained in good condition until they were killed three months after inoculation. The tumours at the seats of inoculation and the lesions in the prescapular glands were like those seen in calves inoculated with bacilli of human type, but the lungs were affected more severely than those of any calves inoculated with bacilli of that type, and there were somewhat widespread lesions in the lymphatic glands and, in two cases, tubercles in the spleen. These lesions were of a chronic type, and showed a marked tendency to calcification.

A culture grown from a lesion of one of these animals was injected into four other calves in doses of 10 and 60 mg. with results similar to those just described.

At this point the author, who carried out these investigations for the Royal Commission, was removed to another sphere of activity, and the investigation of the tubercle bacilli concerned in lupus was continued by A. S. Griffith. This observer repeated the investigation of the original strain of bacilli derived from the case, and, in addition to confirming what had already been claimed for it, discovered an additional fact of fundamental importance, namely that the virulence of the strain for the monkey —an animal which the reader will remember is susceptible

[1] *R.C.T. Fin. Rep.* App. vol. 1, pp. 38 and 164.

to both of the mammalian types of tubercle bacilli—was lower than that of either the bovine or the human type. This fact disposed of the suggestion that the strain was transitional and formed a link between the two types; for while it was possible to regard it in this light so far as calves and rabbits were concerned, the view clearly failed to explain its low virulence for an animal which is just as susceptible to infection with the human as with the bovine bacillus. Clearly it was a case of attenuation affecting virulence for all these animal species, and not merely of change from the wider range of virulence of one type to the narrower range of the other[1].

Griffith then proceeded to investigate for the Commission twenty additional cases of lupus. From one of these no strain of tubercle bacilli could be obtained in culture, but in the case of all the rest the attempt to cultivate the bacilli was successful. There were consequently nineteen new strains of tubercle bacilli, besides that from the original patient. From the latter a second strain was acquired three and a half years after the first, and from two other cases also second strains were grown from material removed six months and two and a half years respectively after the first had been received. There were therefore, in all, available for this investigation, including the strain from the original case, twenty-three strains of tubercle bacilli from twenty cases of lupus.

The cultural characters of these strains, and the particular degree of virulence which each of them possessed for various species of animals was very thoroughly studied, the experiments being repeated many times in order that any errors which might

[1] The human type of tubercle bacillus should, as we have attempted to show elsewhere, not be regarded as *less virulent* than the bovine, but as *having a more limited range of virulence* for various animal species. For certain species it is every bit as virulent as the bovine type itself, and for man perhaps more so. This point has been discussed already (on p. 212), but in view of its pertinence to the present question the reader will pardon its repetition.

The low virulence of this strain of bacilli for the monkey was placed beyond any doubt whatever by numerous experiments. Three monkeys were infected by feeding, and no less than eight by injection with carefully measured doses of culture. "Total general tuberculosis indistinguishable from that set up by either human or bovine bacilli was indeed caused in these animals," as Griffith tells us, "but the duration of life was much longer." loc. cit. Fin. Rep. vol. II, p. 43.

arise in consequence of variations of resisting power of different individual animals should be avoided.

The main results of this investigation were as follows: According to their cultural characters some of the strains corresponded to the human type and others to the bovine type. Twelve strains (from eleven cases) belonged to the former (eugonic) type and eleven strains (from nine cases) belonged to the latter (dysgonic) type. The dysgonic strains varied in luxuriance of growth, just as do those obtained from other kinds of human tuberculosis or from the ox itself, some growing very sparsely indeed, and others approximating in luxuriance of growth more or less closely to the human type. These dysgonic lupus strains Griffith classed in three groups, just as he had done the strains of bovine origin. Three of them found a place in Class I, among the least luxuriant of the bovine bacilli, four in Class II, and four in Class III among the more easily-growing strains of bovine origin. The twelve eugonic strains, like the typical bacilli of human type which they resembled in cultural characters, did not differ in manner of growth materially from one another.

While these twenty-three strains of lupus bacilli were identical in their manner of growth with one or other of the two well-recognized types into which mammalian tubercle bacilli are divided, in virulence they deviated (as H 53 had done) for the most part from those types. Only four strains (two dysgonic from the same patient and two eugonic) possessed the full virulence of the type to which in cultural characters they severally corresponded. The rest fell definitely, but to a variable extent, below the standard of their type.

Thus of eleven lupus strains which grew like bovine bacilli nine were less virulent than those bacilli for calves and rabbits. The default of virulence varied, as we have said, in different strains; some produced in these animals general disease like that caused by the bovine bacillus, only not so severe and not fatal, or fatal only after a much longer period than usual; others produced slight disease differing little if at all from that caused by bacilli of human type. But the latter strains, while resembling the human type of bacillus in this respect, differed from it, not in cultural characters only, but in being less virulent for the monkey, and, one may add in the case of some of them, the guinea-pig also.

Of the twelve strains which grew like the human type only two, as we have said, had the full virulence of that type. The other ten fell short of this standard, and produced in animals for which the ordinary strains of human type are virulent (namely monkeys and guinea-pigs), a less severe disease. It is true that in these species even the least virulent of the viruses produced progressive tuberculosis, but in all of the animals inoculated with each of the ten viruses in question it was evident that the disease was less severe and ran a slower course than that caused in similar animals by ordinary strains of bacilli of human type obtained from other kinds of tuberculosis.

Thus most of the strains which nearly resembled the human type were less virulent than that type. They were therefore to be regarded either as attenuated members of the type, or as constituting an entirely new type. Of these alternatives the former is to be preferred because the strains varied among themselves, and in fact seemed to form a series which at one end merged, without a break, in the normal members of the type, and even at the other did not diverge very greatly from them. The evidence therefore compels one to regard them as strains, essentially of human type, in which attenuation had occurred, and had been carried to various lengths.

If this is the right view to take of the eugonic strains, and there can hardly be any doubt that it is, then it seems reasonable that a similar view should be adopted concerning the dysgonic strains also which resembled more or less closely the bovine type. Their deviation from that type in the matter of virulence was often greater than the deviation of the eugonic strains from the human type; but here again we seem to be dealing with a continuous series with various grades of virulence including that of the type itself.

It was perhaps tempting at first to regard the dysgonic strains, the virulence of which for calf and rabbit was less than that of the bovine type but higher than that of the human type, as forming a link between these types; but, as we have seen, this transitional view was untenable owing to the fact that their virulence for monkeys and guinea-pigs was lower than that of the human type; and moreover, even if this view were to be accepted in explanation of the dysgonic strains, there would still remain the eugonic strains, the virulence of which for all species was lower than that of the human type, to be accounted for. The attenuation hypothesis, on the other hand, has the advantage that it is the only one which accounts for *both* the eugonic and the dysgonic strains of low virulence. It seems certain then that we have to do with attenuation—an attenuation which affects the majority of strains coming from lupus, whether they belong essentially to the human or to the bovine type.

Whether the bacilli are attenuated before they cause lupus, or become so during their residence in the human skin, is a question which will be discussed presently; but we may point out in passing that the fact that some of the strains show no default of virulence at all, while others show various grades of attenuation is in favour of the latter rather than of the former alternative.

These conclusions are not yet accepted abroad; but so far no foreign work on the scale of Griffith's investigations for the Royal Commission has been published; and they have been greatly supported and extended by a second investigation which he carried out at Cambridge after the termination of the labours of the Commission. This second investigation will have to be reviewed in detail, but perhaps we may be allowed to defer its consideration for a moment, while we pass on to examine the bearing of the first research on the various problems connected with lupus. This done we shall be better able to follow with interest the second research, and to see how it supports or modifies the deductions drawn from the first one. If this method seems redundant the writer must plead in excuse that it was, of necessity, the method which he himself followed; and that it seems to him to be the least tedious and best way to grasp the true significance of the facts brought out by the experiments.

Is Lupus caused by an Attenuated Bacillus, or do the Bacilli found in its lesions lose some of their Virulence during the course

of their Residence in the Human Skin? One reason in favour
of the latter hypothesis has already been mentioned: lupus
bacilli show varying degrees of attenuation, and some of them
are as virulent as the normal members of the types they
represent; if lupus with all its peculiarities can in some cases
be caused by an ordinary tubercle bacillus, it is clear that its
low virulence and chronic course do not demand an abnormal
bacillus in other cases clinically identical; consequently one
reason for believing that the bacilli which cause lupus must
be attenuated bacilli falls to the ground.

We have now to consider another argument. If these lupus
strains of low virulence are rightly to be regarded as attenuated
members of one or other of the two well known types of mammalian tubercle bacilli, as we have endeavoured to show, and
if the attenuation has occurred in the course of the disease in
the individuals from whom the bacilli have been obtained, one
might reasonably expect that the low degree of pathogenicity
thus recently attained would not be fixed unalterably, and
that virulence would be restored by returning each strain to
such conditions of growth as are normal to its type. In other
words one might expect the attenuated dysgonic strains to
become ordinary virulent bovine strains on *passage* through
the calf, and the attenuated eugonic strains to become ordinary
virulent human strains on *passage* through the deep-seated
tissues of man—if this could be done—and perhaps also through
those of the guinea-pig or monkey. And we might go further
and expect that the readiness with which virulence was restored
would be greater in the less attenuated strains, and in those
which had resided for the shortest period in the skin of their
human host.

Passage Experiments. With the object of following out
this line of argument experimentally the strain H 53 was tested
after residence in the calf, but no increase of virulence was
detected[1]. Griffith also subjected several of the attenuated
strains to the conditions of life in bovine tissues, and afterwards retested their virulence. The results were somewhat
inconclusive. Six of the dysgonic strains were passed through

---

[1] See *R.C.T. Int. Rep.* App. vol. II. table on p. 883.

come from cases in which the disease had had the longest duration. Now we have seen that Griffith classified his strains of bacilli, after dividing them into the two main groups, into subgroups according to their virulence. We have therefore only to place the information thus expressed side by side with the duration of the disease to see whether these two factors march hand in hand. The following table gives these facts.

Degree of Virulence and Duration of Disease[1].

Dysgonic type			Eugonic type		
Strain	Grade of virulence	Duration of disease	Strain	Grade of virulence	Duration of disease
110 a	I	4 years	99	I	Unknown*
110 b	I	4½ ,,	92	I	1⅔ years
100	II	17 ,,	109	II	3 ,,
105	II	1 year	112	II	7–8 years
53 b	II	13–15 years	71 a	II	9 years
107	II	8 years	71 b	II	11 ,,
108	II	5 ,,	101	II	36 ,,
53 a	II	10–12 years	114	II	15 ,,
85	II	3 months			
111	III	10 years	103	III	24 ,,
			106	III	20 ,,
			84	III	15 ,,
			102	III	15 ,,
91	IV	3½ ,,			

* The patient was eight years old.

[1] Perhaps the first thing which strikes one on looking at the tables is the greater average duration of the disease in those cases which yielded eugonic strains as compared with those which yielded strains of dysgonic type. The average duration is actually twice as long in the one case as in the other. This at first sight might seem to give colour to the view that dysgonic bacilli tend to become eugonic bacilli by long residence in the human body. And one must remember in this connection that these cases of lupus are long in proportion to other kinds of tuberculosis, and therefore that such a change, if it takes place at all in any kind of human tuberculosis is likely to occur in lupus. But the correlation of type of bacillus and duration of disease apparent in this table is almost certainly fortuitous, for it is not borne out in Griffith's second series of cases where the average duration of disease is precisely the same in each group. (See p. 639.)

The first two strains in each table are typical examples of the bovine (dysgonic) and human (eugonic) types respectively. The rest resemble, more or less closely, those which they follow, the least virulent being at the bottom of each list.   It will be obvious therefore that if virulence diminishes progressively as the disease advances the most recent cases should come first in the list and the oldest ones last.   Now if we look at the tables to see whether this is so or not we cannot detect among the dysgonic strains any relation of this kind whatever. Strains from cases of comparatively short duration occur at both ends of the list, and others from cases of long duration are to be found in the middle, or even near the top   Among the eugonic strains, however, there is some relation apparent between the length of the disease and the degree of attenuation.   For example, one of the two strains which possessed the full virulence of the type came from the most recent case of all, in which the disease had commenced less than two years previously, and the six least virulent strains (at the bottom of the list) all came from very old cases, in which the disease had been in existence for from fifteen to thirty-six years.   There is however no great regularity, and it seems probable that the relation in question is complicated by another factor.

Has Progressive Attenuation been observed in any given Case? Three of the cases were examined more than once; with the following results: Strain 110, when first obtained, after the disease had existed for four years, was a typical example of the bovine type, and its virulence was that of its type.   A second strain, taken only six months after the first, showed no change. The interval possibly was too short.   In the next case, H 71, the strain was already somewhat less virulent than its type when first examined after residing nine years in the human skin. Two years later it was unaltered.   In the case of H 53 the second strain was even a trifle *less* attenuated than the first; but the disease was already of ten or more years' duration when the first investigation was commenced, and the interval between the two investigations—three and a half years—is not a large fraction of the whole period.

Thus the evidence derivable from repeated investigation fails to reveal any progressive attenuation. But it is very scanty, and the cases for the most part too old at the first investigation. One would like to know the result of a third investigation of H 110 after several years, or of a second investigation of H 92. But for. such information we must wait. In the meantime the evidence may perhaps be regarded as inconclusive rather than negative.

Possible Causes of Attenuation which may act in One Case and not in Another. We have seen reason to think that attenuation takes place in the human skin, but it is not always proportionate to the length of residence there. To this point we must return again when we are in possession of further facts for consideration. In the meantime let us assume that this is so, and see whether we can find any cause or causes which should act more in one case than in another. Two possible suggestions present themselves. Attenuation may, very possibly, be due to daylight, and may, perhaps, vary greatly in different cases according as the lesions are situated on parts of the body more or less exposed to its action; in other words, it may depend upon the intensity as much as on the duration of illumination. This suggestion we shall consider in a moment. The other is that attenuation may perhaps be due to therapeutic agents, especially X-rays or Finsen's light; and to this we will first give our attention.

A. S. Griffith has informed the writer that some of his strains of low virulence came from cases which had previously received no treatment of any kind. But in such a matter it is difficult to learn the exact truth; for patients sometimes conceal from their physicians the fact that they have been in the hands of another doctor, and are reluctant to admit that they have already received any expensive form of treatment lest, if it were known to have been tried without success, a repetition of it would be denied to them. The patient from whom came the strains H 53 *a* and *b*, is known to have been treated with Finsen's light in the interval between the two investigations, and yet the second strain of bacilli was, as we have seen, if anything a little less attenuated than the first.

But the treatment was applied soon after the first investigation was begun, and between this and the commencement of the second investigation there was an interval of three and a half years. During the early part of this time there was a temporary improvement following the light treatment, but it did not persist, and the disease continued to spread widely and affected new regions[1]. Conceivably the bacilli of the second strain may have sprung from a line of ancestors which at the time the treatment was applied entirely escaped its direct action. It is impossible therefore to draw any inference from this case.

In another case X-ray treatment is known to have been applied, and the strain of bacilli (H 102) was one of the most attenuated of the eugonic group, but the disease had already lasted for fifteen years and it is by no means evident that the treatment had anything to do with the low virulence.

Before we leave this point mention may be made of a German case of tuberculosis of one of the bones in the hand of a child. In this case, almost alone among instances of tuberculosis other than lupus, some attenuation of virulence was observed; and on this account the case excited so much interest at the Gesundheitsamt that no less than five separate investigations of the bacilli were made at different times. The case was first investigated by Oehlecker in 1905[2], and afterwards on four occasions by Weber and Steffenhagen, who published full details in 1912[3]. It will not escape the notice of the reader that here also, as in lupus, we have to do with a lesion sufficiently near the surface to be not altogether inaccessible to the possible action of daylight.

The following is a brief outline of the case. Tuberculous disease started in a metacarpal bone in the second year of life, and had persisted for six years when the first investigation of the tubercle bacilli was begun. From this case during the next four and a half years four additional strains of tubercle bacilli were isolated. The original strain was, as we have said, studied by Oehlecker who regarded it as an ordinary example of

---

[1] *R.C.T. Fin. Rep.* App. vol. II, p. 43.
[2] *Tub. Arbeit. etc.* Heft 6, p. 117.   [3] *Ibid.* Heft 11, p. 1.

the bovine type, with the normal virulence of that type. It was only in subsequent strains that any defect of virulence was detected. The second strain was obtained two years after the first by Weber and Steffenhagen, and was recognized to be attenuated. It produced much less severe disease in calves and rabbits than is caused by equivalent doses of typical bovine bacilli, but in other respects it conformed to that type. The third strain was obtained two months after the second and was of similar character. It also possessed low virulence for the ox; ·5 mg. intravenously injected failing to produce a fatal result, though the same dose of the original culture had caused death in twenty-four days. On the other hand it appeared a little more virulent for rabbits than the previous strain. The fourth strain was obtained fifteen months after the third. Its virulence for calf and rabbit was low, like that of Strain No. 3. By intravenous injection its effect was about the same as that of this strain, but by subcutaneous injection it was rather more severe. Such differences are however probably referable to differences of resisting power among the individuals which constituted the test animals. The fifth and last strain, taken eighteen months after the fourth, was unlike all the others except the original strain; for it showed no sign of attenuation, "the result of animal experiments" being "approximately the same as those usually obtained with bovine bacilli."

The authors discussed the significance of the facts revealed by this investigation. They dismissed the suggestion that an originally bovine bacillus was by long residence in the human body in process of becoming converted into a bacillus of human type; for the bovine cultural characters were retained throughout, and the virulence, though it fell off for a time, ended by regaining the bovine standard. The authors concluded that the strain of bacilli, in spite of long residence in the body of man, retained its bovine type, but with notable fluctuations of virulence. "These fluctuations," they say, "may be expressed by a curve which at first falls somewhat; and again rises little by little to its original height." They admit that these fluctuations of virulence far surpassed those observed in other strains of tubercle bacilli, but they suggest that they may have been caused by treatment by bactericidal chemicals, Röntgen rays or Finsen light to which the child had been subjected. No details however are given of this treatment.

Is the Low Virulence of the Majority of Strains of Tubercle Bacilli from Lupus related to the Degree of Accessibility of the Lesions to Daylight? We now turn to the question whether it is daylight which is the cause of the low virulence of the tubercle bacilli found in so many cases of lupus. One does not need to labour the argument that alone of all the lesions caused in man by tuberculosis those of lupus frequently yield bacilli of low virulence, and that equally alone of all these lesions those of lupus are superficial and accessible to daylight.

But the lesions of lupus are not *equally* accessible to light; some are on the face, others on parts habitually covered with clothing, others again in even darker places such as the nasal and buccal cavities. Neither are the strains of tubercle bacilli equally attenuated. We have now to see whether the most exposed lesions yield the most attenuated bacilli, allowance being made, of course, for the time the lesions have been in existence.

Such facts as seem to bear on the problem we are now considering have been extracted from Griffith's report and are set out in the following table. The various strains of bacilli are as before placed in two groups, the eugonic and the dysgonic, and arranged as far as possible in the inverse order of accessibility to light of the lesion which furnished the bacilli. Other details such as the sex and age of the patient and the distribution of the lesions on the surface of the body are added. Finally the grade of virulence is set out in the last column according to the scale drawn up by Griffith, No. I representing full virulence of the class to which the strain is assigned on account of its cultural characters, and the succeeding numbers representing diminishing grades of virulence. Hence, if accessibility to light is the determining factor in attenuation, and if we have assessed it correctly in each case, then the grades of virulence (as shown in the last column) should diminish from above downwards. In other words those strains with unattenuated virulence (Grade I) should come from the cases with lesions least accessible to light, and should therefore appear at the top of each list, and those with the lowest virulence should come at the bottom.

It must be admitted that this is not the arrangement shown in the tables. It is true that the only fully virulent dysgonic strains H 110, *a* and *b* (from a single patient), came from a covered site, but, on the other hand, the only two fully virulent eugonic strains, H 92 and H 99, came from the face. Again, while the most attenuated of the dysgonic strains, H 111, and H 91, came from the exposed situations, neck and chin, three of the most attenuated of the eugonic strains, H 102, H 103 and H 106, came from the more or less covered sites, arm, leg and elbow. To some extent the time factor may be brought in to explain away these departures from expected rule—the last three examples just mentioned, for example, came from cases of very old-standing disease, and one of the strains, H 92, which came from an exposed site and which nevertheless was not attenuated in any degree, was from a case of very recent disease.

Nevertheless it must be admitted that the evidence does not suffice to afford any substantial support to the hypothesis that daylight is the cause of the attenuation found in the tubercle bacilli from many cases of lupus. But it does not disprove that hypothesis. For the problem is not so simple as it seems at first sight. Several factors combine to complicate it. The bacilli investigated are, naturally, taken from actively growing margins, and not unfrequently from entirely new lesions. They may therefore have acquired their peculiar degree of virulence when their forbears were living in some other situation where the conditions as regards exposure to daylight were quite different from those of the part last occupied by them. The history of the case must therefore be taken into consideration. Moreover it is just possible, if the conditions of life in human skin tend to cause attenuation, that virulence may be lost while the lesions remain quiescent, and may be regained in active lesions where the bacilli are rapidly multiplying.

But to return to simpler considerations: the degree to which the bacilli have been exposed to light is most difficult to estimate; for it will vary much according to circumstances.

is the degree of attenuation of the bacillus related to the site of lesion?

No. of case	Sex	Age	Duration of disease in years	Situation of lesion or lesions	Site of material examined	Age of lesion examined	Grade of virulence
Dysgonic type							
53 a	F	15	10–12	Hip	Hip	—	V
53 b	,,	18½	13–15	,,	Ant. Sup. Spine of Ilium	—	III
110 a	M	10	4	Face and trunk	Flank	1 month	I
110 b	,,	10½	4½		Thigh	Of old standing	I
100	F	37	17	Arm	Arm	—	II
107	M	17	8	Face, neck, arms	Elbow	—	IV
108	,,	8½	5	Face, arms, buttock	Arm	—	IV
111	,,	17	10	Neck	Side of neck	—	VII
91	,,	9½	3½	Chin	Under surface of chin	1½ years	VII
85	,,	5	3 months	Nose	Nose	—	VI
105	F	15	1	Palate, nose, lip, cheek	Tip of nose and cheek	—	III
Eugonic type							
103	F	28	24	Leg	Outer side of leg, just below knee	—	V
112	F	16	7–8	Arm	Post. aspect, upper arm	—	III
71 a	,,	14	9	Face, neck, back	Post. int. aspect of arm	? 2 years	III
71 b	,,	16	11	arm, leg			III
101	,,	53	36	Cheek, nose, arm, wrist	Arm	18 months	III
109	,,	5	3	Elbows	Elbow	Fresh growth	II
106	,,	27	20	Face, ear, neck, arm	Elbow	—	V
102	,,	33	15	Face, arm	Arm	—	VI
114	,,	16	15	Nose, neck	Neck	—	IV
92	,,	3¾	1⅞		Cheek	—	I
84	,,	68	?20		,,	—	V
99	,,	8	?	Upper lip, nose, neck	Upper lip	—	I

The occupation and place of residence of the patient will not be without influence, and on the sex, and even the temperament, of the patient will largely depend the amount of light which reaches the bacilli. One must remember that light penetrates more or less through bandages and clothing, and that after all it may be of more importance, in this consideration, on which surface of a limb a lesion is situated, than whether it is situated on that limb or on some other part of the body. Even in the case of a lesion situated on the chin, it will make a considerable difference to the intensity of the illumination it receives whether the lesion is upon the upper or the lower surface of that prominence.

The investigation then is not free from difficulty; and if the results are inconclusive it is perhaps no more than might have been expected. Under the circumstances the most just verdict to pronounce concerning the charge brought against daylight would seem to be not proven rather than not guilty.

It seems to be permissible therefore still to believe in the possibility of light being after all the cause of attenuation, though we have been unable to prove it. A direct experimental investigation of the problem would seem to be desirable. Strains of tubercle bacilli might be grown in duplicate series—one in the dark, in the ordinary incubator, and the other in an incubator provided with a glass door through which regulated amounts of daylight might be admitted. After cultivation in this manner for considerable periods of time the virulence of the two series of cultures might be determined and compared. In this way one might learn whether light is capable of causing attenuation.

A. S. Griffith carried out some preliminary experiments on the action of artificial light on tubercle bacilli, and showed, as was to be expected, that exposure to intense light inhibited growth[1]; but he did not touch the problem of its effect upon virulence[2].

[1] *R.C.T. Fin. Rep.* App. vol. II, p. 9. Griffith made seven experiments with Finsen's apparatus and three with Kromeyer's.

[2] A curious point may be noticed in the preceding table which may or may not be merely a coincidence. All the eugonic strains, corresponding more or less to the human type, came from females, while the dysgonic, or **bovine**, strains

Griffith's Second Investigation.

When the existence of the Royal Commission had come to an end A. S. Griffith continued in Cambridge his investigation of the tubercle bacilli from lupus. These researches are not yet concluded; and we must yet await his last word. But in the meantime a substantial addition to the evidence, in the report of twenty-five additional cases, has been published[1]. This report confirms and extends the results of the first investigation. Twelve cases yielded tubercle bacilli culturally identical with the bovine type, and thirteen yielded tubercle bacilli culturally identical with the human type—almost exactly the same proportion as before. Only two of the bovine and three of the human strains possessed the full virulence of the type to which by their cultural characters they appeared to belong. Some of the bovine strains were as little virulent for calf and rabbit as ordinary strains of human type.

All the strains were tested for virulence on rabbits and guinea-pigs. And in addition eight of the dysgonic strains were tested on calves, and the rest on goats. Three strains were tested on both calves and goats. Three of the dysgonic and six of the eugonic strains were tested on monkeys also. Thus the degree of virulence of each of the strains of bacilli for a number of different species of animals was very closely determined. The determination of the cultural characters was no less thorough.

Classification of the Anomalous Lupus Bacilli. Evidence of Attenuation. Griffith himself, referring to the interpretation

were distributed among six males and three females. This raises the question: Can it be that males have facilities for acquiring infection with bovine bacilli which are absent in the case of females? No such correlation however between sex of patient and type of bacillus is seen in Griffith's second series.

First Series.   Males 6 = Bov. 6 + Hu. 0.   Females 15 = Bov. 4 + Hu. 11
Second Series. Males 11 = Bov. 4 + Hu. 7.   Females 14 = Bov. 8 + Hu. 6

Total   Males 17 = Bov. 10 + Hu. 7.   Females 29 = Bov. 12 + Hu. 17

Nevertheless, taking both series together, there is a greater proportion of bovine infections among the males (59 per cent.) than among the females (41·4 per cent.). This raises the question whether in other kinds of tuberculosis there is more bovine tuberculosis among males than females. We may test this question by means of Griffith's recent investigation of cervical gland tuberculosis. Sixty-six per cent. of the males were infected with bovine bacilli and only 43 per cent. of the females. This is rather curious and deserves more attention.

[1] *Journ. of Pathol. and Bacteriol.* 1914, vol. XVIII, p. 591.

of the facts elicited by this investigation, discusses the relative importance of cultural characters and virulence respectively as a guide to affinities of type; and attaches great importance to the former. He points out that there are two kinds of tubercle bacilli which are anomalous; the one which grows like the human type, and yet has the range of virulence of the bovine type, and the other which grows like the bovine type but lacks the virulence of that type for calves, rabbits and certain other animals. The latter so far as they have been met with in human tuberculosis, if we except the strain from the case of metacarpal bone disease, and Eastwood and F. Griffith's strain already mentioned, have occurred only in lupus. Among animals they have been obtained two or three times from the horse, and three times from the pig. As to the strains which grow like the human type and yet have much the same virulence (for calves and rabbits) as the bovine type, Griffith justly points out that they have always turned out on adequate investigation to be mixtures of the two types. But those which have the cultural characters of the bovine type but less than its standard virulence cannot be disposed of so easily. Either they are to be regarded as bovine strains with attenuated virulence, or human strains with aberrant cultural characters. Which of these views is adopted will depend very much on the importance which we attach to cultural characters, and on our faith in the possibility of their definite determination. Now we have pointed out in another chapter that there are difficulties in the way of accurately determining cultural characters. Various kinds of media, do what we will, refuse to give uniform results. As Griffith himself admits that if you sow two cultures of a given strain on two identical tubes of the same medium the results may be different. Virulence tests, in spite of susceptibility varying in different individual animals, give more constant, and, let us add, more objective, results. The natural attitude, therefore, for the plain man to adopt, when confronted with a strain of bacilli which has the limited virulence of the human type and yet will not grow as luxuriantly on artificial media as that type, is to suspect that through some means there has been a failure to bring to light the true cultural characters, and to rely rather on the results of animal inoculation than on those of artificial cultivation. In this Griffith thinks he would be wrong. Cultural characters, he holds, are of fundamental importance, and can be brought out with certainty by thorough and competent investigation[1].

Some of the strains of lupus bacilli which Griffith classifies as bovine have, in Griffith's own words "no higher virulence for the rabbit (inoculated subcutaneously) than human tubercle bacilli[2]." These strains, as Griffith points out, would be regarded by the observer who attaches more importance to virulence than to cultural characters as strains of human type the cultural characters of which were either abnormal or insufficiently determined.

But in considering the evidence for attenuation we can afford to leave these extreme instances out of count for a moment[3]; for they are in a minority, and if we exclude them there remain plenty of dysgonic strains of low virulence which clearly must belong to the bovine type and which amply suffice to serve as evidence of attenuation. The virulence of these, though low, is not limited like that of the human type, but has the *range* for different animal species which is the peculiar possession of the bovine type, though it falls short in *intensity* of the standard of that type. In plain words these strains cannot belong to the human type because they are more virulent for calf, goat, pig and rabbit than that type. They are either attenuated strains of bovine type, or a new type altogether. The latter alternative is ruled out because these strains form a continuous series with varying grades of

---

[1] Griffith himself took infinite pains. "The testing of a strain," he tells us, "began with the early generations and continued with later ones until it was certain that the cultural capacities had been fully brought to light. Young and vigorous cultures only were used for sowing the test media. The latter were very carefully prepared, and all batches which did not give completely satisfactory results to initial tests were rejected." The cultural characters were tested not on a restricted number of media, but on all the media used in the laboratory.

[2] *loc. cit.* p. 599.

[3] From quite another point of view the matter is very important (see footnote, p. 639).

virulence, verging at one end of the scale into the standard virulence of the bovine type; they are therefore attenuated strains of bovine type, or at least strains of low virulence belonging to that type. It is hardly possible to hold any other view with regard to such a strain as for example H 53, and if we admit the hypothesis of attenuation, or agree that bovine strains may be of various degrees of virulence, to explain such strains as this, we may surely go a little further, and postulate greater degrees of attenuation, or lower degrees of virulence, to explain the extreme cases.

The conclusion that there exist among lupus bacilli dysgonic strains which belong to the bovine type, and which yet possess lower virulence than the ordinary bovine bacilli is supported by the fact that there are also eugonic strains of lower virulence than that of the human type. These clearly must belong to the human type, or else constitute a type by themselves, for there is no other type to which they approximate; and the latter alternative is excluded as before because they too form a continuous series of varying virulence merging at one end into that of the type itself.

Thus we are led, as before, to the conclusion that certain strains of bacilli derived from lupus belong some to the bovine and others to the human type, and yet possess grades of virulence less than that of their type. Whether these have sustained their loss of virulence during their residence in the human skin, or whether they are to be regarded as strains of previously low virulence is another question. But the fact that they have rarely been found except in lupus, to say nothing of the results of the passage experiments which we have already discussed, is in favour of the former of these alternatives. Let us assume for the moment that they are attenuated, and let us see whether we can find any cause for their attenuation.

Search for the Cause of Attenuation. If now we proceed to analyse Griffith's second series of cases, as we did the first, in order to see whether they afford any evidence as to the cause of the low virulence of the majority of the lupus strains of bacilli, the outcome is, as before, inconclusive.

With respect to the question whether there is any correlation between the degree of attenuation and the duration of the disease the results are like—and curiously like—those obtained in the previous investigation. For, just as before, while there is, as Griffith points out, no correlation evident in the dysgonic (or bovine) group, in the eugonic (or human) group there is again some indication that attenuation goes hand in hand with duration of disease. Why there should be this relation

Degree of Virulence and Duration of Disease.

	Dysgonic type			Eugonic type	
Strain	Virulence*	Duration of disease	Strain	Virlence*	Duration of disease
160	Standard Bovine	10 years	165	Standard Human	1 year
155	,,	10 ,,	180	,,	1½ years
			162	,,	6 ,,
176	Attenuated Bovine	9 ,,			
159	,,	23 ,,	179	Attenuated Human	4 ,,
152	,,	3½ ,,	175	,,	11 ,,
173	,,	14 ,,	168	,,	½ year
174	,,	16 ,,	156	,,	6 years
178	,,	10 ,,	151	,,	7 ,,
153	,,	22 ,,	170 a	,,	6 ,,
158	,,	19 ,,	170 b	,,	6⅛ ,,
154 a	,,	8 ,,	157	,,	11 ,,
154 b	,,	8½ ,,	163	,,	38 ,,
172	,,	8 ,,	166	,,	20 ,,
			161	,,	40 ,,

* This is arranged as nearly as possible in "order of merit," the most attenuated viruses coming last. The order of virulence is taken from Griffith's tables IX, X, and XI, *loc. cit.* pp. 617, 621 and 622.

apparent in one group, but not in the other it is difficult to say, and it is possibly only a coincidence; but it is, in that case, remarkable that precisely the same coincidence should have occurred in Griffith's earlier series of cases[1].

[1] The investigation is, moreover, rendered exceedingly delicate by complication introduced by the existence of two types of bacilli; for a few mistakes as to type would reduce the strongest evidence to chaos. Suppose, for example,

But what is the evidence exactly of this relation between duration of disease and low virulence in the eugonic group of bacilli? Let us turn to the table again and see. Two of the three strains which showed no attenuation but had the full virulence of the human type came from comparatively recent cases. The strains of bacilli concerned had been living in human skin for one year and one year and a half respectively. At the other end of the scale we find three strains, the most attenuated of all, coming from very old cases, in which the disease had persisted from twenty to forty years. But beyond this there is no regularity. An unattenuated strain came from a case of six years' duration, and one which showed a moderate degree of attenuation came from the most recent of all the cases, in which the disease had lasted but six months. Thus we may say again, as we did before when reviewing Griffith's earlier series of cases, that there is some relation between degree of attenuation and duration of disease visible in the eugonic group; but it is not constant, and would appear to be complicated by some other factor.

a strain of bacilli which belongs to the human type, and which has the normal virulence of that type, to fail, for one reason or another, to reveal its full cultural potentialities and to be wrongly classified in the dysgonic or bovine group instead of in the eugonic or human, or, again suppose the strain to be really one of those "dysgonic humans," of which we have reason to suspect the existence (see p. 649, also App. III, p. 680), and to have got classified among the bovines. Consider what would be the result of such a very natural mistake. The result would be to make a strain which is in no degree attenuated to appear as one very highly attenuated; and instead of figuring at the top of one list it would come at the bottom of the other. Under these not impossible circumstances we should be at a loss to account for an attenuation which had never taken place.

In order to see what would be the effect of such a mistake on the problem we are now considering let us assume for the moment that H 172 and H 154 belonged really to the human type and were either "dysgonic humans" or that for some reason their true cultural potentialities remained unrevealed. Their virulence for the rabbit, and in one case the calf also, was no higher than that of the human type. (See Griffith, *loc. cit.* p. 617.) Placed on the bovine side these strains appear highly attenuated, and form a marked contrast to less attenuated strains from much older cases. But if these could be transferred to the human side, their virulence would appear to correspond with the duration of the disease in the patients from whom they came. Similar considerations might be applied in the case of strains 85 and 91 in the table which shows the relation of virulence to duration of disease in Griffith's first series (p. 626).

Action of Daylight. Attenuation and Site of Lesion. Turning now to the question whether there is evidence of correlation between the probable intensity of exposure to daylight (as indicated by the site of the lesion) and the degree of attenuation of the bacilli we meet with the same difficulties as before. Moreover the series of cases is not the best possible for the purpose in that it contains no extreme cases. That is to say there are no cases which furnished bacilli from what we may regard as the darkest regions, namely the mucous membranes, and few from the lightest, such as the nose and other parts of the face. The majority came from cutaneous surfaces which are commonly covered, or from such situations as the arm or neck concerning which the amount of exposure is difficult to assess correctly, depending as it does so much on sex, occupation and temperament of the patient, and on the precise part of the limb affected. Such as they are the results are set out in the table on p. 642.

In this table the various strains of bacilli are again divided into two main groups, namely the dysgonic, which have the cultural characters of the bovine type, and the eugonic, which have the cultural characters of the human type. In each group the strains are arranged as much as possible in the inverse order of accessibility to daylight of the site of the lesion which furnished the material removed for investigation; thus the strains from sites which are considered the least accessible, such as the leg or trunk, are placed first, and those from the most accessible sites, such as the face or hand, last. The virulence of the strains, as nearly as possible as determined by Griffith, is given in the last column, I representing the highest grade of virulence[1]. It is therefore evident that if low virulence is correlated with accessibility to daylight the strains which are placed first on the lists, coming as they do from the darkest situations, should be the most virulent, and those which are

---

[1] It must be pointed out that the virulence of the dysgonic strains is graded in four classes and that of the eugonic strains in two only. This is as closely as may be in accordance with Griffith's tables IX and X (*loc. cit.* pp. 617 and 621). Thus in the eugonic group Grade II is the equivalent, not of Grade II of the dysgonic group, but of the dysgonic Grades II to IV.

Is the Degree of Attenuation related to the Site of the Lesion?
(A. S. Griffith's Second Series of Cases of Lupus.)

Type	No. of case	Sex	Age	Duration of disease (years)	Situation of lesion or lesions	Site of material examined	Treatment	Grade of virulence
Viruses of Bovine type	173	M	26	14	Chest and neck	Chest	"A good deal of X-ray treatment"	IV
	154 a	F	14	8	Chest, neck, face	Chest	—	IV
	154 b	"	14½	8½	—	Chest	"At one time X-ray treatment 3 times weekly"	IV
	158	M	19	12	Axilla, neck, face	Axilla	—	IV
	176	"	12	9	Arm	Arm	—	I
	152	F	36	3½	Arm, face	Arm	Hg	III
	178	"	10	5 or 6	Arm and generalized	Arm	—	III
	153	"	22	15	Arm, face, neck, toe	Arm	—	IV
	172	"	16	8	Arm, chest, face, palate	Arm	—	IV
	160	"	16	10	Forearm	Forearm	—	I
	155	M	14	10		,, Neck	—	I
	159	F	28	23	Neck, face	Neck	—	II
	174	"	16	2	Ear	Ear	CO_2*	II
Viruses of Human type	157	M	22	11	Chest, arm, neck, chin	Chest	—	II
	156	"	18	6	Thigh, neck, face	Thigh	—	III
	179 a	F	10	4	Leg	Leg	—	III
	170 a	M	9	6	Arm, face, legs	Arm	—	III
	170 b	"	9	6½	—	,,	Had X-ray treatment	III
	151	F	15	7	Arm, face, legs	,,	—	III
	163	"	46	38	Arm, face	,,	—	III
	161	M	50	40	Neck and face	Neck	—	III
	175	F	19	11	,,	,,	—	III
	166	M	71	20	—	,,	—	III
	162	F	13	6	Ear, face, hand	Ear	—	I
	165	M	57	1	Hand	Hand	—	I
	180	"	35	1½	Thumb	Thumb	—	I
	168	,, F	15	½	Nose	Nose	—	II

I = standard virulence of the type.   II, III, IV = various grades of virulence lower than this standard.   Grade II in the eugonic group must not be taken as equivalent of Grade II in the bovine group but as equal to Grades II, III and IV combined.

placed last should be the least virulent.   In other words Grade I of virulence should be first, and the others should follow in numerical order.

A glance at the table is sufficient to show that this is not the case.   There is, in fact, to be found there no evidence that the degree of attenuation goes hand in hand with the intensity of illumination.   Rather it would seem that the opposite is the case; and though this is probably fortuitous it nevertheless emphasizes the absence of evidence in favour of the hypothesis which is on trial.

We can however, at best, only expect that the degree of attenuation should be proportional to the intensity of illumination when the duration of the disease is constant; and this of course is not the case, but very much the reverse.   We must therefore look to see whether in particular cases which are conspicuous exceptions to the expected rule the duration of disease, either short or long, has overborne the influence of the intensity of illumination.   It must be confessed we get little help from this source.   Two of the normal eugonic strains from exposed sites (H 165 and H 180) came, it is true, from recent cases, and there may not have been time for attenuation to occur; but, on the other hand two of the dysgonic strains (H 160 and H 155) which were equally unattenuated, and which were obtained from the forearm—a site which we must consider (remembering that thin clothing is penetrable) as moderately exposed to light—came from cases in which the disease had already lasted ten years.   Lastly another dysgonic strain (H 159) of comparatively high virulence was cultivated from a lesion in the neck of a patient in whom lupus had already persisted for twenty-three years!

We must confess therefore that the result of this examination of the results of Griffith's second series of lupus cases is, like that of the first, disappointing to those who had hoped to obtain evidence of the view that daylight is the cause of the low virulence of most of the tubercle bacilli found in the lesions of lupus.   But again we must call attention to the difficulties of the inquiry.   The case is not so simple as it first appeared. It is almost impossible correctly to assess the relative amount of illumination received by the lesions of the various cases. And moreover very few mistakes in rightly placing a human strain whose cultural characters had been insufficiently brought to light, or the classification of a dysgonic human strain as an attenuated bovine strain, would seriously confuse the evidence[1]. Therefore while we grant that the hypothesis in question has been far from established, we do not admit that it has been disproved, and in the absence of any better one, we shall continue to incline to the belief that the long continued action of daylight is the most probable explanation of the attenuation of the tubercle bacilli found in the majority of the cases of lupus[2].

Action of Therapeutic Radiation. Turning now to the question whether attenuation may be the result of treatment with X-rays or artificial light we find it very unlikely that this was so in our cases because in the great majority no such treatment seems to have been applied. It is true however, as we have pointed out already, that there is some difficulty in learning what treatment was received by a patient before he came into the hands of the medical man who furnished the material for the bacteriological investigation. But even if we make a liberal allowance for reticence on the part of the patient treatment by X-rays or Finsen's light does not seem to be in such common use as could possibly account for the attenuation of the large proportion of strains of lupus bacilli which fall in virulence below the standard of their types.

The information concerning the treatment of the patients who furnished the material for Griffith's investigation is given in the penultimate column of the table. It is, as we have said, very scanty; only a few patients are known to have received any. But, such as it is, it is not adverse to the view that such treatment may be a cause of attenuation. It is perhaps significant that no X-ray or light treatment is recorded in any case which yielded a virulent strain of bacilli, and that from the three patients in whose cases X-rays are known to have been employed bacilli were obtained which were more or less

---

[1] P.S. No error of this kind however will explain the possession of full (bovine) virulence by viruses after residence of 10 years in forearm.

[2] See note on the therapeutic action of daylight, at the end of this chapter.

attenuated—in two of them indeed (H 154 and H 158) highly attenuated. But the evidence is too scanty to be of much value.

Is Lupus caused by a Tubercle Bacillus the Virulence of which is already of Low Grade? Now that we have examined the evidence in favour of the view that attenuation of the virulence of lupus bacilli takes place during their residence in human skin, and have found it not very satisfactory, and have failed entirely to demonstrate any cause which might produce such attenuation (though the action of daylight has not been put entirely out of court), let us turn to the other alternative and see whether any case can be made out for the hypothesis that lupus is caused by a bacillus already of low virulence before it takes up its residence in the human skin.

Where could such attenuated bacilli come from? They have been found only very rarely, in cases of tuberculosis other than lupus. One very slightly attenuated strain has indeed been recorded, as we have seen, by German writers from a metacarpal bone; and a second strain which had the virulence of the human type and the cultural characters of the bovine type was as has been said already obtained by Eastwood and F. Griffith from a mesenteric gland found in a boy who died of spinal caries. But these stand alone[1]. They are almost the only strains of human origin known to the writer, other than those from lupus itself, which possess a virulence less than that of the type to which they obviously belong. There is practically no evidence that lupus spreads as such from one case to another. We are therefore unable to find a human source of bacilli of low virulence like those which are found so commonly in lupus.

Let us see whether such a source can be found in any of the lower animals. The reader will remember that several of the strains of tubercle bacilli from the horse which have been investigated and three from the pig possessed, together with bovine cultural characters, a low degree of virulence, and these are almost the only bacilli which can be compared with those which have come from so many cases of lupus. Can it be that lupus is contracted from the horse? It must be admitted at once that this is very unlikely. Cases of lupus are probably at least as common

---

[1] P.S. Others have been added since. (See p. 680.)

as cases of equine tuberculosis. Lupus is, apparently, no more frequent among those who have to do with horses than among others who have not. It is indeed a good deal commoner among women than among men. Horse flesh is not used for human consumption in this country; and bacilli with the cultural characters of the human type—which cause at least half the cases of lupus—have hardly ever been found in the horse[1]. It seems impossible then that lupus should come from the horse. No better case can be made out for the pig.

There remains the fowl. Avian tubercle bacilli are commonly believed to be non-virulent for man; yet this doctrine is not held universally, and Rabinowitsch has described a case which she believes to have been caused by an avian bacillus[2]. A. S. Griffith has a curious statement concerning the "atypical, subacute, general tuberculosis which is met with in the great majority of guinea-pigs inoculated intraperitoneally with attenuated (lupus) bacilli (in doses of 0·1 mg.). He says "this form of tuberculosis has very distinct features and resembles that which follows intraperitoneal inoculation of this animal with avian tubercle bacilli[3]." It is tempting therefore to speculate whether after all some cases of lupus may not be caused by avian bacilli. The question has perhaps not received all the attention it deserves, but an affirmative answer would seem to be improbable. None of Griffith's strains grew like avian bacilli and nine of them were injected into fowls without causing progressive tuberculosis[4].

Thus we are unable to find any source of bacilli similar to those which are commonly found in lupus; and we are driven back to the hypothesis that lupus bacilli acquire their peculiar

[1] One strain of tubercle bacilli of human type is mentioned by Möllers as having been obtained from the horse, in the R. Koch Institute for Infectious Diseases in Berlin. *Report of the Tenth International Tuberculosis Conference*, 1912, p. 99.

[2] *Virchows Archiv*, Beiheft z. Bd. 190, p. 476. Löwenstein claims to have found avian bacilli in sputum, in two cases of kidney trouble in children and also in Lipschütz' fatal case of tuberculosis of skin and mucous membranes.

[3] *Journal of Pathology*, vol. XVIII, p. 612.

[4] *R.C.T. Fin. Rep.* App. vol. I, pp. 47 and 259–263. Some of the injections produced "acute tuberculosis" but this occurred in one fowl also injected with sputum bacilli.

properties during their residence in the human skin. Three arguments may be advanced finally in support of this view. First the fact that bacilli of abnormally low virulence are found belonging *both* to the bovine and the human types makes it more likely that a common environment has produced the abnormality than that there should be, independently of lupus, bacilli belonging to two distinct types, and yet possessing the common property of abnormal virulence and the capacity to cause in man that form of tuberculosis and no other. Secondly if the peculiar slow but persistent character of lupus and its little tendency to attack internal organs seems to demand, as Straus thought, a bacillus of low antecedent virulence, we should expect a bacillus of low virulence to be present in *every* chronic case of that disease. But this we have seen is not the case; of the bacilli derived from lupus about one strain out of every five has proved to be a fully virulent example of one or other of the two mammalian types of tubercle bacilli; and the cases which have yielded these strains have not shown any clinical peculiarity.

Still another argument may be brought forward in favour of the view that lupus is caused by bacilli which possess the normal virulence of their types. Many cases of lupus have been secondary to disease in cervical glands. About 12 per cent. of Griffith's cases were of this kind, and all of these, with one exception, yielded bacilli of low virulence. Yet there is no reason to believe that the bacilli were of low virulence while they were living in the cervical glands. Griffith himself, when he attacked the problem of cervical gland tuberculosis, had for one of his objects the search for bacilli of low virulence such as he had found in lupus. But he failed to find them in the sixty-eight cases of cervical gland tuberculosis which he investigated. We must therefore conclude that when lupus is secondary to cervical gland tuberculosis it has been caused originally by a fully virulent bacillus; and if this is true of such cases it is not improbable that it is true also of the others which do not begin in cervical glands.

Continental Investigations of the type of tubercle bacilli concerned in lupus have been few; and of some of them we have, at present, only preliminary reports. Italian observers seem to have noticed that the virulence of the bacilli was abnormally low, but there is not universal recognition of the fact that the majority of lupus strains are attenuated. The proportion of bovine infections is generally much lower than that found by Griffith.

Professor Gosio, at the Tenth International Tuberculosis Conference held at Rome in 1912, briefly reported, among other cases of tuberculosis investigated at the Italian Board of Health, ten instances of lupus. All of these he found were caused by bacilli belonging to the human type. Their virulence was abnormally low. There was in addition a case of *tuberculosis verrucosa cutis* caused by a bacillus of bovine type.

Möller, 1904, isolated a strain of tubercle bacilli from a guinea-pig infected with lupus material; but the description of its characteristics is not sufficiently complete to determine the type to which it belonged.

Weber and Taute, 1907, obtained a culture from another case, and found it identical, in morphological and cultural characters, and in its virulence for the rabbit, with the human type.

Rothe and Bierotte[1], 1913, have issued, from the Institute for Infectious Diseases in Berlin, a preliminary report on an investigation of the type of tubercle bacilli found in lupus. The report deals with twenty-eight cases. From twenty-three of these were obtained bacilli of human type; from four bacilli of bovine type alone; while from the remaining case, in which the disease had attacked two separate regions, bacilli of bovine type were cultivated from the nose, and bacilli of human type from the nates. The observers do not seem to have found anything abnormal about the virulence of these strains of tubercle bacilli.

It is rather remarkable that they did not find a larger proportion of bacilli of bovine type. They ascribed, as we have seen, only five strains out of twenty-nine to this type, or rather more than one in six (17·2 per cent.), while Griffith

[1] Rotte and Bierotte (1913), "Untersuchungen über den Typus der Tuberkelbazillen bei Lupus Vulgaris," 1te Mitteilung, *Veröffentlichen der Robert Koch-Stiftung zur Bekämpfung der Tuberkulose*, Heft VIII and IX. A preliminary communication appeared in the *Deutsch. med. Wochenschr.* 1912, p. 1631.

placed nearly half of his (47 per cent.) in this category. Thus
it would appear that bovine infection in lupus is almost three
times as common in England as it is in Germany. Some not
inconsiderable difference was to be expected after studying
the results obtained in cervical gland tuberculosis, but hardly
so great as this; and when we remember that the English
observer found attenuation and the German observers did not,
we cannot but consider it possible that the one side classed
as strains of human type what the other would have regarded
as attenuated strains of bovine type. The discrepancy may
in fact be due to a difference in the relative value attached to
cultural characters and virulence respectively by the two
schools. It is, for example, just conceivable that some of
Griffith's dysgonic strains of low virulence were really human
strains the cultural potentialities of which had not been fully
brought to light, or, what seems less improbable, that they
belonged to a new sub-class of tubercle bacilli which seems to be
gradually emerging from obscurity, and combines the sparse
growth of the bovine with the limited virulence of the human
type—a class which perhaps we may, for convenience, term the
"dysgonic human" class[1]. On the other hand it may be that the
Germans treated as of secondary importance the failure of some
of their strains to grow up to the standard of the human type
and so classified as belonging to the human type, what Griffith
might possibly have regarded as belonging to the bovine type[2].

[1] See Appendix III, p. 680.

[2] As a matter of fact two of the strains which they classed as human grew
badly. These are Nos. 5 and 18 (loc. cit. pp. 109 and 115). The authors themselves state that the cultural characters of these strains were undetermined
and yet they are included in the general classification from which we have
quoted (loc. cit. p. 97). Elsewhere in referring to new material not fully
worked out at the date of the report they mention two older cases in which
the determination of the cultural characters presented difficulties. These
they relegate to their next report (loc. cit. p. 91).

But about the majority of the strains there could have been no mistake
as to the type; and it may seem remarkable that the Germans did not
notice in these any defect of virulence. But it is to be observed that
they used the rabbit for the determination of virulence, and this animal is
not well suited to reveal small differences of virulence among strains of bovine
type on account of its extreme susceptibility. Thus in the Royal Commission
research the low virulence of H 53, the first of the lupus strains, would probably
have been missed if it had been tested only on rabbits and not upon calves also.

Burnet, 1915, has quite recently sought for attenuated tubercle bacilli in various kinds of cutaneous tuberculosis, not including such as were secondary to tuberculous disease in subjacent bones or glands; and has reported, very briefly, that he has found four strains definitely attenuated among fourteen which he isolated from various cutaneous lesions. The series of cases included four instances of lupus, and two of these yielded attenuated strains of bacilli. All the four attenuated strains belonged to the human type; but the type of the remaining ten does not seem to have been determined.

Passage of one of the attenuated strains through guinea-pigs and a rabbit did not result in any increase of virulence; but from rhesus monkeys infected with it tubercle bacilli were obtained which possessed the normal virulence of the human type.

Attempts to Produce Lupus Experimentally. Some observers have tried to cause lupus to develop in monkeys by inoculating tubercle bacilli into scarified areas of skin; but with very partial success. Griffith made one experiment of this kind in a chimpanzee, but failed to cause lupus[1]. The tubercle bacilli employed had come from a case of lupus, and were of the bovine type and slightly attenuated. The dose was 0·01 mg. of bacilli, spread over a scarified area of 5 cm. The infected patch scabbed over and the skin quickly resumed its normal state, but an abscess formed in the axilla, burst five months after the inoculation, and left a discharging ulcer. The animal died soon after from an unascertained cause. The skin at the site of inoculation was then normal; there was an ulcerated discharging gland in the right axilla, and no sign of disease elsewhere. Two guinea-pigs inoculated with caseo-pus from the ulcer developed tuberculosis; and of two guinea-pigs inoculated with an emulsion of the spleen one became tuberculous. Cultures obtained from these guinea-pigs exhibited the characters of growth of the original strain.

On the other hand Kraus and Kren (1905), Baermann and Halberstaedter (1906), and Kraus and Grosz have been more successful, and have been able to produce some kind of cutaneous

[1] *R.C.T. Fin. Rep.* App. vol. IV, p. 18.

tuberculosis in monkeys, with both human and bovine tubercle bacilli[1], and even, according to Rabinowitsch, with avian bacilli; but in the latter case the effect was transitory. The disease thus caused, however, did not resemble lupus very closely. It lacked its persistent character and showed little tendency to spread. That caused by the human type of bacillus is said to have remained limited in extent and to have tended to heal, while the disease caused by the bovine bacillus was progressive and fatal. Kraus and Grosz make the surprising remark that in the cutaneous lesions caused by the bovine type of micro-organism very few bacilli, or scarcely any, are to be found, while in the retrogressive lesions produced by the human type bacilli are present in enormous numbers, as in the lesions of leprosy. A similar abundance of bacilli may also be seen in the fugitive lesions caused by avian bacilli.

Summary and Conclusions.

Both the human and the bovine types of tubercle bacilli take part in the causation of lupus.

The avian type of bacillus has not been found in that disease.

In this country about 47 per cent. of the cases investigated have yielded bacilli judged to be of bovine type. On the Continent the proportion of cases recognized to be caused by this type of bacillus is much smaller.

The majority of strains of tubercle bacilli from lupus have a lower virulence for animals than that which is normal to their type. Some, however, are quite typical examples of one or other of the two mammalian types.

The degree to which virulence falls short of that which is normal to the type varies; so that we have two groups of strains—a bovine and a human—each of which forms a series of varying grades of virulence, beginning with that normal to the type itself.

Concerning the greater number of strains of tubercle bacilli there can, in spite of low virulence, be no reasonable doubt as to the type to which they belong. But there are a few strains which it is difficult to classify, and which might be regarded

---

[1] Quoted from Rabinowitsch, *Virchows Archiv*, Beiheft z. Bd. 190, p. 215.

by one school as highly attenuated bovine strains, and by another as human strains with aberrant cultural characters.

Which of these views is adopted will depend on the relative importance attached to cultural characters and virulence; and it is probable that such discrepancy as there is between English and Continental findings may be due partly to a difference in the value attached to these indications here and abroad.

Nevertheless it is probable that there is in lupus, as in other forms of human tuberculosis, a real difference in the relative frequency of infection with bovine bacilli in this country and on the Continent respectively.

It must be admitted that our inquiries concerning the cause of the low grade of virulence possessed by the majority of strains of tubercle bacilli obtained from the lesions of lupus have proved inconclusive. The most that one can venture to say is that it seems probable that the bacilli which cause lupus are fully virulent tubercle bacilli at the start, and that, as a rule, their virulence becomes attenuated during the course of the disease. The fact that varying grades of virulence exist, both in the human and bovine groups of bacilli, is consonant with this view.

The alternative hypothesis that lupus is caused by bacilli *already* of low virulence, much as it accords with the clinical characters of the disease, seems to be untenable for several reasons, but chiefly owing to the absence of any known and sufficient source of such bacilli.

While we believe that attenuation takes place during the course of the disease we freely admit that the degree of attenuation reached in any given case is by no means always proportionate to the duration of the disease. This is the case even in the human group of viruses, while in the bovine group there is no evidence at all of any relation of this kind.

If however we were to adopt a slightly different estimate of the relative values of cultural characters and comparative range of virulence as criteria of type, and were to classify afresh some of the most extreme examples of the strains hitherto regarded as attenuated bovines and concerning the type of which some difficulty might reasonably be admitted, if, in fact, we were to regard these as "dysgonic humans" or strains of human type whose cultural potentialities had not fully come to light—if this were done then the want of correlation between the degree of the degradation of virulence of the bacillus below the standard of its type and the duration of the disease in the patient which furnished it (which was so peculiar a feature of the dysgonic (bovine) as contrasted with the eugonic (human) group of viruses in each of Griffith's series of cases) would largely disappear, and the one group would come into line with the other.

As to the cause of attenuation nothing definite can be affirmed. Treatment with X-rays or Finsen light, though possibly one cause of this change, is not employed in a sufficiently large proportion of cases to account for the low virulence which is found in eight out of ten of the strains of tubercle bacilli which have been isolated in this country from lupus. There remains the action of daylight and in the absence of any more probable explanation it seems to us permissible to hold tentatively that this may be the cause of the attenuation. At the same time there is no *proof* of this, and it is only right to emphasize the fact that the most attenuated viruses have not come as a rule from the most exposed parts of the body.

If lupus is caused by ordinary tubercle bacilli which at the outset are fully virulent, it may be asked, how is it that the disease runs a course so different from that of other kinds of tuberculosis—why, on the one hand, does it show so slight a tendency to spread deeply to lymphatic glands and internal organs and is so seldom fatal, and yet, on the other, is so persistent and intractable? We have seen that the explanation is not to be found in any special properties of the bacillus; it must therefore be sought for in the patient.

Perhaps the explanation lies hidden in some anatomical peculiarities of the skin which only permit the bacilli to multiply with extreme slowness—for lupus lesions are notoriously poor in bacilli—and consequently restrict the chances of a general infection until the patient has acquired some degree of immunity. But why then is the disease so persistent? Perhaps the skin possesses only imperfect mechanisms for bacterial destruction. But this can hardly be so; for no bacteria other than tubercle bacilli exhibit any special persistence when they invade the skin[1].

Thus we are led to entertain the idea that the skin in certain individuals has a special weakness which allows tubercle bacilli to remain in it in comparative security. If this is true, and there is some physiological idiosyncrasy of the individual subject to lupus, we may well believe that the disease is not necessarily the result of a local external inoculation, but may be caused by bacilli which have entered the body by some other portal and have been carried to the skin by the blood-stream[2].

It must be admitted that in spite of much good work and some remarkable discoveries the etiology of lupus remains obscure.   Does lupus attack the skin because of local accident of inoculation, or because of some peculiar weakness in the skin

[1] There can hardly be any doubt that in its relation to bacterial invasion the skin exhibits very special properties.   One thinks at once of erysipelas, caused apparently by the ordinary *Streptococcus pyogenes* and yet running a course very different from that of the pyogenic lesions produced by this micro-organism elsewhere.   But erysipelas shows no particular persistency as compared with the other activities of the streptococcus.   Several other skin infections besides erysipelas present the peculiarity of spreading at one margin and healing at another which we see also in lupus.

[2] Senn, in his *Principles of Surgery*, 1890, stated, rather dogmatically, that "lupus vulgaris, and probably other varieties of this affection of the skin, are nothing more or less than cases of cutaneous inoculation-tuberculosis" (*loc. cit.* p. 459).   But he admits that a diffuse tuberculosis of skin and mucous membranes occurring as a sort of secondary localization in patients suffering from advanced tuberculosis has been described by several authors (*loc. cit.* p. 462), but this is not what one ordinarily regards as lupus.

At the International Conference at Rome in 1912 the view that lupus in the great majority of cases is not due to direct infection from the outside, but is the result of metastasis from some older focus, was supported by Neufeld.

One knows, of course, that many cases of lupus are secondary to disease in subjacent glands or bones, but this is not metastasis but direct infection in continuity of tissue.   The view that is attracting attention now is that lupus ordinarily may not be a direct infection at all, but may be due to blood-borne bacilli in persons whose skins are peculiarly susceptible.   Treves in his *System of Surgery* (vol. I, p. 717) mentions among the complications of lupus the occurrence of a widespread outbreak of lupus nodules on many parts of the body, quite remote from the primary patch.   "This curious fact, observed most often in children, can," he says, "only be explained by infection through the blood."

of the individual? We cannot say. Is it caused by a bacillus already attenuated, or by a bacillus of standard virulence which becomes attenuated afterwards? Probably the latter. What is the cause of this attenuation? We do not know. We can only guess that it is daylight, but can bring nothing but probability in support of our hypothesis. Why is lupus at once so mild constitutionally and yet persistent almost to the point of malignancy? None of these questions can be answered; at best we have only been able to suggest some more or less plausible solutions to some of them.

One thing is certain: lupus presents problems of the greatest interest to the pathologist, and more work is needed to elucidate them. . That which has already been done has obtained splendid results, but it has not exhausted the subject.

Note on the Influence of Sunlight on Surgical Tuberculosis.

The therapeutic influence of sunlight on surgical tuberculosis has been attracting considerable attention in recent years, and direct exposure to the sun's rays has been deliberately employed at Leysin in the Swiss mountains and elsewhere. In 1912 Dr F. Morin reported very favourably to the Tuberculosis Congress in Rome on the results of this treatment in cases of tuberculosis of glands, bones and joints and skin (*Brit. Med. Journ.* 1912, I, p. 962), and shortly afterwards, M. Armand Delille related equally encouraging experiences to the Société de Pédiatrie in Paris. His remarks were confirmed by others present. Quite recently Dr A. Rollier has published a remarkable book, full of pictures of the results produced at Leysin. The little patients, after a period of progressive acclimatization, live for part of the day in the open air, entirely without clothes other than a loin cloth. In this garb they are shown attending school under a tree with the snow around them, and they may even be seen skating and skiing with no additional protection other than their boots. Some of the cures shown in the illustrations appear almost miraculous; and it is distinctly encouraging to turn from a picture of an emaciated child covered with numerous superficial tuberculous lesions, to other pictures of the same child showing how he became the champion of the boys and the leader of their sports. The cases found most suitable for the treatment were those formerly known as "strumous," namely tuberculosis of lymphatic glands, joints and skin. Now in these the lesions are more or less superficial, and it is not impossible that the beneficial influence of sunlight may be exerted directly on the bacilli, though this does not seem to be Rollier's opinion, and indeed it is evident that we cannot disassociate the direct effect of sunshine from the constitutional influence of the climate and of the other treatment they receive. (*La Cure de Soleil*, Dr A. Rollier, Baillière et fils, Paris, 1915.)

Dr Lynn Thomas has written to the *British Medical Journal* to say that treatment with sun's rays has been recently employed with success at the Glan Ely Sanatorium in Wales. See also Holmboe on heliotherapy in Norway. Abst. in *Lancet*, 1916, I, p. 199.

Note on Cutaneous Tuberculosis in Birds.
Tuberculosis in the parrot often takes the form of a cutaneous affection, and is caused as a rule by the human type of bacillus. Cutaneous lesions are sometimes seen in other birds also, and are then caused by avian bacilli. So far as the writer is aware no defect of virulence has been observed in the bacilli of either type obtained from cutaneous lesions in birds, but it would be interesting to subject them to a more critical examination than they have probably as yet received, and to see whether any of them are attenuated as are the tubercle bacilli from the majority of cases of lupus.

REFERENCES. XVII

(Chapter xxv)

Lupus.

Baermann and Halberstaedter (1906) (Java Expedition von Neisser). Experimentelle Hauttuberkulose bei Affen. *Berl. klin. Wochenschr.* No. 7.

Burnet, Et. (1915).   Sur la Virulence des Bacilles Tuberculeux. *Ann. de l'Inst. Pasteur*, vol. xxix, p. 221.

Cobbett (1907).   *R.C.T. Int. Rep.* App. vol. ii, pp. 16, 884, 1029, 1059 and 1129.

Griffith, A. S. (1911).   *Ibid. Fin. Rep.* App. vol. ii.   Investigation of Viruses obtained from Cases of Lupus.

—— (1914).   Further Investigations of the Strains of Tubercle Bacilli isolated from Cases of Lupus. *Journ. of Pathol. and Bacteriol.* vol. xviii, p. 591.

Koch, R. (1884).   *The Etiology of Tuberculosis.* Eng. trans. *Microparasites in Disease.* New Syd. Soc. pp. 122, 161 and 180.

Kraus and Kren (1905).   Ueber Erzeugung von Hauttuberkulose bei Affen. Quoted by Rabinowitsch, *Virchows Archiv*, Beiheft zum Bande 190, p. 215.

Kraus and Grosz (1907).   Ueber experimentelle Hauttuberkulose bei Affen. *Wiener klin. Wochenschr.* vol. xx, No. 26, p. 795. Quoted by Rabinowitsch, *loc. cit.* p. 215.

Lipschütz (1914).   Über ein eigenartiges durch den Typus gallinaceus hervorgerufenes Krankheitsbild der Tuberkulose, etc. *Archiv f. Dermatol. u. Syphilis*, vol. cxx, p. 387.

Löwenstein (1913).   Ueber das Vorkommen von Geflügel-Tuberkulose beim Menschen. *Wiener klin. Wochenschr.* p. 785.

Möller (1904).   Vergleichende experimentelle Studien über Virulenz verschiedener Tuberkelbazillenstämme menschlicher Herkunft. *Zeitschr. f. Tuberkulose*, vol. v, p. 5.

Rothe and Bierotte (1913).   Untersuchungen über den Typus der Tuberkelbazillen bei Lupus vulgaris, 1te Mitteilung. *Veröffentlichungen der R. Koch-Stiftung zur Bekämpfung der Tuberkulose*, Heft viii and ix.   *Deutsch. med. Wochenschr.* 1912, No. 35.

Straus (1895).   *La tuberculose*, p. 725.

Weber and Steffenhagen (1912).   Was wird aus den mit Perlsuchtbazillen infizierten Kindern, und welche Veränderungen erleiden Perlsuchtbazillen bei jahrelangem Aufenthalt im menschlichen Körper. *Tub. Arbeit. a. d. Kaiserl. Gesundheitsamte,* Heft ii, p. 1.

Weber and Taute (1907).   Weitere Untersuchungen über Tuberkelbazillen verschiedener Herkunft, etc.   *Ibid.* Heft 6, p. 15.

CHAPTER XXVI

THE PART PLAYED BY BOVINE INFECTION IN HUMAN TUBERCULOSIS

We have now arrived at the point from which it is desirable to take a comprehensive view of the relative importance of infection with human and bovine tubercle bacilli respectively in human tuberculosis. No doubt we do not yet possess the evidence which will enable a final verdict to be pronounced; certain questions concerning atypical strains await solution, and the last word has not yet been said on the question of stability of types of tubercle bacilli. Under these circumstances all that can be done is to produce some sort of provisional estimate based upon such evidence as is at present available; and this with the caution that it stands or falls upon the doctrine that the various types of tubercle bacilli are stable, or at least so far stable that they do not change during the period of the disease in any one individual. If this doctrine should in the future be found to be untenable—an event which appears to us to be improbable—the estimate will have to be profoundly modified.

This estimate may be arrived at in the following way. Among grown up people fatal bovine infections are, statistically speaking, almost negligible; among children over five years of age they are so few as to make very little difference to the result; the great majority of deaths from infection with bovine bacilli occur in children under five years of age. Let us then proceed to estimate the amount of fatal bovine infection in children under five, and we shall arrive at a measure, somewhat, but not much, below the truth, of the total mortality caused by bovine bacilli at all ages.

Now we have already estimated to the best of our ability, and according to the information available, the proportion of bovine infections in each of the classes into which tuberculosis is clinically divided, and the figures published by the Registrar-General afford us a means of calculating the percentage of the total deaths among children under five from tuberculosis of all kinds provided by each of these classes. From these two sets of data we can deduce the percentage of deaths from tuberculosis of all kinds in children under five which is caused in each class by the bovine bacillus. We have only to add these together to get the proportion of deaths from tuberculosis of all kinds at this age period which is caused in all classes together by the bovine bacillus. This we calculate is about 33 per cent., or one-third. The following table shows how this figure is arrived at.

Proportion of Deaths attributable to Bovine Infection in 100 *Children under Five Years of Age, dying of Tuberculosis of all kinds.*

Class of tuberculous disease	Number of deaths in each class (Reg. Genl. Rep. 1911)	Percentage of total deaths attributed to each class	Proportion of deaths in each class caused by the Bovine Tub. Bac.	Percentage of total deaths in children attributed to Bov. Tub. Bac. in each class
Pulmonary tuberculosis	1448	16·3	$\frac{1}{6}$	2·7
Tuberculous meningitis	3347	38	$\frac{1}{8}$	4·75
Abdominal tuberculosis	2700	30·2	$\frac{3}{4}$	22·5
General tuberculosis	1185	13·2	$\frac{1}{6}$	2·17
Tub. of bones and joints	83	1	$\frac{1}{4}$	·25
Tub. of other organs	114	1·3	?	say ·63
	8877	**100·0**	—	**33·00**

Now the deaths from tuberculosis of all kinds among children under five years of age constituted, at the date of the last Report of the Registrar-General, one-seventh of the deaths from the same cause at all ages. If we may assume for the moment, as a very rough approximation, that *all* deaths from tuberculosis which are caused by infection with bovine bacilli occur under five years of age, and that all which take place after this period are caused by infection with bacilli of human type, then we should conclude that one-seventh of 33 per cent.—or 4·7 per cent.—of all the deaths from tuberculosis at all ages is due to infection with bovine bacilli. Let us, for the sake of round numbers—since we are only dealing with broad approximations—call this 5 per cent., and let us take this figure as the basis of our calculation. To it we must add something for the deaths from bovine infection which occur after five years of age. The estimation of this allowance is more or less guesswork, but we have shown that it must be, relatively, a small one. If we put it at 1 per cent., this will probably be a liberal allowance. Thus we arrive at the estimate that the mortality caused by infection with the bovine type of tubercle bacillus at all ages is 6 per cent. of that caused by both types of tubercle bacilli combined. This, on the basis of our latest returns, would amount to 3180 deaths per annum.

We might have based our estimate on the proportion of bovine infections in each kind of tuberculosis at all ages instead of in children under five as we have done. In that case the estimate would have worked out rather higher, namely at about $7\frac{1}{2}$ per cent. But we prefer the former method as more accurate, because so much of the work has been carried out on material obtained from this early age period.

Of other forms of tuberculosis not included in our calculation, such as tuberculosis of cervical glands and lupus, the proportion of bovine infections is very much higher, probably approximating to 50 per cent. But these forms of tuberculosis are not fatal as such, and when they lead to death it is by the implication of the great internal organs, and the deaths fall into other categories. They are therefore not really excluded from our estimate.

Is Infection with Bovine Bacilli more curable than that with Human Bacilli? This question does not admit of a precise answer. We can here only deal with probabilities and arguments; for once an infection is cured it is not possible to tell what type of bacillus has caused it. Nevertheless there are two good reasons for believing that the human type of tubercle bacillus is more virulent for man than the bovine, and that infection with the latter is not followed by death in so large a proportion of cases as infection with the former. The first of these reasons is afforded by the fact that while bovine bacilli are found very commonly in very young children, they become less frequently seen as age advances, and are rare in adult life.

42—2

This fact admits of only two solutions: either the bovine bacilli slowly turn into human, a conclusion which we have shown elsewhere is not borne out by the best investigations, or the bovine bacillus, while it readily invades the bodies of children, is scarcely able to infect the more resistant adult, while the human bacillus can easily do so.

The second reason is based upon the allegation that infection with bovine bacilli is especially frequent in the more curable kinds of tuberculosis. Let us see how far this is supported by evidence. In the first place we have seen that bovine infections are particularly common in abdominal and cervical gland tuberculosis, neither of which is so commonly fatal as pulmonary tuberculosis which is almost always caused by the human type of bacillus. But perhaps it may be objected that this is because the lungs are more vital and delicate structures than lymphatic glands or peritoneum.

The argument may be supported by the case of tuberculous peritonitis. One remembers the surprise felt in the Medical Profession when, in cases in which tuberculous peritonitis had been rendered directly visible by abdominal section, the disease was, not very uncommonly, found to end in recovery. At the present day, we may safely say, tuberculous peritonitis is regarded as more curable than pulmonary tuberculosis, and we now know that the former is frequently, and the latter hardly ever. caused by the bovine type of bacillus.

Further evidence may be obtained from the striking fact that has come to light, in recent years and in many quarters, that quite a notable number of tuberculous lesions—not calcareous ones only, but often caseous and containing well-formed bacilli—are incapable of infecting guinea-pigs or of yielding cultivations. Such lesions may be regarded as cured—at least the infection is at an end—and the evidence referred to rests on the fact that such cured lesions have been found more commonly in those sets of glands, such as the cervicals and mesenterics, which are frequently infected with bovine bacilli than in the bronchials which are far less often infected with this type of micro-organism. Let us examine this evidence in detail.

Weber and Taute[1] reported no less than thirty instances in which mesenteric or other abdominal lymph glands, obviously calcareous or caseous, were emulsified and injected into guinea-pigs without causing tuberculosis.

Among the Royal Commission cases were ten in which glands obviously tuberculous failed to infect guinea-pigs injected with them. In seven of these cases the affected glands were mesenteric, in one cervical and inguinal, in one axillary, and in one bronchial[2].

Eastwood and F. Griffith recorded sixteen cases in which lesions obviously tuberculous, many of which contained visible tubercle bacilli, failed to infect guinea-pigs injected with them. In one of these cases the point of origin seemed doubtful. In seven it was alimentary, and in eight respiratory[3].

A. S. Griffith met with five similar cases. In four the tuberculous disease was localized in the mesenteric glands and in the fifth in the bronchial glands, only one set of glands in each case being implicated.

Again, in his study of cervical gland tuberculosis, A. S. Griffith found that among the glands removed from 110 children those from twenty-nine, though definitely tuberculous to the naked eye, failed to infect guinea-pigs. Fifty guinea-pigs in all were injected, and in two cases the investigation was repeated. Moreover direct culture was tried in twenty-six of the cases and failed every time. The bacilli were therefore not attenuated; they were dead. In fifteen of these cases tubercle bacilli were seen in the emulsions and in seven of these the bacilli were numerous or moderately numerous, and were short and well stained. Griffith himself is inclined to regard the morphological character and the number of bacilli as presumptive evidence of bovine infection.

Lastly, one may mention a case of infection with bovine

[1] *Tub. Arbeit. etc.* Heft 6, p. 43.

[2] *R.C.T. Int. Rep.* App. vol. II, p. 17, and *Fin. Rep.* App. vol. I. pp. 14 and 103.

[3] Of caseous or calcareous glands, five bronchials and seven mesenterics were injected without result.

bacilli in which it was twice proved that the disease had died out locally. The case was as follows:

> C. L.[1], when a little more than a year old, came under observation for tuberculosis of cervical and inguinal glands. Two glands removed from the neck were found to be caseous and purulent. From them a strain of bovine bacilli was cultivated which proved to be dysgonic and highly virulent for calves and rabbits. Fifteen months later two more cervical glands were removed. They are described as being as large as gooseberries and containing softened caseous matter. They were emulsified and injected into guinea-pigs, but failed to cause tuberculosis. Cultures also were attempted, but no growth occurred. The infection had come to an end, in these glands at any rate. About two and a half years later a tuberculous inguinal gland was removed. It was caseous and calcareous and a few tubercle bacilli were demonstrated by microscopic examination; but guinea-pigs and rabbits which were injected with it failed to develop tuberculosis, and no cultures could be grown directly from it. The child which had been in very poor health at the time of the first operation was quite well and healthy looking when last seen.

Taking all these investigations together, we find that there are a large number of instances on record of healed tuberculosis in cervical and mesenteric glands, organs which are frequently attacked by bovine bacilli, and only a few instances of healed tuberculosis in bronchial glands, which are seldom attacked by bovine bacilli, and very commonly by human bacilli. It is true that we have not any strictly uniform series of observations on glands of the two classes to compare with one another, and that much more numerous investigations have been made with the one class of gland than with the other. We have not even been able to work out a percentage in each case, and the results of Eastwood and F. Griffith suggest caution. But at the same time the very large number of healed tuberculous lesions in such lymphatic glands as are known to be frequently the seat of disease caused by bovine tubercle bacilli is imposing, and though not proof that lesions caused by bovine bacilli are more curable than those caused by human bacilli, is at any rate presumptive evidence of this hypothesis.

[1] *R.C.T. Int. Rep.* App. vol. ii, p. 621, and *Fin. Rep.* App. pp. 12 and 108.

CHAPTER XXVII

GENERAL SUMMARY AND CONCLUSIONS

We have now arrived near the end of our task, and there remains nothing to be done but to gather together in concise form the various conclusions which may, we believe, justly be drawn from this inquiry.

We have studied the grounds for dividing tubercle bacilli into several "types," and have inquired to what extent the latter are stable. We have followed the distribution of the types in various animals. We have, in greater detail, surveyed the domain of human tuberculosis and sought to discover in each of its subdivisions the parts, if any, played by these types. Our conclusions may therefore be divided into two divisions: one which concerns the classification of tubercle bacilli, and the other which deals with their distribution among various animal species, and more especially in the different forms of tuberculosis as it occurs in man.

I. *General Conclusions concerning the Classification of Tubercle Bacilli.*

1. Tubercle bacilli are of three kinds or "types," known respectively as the human, the bovine and the avian.

2. These types each present peculiarities of growth and virulence. It is not correct to say that one is more virulent than another, though this may be true of their virulence towards a given species of animal; the difference may be more accurately defined by stating that one type is virulent for a large group of animals, and another for a smaller group.

3. Though these three kinds of tubercle bacilli have doubtless descended from a common ancestral type, yet the special characters, which they have acquired by adaptation, each to a particular species, or group of species, of animal, and which distinguish them from one another, have become

fixed, and are now stable; that is to say they are stable to the extent that the types do not tend to change one into another when the conditions of life are altered and made as favourable as possible for such a change (as for example when bacilli of human type are made to live in the ox). We do not, of course, mean to assert that this stability of type is absolute, and would continue if the new conditions were to be prolonged indefinitely, but merely that no alteration of type becomes evident when such change of environment is continued for so long a time as that to which laboratory experiments can reasonably be extended. There is therefore reason to believe that bovine tubercle bacilli when they attack man do not, in the course of the disease in any one individual, become changed into bacilli of human type.

4. This conclusion is supported by the fact that when bacilli of bovine type are found in human tissues, even in cases where the disease is of very old standing (cases of lupus excepted) they show no deviation of any kind from their type; but are as virulent for calves, goats and rabbits (animals which resist infection with the human type of bacillus), and grow as sparsely on artificial media (which is characteristic of bovine bacilli) as do the bovine bacilli from the ox itself.

5. The doctrine of stability of type is in harmony with the fact that atypical strains (which might be regarded as transitional) are rare. Moreover one class of these—which we may perhaps venture to call the *eugonic virulents* because they combine the free growth, on artificial media, of the human type with the wide range of virulence of the bovine type—have often been proved to be mixtures. Of atypical strains there remain then only a few which combine the dysgonic growth of the bovine type with the limited range of virulence of the human type[1] (a class which might be called the *dysgonic human* type), and some others which resemble the human and bovine types except that their virulence is not so high.

6. These latter are believed to be attenuated members of the bovine and human types. They resemble, in cultural

[1] *E.g.* strain No. 99, Eastwood and F. Griffith, see p. 604 of this volume, and others, for which see App. III, p. 681.

characters and in range of virulence for various animal species, one or other of these types, but they differ from them in degree of virulence, and this to a variable extent.

II *a*. *Distribution of the Three Types of Tubercle Bacilli among Various Animal Species.*

1. *The Bovine Type of Tubercle Bacillus* is found in the tuberculous lesions of the ox,· pig, goat, sheep, horse, camel, cat, dog, monkey and, in a certain proportion of cases, man.

Atypical strains, resembling the bovine type in cultural characters, and more or less also in the wide range of their virulence, but falling short of the bovine standard in the severity of the disease which they cause, have been found several times in the horse and pig. They have also occurred rather frequently in man, in cases of lupus.

2. *The Avian Type of the Bacillus* has been found in the tuberculous lesions of the common fowl and in those of most of the domesticated birds. It has been demonstrated in the rabbit living in captivity with fowls, in rats and mice caught in the poultry yard, and in localized glandular tuberculosis in the pig. It has been described but rarely in human lesions, and it is probable that it plays no important part in human tuberculosis.

3. *The Human Type of the Bacillus* is the most limited in its distribution of the three. It is found in the great majority of cases of human tuberculosis, in perhaps more than one half of the rather uncommon instances of tuberculosis in the dog, and, sometimes, in the localized glandular tuberculosis of the pig. It is said to have been found once in the horse. It is found also in the tuberculous lesions of the captive monkey and the caged parrot, and, rather curiously, in many of the instances of tuberculosis which occur in the mammals of zoölogical gardens—it has been found, for example, in the antelope, elephant and lion.

Atypical strains, closely resembling the human type, but falling short of the standard of this type in virulence, have been found rather frequently in cases of lupus.

II *b*. *Distribution of the Various Types of Tubercle Bacilli in Human Tuberculosis.*

1. The great majority of the fatal cases of tuberculosis in man are caused by the human type of tubercle bacillus. This majority has been roughly estimated at 94 per cent. The remaining 6 per cent. of the fatal cases are caused by the bovine bacillus.

The avian bacillus has practically no share in this mortality.

2. Of non-fatal cases of tuberculosis, and particularly of such as involve cervical or mesenteric lymphatic glands, the bovine bacillus claims a much larger share, which, in very round numbers, may be put somewhat above 50 per cent. A smaller, but still large, proportion of cases of lupus also are caused by this type of bacillus.

3. Infection with bovine bacilli is commonest in infancy, uncommon after five years of age, and rare in adult life.

4. The kind of tuberculosis for which the bovine bacillus is responsible in mankind may be defined in more detail. It is in fact mainly connected with the alimentary canal. It includes tuberculosis of mesenteric glands, with or without ulceration of intestine, and, arising out of this, tuberculous peritonitis and certain instances of meningitis and general tuberculosis. To these may be added tuberculosis of tonsils and various groups of lymphatic glands in the neck, and lupus.

5. The kind of tuberculosis for which the human type of bacillus is responsible is mainly pulmonary, and such as arises from bacilli which enter the tissues through the respiratory passages. It includes also, as we have just seen, somewhat less than half the cases of abdominal and cervical tuberculosis and more than half the cases of lupus. It is responsible for the great majority of instances of general tuberculosis and meningitis.

From a few adult cases of pulmonary tuberculosis in this country and elsewhere only bovine bacilli have been obtained; but it is probably not too much to say that such cases are very exceptional, and that the immense majority of the instances of disease which are classed as phthisis are caused by the human type of tubercle bacillus.

6. Concerning the share taken by each of the two mammalian types of tubercle bacilli in bone and joint tuberculosis an opinion which is strangely in contrast with that received generally has lately been expressed in Edinburgh. This represents the proportion of such cases caused by infection with bovine bacilli, in that city, at considerably more than 50 per cent. (58·6 per cent.). Elsewhere, however, the Royal Commission in this country, the Gesundheitsamt in Berlin, and the Department of Health in the City of New York agree in finding the part played by bovine bacilli in this kind of tuberculosis only a small one. The question cannot as yet be considered as settled[1].

7. There is evidence that the share taken by the bovine bacillus in causing tuberculosis differs in different countries. It would appear to be highest in Scotland, and lowest in Germany. Evidence of this has been obtained mainly in the domain of cervical gland tuberculosis, in lupus, and in that of bone and joint tuberculosis; and it is in this latter that the greatest discrepancy in the results has been obtained. The matter however must still be considered *sub judice*. Probably there *is* some difference in different countries; possibly it is considerable; but the evidence of this is at present rather new, and it needs confirmation before it can be accepted as final.

8. It is probable that the bovine bacillus is less virulent for man than the human bacillus. If this is the case man stands in this respect alone among mammals, for, with the exception of the apes and monkeys which are equally susceptible, and the dog which is equally resistant to either type, all other species, so far as is known, are more severely affected with the bovine than with the human bacillus. Nevertheless this exception to the rule need not surprise those who believe that the human type of bacillus has been evolved in the body of man, and has gradually adapted itself specially to the conditions of life in his tissues. The bovine bacillus, on the other hand, probably passes frequently from one species to another, and has

[1] For some quite recent work see Appendix, p. 679.

become adapted to living in a group of animals rather than in any one of the species which constitute that group[1].

9.   The evidence that the human type of bacillus is more virulent for man than the bovine type rests mainly on two facts: (1) that bovine bacilli are common in children and rare in adults; and (2) that the tendency to cure seems to be greater in those kinds of tuberculosis in which bovine infection is common than in others in which it is rare.

10.   The importance of tuberculosis is not to be measured only by the fact that it causes, in England and Wales alone, the deaths of over fifty thousand persons each year, large as this number is.   A very considerable proportion of those deaths occur in the prime of life, or only a little earlier; and in addition to these deaths tuberculosis produces a great number of cripples.

11.   This mortality, large though it is now, is smaller than it was half a century ago.   Since that time the number of deaths caused each year by tuberculosis has diminished steadily and substantially, and the ratio of deaths to population has fallen by more than 50 per cent.

This death-rate is now declining rapidly, and at an ever-increasing velocity.   It is not too much to say that if this decline should continue to progress more or less along the line it has followed in the recent past tuberculosis will have become a rare disease before the end of the century.   The eyes of some indeed discern already on the far away horizon signs of its complete eradication.   The vision may prove to be a delusion;

---

[1] The bovine type of bacillus probably seldom passes from man to other mammals, or from one man to another, because the type of disease it causes is hardly ever of such a kind as to disseminate bacilli in an assimilable manner.

Adaptation of the bacillus to its host or hosts is only one-half of the story; development of special resisting power on the part of those species liable to attack is the other.   Thus it is that while we see the domesticated mammals for the most part susceptible to the infection only with the bovine type of bacillus, which may be considered to have specially adapted itself to attack them, we see also the wild mammals in captivity, which have never been forced to develop any special powers of resistance against tubercle bacilli, susceptible to invasion by the human type of bacillus as well as (for all we know to the contrary) to that of the bovine type of bacillus.

but at any rate even the most matter-of-fact of us may look
forward with confidence to a time, at no very distant date,
when society will be relieved of a large portion of this incubus,
which at present causes the death of one person in every ten
in this island, and cripples and disfigures many another.

12. The cause of the decline is not clearly known. It is
probably complex. Changes which may be summed up in
the phrase "amelioration of social conditions" are certainly
among the most important of the factors.

13. That partial immunization of the human race by means
of minimal infections with bovine or other types of tubercle
bacilli has played any part in this decline cannot be asserted
because there is no evidence that such infections have been more
frequent in recent years than in earlier ones. But that the human
race owes a good deal of its capacity for resisting tuberculosis
to this cause is not improbable In support of this view we
may adduce the following facts: we know that small doses
of bovine tubercle bacilli are repeatedly swallowed by children
and others in milk and butter, and that small doses of human
bacilli must frequently be inhaled[1]. We know also that a
proportion of people, variously estimated but which is probably
a good deal over 50 per cent., contain in their bodies, in the
form of calcareous or caseous nodules, or scars in the apices
of the lungs, evidence of abortive tuberculous infection; we
know that small doses of tubercle bacilli produce far less
severe results than those caused by large ones, especially in
animals which, like man, are not without considerable powers
of resistance; we know that some degree of increased resistance
to tuberculous infection, or "immunity," may be induced
artificially in animals by the administration of small doses of
tubercle bacilli, especially of such as are not virulent for the
species; we therefore cannot avoid concluding that much of
this abortive tuberculosis must be caused by these small and

[1] Burnet believes that no inconsiderable amount of immunization is
brought about by abortive infection with bacilli "attenuated," or perhaps
one would prefer to say impaired as to their vitality, by influences, such as
daylight, acting on them after their escape from the body (*Ann. de l'Instit.
Pasteur*, vol. XXIX, p. 220).

repeated doses of tubercle bacilli, and probably to a very large extent by those which are swallowed in milk. It appears to us therefore difficult to believe that the resistance of the population as a whole can remain uninfluenced by these very frequent abortive and repeated infections, and we are therefore inclined to believe that the resistance of the race to more serious tuberculous infections is considerably enhanced by them.

14. Under these circumstances what is to be done about tuberculosis in cattle? Are we to attempt to reduce or eradicate it in the hope of preventing a large proportion of the tuberculosis among children? Or should we be worse off after all if such attempts were made, and were successful?

The answer would seem to depend on the following considerations: the harm done by the bovine bacillus is certain, the benefit it confers is problematical. As to the extent of the harm, we can measure that approximately. It amounts, according to our estimate, to rather more than three thousand deaths per annum (mostly of infants and young children), together with a large amount of suffering and disfigurement. As to the benefit, it is not calculable, but it may perhaps be not inconsiderable. The deaths and suffering due to tuberculosis derived from bovine sources might undoubtedly be saved, provided the nation would find the necessary money; but at what additional cost, if any, of life due to the increased ravages of the tuberculosis contracted from human sources?

If the question is thus rightly stated, two principles would seem to be clear: on the one hand we ought not to lose the bone for the shadow; we should not hesitate to attack the certain evil for fear of the problematical consequences; and on the other we should be unwise to ignore the latter altogether. Bovine tuberculosis therefore should be dealt with firmly but tentatively, the result of each measure being watched before the next is attempted.

The lines of procedure should be determined by the acceptance of the proposition that in general the severity of infection varies with dose—a proposition which is abundantly supported by experiment. The harm is done mainly by large doses of bacilli, and these are likely to be taken when milk from a tuberculous udder is consumed unmixed with other milk. Small doses are less likely to be harmful, and it is to these, if to any, that the immunization is to be credited. Such doses are taken when the milk from many cows is mixed before consumption. It follows therefore that the sale of milk from single cows or from small herds should be discouraged, and that every effort should be made to discover and eliminate cows with tuberculous udders. We need hardly fear that any efforts which may be made in this direction will be attended with such complete success as to endanger the quality of resistance which at present sets a limit to the ravages of tuberculosis among mankind.

15. The same principle should guide our administrative dealings with sources of infection with tubercle bacilli of human type. These sources are almost all confined to cases of phthisis; for other forms of tuberculosis seldom cause lesions from which tubercle bacilli escape in such a form as to prove dangerous. Let us accept the principle, in respect of the human type of bacillus which we have already proposed in the case of the bovine, namely that in the main it is the large doses of bacilli which are dangerous, and that small ones are often harmless or even beneficial by increasing resistance. If this be granted the course is clear: infection from dust in the street—indeed all infection at a distance—does not so much need to be dealt with, as the infection in the immediate neighbourhood of the consumptive person. Consumptive children should be sent to special schools, and should not be given the care of babies. Special cases of phthisis, as for example in overcrowded households, should be segregated. But the principal desideratum is that the public should learn that tuberculosis is contracted from consumptive patients, and without panic and without inflicting unnecessary hardship, should in the light of this knowledge take steps to protect themselves and their children.

APPENDIX

I

It was at one time the intention of the author to add a chapter on immunization but he found it impossible to compress the subject into sufficiently small compass and so the intention was abandoned. Some incidents however, which would have been included in this chapter, have a definite bearing on points already discussed; and these will be described in the following notes.

1. *General Dissemination of Tubercle Bacilli after Subcutaneous Injection.*

Mention has already been made (p. 253) of the fact that it was found during the work of the Royal Commission that, in about half the calves injected subcutaneously with tubercle bacilli of human type, minute, non-progressive, grey tubercles appeared in small numbers in the lungs, and occasionally in the lymphatic glands, and even in some of the other organs. The repeated appearance of these little foci seemed to point to a dissemination of tubercle bacilli by the blood-stream shortly after injection, and before the body had had time to organize its local defences and confine the invaders. For experience had abundantly shown that these bacilli are incapable, in moderate numbers, of causing destructive lesions in the ox species, and it seemed unlikely that they could have won their way to the blood-stream by breaking down the barriers interposed in their course by the lymphatic glands. Rather, it seemed, the dissemination must have occurred very early, when, we may suppose, the lymphatic glands, as yet intact, failed to arrest all the bacilli brought to them on account of the overwhelming numbers with which they were required to deal after an injection of 50 mg., and when as yet no barrier had been built about the invaders in the form of a local lesion.

This question seemed sufficiently interesting to be put to the test of experiment. Some calves were therefore injected in the usual way, subcutaneously with 50 mg. of bacilli of human type, and having been killed after intervals varying from three days upwards, their blood and tissues were searched for tubercle bacilli by the method of guinea-pig inoculation[1].

The results of these experiments confirmed expectation, and showed that within three days of subcutaneous injection tubercle bacilli may be found in all the organs and lymphatic glands. In one case they were proved to be in the blood eight days after the injection.

A. S. Griffith and F. Griffith[2] repeated these experiments and greatly extended their range, employing various species of animals, including the ox, pig, cat, rabbit, guinea-pig, rat, chicken and monkey, and reducing the interval between injection and examination. Their experiments confirmed the results already obtained, and showed that the dissemination takes place within twenty-four hours and occurs in every species, and quite independently of the virulence of the microbe for the animal concerned.

2. *Persistence of Tubercle Bacilli of Human Type in the Tubules of the Cow's Udder.*

If tubercle bacilli of human type are introduced through the ducts of the teats into the unwounded sinuses and tubules of the functional mammary gland of the cow no tuberculosis occurs either there or elsewhere, but the bacilli persist for a very long time and continue to be excreted in the milk, so that it is practically certain that they take up their abode there and multiply. The cow usually develops a capacity to react to tuberculin, but this is often transient, or irregular. The evidence for these statements is as follows:

In the very early days of the Royal Commission (1902–3) six cows were inoculated in the mammary gland after the manner described above, five with emulsions of tuberculous tissues and one with culture. Four of them reacted to tuberculin at one time or another after the inoculations. It may be said that,

---

[1] Cobbett, *R.C.T. Int. Rep.* App. vol. III, p. 221.
[2] A. S. and F. Griffith, *Ibid.* p. 235.

with one notable exception[1], no structural change occurred in the udder beyond a little induration and fibrosis; even this was not constantly present. The supra-mammary lymphatic glands were not affected. The author well remembers repeatedly testing the milk from the separate quarters of the udders of these cows by injection of guinea-pigs and how strongly he was impressed by the persistence of the tubercle bacilli in the milk of the infected quarters, while that from the other quarters always yielded negative results. The records of these injections, however, have not been preserved and he is unable to state exactly how long in each case the milk remained infective.

Similar observations were evidently being made about the same time in the United States, for Schroeder and Cotton[2] in 1906 stated that a cow which they had injected in the milk sinuses with "tubercle bacilli of low virulence" (by which expression we may, at the present day, infer tubercle bacilli of human type) continued to excrete living tubercle bacilli for four years and ten months.

3. *Danger of Immunizing Milch Cows with Living Tubercle Bacilli.*

It has already been shown that after subcutaneous injection some of the bacilli injected become distributed by the blood-stream to various glands and organs. The same thing occurs, of course, to an even greater extent after intravenous injection. It may be that the bacilli thus distributed are retained chiefly in those organs which possess a phagocytic capillary endothelium, and that we are therefore not entitled to assume the presence of

---

[1] The exception was Cow 3 injected with culture of human type. Some considerable changes undoubtedly took place in the inoculated quarters of the udder of this cow which were thought at the time to be tuberculous. These quarters are described in the post-mortem notes (for which the author is not responsible, though they appear in a volume under his name) as having lost all their normal structure and come to consist of "numerous yellow gelatinous-looking nodules which varied in size from 1 to 5 mm. or more," and of which some were "caseous." The conclusion arrived at was "universal tuberculosis of the inoculated quarters of the mamma." If this conclusion was correct the case was most unusual, for in no other was a like effect produced, and it is remarkable that the supra-mammary gland was not tuberculous. (*R.C.T. Int. Rep.* App. vol. II, p. 30.)

[2] *U.S. Bureau of Animal Industry, Bulletin* 93, p. 11.

the bacilli in any organs in which they have not been actually demonstrated. In the experiments described in the earlier part of this appendix, so far as they relate to heifer calves, the bacilli must have been carried to the immature mammary glands. But that they *lodged* there we do not actually know, because these glands were not tested; the significance of their presence not being perceived at the time. Nevertheless the experiments showed a *possibility* that they may lodge and persist there, and the question naturally arose whether under such circumstances they may endure in this situation until the mammary gland becomes functional.

But even if this were so another step in the full tale of evidence would still be wanting before one could be sure that the process of immunizing with living bacilli was attended by danger of the milk becoming infective, for one could not be sure that tubercle bacilli of human type, and others of low virulence for the ox (which are incapable in small numbers of causing a destructive lesion), would, even if they remained in the mammary gland long enough, make their way from the spot to which they had been carried by the blood-stream into the milk itself. The evidence of this transition, however, was soon forthcoming; for in 1907 Weber and Titze related the following very instructive experience[1]:

A heifer calf when eight months old was given an intravenous injection of tubercle bacilli of human type on Oct. 15, 1903. About a year later the animal, now a young heifer, was sent to the bull, with the object, should opportunity arise, of ascertaining whether any immunity a mother might acquire would be transmitted to the offspring.

For the purpose of increasing the resisting power of the prospective mother further injections of human tubercle bacilli were administered subcutaneously to the heifer while she was in calf: namely on Jan. 6th, on Feb. 11th and on April 20th, 1905.

On July 30th a calf was duly born and was allowed from its birth to be suckled by its mother.

---

[1] "Die Immunisierung der Rinder gegen Tuberkulose," *Tub. Arbeit a. d. Kaiserl. Gesundheitsamte*, Heft 7, p. 9.

The milk was subsequently tested by inoculation of guinea-pigs and found to be infective. Later on, in 1906, it was demonstrated repeatedly that the tubercle bacilli were present only in the milk of the right hind quarter, that from the other three quarters causing no tuberculosis in the guinea-pigs injected with it.

Cultures were obtained from the milk of the right hind quarter and found to be of human type.

On Feb. 21st and March 20th, 1907, the milk of the right hind quarter was injected with negative results. The udder had ceased to yield infective milk, and on July 4th the cow was killed. Post-mortem examination failed to show any sign of tuberculosis either in the udder or elsewhere; there was however some atrophy and fibrosis of the quarter which had so often yielded tubercle bacilli.

Meanwhile the calf had died, when eight weeks old, of some intercurrent disorder; and at the post-mortem examination there was found in a mesenteric gland a little tuberculous nodule about the size of a bean containing some caseous foci as large as pins' heads. From this nodule tubercle bacilli of human type were cultivated.

About the same time in the laboratories of the Royal Commission, A. S. Griffith[1] was investigating the question whether tubercle bacilli, present for any reason in the body of an animal during lactation, may get into the milk. For this purpose cows and goats were injected, subcutaneously and intravenously, with various types of tubercle bacilli, and the milk was tested from time to time by the inoculation of guinea-pigs. These experiments clearly showed that after artificial inoculation bacilli may appear in the milk without any lesion whatever being discoverable in the udder. Incidentally they revealed the fact that if bacilli were injected for the purpose of immunization, not only might some of them get carried to the udder, but also that even such as are of human type might make their way through the epithelium and gain access to the milk itself.

These experiments, then, like that of Weber and Titze,

[1] "The Excretion of Tubercle Bacilli in the Milk of Cows and Goats," *R.C.T. Fin. Rep.* App. vol. III, p. 81.

conclusively demonstrated that it was dangerous to inject living tubercle bacilli into milch cows and goats *during pregnancy* or *lactation*.   But injection for the purpose of immunization was being practised, not on cows, but on calves, and it remained to be seen whether tubercle bacilli of human type will when injected *into the heifer calf* gain entrance into the immature mammary gland, and if so whether they may remain there long enough to infect the milk subsequently when the calf becomes a cow, and reaches the period of lactation.

The first part of this problem was solved by A. S. Griffith in collaboration with his brother F. Griffith[1].   For this purpose they inoculated subcutaneously eleven heifer calves and an adult and pregnant goat.   Various types of bacilli were selected for these experiments including, in several cases, the attenuated bovine bacilli from cases of lupus; but what more particularly concerns us now is that two calves and the goat were injected with bacilli of human type.

The calves were killed several months after inoculation and the contents of their immature mammary glands tested for tubercle bacilli by the injection of guinea-pigs, and the sowing of tubes of culture media.

The contents of the tubules of the mammary glands were obtained as follows: some sterile salt solution was first injected into the milk sinuses through the ducts of the teat, and after massage was recovered together with whatever it had succeeded in washing from the ducts and tubules.

The results demonstrated that in seven out of the eleven heifer calves, including the two injected with bacilli of human type, the bacilli were present in the secretion of the glands. In the case of the goat the milk was tested after parturition but with negative results.

The second part of the problem stated above, namely whether tubercle bacilli of human type having reached the immature udder may persist there long enough to contaminate the milk when at some subsequent period lactation ensues, has now been solved completely.   A curious experience which occurred in Cambridge in 1908 seems pertinent to our inquiry and worth relating.   A calf belonging to a neighbouring herd had given a

---

[1] *R.C.T. Final Report*, App. vol. III, p. 94.

very definite reaction to tuberculin and, having been condemned, was sent to the Pathological School to be killed and examined. The post-mortem examination was conducted by the writer in the presence of A. S. Griffith. Nothing suspicious was found until the mesenteric glands were reached, when, after careful search, a little nodule, scarcely as large as a pea, was found in one of these glands. The nodule was obviously tuberculous and contained acid-fast bacilli which Griffith at the time pronounced to be abnormally long for bovine bacilli. They were subsequently recovered in pure culture from a guinea-pig which was injected with an emulsion of the nodule, and in due course proved to be ordinary tubercle bacilli of human type.

How had human tubercle bacilli gained entrance to this calf? This question cannot be answered with certainty; but a solution may be suggested with some confidence. It was ascertained that at the farm where the calf was born an attempt to immunize the herd had been made some time previously, and it is possible, though this cannot be definitely asserted, that the mother of this calf had been one of the animals which had received an intravenous injection of human tubercle bacilli, and that these had got into the milk and subsequently infected the calf, just as is known to have occurred in Weber and Titze's case.

Shortly after this experience Griffith[1] had the opportunity of examining the milk of two heifers from the same herd. These animals were known to have received immunizing injections of tubercle bacilli of human type, intravenously some two years previously. The results of this investigation showed that the milk of one of these animals was capable of transmitting tuberculosis to guinea-pigs injected with it; and from some of these guinea-pigs were obtained cultures of tubercle bacilli of human type.

It is true that similar experiences do not seem to have been met with in Germany where two selected strains of tubercle bacilli, known as tauruman and bovo-vaccin respectively, have been used for immunizing cattle: for Weber and Titze tested

[1] "Human Tubercle Bacilli in the Milk of a Vaccinated Cow," *Journ. of Pathol. and Bacteriol.* 1913, vol. XVII.

the milk of 79 heifers injected when calves with one or other of these strains without finding tubercle bacilli in any sample[1] Nevertheless the evidence given above is sufficient to show that it will not do to inject living tubercle bacilli into heifer calves which are destined to become milch cows. Whether it is permissible to immunize in this way calves intended for the butcher is another question. It is obvious of course that the danger arising from contamination of meat is as nothing compared with that arising from contamination of milk; for the former is cooked and the latter consumed raw, and, moreover, frequently given to babies. Nevertheless, even if it were considered safe to practise immunization in this way with certain regulations and restrictions, it is doubtful whether it would be worth while if brood stock had to be excluded. The fact is that whatever be the method of immunization employed the immunity produced is not of a high order, and is variable and somewhat transient; and it is probable that the suppression of bovine tuberculosis may be brought about, not only more safely, but more surely, by Bang's method of removing the calves from their mothers and bringing them up on sterilized milk or on that taken from non-reacting cows.

II

Tubercle Bacilli from Bone and Joint Tuberculosis.

Two important papers on this subject, by Eastwood and F. Griffith and by A. S. Griffith respectively have been written since the rest of this book was in paged proofs. As it is impossible to incorporate the results in the chapter dealing with the subject, a summary will be given here.

Eastwood and F. Griffith[2] examined material obtained by surgical operation from 313 English cases. Forty-seven of these gave negative results, neither causing lesions in guinea-pigs, nor yielding cultures when the spleens of the inoculated animals were sown on tubes of egg medium. From five cases the

[1] *Tub. Arbeit. a. d. Kaiserl. Gesundheitsamte*, Heft 10, pp. 171, 183.

[2] "The Characteristics of Tubercle Bacilli in Human Bone and Joint Tuberculosis," *Journal of Hygiene*, 1916, vol. XV, p. 257.

material was not obtained from the joints or bones affected but from some distant site. These are put on record, but are not included in the statistics of the types of bacilli found in bone and joint tuberculosis. All five cases yielded bacilli of human type.

There remain 261 cases from which cultures of tubercle bacilli were obtained through guinea-pigs inoculated with material removed directly from an affected bone or joint or from an abscess in the neighbourhood of such a lesion.

The cultures obtained from these cases were after due investigation classified as follows:

Types of Tubercle Bacilli at Different Age Periods.

Age Period	No. of Cases	Human	Bovine	Atypical
0–5 years	47	**31**	**14**	**2**
5–10 ,,	108	**75**	**31**	**2**
10–16 ,,	62	**52**	**7**	**3**
16–25 ,,	15	**12**	**3**	—
over 25 ,,	29	**26**	**0**	**3**
Total	261	**196**	**55**	**10**

The percentages of bovine infections are:

All ages (55 out of 261) ... 21·1 per cent.
Under 10 years (45 out of 155) 29·0 ,, ,,
Over 10 years (10 out of 106) 9·4 ,, ,,

A. S. Griffith has kindly communicated to the writer for inclusion in this summary the results of his investigation, which at the moment of writing have not yet appeared in print. The investigation embraces 136 completed cases, 27 being from Scotland and the rest, 109 in number, from England. Together they yielded 18 per cent. of bovine bacilli.

The following analysis shows how the bovine infections were distributed between the Scotch and English cases and among the children of different ages.

Type of Tubercle Bacilli found in Bone and Joint Tuberculosis.

England.

Age Period	No. of Cases	Human	Bovine	Atypical	Percentage of Bovine Infections
0–5 years	21	16	5	0	*23·6*
5–10 ,,	55	42	10	3	*18·2*
10–16 ,,	27	24	1	2	*3·8*
16 and over	6	6	0	0	*0·0*
Total	109	88	16	5	*14·7*

Scotland.

Age Period	No. of Cases	Human	Bovine	Atypical	Percentage of Bovine Infections
0–5 years	16	10	6	—	*37·5*
5–10 ,,	6	4	2	—	*33·3*
10–16 ,,	3	3	0	—	*0·0*
16 and over	2	2	0	—	*0·0*
Total	27	19	8	—	*29·6*

In view of the results of these two recent and comprehensive investigations, carried out in the laboratories of the Local Government Board and of Cambridge University respectively, it is clear that the estimate hitherto entertained of the part played by bovine bacilli in human bone and joint tuberculosis must be revised. Whatever may be the proportion of bovine infections in foreign countries, and as to this we cannot yet speak with any confidence, in England at any rate, it would appear that bone and joint tuberculosis is caused by the bovine tubercle bacillus in about one case in five, taking cases at all ages, and, among children under ten years of age, in more than one in every four. In Scotland, it can hardly be doubted, the proportion of bovine infections is considerably higher, amounting in Griffith's series of cases to a little over one in three in children of this age. But the extremely high proportion of bovine infections claimed by Fraser (namely almost two out of every three) has not been confirmed.

III

A New Sub-type of Tubercle Bacilli.

In their recent investigation of bone and joint tuberculosis, which we have just reviewed, Eastwood and F. Griffith met with strains of tubercle bacilli which they considered to be atypical. No less than 10 of these strains were obtained from 261 cases. They are said to have resembled others which the authors had already studied, namely two from the pig (see p. 406) and one from a child with tuberculosis of the vertebral column (see p. 604). These strains possessed the virulence for the rabbit of the human type and the cultural characters, more or less, of the bovine type.

The authors divided these 13 atypical strains into two groups which were to be distinguished from each other by their growth on serum (*loc. cit.* p. 295). While all were dysgonic on agar, potato and broth, seven produced yellow pigment when grown on suitable serum—a characteristic of the human type (see p. 209)—while six did not. Thus the former would seem to be more closely allied to the human and the latter to the bovine type. The former are perhaps "dysgonic humans" and the latter "attenuated bovines." The authors however do not go as far as this, but confine themselves to a statement of the facts.

A. S. Griffith also has met with these dysgonic human strains (to which we have already alluded on p. 649). Four of them were described by him in his recent report on tubercle bacilli derived from sputum[1]. These strains are said to have produced in the rabbit and guinea-pig the pathogenic effects of standard human tubercle bacilli, and to have resembled human bacilli also in their mode of growth on serum and glycerin-serum. It was in respect of their growth on glycerin-agar, glycerin-potato and glycerin broth that they were atypical. "On these media," Griffith says, "they were dysgonic, and displayed characters which would have entitled them to classification with bovine tubercle bacilli."

[1] *Lancet*, 1916, I, p. 721.

Both Eastwood and F. Griffith and A. S. Griffith found that the anomalous characters of growth of these strains were stable and appeared constantly on repeated cultivation continued over two years and more.   A. S. Griffith states that he regards them as "stable new varieties of the tubercle bacillus" and "on account of their closer resemblance to the human than the bovine type" he provisionally classifies them as "atypical human tubercle bacilli."

With respect to pigment production A. S. Griffith points out that the production of orange-yellow pigment by bacilli of human type does not occur on every serum, but only on such as is itself of a rich golden colour.   On paler samples of ox serum the colour is variable, and on colourless serum, such as is usually obtained from the calf, pig, goat or horse, the cultures of human tubercle bacilli are greyish and not pigmented.

Griffith attaches considerable importance to this pigment production, and points out that care should be taken to employ a serum which has been found to give a good orange-yellow colour with cultures of human type.   He himself always used serum from the same cow, which was bled at intervals for the purpose of affording a culture medium.   If attention had not been directed to this point "these strains," as Griffith himself points out, "would have been classified as dysgonic with the pathogenicity of standard human tubercle bacilli."

The possibility of arriving at such a conclusion in the case of strains of this kind and, consequently, of regarding them as attenuated examples of the bovine type rather than dysgonic examples of the human type has an important bearing on the problems we were discussing in the chapter on lupus (see footnote p. 639).   In lupus it is fairly clear that we have to deal with strains of bovine (as well as of human type) with attenuated virulence, and if as seems possible we may sometimes meet with dysgonic strains of human type also from this source the classification of the bacilli into bovine and human becomes very difficult.   To this difficulty perhaps some of our ill-success in seeking the cause of attenuation of lupus bacilli is to be ascribed.

A. S. Griffith has informed the writer that in his as yet un-published investigation of bone and joint tuberculosis he has found five additional atypical strains similar to those described above. In addition he has met with one strain from an abscess in the thigh in a case of cervical gland tuberculosis which differed from other atypical strains in growing like the human type and possessing attenuated virulence; thus resembling the attenuated strains of human type obtained from lupus.

Atypical strains, more or less conforming to the human type, but growing badly on broth have been described both by Ungermann and by Burckhardt (p. 230). These were probably similar to the atypical strains now under consideration.

What is to be the place in our classification of tubercle bacilli of this new kind of bacillus which has lately emerged from obscurity? Is it to be looked upon as a new sub-type, a solution towards which Griffith tends to incline, or should it be regarded merely as a variant of the human type? It is too early to attempt to answer this question; but we would point out that while three grades of cultural potentialities have been credited by Eastwood and by A. S. Griffith to the bovine tubercle bacillus, but two have been allowed to the human type (p. 357). Perhaps the simplest solution would be to allow the same number of grades of cultural characters to *each* of the types, and to regard these so-called "atypical" strains as dysgonic variants of the human type. This solution may possibly be objected to on the ground that it gives too much weight to differences of pathogenicity and too little to those of vegetative capacity. And it must in all fairness be admitted that if this solution were to be accepted, the cultural characters of the two types would overlap, and we should be faced with the further difficulty that in each type we should have to admit the existence of attenuated members.

Are we then driven to conclude that growth, characters and virulence are both unstable? If so what becomes of the distinction between the types themselves?

That the types really exist, in the main clear and distinct, can hardly be doubted. These anomalous strains, it must be remembered, are the *exception*; and, whatever we may think of them, they cannot upset the broad distinctions which separate the great majority of tubercle bacilli into three types.

IV

The Use of Antiformin for raising Primary Cultures.

A. S. Griffith now reports favourably on his newer method (mentioned on p. 219). It will be remembered that he found that the presence of a little antiformin in the fluid actually used for sowing the cultures was not detrimental to the growth of the bacillus, and, moreover, that it was inadvisable to wait until an antiformin-sputum mixture had become so fluid that it was possible to centrifuge it. He therefore dispensed with the centrifuging altogether, and merely sowed successive cultures from a mixture of sputum and antiformin after varying intervals of time.

This method succeeded in 26 out of 31 experiments. The secret of success is the sowing of a series of cultures after various periods of exposure to the antiformin. For with too short an exposure the extraneous bacteria are not all killed and will overgrow the tubercle bacilli, and with too long an exposure the tubercle bacilli are rendered incapable of growing. Griffith at first used an addition of 5 per cent. of antiformin to the sputum, and even with this weak mixture he found that, in 13 out of the 26 successful experiments, although after 10 minutes exposure cultures sown yielded pure growths of tubercle bacilli, after a further exposure of 5 or 10 minutes the tubes sown remained completely sterile. In one case a tube sown 5 minutes after making the mixture yielded abundant growth of ordinary micro-organisms, one sown after 10 minutes gave a pure culture of tubercle bacilli, while tubes sown after 15 and 20 minutes remained sterile. Thus the limits of time available for successful culture may be brief. Griffith thinks that this is especially the case with thin sputa; with thick sputa, on the other hand, tubercle bacilli may sometimes be cultivated from mixtures after 24 hours[1].

What is the best percentage of antiformin to add? Should we add little and allow long intervals between the successive sowings, or add much and sow the tubes in quick succession?

[1] *Lancet*, 1916, I, p. 723.

Griffith got good results with a 5 per cent. addition, but his more recent experience, which has been made with tuberculous animal tissues as well as with sputum, has led him to the conclusion "that it is more advantageous, especially when dealing with tenacious sputum, to use high percentages of antiformin with short exposure than low percentages with long exposure." A similar opinion has been expressed by McFadyean and Knowles[1]. For routine use with sputum Griffith now recommends an addition of 15 per cent. of antiformin. "The first sowing should be made one or two minutes after mixture according to the consistency of the sputum, and three tubes at least ought to be sown within the first five minutes. Thereafter the intervals may be longer—about five minutes, especially if the sputum remains undissolved and mucinous. There is no need to sow tubes after twenty minutes or after the sputum has completely dissolved."

[1] *Journ. of Comp. Pathol. and Therap.* vol. XXVII, part 2.

INDEX OF SUBJECTS

Abbreviations, T.=tuberculosis, t.b.=tubercle bacilli,
f=footnote

Abdominal tuberculosis, types of t.b. found (man) 580, table 583; abdominal origin of pulmonary tuberculosis 141; summary 176; T. of mesenteric glands in cases of phthisis 174

Abortive infections 21, 65, 69, 669

Acid-fast group of bacilli 198; acid-fast bacilli in milk 199; in tuberculous lesions in swine 404; in Johne's disease 388; acid-fast streptothrices 199

Acid-fastness, degrees of 199; may be dependent on composition of the culture medium 199

Adaptation of t.b. to conditions of artificial culture 203, 226, 286; (on broth) 209, 236; conclusion 242

Age when infection occurs (in man) 131; (in the ox) 381

Air passages, freedom of entry of air-borne bacteria into 148

Antelope, instances of T. in 482

Anthracosis, a chronic process 148; portal of entry of the carbon: natural anthracosis in the guinea-pig 147; experimental 145, 149

Antiformin, use of in raising cultures of t.b. from sputum, etc. 218, 684

Argentine Republic, frequency of swine T. 396 f, 398

Arkansas, Oklahoma and Texas, rarity of tuberculosis in swine allowed to run wild in the forests 396

Aspiration of t.b. into the lung, a source of error in feeding experiments 160, 162, 165, 327, 500, (in apes) 517 f

Ass, rarity of T. in 447; experimental infection 478; is it more susceptible to infection with equine bacilli? 481 f

Assortative mating 82

Attenuation of t.b.—see "Stability of type"

Atypical t.b. 214, 301 f, 354, 356, 369; from the pig 362, 406, 681; from the horse 364, 406, 470; from man, phthisis 212 f, 681; bone and joints 604, 629, 681; lupus 617, 620, 627, 635, 636, 649

Avian tubercle bacilli—see under "B. tuberculosis"

B. prodigiosus, inhalation expts. 148; feeding expts. 163

B. tuberculosis. Discovery 57; relation to other acid-fast bacteria, and to the diphtheria and streptothrix groups 198

    Morphological characters 198, 224; branching 199; comparative length of human and bovine t.b. under various conditions 201; short forms sometimes in sputum 224

    Cultural characters 202, 204, 209, 225; pigmentation 205, 681, 682, 685; diagnostic value of 231; relative importance of cultural characters and virulence 636, 683

    Virulence for various animal species 211 et seq., table 248

    Classification 196, 299, 663, 683; atypical strains—see under "Atypical"; a new sub-type 680; difference of virulence of human and bovine types no mere difference of degree 212, 619 f, 684

    Methods of staining 199; of cultivating 218, 685

C.   44

INDEX OF AUTHORS

investigation (at Cambridge) 635; tabular summaries of results 639,
642; action of artificial light on t.b. 634
Griffith, A. S. and F. *Stability of type of tubercle bacilli*—modification experiments
with bovine t.b. in (1) the monkey and chimpanzee 350; (2) dog 351
Swine tuberculosis. Types of tubercle bacilli found in the pig 403;
localized tuberculosis 402, 399; T. in the mammary gland of the
sow 385 f; t.b. in the joints 400; intestinal origin of T. 402.
Dissemination of t.b. after subcutaneous injection 673; do t.b. in the
blood get into the milk without lesion of mammary glands? 677;
T. in a sparrow 528
Griffith, F. *Duration of life* of cultures of tubercle bacilli 221
Stability of type of t.b. Modification experiments with (*a*) avian t.b.
in the (1) calf 310; (2) various animals 311, 312; (*b*) mammalian
t.b. in the fowl 309; bovine t.b. in the dog 352
Virulence of avian t.b. for goat 419, 420; pig 412; horse 474, 475, 476;
guinea-pigs 440; rabbit 428; monkeys 518; chimpanzee 519;
dog 501; cat 509; rat 449; mouse 456
Horse. Types of t.b. found in the horse—atypical strains 469 *et seq.*;
experimental infection 475
Chimpanzee and other monkeys. Types of t.b. found in spontaneous
tuberculosis 511
Rabbit. Spontaneous infection with avian bacilli 427
Wild animals kept in captivity, instances of T. in 482
Parrot 538
Grober. Portals of entry in phthisis—indian-ink experiment 175
Grund. Growth of bovine t.b. on broth 227; the reaction curve 234, 236

De Haan. Immunity of wild monkey from T. 510; rarity of T. in cattle of
Java 375
Haldane, Martin and Thomas. T. in tin-miners 97 f; low infectiveness of
miners' phthisis in Cornwall 100
Hamburger. Frequency of infection at various periods of early life 130
Hamel. Relative number of deaths from pulmonary and other kinds of T.
in various countries 550 f
Hamilton. Nature of phthisis caused by stone dust 104
Hammond Smith. T. in a kestrel 528
Harbitz 176
Harden. Bio-chemistry of *B. tub.* 239
Hay, Matthew. Deaths from phthisis attributed to bronchitis 2 f, 13 f;
decline of T. 17 f; greater liability of girls than boys to phthisis 39
Heberden. Infectiousness of phthisis 49
Héricourt and Richet. Effect of avian t.b. on monkey 517; therapeutic
use of dog's blood in tuberculosis 486, 461
Heymans. Reactivation of lesions due to human t.b. in the rabbit 277
Hippocrates 47
Hobday and Belcher 491 f
Holth. Johne's bacillus 389
Humphry, Sir George. Collective investigation of infectiousness of phthisis
53, 80
Hutchens, Prof. H. Comparative length of human and bovine t.b. 200
Hutchinson, Sir Jonathan 68
Hutyra and Marek. T. in the parrot 538

Jensen. T. in the dog 489; in the cat 503
Johne. Expt. T. in the ass 478
Johne and Frothingham 388
De Jong. Spontaneous T. in the mouse 451
De Jong and Stuurmann. Case of pulmonary tuberculosis alleged to be
caused by bovine bacilli 559; summary of the case 565

Kelly 24

mortality from T. in various towns 91; influence of flats on outdoor exercise 95

Sehlbach. Frequency of infection in the first year of life 130

Shattock. Human mammary tuberculosis 384 f

Shattock, Seligmann, Dudgeon and Panton. Stability of type of mammalian t.b. in the fowl 307; T. in the birds of the Zoölogical Gardens, London 526; no T. in the wild pigeon 528; instance of T. in a wild bird 527; T. in the parrot 535; insusceptibility of fowls and pigeons to mammalian T. 541, 542

Sibley. T. in the birds of the Zoölogical Gardens, London 526; no T. in the wild pigeon 528; peculiarity of the lesions of T. in birds 529 f

Siedamgrotsky. T. in cattle of Saxony 378

Silvius, Franciscus. First description of tubercles 47

Smith, G. Elliot and Ruffer. Tuberculosis in an Egyptian mummy 46

Smith, Theobald. Differentiation of human and bovine t.b. 189; reaction curve 231, 234, 236, 238

Smith, Th. and Brown. Types of t.b. in cervical gland tuberculosis 591

Sprigge. Spread of infection from a case of phthisis in a dress-maker to her assistants 53

Steinmeyer. Relation of meningitis to general tuberculosis 570 f

Sticker. Experimental T. in the dog 501

Stockman. Experimental T. in the ass 478; T. in the dog 487; Johne's disease in the sheep 388

Straus. Pulmonary T. in the pig 401; expt. T. in the mouse 452; T. in the dog 487; canine T. mainly a pulmonary disease 489; a forecast of the type of t.b. found in lupus 615; portal of entry in lupus 615 f

Straus and Gamaléia. Differentiation of avian and mammalian t.b. by means of the dog 246, 501; fate of avian t.b. in the guinea-pig 313; effect of avian t.b. injected into guinea-pigs 438; insusceptibility of the fowl to infection with mammalian t.b. 540

Stuurmann. Johne's disease believed to be caused by the avian bacillus 388 —see also de Jong 559, 565

Summons. Miner's phthisis and pulmonary tuberculosis in S. Africa 106

Symmers. On the intestinal origin of phthisis 142; experimental anthracosis 146

Tappeiner. Feeding expts. on dogs 492

Tatham. Reliability of statistics 10 f; occupational mortality among females 43 f; potter's phthisis 106

Templeman. Female occupation and child mortality in Dundee 95

Thomas, Dr Lynn. Therapeutic influence of sunlight 655

Thomassen. T. in the dog of a butcher 49

Thompson. Frequency of tuberculosis in the goat 414

Thorne Thorne. Subsoil drainage 24

Thucydides. Belief in the contagiousness of plague 47

Titze. Feeding expts. with avian t.b. on pigs 411; on a foal 475

Titze and Weidanz. Expts. on the dog 494, 499; exceptional result on a feeding experiment 500

Todd. Views on development of the fœtus 50

Tonking. T.b. in the sputum of phthisical Cornish miners 102

Transvaal Medical Society. Fibroid phthisis and pulmonary tuberculosis 106; T.b. in the sputum of gold-miners 102

Treves. On the escape of the lymph glands in lupus 615 f

Trousseau 19

Trudeau. Attenuation of t.b. 288

Twort. Dead bacilli or their extracts as constituent part of culture media for bacteria which grow with difficulty 216, 219

Twort and Ingram. Cultivation of Johne's bacillus 216, 389

Ungermann. Proportion of deaths of children caused by T. 11 f; frequency of infection in early life 130; relative frequency of infection of various groups of glands 170; exam. of the glands of a newly born infant 128;

www.ingramcontent.com/pod-product-compliance
Ingram Content Group UK Ltd.
Pitfield, Milton Keynes, MK11 3LW, UK
UKHW040701180125
453697UK00010B/325